Acute liver failure (ALF), or fulminant hepatic failure, is a distinct clinical syndrome which crosses medical disciplines. ALF advances rapidly, unexpectedly, and with devastating physiologic consequences including multiorgan failure. Though a relatively rare condition, ALF is a major focus of clinical and research attention, and with the option of transplantation the importance of understanding pathogenesis, management, and prognosis for ALF has taken on a new urgency.

This is the first book dedicated to ALF. The editors are international authorities in liver study who bring together a distinguished team of contributors to describe the etiology, pathology, and treatment of this important syndrome. Also covered are consensus techniques in liver transplantation in ALF patients, as well as descriptions of artificial and bioartificial liver assist devices. A section on future treatments includes hepatocyte transplantation, auxiliary grafts, and other temporary liver support.

Notable for the high level of technical and clinical expertise of its authors, and its comprehensive coverage, this volume will prove invaluable to internists, hepatologists, gastroenterologists, surgeons, intensive care providers, and other clinicians involved in the diagnosis and treatment of ALF.

Acute Liver Failure

Acute Liver Failure

Edited by

WILLIAM M. LEE
University of Texas Southwestern Medical School, Dallas

and

ROGER WILLIAMS
King's College School of Medicine and Dentistry, London

Foreword by

Jean-Pierre Benhamou
and
Jacques Bernuau

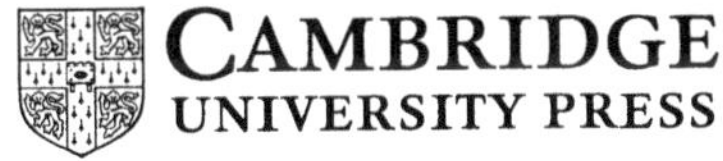

CAMBRIDGE UNIVERSITY PRESS
Cambridge, New York, Melbourne, Madrid, Cape Town,
Singapore, São Paulo, Delhi, Tokyo, Mexico City

Cambridge University Press
The Edinburgh Building, Cambridge CB2 8RU, UK

Published in the United States of America by Cambridge University Press, New York

www.cambridge.org
Information on this title: www.cambridge.org/9780521188944

First published 1997
First paperback edition 2011

A catalogue record for this publication is available from the British Library

Library of Congress Cataloguing in Publication data

Acute liver failure / edited by William Lee, Roger Williams.
p. cm.
ISBN 0–521–55381–4 (hardback)
1. Liver—Failure. I. Lee, William M. II. Williams, Roger,
1931–
[DNLM: 1. Liver Failure, Acute. WI 700 A1895 1997]
RC848.F27A28 1997
616.3′62—dc20
DNLM/DLC
for Library of Congress 96–16709 CIP

ISBN 978-0-521-55381-0 Hardback
ISBN 978-0-521-18894-4 Paperback

Additional resources for this publication at www.cambridge.org/9780521188944

Dedication

This volume is dedicated to our wives, Liza and Stephanie.

''All other goods by fortune's hand are given,
a wife is a peculiar gift of heaven.''

Alexander Pope, 1688–1744

Contents

Part Six Other Applications

Preface

This book is the outgrowth of two previous efforts to review current knowledge in acute liver failure. The first was the 1990 symposium/workshop entitled *Acute Liver Failure*, which was published by the British Society of Gastroenterology as a short monograph, and the second was a review with the same title in the *New England Journal of Medicine* in 1993. We became aware that there was no definitive text covering this topic. Although a relatively rare condition, none is so dramatic or devastating as acute liver failure, and this may explain the interest of so many clinical and research groups in a relatively uncommon problem. There are few other conditions in medicine in which young healthy patients can evolve to coma, intensive care and organ transplantation (or death) more rapidly, or for which the careful, considered, but rapid judgement of attending physicians is more important. We have used the term "acute liver failure" predominantly in this book where others frequently use the terms "fulminant hepatic failure" or "fulminant hepatitis." When talking about the topic as a whole, we use acute liver failure as an umbrella term, while reserving fulminant hepatic failure for one form of acute liver failure having specific time limitations (see Chapter 1).

One of the main tenets of this book is that when liver failure occurs rapidly, it affects every organ of the body. As a result, many medical subspecialists become involved, from liver and gastrointestinal physicians, to nephrologists, intensivists, surgeons, neurosurgeons, as well as cell biologists, and those interested in biomechanical liver support. The disease incorporates fascinating physiologic changes such as cerebral edema which are as yet largely unexplained. The present text is an effort to pull together the diverse parts of acute liver failure, and to present them in a comprehensive fashion: etiology, pathophysiology, management, transplantation issues and future options. We have assembled the best authorities in the field from Europe and from North America, and have tried to balance, where necessary and appropriate, opposing views and ideas on specific aspects of the subject.

Of necessity, multiauthor books may have omissions, as well as overlaps. In most instances, we have been able to at least limit the amount of redundant material. With some topics, for example in considering management, we resisted the temptation to prune severely in favor of presenting several viewpoints since this is probably a more realistic approach to the subject.

There are very few absolutes in acute liver failure. It is clear however, that experience in caring for patients with acute liver failure is vitally important to optimal survival of this fragile patient population. Our sincere hope is that this book will be of value to all medical specialties concerned in the care as well as research of this rare condition, and that it will provide a firm basis on which evolving new ideas and results can be developed further.

William M. Lee, MD
Roger Williams, CBE, MD

Foreword

Acute liver failure is a highly complex syndrome arising when acute liver cell damage causes the breakdown of vital functions of the normal liver within a few days or weeks. Clinical encephalopathy, which is usually considered to be the hallmark of the syndrome, is always preceded by a rapid decrease in coagulation factors.

The incidence of the syndrome has been estimated to be 2000 cases a year in the United States and roughly 150 cases a year in France. Such a low incidence explains why, in all too many patients, the diagnosis of acute liver failure is so often delayed. The complexity of the syndrome is reflected in the numerous designations used by hepatologists and is due both to its multiplicity of effects on various organs – mainly brain and kidney – and the diversity of the causes.

Although acute viral hepatitis is the predominant cause worldwide, there are numerous other causes. Some of these, for example Wilson's disease, autoimmune hepatitis, and acute fatty liver of pregnancy, are uncommon, but their early recognition and specific treatment prevent acute liver failure, and this is undoubtedly the best strategy to adopt.

Acute liver failure often develops in previously healthy young adults or even children. The particular difficulty in the clinical management of such patients is determining whether they belong to that 25% on average who will recover spontaneously. Therefore, when presented with acute liver failure, many questions arise that need to be answered as quickly as possible without adding the further complication of iatrogenic aggravation: What is the cause? What is the prognosis? What needs monitoring? What clinical management is best? To transplant or not to transplant?

All these difficult questions and their answers have been brought together by William M. Lee, Roger Williams and the 38 co-authors of this remarkable volume. The resulting book offers the reader a state-of-the-art commentary on the many facets of the syndrome of acute liver failure and the recent advances in its management, detailing what and what not to do when treating these extremely fragile patients. Emergency medicine is not easy and we support the point made in several chapters that uncertainty – a daily companion of physicians – still predominates in numerous areas (mainly pathophysiology, monitoring, prognosis and therapeutics) within the field of acute liver failure.

In full agreement with the authors, we warmly recommend the *early referral* of patients with acute liver failure – *and also of those with acute liver disease without clinical encephalopathy but with severe coagulopathy* –

to liver units experienced in their clinical management. Recent experience with acetaminophen-induced acute liver failure at King's College Hospital and our experience with non-acetaminophen-induced acute liver failure at Beaujon Hospital confirm that such early referral improves the overall survival rate.

The coverage of the topic of emergency liver transplantation, including auxiliary liver transplantation, is one of the most outstanding aspects of this book. Still a dream 25 years ago, emergency liver transplantation is now an actual treatment that has undoubtedly, within the past 10 years, improved the overall survival rate of patients with presumed fatal acute liver failure, even if some of them have probably been overtransplanted. However, behind the scenes, the lives of patients after emergency total liver transplantation, even if often considered to be "normal", are dependent upon lifelong immunosuppression. Accordingly, doctors as well as patients' families will tell you that spontaneous recovery with the patient's own liver is always preferable, and is the gold standard of any therapeutic strategy in patients with acute liver failure.

This book also points the reader towards the future in the treatment of acute liver failure: namely, the "bioartificial liver". Do we already have an extracorporeal device filled with living hepatocytes that actually works, even for few hours, as liver parenchyma? Although preliminary results look encouraging, a positive answer to this question is far from certain.

The present book is unique and will become a must in the field of acute liver failure. It will provide help to physicians in the most difficult moments they will share together with their patients who are affected by acute liver failure. Reading these 23 chapters after having taken care of almost 800 patients with acute liver failure reinforced our personal understanding of the syndrome. *Acute liver failure attests the failure in preventing both the cause and the aggravation of the initial liver disease.* Prevention against acute liver failure should be a major goal of the near future. Prevention of the most frequent causes is at hand: with a more widespread use of vaccination, the incidence of fulminant hepatitis B and that of fulminant hepatitis A are likely to decrease significantly, at least in the Western countries. Improving the education of doctors in the prevention and the early detection of drug-induced toxicity should help to prevent life-threatening accidents of drug-induced hepatotoxicity. Prevention of the aggravation of the initial liver disease requires mainly the immediate cessation of the use of xenobiotics at the very onset of any acute liver disease, and also the early diagnosis of some rare, but treatable, causes of acute liver failure.

Jean-Pierre Benhamou, MD
Jacques Bernuau, MD
Service d'Hépatologie,
Hôpital Beaujon,
Clichy, France

Acknowledgments

The editors would like to thank first all the authors who toiled tirelessly to make this volume what it is. No multiauthor book is better than its individual chapter authors, and we have assembled the best group here. Special thanks to Renate Davis for editorial assistance in the United States, Scott Bodell for assistance with the illustrations, Eileen Withrington, Editorial Assistant in the Institute of Liver Studies, King's College Hospital, and to Richard Barling and Andy Leinicke of Cambridge University Press for their careful editing and monitoring of our progress.

Contributors

Evren Atillasoy,
The Mount Sinai School of Medicine, Division of Liver Diseases, One Gustave L. Levy Place, New York, NY 10029, USA

William F. Balistreri,
Division of Pediatric Gastroenterology & Nutrition, Children's Hospital Medical Center, 3333 Burnet Avenue, Cincinnati, Ohio 45229-3039, USA

Paul D. Berk,
Department of Medicine, Division of Liver Diseases, The Mount Sinai Medical Center, One Gustave L. Levy Place, Box 1039, New York, NY 10029, USA

Henri Bismuth,
Centre Hepato-Biliaire, Hôpital Paul Brousse, 94800 Villejuif, France

Andres T. Blei
Medical School Northwestern University, Northwestern Memorial Hospital, Chicago, Illinois 60611, USA

Karim Boudjema
Centre de Chirurgie Viscérale et de Transplantation, Hôpital Universitaire de Hautepierre, Avenue Molière, 67098 Strasbourg Cedex, France

Marie-Pierre Chenard-Neu
Service d'Anatomie Pathologique Generale, Hôpital Universitaire de Hautepierre, Avenue Molière, 67098 Strasbourg Cedex, France

James M. Courtney
Bioengineering Unit, University of Strathclyde, 106 Rottenrow, Glasgow G4 0NW, UK

Ian D. D'Agata
Children's Hospital Medical Center, Cincinnati, Ohio 45229-3039, USA

John Devlin
Institute of Liver Studies, King's College Hospital, London SE5 9RS, UK

Antony J. Ellis
Institute of Liver Studies, King's College School of Medicine & Dentistry, Bessemer Road, London SE5 9PJ, UK

Nelson Fausto
Department of Pathology SM30, University of Washington School of Medicine, Health and Science Bldg, Rm C515, Seattle, Washington 98195, USA

Ira J. Fox
Department of Surgery, University of Nebraska, 600 S 42nd Street, Omaha, Nebraska 68198-3280, USA

Jörg Gerlach
Medizinische Fakultät der Humboldt, Universität zu Berlin, Forschungshaus Virchow-Klinikum, Augustenburger Platz 1, D-13353 Berlin, Germany

Bent Adel Hansen
Medical Department A, Rigshospitalet, Copenhagen, Denmark

Robin D. Hughes
Institute of Liver Studies, King's College School of Medicine & Dentistry, Bessemer Road, London SE5 9PJ, UK

Daniel Jaeck
Centre de Chirurgie Viscérale et de Transplantation, Hôpital Universitaire de Hautepierre, Avenue Molière, 67098 Strasbourg Cedex, France

Neil Kaplowitz
Division of Gastrointestinal and Liver Diseases; USC Center for Liver Diseases, University of Southern California School of Medicine, Los Angeles, CA 90033, USA

James H. Kelly
Amphioxus Cell Technologies and Baylor College of Medicine, PO Box 1633, Stafford, Texas 77497-1633, USA

Fin Stolze Larsen
Medical Department A, Rigshospitalet, Copenhagen, Denmark

William M. Lee
Clinical Center for Liver Diseases, University of Texas Southwestern Medical Center at Dallas, 5323 Harry Hines Boulevard, Dallas, Texas 75235-8887, USA

Gary A. Levy
University of Toronto, The Toronto Hospital – General Division, Multi Organ Transplant Program, 621 University Avenue, 10 NU-151, Toronto, Ontario M5G 2C4, Canada

Alistair J. Makin
Institute of Liver Studies, King's College School of Medicine & Dentistry, Bessemer Road, London SE5 9PJ, UK

Kevork M. Peltekian
Dalhousie University, Queen Elizabeth II, HSC, 4088–1278 Tower Road, Halifax, Nova Scotia, B3H 2Y9, Canada

John Philpott-Howard
Department of Medical Microbiology, King's College Hospital, Bessemer Road, London SE5 9PJ, UK

Bernard Portmann
Institute of Liver Studies, King's College School of Medicine & Dentistry, Bessemer Road, London SE5 9PJ, UK

Caroline A. Riely
University of Tennessee Memphis, 951 Court Avenue, Room 555D, Memphis, Tennessee 38163, USA

Nancy Rolando
Institute of Liver Studies, King's College School of Medicine & Dentistry, Bessemer Road, London SE5 9PJ, UK

Namita Roy Chowdhury
Albert Einstein College of Medicine, 1300 Morris Park Avenue, Bronx, New York 10461, USA

Jayanta Roy Chowdhury
Albert Einstein College of Medicine, 1300 Morris Park Avenue, Bronx, New York 10461, USA

Didier Samuel
Centre Hepato-Biliaire, Hôpital Paul Brousse
94800 Villejuif, France

Romil Saxena
Department of Pathology,
Montefiore Medical Center and
Albert Einstein University,
111 East 210th Street, Bronx,
NY 10467-2490, USA

Byers W. Shaw Jr
Department of Surgery, University of Nebraska,
College of Medicine, Omaha,
Nebraska 68198-3280, USA

Norman L. Sussman
Amphioxus Cell Technologies and
Baylor College of Medicine,
PO Box 1633, Stafford, Texas 77497-1633, USA

Gloria Sze
Division of Gastrointestinal and Liver Diseases,
University of Southern California School of
Medicine,
Los Angeles, CA 90033, USA

Dwain L. Thiele
University of Texas Southwestern Medical Center
at Dallas,
5323 Harry Hines Boulevard,
Dallas, Texas 75235-9151, USA

Niels Tygstrup
Medical Department A, Rigshospitalet,
Copenhagen,
Denmark

Mark D. Uhl
University of Tennessee Memphis,
951 Court Avenue, Room 555D,
Memphis, Tennessee 38163, USA

Julia A. Wendon
Institute of Liver Studies,
King's College Hospital and King's College
School of Medicine & Dentistry,
Denmark Hill, London SE5 9RS, UK

Roger Williams
Institute of Liver Studies,
King's College Hospital,
London SE5 9PJ, UK

PART ONE Clinical Syndrome and Etiology

1 Classification and clinical syndromes of acute liver failure

Roger Williams

INTRODUCTION

Acute liver failure (ALF) describes a constellation of clinical symptoms associated with sudden cessation of normal hepatic function (Hoofnagle et al. 1995). The defining state is hepatic encephalopathy and the development of a coagulopathy with subsequent jaundice. In many cases this clinical picture is associated with cerebral edema, renal impairment and multiorgan failure. All of these clinical features need not develop in every case and are not specific to the etiology of the ALF. Patterns may be discerned which can indicate the etiology, for example those with acetaminophen (paracetamol) overdose often present with encephalopathy and severe coagulopathy which may progress rapidly to cerebral edema although the patient may not be jaundiced, whereas patients with non-A non-B hepatitis more often present with deep jaundice but are less likely to develop cerebral edema. First described as acute yellow atrophy, acute liver failure has continued to challenge clinicians and, in spite of many advances, it still carries a significant mortality.

In 1946 Lucke and Mallory reported the rare occurrence of fatal hepatitis as a consequence of epidemic hepatitis (Lucke and Mallory 1946). They distinguished two clinical courses: fulminant, with a rapidly fatal outcome, and a subacute form with a slower course but equally poor prognosis. The first attempt at a formal definition was by Trey and Davidson in 1970, who described fulminant hepatic failure as "a potentially reversible condition, the consequence of severe liver injury, with the onset of hepatic encephalopathy within eight weeks of the first symptoms and in the absence of pre-existing liver disease" (Trey and Davidson 1970). Within that definition lies the recognition that patients may present unwell before any clinical evidence of liver damage. Although in many instances there will be a clear history of symptoms compatible with an acute viral hepatitis, many of these are non-specific which makes the precise timing of the onset of illness difficult. In 1986, Gimson et al., in describing an even rarer type of ALF, defined late onset hepatic failure as the development of hepatic encephalopathy between eight and twenty-four weeks from the onset of jaundice (Gimson et al. 1986), use of the latter being more readily identified by both patients and clinician and allowing more accurate timing of the illness. Workers in France, however, in using a different set of definitions have based these on the interval from the onset of jaundice to the development of encephalopathy. The term fulminant hepatic failure is used to categorize patients with encephalopathy developing within two weeks of the onset of jaundice and the term subfulminant hepatic failure to describe those who develop encephalopathy between two and twelve weeks from the onset of jaundice (Benhamou 1991).

Hyperacute, acute and subacute liver failure

The time considerations, it has become clear, are of considerable importance in indicating likely prognosis. Paradoxically, it is the group of patients with the most rapid onset of encephalopathy who have the best chance of spontaneous recovery (Gimson et al. 1986; Benhamou 1991). To take account of this, we have recently proposed a new classification in which ALF is taken as an umbrella term with subgroups of hyperacute, acute and subacute to reflect different clinical patterns of illness, etiology and, most importantly, prognosis (O'Grady et al. 1993) (Table 1.1). Hyperacute hepatic failure is used to describe those patients who develop encephalopathy within eight days of the onset of jaundice. The majority of those in this group have acute acetaminophen poisoning but a proportion of those with acute hepatitis A or B may also present in this way. Acute hepatic failure includes those with a jaundice to encephalopathy time of eight to twenty-eight days. The majority of those with viral hepatitis as the cause present in this window. Subacute hepatic failure describes those with a jaundice to encephalopathy time of four to twenty-six weeks. Most of these patients have so called non-A non-B hepatitis where no viral agent can be identified (Gimson et al. 1986; O'Grady et al. 1993).

Table 1.1. *New classification of acute liver failure, based on time from first sign of jaundice to appearance of encephalopathy, with frequency of different etiologies in the three groups (from O'Grady et al. 1993)*

	Frequency (%)		
	Hyperacute 0–7 days	Acute 7–28 days	Subacute 5–26 weeks
Hepatitis A	55.2	31	13.8
Hepatitis B	62.5	29.2	8.3
NANB hepatitis	13.6	38.8	47.6
Idiosyncratic drug reactions	35.3	52.9	11.8

Epidemiology and geographical variations

Acute viral hepatitis accounts for up to 50 percent of cases of ALF seen in North American and European centers although in many cases, as already referred to, no specific infective viral hepatitis agent can be identified despite a clinical picture compatible with viral hepatitis (Fagan and Harrison 1994 and Chapter 2). The contribution of the newly described hepatitis virus GB agents in fulminant viral hepatitis is not yet defined. In India, a high proportion of cases present with subacute liver failure of the non-A non-B type. Hepatitis E is also more frequently encountered in subtropical areas and is associated with high mortality, particularly in pregnant women. In most reported series, hepatitis B (HBV) is the most common type of viral hepatitis resulting in ALF, followed by non-A non-B and hepatitis A. This is particularly true in France where 46 percent have HBV and in Japan where 62 percent do. In the UK, non-A non-B is the most common "viral" cause of ALF reflecting the low background prevalence of HBV infection.

In general, the different agents responsible for ALF in each country proportionally relate to the underlying prevalence of those infections in the particular country. Thus, hepatitis B induced ALF is common in the Far East where HBV infection is common but is rare in the UK where HBV infects less than 1 percent of the population. Indeed, in the UK the proportion of all cases with ALF in which a viral etiology is implicated is less than 30 percent with more than half of these having a seronegative hepatitis. This is also a reflection of the high prevalence of acetaminophen-associated ALF in the UK. In France, the proportion of viral-associated ALF is higher, HBV being the major viral agent (Benhamou 1991) and in the USA the figures are similar with viral hepatitis accounting for 62 percent of cases (Hoofnagle et al. 1995).

With respect to hepatitis C, in substantial series of patients from the Western world, instances of infection were either absent or very rarely found (Sallie et al. 1994; Wright et al. 1991; Theilmann et al. 1992; Feray et al. 1993), although there are also some well documented single case reports of fulminant hepatitis C from these regions (Theilmann 1992). In Japan, however, over half of the patients from one series with acute or subacute liver failure had evidence of infection with hepatitis C virus (HCV) (Yoshiba et al. 1994). Evidence of HCV infection was detected in only one patient with HBV-ALF, although in another series from Japan, a number of patients with HBV-ALF had dual infection with HCV-RNA and this was associated with a worse prognosis (Yanagi et al. 1991). The French experience is similar: nearly half of hepatitis B surface antigen (HBsAg) positive patients with ALF had detectable HCV-RNA in serum (Feray et al. 1993). In a recent study from Taiwan, HCV-RNA could be detected in a significant number of patients with all types of fulminant hepatitis, and the authors of this paper suggest that 40–50 percent of cases of fulminant viral hepatitis in their region are related to HCV infection (Chu et al. 1994).

The etiology and number of cases of ALF progressing to grade III and IV coma admitted to the Liver Failure Unit at this Institute over a recent two-year period are given in Table 1.2.

Table 1.2. *Etiology of 342 cases of acute liver failure admitted to the Liver Failure Unit, King's College Hospital, 1993–1994*

Overdose	
Acetaminophen	250
Ecstasy	2
Viral hepatitis	
A	8
B	8
Non-A, B, C, D, E	28
Other causes	
Wilson's disease	3
Fatty liver of pregnancy	7
Lymphoma/malignant infiltration	7
Sepsis	2
Budd–Chiari syndrome	5
Ischemic hepatitis	9
Miscellaneous	6
Idiosyncratic drug reactions	
Lamotrigine, cyproterone, nonsteroidal anti-inflammatory drugs, chloroquine, Rifampicin/Isoniazid, Halothane, Flucloxacillin	7

BASIS OF CLINICAL SYNDROME

Most of the damage to the liver has already been done by the time of presentation and pathologic examination of the liver at this phase of the disease process will show areas of collapsed hepatic parenchyma in which all viable hepatocytes have been destroyed and, depending on time after onset, areas of regeneration. The clinical signs and pattern of illness depend on the balance between three factors: the liver's ability to regenerate, the adverse metabolic consequences of loss of a functioning liver, and the wide range of toxic substances released into the serum from the necrotic liver.

Characteristically there is evidence of multiorgan failure. Although symptoms and signs of the different organ involvement are often considered separately, when it comes to treatment it is imperative to realize their interdependence and the central driving force of the primary liver injury, as illustrated in Figure 1.1. As an immediate consequence of the acute

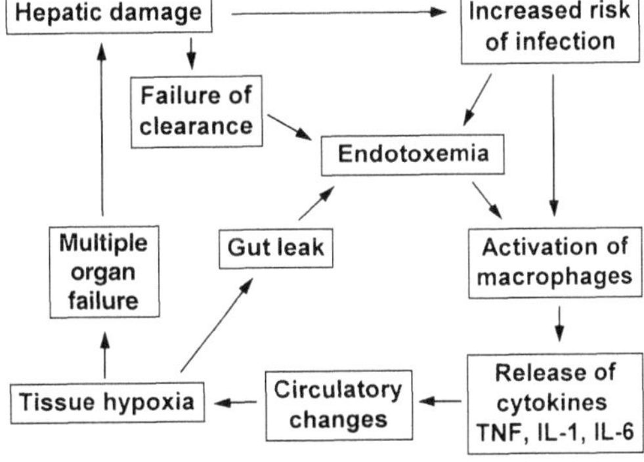

Figure 1.1 Vicious cycle of events in pathogenesis which provide the basis for multiorgan failure.

liver injury, host defenses to infection are severely compromised and with secondary bacterial infection there is endotoxemia, activation of macrophages, and release of cytokines and tumor necrosis factor. The resulting clinical picture is similar to that of septic shock with hypotension and other circulatory changes leading to tissue hypoxia and damage to a number of organs as well as the gut, and with further ischemic injury of the liver: a vicious cycle indeed.

Nevertheless, as a result of a better understanding of the basis of multiorgan failure and the development of intensive liver care, quite apart from the introduction of liver transplantation for 15–20 percent of the most severe cases, survival results over the years have steadily improved (Figure 1.2).

Encephalopathy and cerebral edema

For those patients with ALF whose encephalopathy does not progress beyond grades I–II the prognosis is excellent, whereas in grades III–IV the mortality is very much higher dependent on clinical pattern of onset and etiology (Lee 1993). Until recently about 80 percent of patients with grade IV encephalopathy progressed further to develop cerebral edema (O'Grady et al. 1988), but the frequency of cerebral edema has decreased recently, possibly as a result of better treatment of microcirculatory disturbances and of infection. The pathogenic mechanisms that result in hepatic encephalopathy and brain edema in patients with ALF remain incompletely understood. Possible etiological mechanisms include the presence of benzodiazepine agonists, altered gamma aminobutyric acid (GABA) status, increased aromatic amines, ammonia and mercaptans. Joint studies with workers at the US National Institutes of Health have demonstrated recently the presence of raised brain concentrations of 1,4-benzodiazepines in patients with ALF (Basile et al. 1991). It would appear that a combination of both vasogenic (extravasation of protein and extracellular edema in the presence of a damaged blood brain barrier) and cytotoxic (intracellular edema) factors are responsible for the cerebral edema in ALF. The clinical signs of the resulting increase in intracranial pressure (ICP) are those of systemic hypertension, decerebrate posturing, abnormal pupillary reflexes and ultimately impairment of brain stem reflexes.

Although some studies of patients in grade IV encephalopathy have shown raised cerebral blood flows (CBF) contributing to the elevation in ICP, more recent work suggests that this is not the case. Indeed CBF has been shown to be low (Almdal et al. 1989; Sari

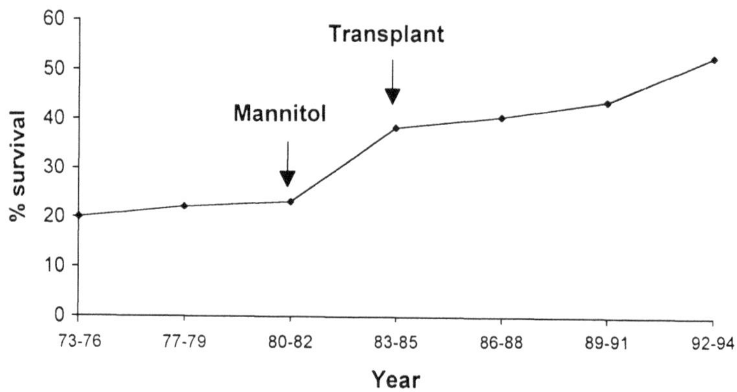

Figure 1.2 Survival percentages for all etiologies of acute liver failure (grades 3–4 encephalopathy only), since the Liver Failure Unit opened in 1973. Total of 1,231 patients shown.

et al. 1990), and it has been postulated that cerebral ischemia may be an important factor in the cerebral damage. In particular it may underlie the development of epileptiform activity. This is difficult to detect clinically in the paralyzed, ventilated patient, and an EEG monitor is of considerable value. The early recognition of this complication and its control by diazepam and/or phenytoin is of vital importance in minimizing the likelihood of secondary cerebral edema. With seizure activity, the jugular bulb oxygen saturation is decreased as a result of an increase in oxygen consumption in the brain (Table 1.3).

Table 1.3. *Changes in jugular venous saturation with seizure activity*

			With phenytoin:
Jugular venous saturation	59	→	83%
Mean arterial pressure	70	→	75 mmHg
Intracranial pressure	17	→	14 mmHg
Cerebral perfusion pressure	53	→	61 mmHg
Pupils fixed			Pupils reacting

Metabolic disorders and renal impairment

Hypoglycemia is seen early in the clinical course and is a consequence of an increase in circulating insulin, and impaired gluconeogenesis along with an inability to mobilize glycogen stores. Another common metabolic abnormality also occurring early is hypophosphatemia, seen especially in those who maintain urine output.

Metabolic acidosis is a relatively frequent finding which, had been attributed solely to liver dysfunction and impaired lactate metabolism. It has, however, been demonstrated that much of the acidosis is related to the presence of tissue hypoxia and increased peripheral lactate production (Bihari, Gimson, Lindridge and Williams 1985). This work also demonstrated a strong negative correlation between systemic vascular resistance and oxygen extraction ratio, suggesting that the greater the degree of microcirculatory disturbance, and hence tissue hypoxia, the higher the blood lactate.

A urine output of less than 300 ml per 24 h and serum creatinine of greater than 300 mmol/1, in the presence of adequate intravascular filling pressures occurs in about 70 percent of patients with acetaminophen overdose and in about 30 percent of other cases of ALF (O'Grady and Williams 1986). The renal failure that is seen in association with ALF invariably recovers either when the patient's liver function improves spontaneously or after transplantation.

Infection

Infection is common in patients with ALF and is related to compromised immune function with impaired neutrophil and Kupffer cell function and deficiency of opsonins. In the initial studies from this unit, bacterial infection was identified in 80 percent of patients (Rolando et al. 1990). The infecting organisms were Gram-positive in 54 percent of cases, and over 50 percent of these were *Staphylococcus aureus*. Fungal infection, predominantly with *candida* species, is also a frequent occurrence particularly in the later stages of the clinical condition (Rolando et al. 1991). In ALF, Kupffer cell function is impaired, thus limiting clearance of endotoxin and allowing passage of bacteria translocated from the gut into the systemic circulation. The importance of Kupffer cell function is further emphasized by the study by Canalese et al. who demonstrated that survival from ALF in a group of patients with similar degrees of hepatocyte dysfunction, as measured by galactose clearance, was related to maintenance or early recovery of Kupffer cell function (Canalese et al. 1982).

Coagulopathy

Marked prolongation of the prothrombin time is a characteristic finding in ALF and is closely related to the severity of liver damage. Factor V has the shortest half life and is theoretically the more sensitive yardstick for assessing impairment of synthesis of coagulation factors. In addition to decreased synthesis of clotting factors there is also an increase in peripheral consumption consequent on a degree of disseminated intravascular coagulation (DIC) (O'Grady et al. 1986). Both quantitative and qualitative defects in platelet function have been described, with thrombocytopenia, increased adhesiveness and impaired aggregation. The risk of bleeding appears to correlate not so much with prothrombin time but with thrombocytopenia and the presence of overt DIC. Gastrointestinal hemorrhage is normally related to the development of gastric erosions, although the frequency with which this occurs has been much decreased since the routine use of prophylactic H_2 receptor antagonists and agents such as sucralfate.

Cardiorespiratory complications

Arterial hypoxemia is frequently seen in patients with ALF and is multifactorial in origin. Aspiration of gastric contents, bacterial infection, intrapulmonary hemorrhage, atelectasis, ventilation/perfusion (V/Q) mismatch and more rarely the development of adult respiratory distress syndrome are all contributory factors.

Cardiac arrhythmias are rare and usually due to a definable precipitating event: hypo- or hyperkalemia, acidosis, hypoxia or cardiac irritation due to the insertion of lines. The hemodynamic disturbances seen in patients with ALF are similar to those of patients with sepsis, that is an elevated cardiac output and lowered systemic vascular resistance index. The pathophysiology of the hypotension was first investigated by Trewby and Williams 1977, who demonstrated that peripheral vasodilation rather than primary myocardial failure was present and that volume loading frequently resulted in an increase in cardiac output and an improvement in mean arterial pressure. Patients with ALF display similar hemodynamic abnormalities to those seen in patients with sepsis and trauma, including the development of pathologic supply-dependency for oxygen.

Failure to maintain an adequate oxygen uptake to cells is a fundamental problem in the critically ill patient. This appears to be related to a combination of problems resulting in an inability to regulate delivery and extraction of oxygen at a cellular level. In healthy individuals, physiologic supply-dependency of oxygen only occurs when oxygen delivery (Do_2) falls below a level of 330 ml/min/m^2 (Haupt et al. 1985). Any additional fall in delivery below this critical level will result in a decreased tissue oxygen uptake (Vo_2), with the subsequent development of tissue hypoxia, anerobic metabolism and build up of lactate when delivery falls below a critical lower limit. Patients who are critically ill, such as those with severe sepsis, multiple trauma, adult respiratory distress syndrome, and those with ALF display "pathologic supply-dependency" for oxygen (see Chapter 11), Figure 1.3. "Appropriate values" for oxygen consumption in such circumstances are not known: however, levels should perhaps be considerably higher than that seen in normal healthy controls, since the patients have high levels of circulating catecholamines, are pyrexial and hypercatabolic and frequently have an intense localized or generalized inflammatory reaction. Infusion of prostacyclin, a microcirculatory vasodilator, in patients with ALF resulted in significant increases in oxygen consumption secondary to increased delivery (Bihari, Gimson, Waterson and Williams 1985; Bihari et al. 1986). Patients who die from their ALF have lower systemic vascular resistance and oxygen consumption than patients who survive, suggesting a greater degree of microcirculatory dysfunction in nonsurvivors (Bihari, Gimson, Waterson and Williams 1985; Bihari et al. 1986).

OUTCOME AND RELATED FACTORS

In a multivariate analysis of 588 patients with ALF at King's College Hospital, UK, etiology was identified as the single most important independent predictor of outcome. The best prognosis is observed in patients with acute

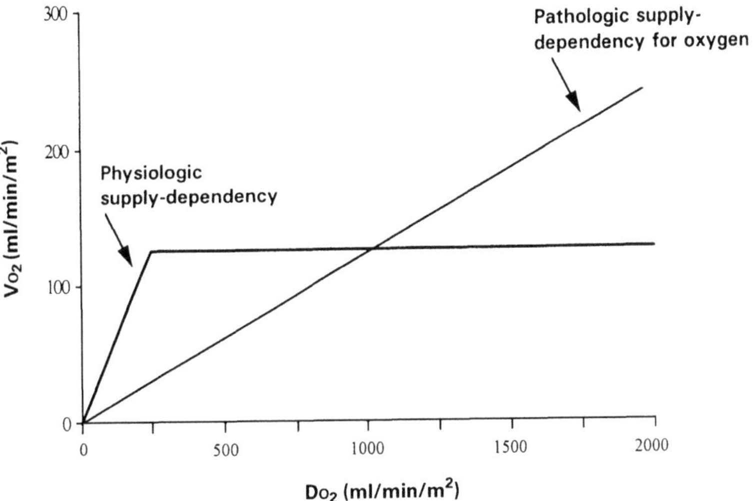

Figure 1.3 Pathologic supply-dependency for oxygen.

fatty liver of pregnancy, whilst amongst the viral causes hepatitis A has the highest survival, hepatitis B intermediate and non-A non-B the worst. The prognosis for drug induced ALF including that of halothane is also poor. The fulminant presentation of Wilson's disease is almost always fatal and the rapid detection of signs pointing to this etiology (hemolysis, splenomegaly and Kaiser–Fleischer rings) is vital so that patients can be listed for transplantation. The rare fulminant presentation of an autoimmune hepatitis also carries a very poor prognosis with medical therapy alone.

Although mortality appears higher in patients who reach deeper grades of coma (III and IV) this is not uniformly so. Patients with slowly progressive or subacute liver failure will often succumb to sepsis and circulatory failure before the development of grade IV coma and the survival of patients with the most rapid progression, as seen in hyperacute liver failure, is better. In an analysis of our series in 1989, the survival for viral hepatitis A and B was 66.7 percent in the absence of cerebral edema, falling to 50 percent when cerebral edema was present, and decreasing further to 30 percent when cerebral edema coexisted with oliguric renal failure (O'Grady et al. 1989). With cerebral death becoming less frequent, infection in association with circulatory failure is now the most common cause of death in our experience.

For all etiological groups, the mortality rate rises with age, and intercurrent illness.

The prolongation of prothrombin time and of the more recently introduced international normalized ratio (INR) was shown in a multivariate analysis of the King's College series to be an independent predictor of outcome in all etiological groups (O'Grady et al. 1989). Although in the acetaminophen overdose group no particular cut off level of INR could be determined, a rise in INR at day 3 to 4 was associated with a 7 percent survival compared with a 79 percent survival in those whose INR fell at that time (Harrison et al. 1990). Assay of specific coagulation factors have been advocated by the French group. In a study of 115 patients with fulminant hepatitis B, factor V levels were lower in those who died and multivariate analysis confirmed this to be the most effective predictor of outcome (Bernuau et al. 1986). However, in a detailed study of 22 patients with acetaminophen-induced ALF carried out in King's College, although factor V levels were lower in the patients who died there was considerable overlap with the survivors (Pereira et al. 1992). In the multivariate analysis already referred to (Bernuau et al. 1986), the height of serum bilirubin was also shown to be an independent predictor of outcome, and was as powerful as the INR in patients with a drug induced or viral etiology. Some patients succumb before the bilirubin has risen significantly and this is more frequently seen in acetaminophen-induced hepatic damage of the hyperacute liver failure type (O'Grady et al. 1993). The presence or development of a metabolic acidosis is the most powerful prognostic indicator in acetaminophen-induced ALF (O'Grady et al. 1989).

With respect to the other possible serum measurements, increases in serum alphafetoprotein are considered to reflect hepatic regeneration and in some series have been associated with an improved prognosis (Murray-Lyon et al. 1976). Determination of unbound group-specific component (Gc) protein concentrations has been shown to have some use as a predictor of prognosis in ALF (Lee et al. 1995). This is an actin scavenger whose levels fall in ALF and, in a retrospective analysis of 42 cases, all fatal cases were correctly identified at two days after admission. However, the test is not widely available at the present time.

REFERENCES

Almdal, T., Schroeder, T. and Ranek, L. 1989. Cerebral blood flow and liver function in patients with encephalopathy due to acute and chronic liver diseases. *Scand J Gastroenterol* 24: 299–303.

Basile, A., Hughes, R., Harrison, P., Murata Y., Pannell, L., Jones, E.A., Williams, R. and Skolnick, P. 1991. Elevated brain concentrations of 1,4-benzodiazepines in fulminant hepatic failure. *N Engl J Med* 325: 473–8.

Benhamou, J.P. 1991. Fulminant and subfulminant hepatic failure; definition and causes. In *Acute Liver Failure: Improved Understanding and Better Therapy*, eds. R. Williams, R.D. Hughes, 6–10. London: Mitre Press.

Bernuau, J., Goudeau, A., Poynard, T., Dubois, F., Lesage, G., Yvannet, B., Degott, C., Bezaud, A., Rueff, B. and Benhamou, J.P. 1986. Multivariate analysis of prognostic factors in fulminant hepatitis B. *Hepatology* 6: 648–51.

Bihari, D., Gimson, A.E., Lindridge, J. and Williams, R. 1985. Lactic acidosis in fulminant hepatic failure. Some aspects of pathogenesis and prognosis. *J Hepatol* 1: 405–16.

Bihari, D., Gimson, A.E., Waterson, M. and Williams, R. 1985. Tissue hypoxia during fulminant hepatic failure. *Crit Care Med* 13: 1034–9.

Bihari, D.J., Gimson, A.E. and Williams, R. 1986. Cardiovascular, pulmonary and renal complications of fulminant hepatic failure. *Sem Liver Dis* 6: 119–28.

Bradley, D. 1992. Hepatitis E: Epidemiology, aetiology and molecular biology. *Rev Med Virol* 2: 19–29.

Canalese, J., Gove, C.D., Gimson, A.E.S., Wilkinson, S.P., Wardle, E.N. and Williams, R. 1982. Reticuloendothelial system and hepatocyte function in fulminant hepatic failure. *Gut* 23: 265–9.

Chu, C., Sheen, I. and Liaw, Y. 1994. The role of hepatitis C virus in fulminant hepatic failure in an area with endemic hepatitis A and B. *Gastroenterology* 107: 189–95.

Fagan, E.A. and Harrison, T.J. 1994. Exclusion in liver by polymerase chain reaction of hepatitis B and C viruses in acute liver failure attributed to sporadic non-A, non-B hepatitis. *J Hepatol* 21: 587–91.

Feray, C., Gigou, M., Samuel, D. et al. 1993. Hepatitis C virus RNA and hepatitis B virus DNA in serum and liver of patients with fulminant hepatitis. *Gastroenterology* 104: 549–55.

Gimson, A.E.S., O'Grady, J., Ede, R.J., Portmann, B. and Williams, R. 1986. Late-onset hepatic failure: clinical, serological and histological features. *Hepatology* 6: 288–94.

Harrison, P., O'Grady, J., Alexander, G. and Williams, R. 1990. Serial prothrombin times: a prognostic indicator in paracetamol-induced fulminant hepatic failure. *BMJ* 301: 964–6.

Haupt, M.T., Gilbert, E.M. and Carlson, R.W. 1985. Fluid loading increases oxygen consumption in septic patients with lactic acidosis. *Am Rev Respir Dis* 131: 912–16.

Hoofnagle, J.H., Carithers, R.L., Shapiro, C. and Ascher, N. 1995. Fulminant Hepatic Failure: Summary of a Workshop. *Hepatology* 21: 240–52.

Lee, W.M. 1993. Acute liver failure. *N Engl J Med* 325: 1862–72.

Lee, W.M., Galbraith, R.M., Watt, G.H., Hughes, R.D., McIntire, D.D., Hoffman, B.J. and Williams, R. 1995. Predicting survival in hepatic failure using serum Gc concentrations. *Hepatology* 21: 101–5.

Lucke, B. and Mallory, T. 1946. Fulminant form of epidemic hepatitis. *Am J Pathol* 22: 867–945.

Murray-Lyon, I.M., Orr, A.H., Gazzard, B., Kohn, J. and Williams, R. 1976. Prognostic value of serum alpha-fetoprotein in fulminant hepatic failure including patients treated by charcoal haemoperfusion. *Gut* 17: 576–80.

O'Grady, J., Alexander, G., Hayllar, K. and Williams, R. 1989. Early indicators of prognosis in fulminant hepatic failure. *Gastroenterology* 97: 439–45.

O'Grady, J.G., Langley, P.G., Isola, L.M., Aledort, L.M. and Williams, R. 1986. Coagulopathy of fulminant hepatic failure. *Sem Liver Dis* 6: 159–63.

O'Grady, J.G. and Williams, R. 1986. Management of acute liver failure. *Schweiz Med Wochenschr* 116: 541–4.

O'Grady, J.G., Gimson, A.E., O'Brien, C.J., Pucknell, A., Hughes, R.D. and Williams, R. 1988. Controlled trials of charcoal hemoperfusion and prognostic factors in fulminant hepatic failure. *Gastroenterology* 94: 1186–92.

O'Grady, J. G., Schalm, S. and Williams, R. 1993. Acute liver failure: redefining the syndromes. *Lancet* 342: 373–5.

O'Grady, J.G. and Williams, R. 1993. Classification of acute liver failure. *Lancet* 342: 743–8.

Pereira, L., Langley, P., Hayllar, K., Tredger, J., and Williams, R. 1992. Coagulation factors V and VIII/V ratio as predictors of outcome in paracetamol-induced fulminant hepatic failure: relationship to other prognostic indicators. *Gut* 33: 98–102.

Rolando, N., Harvey, F., Brahm, J., Fagan, E. and Williams, R. 1990. Prospective study of bacterial infection in acute liver failure: an analysis of fifty patients. *Hepatology* 11: 49–53.

Rolando, N., Harvey, F., Brahm, J., Fagan, E. and Williams, R. 1991. Fungal infection: a common, unrecognised complication of acute liver failure. *Hepatology* 12: 1–9.

Sallie, R., Silva, E., Purdy, M., Smith, H., McCaustland, K., Tibbs, C., Portmann, B., Eddleston, A., Bradley, D. and Williams, R. 1994. Hepatitis C and E in fulminant hepatic failure: a polymerase chain reaction and serological study. *J Hepatol* 20: 580–8.

Sari, A., Yamashita, S., Ohosita, S., Ogasahara, H., Yamada, K., Yones, A. and Vokota, K. 1990. Cerebrovascular reactivity to CO_2 in patients with hepatic or septic encephalopathy. *Resuscitation* 19: 125–34.

Theilmann, L., Solbach, C., Toex, U., Muller, H.M., Pfaff, E., Otto, G. and Goeser, T. 1992. Role of hepatitis C virus infection in German patients with fulminant and subacute hepatic failure. *Eur J Clin Invest* 22: 569–71.

Trewby, P. and Williams, R. 1977. Pathophysiology of hypotension in patients with fulminant hepatic failure. *Gut* 18: 1021–6.

Trey, C. and Davidson, C.S. 1970. The management of fulminant hepatic failure. In *Progress in Liver Failure*, eds. H. Popper, F. Schaffner, 282–98. New York: Grune and Stratton.

Wright, T.L., Hsu, H., Donegan, E., Feinstone, S., Greenberg, H., Read, A., Ascher, N., Roberts, J. and Lake, J. 1991. Hepatitis C virus not found in fulminant non-A non-B hepatitis. *Ann Intern Med* 115: 111–12.

Yanagi, M., Kaneko, S., Unoura, M., Murakami, S., Kobayashi, K., Sugihara, J., Ohnishi, H. and Muto, Y. 1991. Hepatitis C virus in fulminant hepatic failure. *N Engl J Med* 324: 1895–6.

Yoshiba, M., Sekiyama, K., Inoue, K., Okamoto, H. and Mayumi, M. 1994. Contribution of hepatitis C virus to non-A non-B fulminant hepatitis in Japan. *Hepatology* 19: 829–35.

2 Viral hepatitis and acute liver failure

Dwain L. Thiele

INTRODUCTION

Acute liver failure is a rare complication of acute viral hepatitis. Nevertheless, viral hepatitis is the leading cause of fulminant or subfulminant hepatic failure in most hospitals. Each of the well-characterized hepatitis viruses has been implicated in acute liver failure, but the relative frequency of this complication varies widely. Overall case fatality rates of >0.5 percent have been reported among patients with acute, symptomatic hepatitis B or E, whereas acute hepatitis A or C infections are much less commonly implicated (Krawczynski 1993; McNeil et al. 1984; Papaevangelou et al. 1984; Takano et al. 1994). The highest overall incidence of fatal hepatitis has been reported among cases of sporadic acute non-A non-B hepatitis (McNeil et al. 1984; Papaevangelou et al. 1984). Such cases of fatal acute non-A non-B hepatitis are only rarely associated with infection by the hepatitis C or E viruses in the USA and Europe (Feray et al. 1993; Sallie et al. 1994; Theilmann et al. 1992; Wright et al. 1991). Acute hepatitis B alone or in association with other viral co-infections is the most common identifiable cause of fulminant viral hepatitis in developed countries although acute liver failure attributed to acute non-ABCDE hepatitis is equal or greater in frequency. In addition, rare cases of acute liver failure complicate infections by a variety of other viral agents as detailed in Table 2.1.

Table 2.1. *Etiologies of fulminant viral hepatitis*

Hepatitis viruses
Hepatitis B
Hepatitis E
Hepatitis D + B
Hepatitis A
Hepatitis C
non-ABCDE hepatitis?
Hemorrhagic fever viruses
Yellow fever virus
Dengue fever virus
Rift Valley fever virus
Filoviruses (Marburg, Ebola)
Other viruses
Herpesviruses 1, 2 & 6
Varicella-Zoster virus
Cytomegalovirus
Epstein–Barr virus
Adenovirus

FULMINANT HEPATITIS ASSOCIATED WITH ENTERIC HEPATITIS VIRUSES (A AND E)

Although acute hepatitis A is a very common disease world-wide, it rarely causes fulminant hepatic failure in most regions of the world (McNeil et al. 1984; Papaevangelou et al. 1984). Recent data suggest, however, that 20 percent of fulminant viral hepatitis cases from Northwestern Europe can be attributed to acute hepatitis A (Mathieson et al. 1980; Williams and Wendon 1994). These differences likely reflect, in part, evolving changes in the epidemiology of hepatitis A virus (HAV) infection. In particular, along with improvements in personal and public hygiene in developed countries, the epidemiology of HAV has changed from that of a relatively benign, endemic or epidemic disease of childhood to a much rarer, but more virulent sporadic disease of adults (Gocke 1986). The risk of developing acute liver failure appears to rise with increasing age in this and other forms of acute viral hepatitis (McNeil et al. 1984). In addition, other variations on the typically brief clinical course of childhood HAV infections have been reported recently among adults infected with HAV. These include prolonged, cholestatic and/or relapsing courses that in some cases are associated with extrahepatic manifestations such as arthritis or vasculitic skin rashes (Gocke 1986). Persistence of HAV infection has been noted in cases of relapsing or prolonged acute hepatitis A including two cases associated with acute liver failure leading to liver transplantation and subsequent re-infection of liver allografts (Fagan et al. 1990). Thus, in contrast to rapid clearance of viremia in severe acute hepatitis B, unusually severe clinical manifestations of HAV infection in adults have been associated with persistent viremia.

The diagnosis of acute HAV infection in patients with fulminant hepatic failure is usually straightforward, as most patients have high titers of IgM antibodies at time of hospitalization. However, as many as 5 percent of patients tested within several days of onset of symptoms may have undetectable anti-HAV responses (Liaw et al. 1986), suggesting that repeat testing in initially seronegative patients is warranted.

In contrast to the persistence of HAV as a major cause of viral hepatitis in developed countries, the hepatitis E virus (HEV) is limited to underdeveloped countries (Krawczynski 1993) and has only rarely been implicated in fulminant hepatitis in North America or Europe (Feray et al., 1993; Liang et al. 1993; Sallie et al. 1994). However, one of the characteristic features of HEV infections in underdeveloped countries has been the relatively high incidence of severe disease among young adults, especially among pregnant women (Krawczynski 1993). In two large series of cases of enteric non-A non-B hepatitis subsequently associated with HEV infection (Myint et al. 1985; Zhuang et al. 1991), case fatality rates among nonpregnant patients were found to be 0.55 percent and 1.27 percent, respectively. By contrast, fatality rates of 11.9 percent and 13.5 percent were noted among pregnant women and exceeded 20 percent in women presenting during the third trimester (Zhuang et al. 1991). Evidence of HEV infection has been noted in many, though not all, cases of sporadic, fulminant non-A non-B hepatitis in India. Indeed, among 110 consecutive cases of fulminant viral hepatitis in New Delhi, HEV was found to be the most common etiologic agent (Nanda et al. 1994).

IgG and IgM anti-HEV tests have been developed and found to be associated with >90 percent combined sensitivity in detecting antibodies in acute and/or convalescent sera from cases associated with water-borne epidemics. However, the sensitivity of IgM anti-HEV testing during the acute phase of the illness appears to be significantly less (Krawczynski 1993). Thus, additional testing of convalescent samples or use of polymerase chain reaction (PCR) based assays for HEV-RNA may be required to make this diagnosis (Sallie et al. 1994). Unfortunately, anti-HEV testing is not widely available in the USA.

FULMINANT HEPATITIS ASSOCIATED WITH PARENTERAL HEPATITIS VIRUSES

Hepatitis B infection is implicated in many cases of fulminant viral hepatitis in all areas of the world. In the USA, Japan or Europe, acute hepatitis B is the commonest identifiable cause of fulminant viral hepatitis (Mosley 1978; Papaevangelou et al. 1984; Takahashi et al. 1994; Williams and Wendon 1994), whereas in Taiwan chronic HBV infection complicated by co-infection with hepatitis delta virus (HDV), hepatitis C virus (HCV) or unknown agents is the most common cause of acute liver failure (Chu et al. 1994; Wu et al. 1994). USA or European patients with HBV + HDV or HBV + HCV co-infection also appear to have an increased risk of developing acute liver failure (Feray et al. 1993; Govindarajan et al. 1984). In contrast to HBV infections, HCV infections alone have only rarely been implicated as causes of acute liver failure in the USA or Europe (Feray et al. 1993; Liang et al. 1993; Theilmann et al. 1992). Athough HCV infection has been implicated in a higher number of cases of fulminant viral hepatitis in Asian countries (Chu et al. 1994; Wu et al. 1994; Yoshiba et al. 1994), many of these cases involved co-infection with more than one virus or occurred in immunocompromised patients with serious underlying medical problems. All studies of posttransfusion hepatitis have noted a significantly lower incidence of acute liver failure in posttransfusion HCV infections than has been reported among posttransfusion HBV infections (McNeil et al. 1984; Takano et al. 1994; Papaevangelou 1984).

In addition to increased morbidity in patients co-infected with HBV and other viral agents, a variety of immunologic and virologic factors have been associated with an increased risk of developing acute liver failure during the course of acute HBV infection. In contrast to patients with self-limited, uncomplicated acute infections, those with fulminant courses are more likely to be female, to lack detectable serum HBsAg, HBeAg and HBV-DNA at time of presentation and to exhibit enhanced anti-HBsAg responses (Woolf et al. 1976; Brechot et al. 1984; Papaevangelou 1984; Forbes et al. 1988). In at least some geographical areas cases of fulminant hepatitis B are frequently associated with HBV strains possessing mutations encoding precore stop codons that interfere with translation of HBeAg, or mutations in the core promoter that interfere with transcription of the HBeAg coding region (Sato et al. 1995). HBeAg and HBcAg possess significant amino acid sequence identity and HBeAg has been shown to induce T cell tolerance to both HBeAg and HBcAg in mice exposed to this antigen in utero (Milich et al. 1994). The apparent increased severity of hepatitis in neonates or adult humans initially infected with HBeAg negative HBV strains may reflect an enhanced T cell immune response to HBcAg. Finally, a number of cases of HBV-associated acute liver failure have also been reported to develop immediately after completion of courses of cytotoxic drugs or other forms of immunosuppressive therapy (Seeff and Koff 1986). In some cases these episodes have been shown to represent reactivation of chronic HBV infection due to the appearance of increased quantities of HBV-DNA during immunosuppression which set the stage for enhanced immune attack on infected hepatocytes following reconstitution of host immune responses. Thus the available data regarding factors associated with development of fulminant hepatitis following HBV infection argue that enhanced host immune responses play a prominent role in pathogenesis of this complication of HBV infection.

The rapid clearance of viremia in patients with fulminant hepatitis B has important diagnostic implications. Patients with fulminant hepatitis B are more likely to lack detectable serum HBsAg or HBV-DNA and already possess anti-HBs at time of presentation. On the other hand, chronic HBV carriers may present with a picture of acute liver failure precipitated by co-infection with other hepatitis viruses. Therefore, IgM anti-HBc testing is a crucial component of diagnostic evaluation in both patient groups. There has been one report suggesting that a significant fraction of fulminant hepatitis B cases may initially lack all serologic markers of HBV infection and be identified only by the presence of HBV-DNA in liver tissue (Wright et al. 1992). In all cases with markers of HBV infection and, in particular, in patients with a more prolonged or bimodal clinical course, careful assessment for co-infection by other viruses must always be performed.

Both HDV co-infection (simultaneous acute HDV and acute HBV infection) or superinfection (acute HDV in the setting of chronic HBV infection) increase the risk of acute liver failure and account for a significant fraction of cases of fulminant viral hepatitis in many medical centers (Chu et al. 1994; Govindarajan et al. 1984; Saracco et al. 1988; Wu et al. 1994). Paradoxically, however, the mortality rate in fulminant hepatitis related to HDV + HBV infections appears to be significantly less than that in patients infected with HBV alone (Saracco et al. 1988). As HDV infection interferes with replication of HBV and may lead to a fall in the serum titers of HBsAg to below detection levels, antidelta antibody testing should be performed in both HBsAg (+) and HBsAg (−) patients and should be repeated at intervals along with other hepatitis serologies in acute liver failure patients initially seronegative for all hepatitis virus markers.

Although the development of acute liver failure in patients with acute HCV infection alone has only very rarely been reported in Western countries, its role as a co-factor in patients with other underlying causes of liver disease and its potential role as the sole vector in rare cases justifies routine screening for markers of HCV infection. Presently, there are no available IgM anti-HCV tests capable of distinguishing acute from chronic HCV infection (Chau et al. 1991), and it is unclear whether some cases attributed to acute HCV infection might represent patients with chronic hepatitis C and additional superimposed causes of acute hepatitis or flares of chronic hepatitis C precipitated by unusual circumstances. Indeed, in two published cases of acute liver failure complicating posttransfusion HCV infection, severe hepatitis and hepatic encephalopathy were only observed more than four months after initial infection following institution and then abrupt discontinuation of immunosuppressive therapy (Yoshiba et al. 1994). These cases, therefore, are reminiscent of cases of fulminant hepatitis B precipitated by withdrawal of immunosuppressive therapy and suggest a similar role for host immune responses in pathogenesis of hepatic injury. However, other reported cases of fulminant HCV infections are quite different from the typical course of fulminant hepatitis B, being characterized by a more indolent course, multiple serum aminotransferase peaks and a longer time interval between initial signs or symptoms and subsequent development of encephalopathy (Yoshiba et al. 1994). It is thus unclear whether antiviral or even immunosuppressive therapies might be beneficial in these two forms of severe viral hepatitis.

FULMINANT HEPATITIS ASSOCIATED WITH SYSTEMIC VIRAL INFECTIONS

A number of viruses that typically cause extrahepatic disease have been implicated as rare causes of acute liver failure (Howard et al. 1984; Bernuau et al. 1986; Abzug and Levin 1991; Sobue et al. 1991). The majority of these cases of fulminant hepatic failure occur in the setting of disseminated disease and/or develop in immunocompromised hosts. Thus, in most cases the presence of a specific viral infection is strongly suggested by skin rash or mouth ulcers, or the presence of an immunocompromised host. However, in some cases these viral infections have been noted to present with only hepatic manifestations and/or to occur in nonimmunocompromised hosts.

As detailed in Table 2.1, virtually all of the Herpesviruses have been implicated as rare causes of acute liver failure although the etiology of cases attributed to cytomegalovirus or Epstein–Barr virus infections has been questioned (Bernuau et al. 1986). In addition to cases of acute liver failure that present as rare manifestations of viral illnesses common to developed countries, acute liver failure has also been observed during the course of yellow fever and a number of other arbovirus infections common to tropical, underdeveloped countries (Howard et al. 1984). In these cases, acute liver failure usually develops as a late and often preterminal manifestation in patients initially presenting with the clinical picture of hemorrhagic fever.

Diagnosis of acute liver failure induced by infection with viruses other than the classic hepatitis viruses requires close attention to extrahepatic manifestations and epidemiologic clues present in patients without serologic markers of known hepatitis viruses. When liver biopsies can be obtained, unique histologic features may provide additional diagnostic clues.

FULMINANT HEPATITIS ASSOCIATED WITH SPORADIC, NON-ABCDE HEPATITIS

Despite isolation and characterization of HCV and HEV and associated advances in serodiagnostic testing for markers of viral hepatitis, those cases of acute liver failure previously attributed to fulminant non-A non-B hepatitis remain as "non-ABCDE" hepatitis or hepatitis of unknown etiology. Despite the relatively benign nature of parenterally transmitted non-A non-B hepatitis, it has long been recognized that the overall incidence of acute liver failure among serologically negative patients is higher than observed in cases of acute HAV or HBV (McNeil et al. 1984; Papaevangelou et al. 1984). Thus, as detailed in Table 2.2, among consecutive cases of viral hepatitis admitted to infectious disease hospitals in Melbourne, Australia or Athens, Greece, the frequency of fatal, acute liver failure among patients classified as non-A non-B was higher than among those with acute HAV or HBV infections. Although a higher overall incidence of acute hepatitis B was observed in both case series, fulminant non-A non-B hepatitis was actually the commonest cause of fulminant hepatitis in Melbourne, Australia. In the USA, HBV was implicated as the etiologic agent in the majority of cases of fulminant viral hepatitis in reports published during the 1970s (Mosley 1978). However, more recent reports from US liver transplant centers indicate a predominance of non-A non-B cases among patients with fulminant or subfulminant hepatitis (Dodson et al. 1994). Even more impressive is the prevalence of this entity among the large case series reported from King's College Hospital in London where 201 of 329 cases (55.7 percent) of liver failure attributed to viral hepatitis between 1973 and 1993 were classified as non-A non-B hepatitis (Williams and Wendon 1994).

As detailed in Table 2.3, even after extensive assessment for HCV, HEV or "cryptic" HBV infection, the majority of such cases of fulminant or subfulminant non-ABCDE hepatitis remain as diagnostic enigmas. Even in Asia, where HCV or HEV account in different areas for 50 percent or more of cases of fatal acute non-ABCDE hepatitis, evidence of infection by the known hepatitis viruses cannot be found in a significant proportion of cases of acute liver failure (Nanda et al. 1994; Yoshiba et al. 1994).

These seronegative cases of fulminant

Table 2.2. *Fatality rates in patients hospitalized for acute viral hepatitis*

City	Type	Total cases (*n*)	Fulminant hepatitis *n*	Fulminant hepatitis %	Fatal cases *n*	Fatal cases %
Athens, Greece[a]	HAV	286	1	0.35	1	0.35
	HBV	1190	48	4.03	42	3.53
	non-A non-B	338	16	4.73	13	3.84
Melbourne, Australia[b]	HAV	2174	—	—	3	0.14
	HBV	2253	—	—	29	0.84
	non-A non-B	1050	—	—	24	2.29

[a] Papaevangelou et al. 1984.
[b] McNeil et al. 1984.

Table 2.3. *Hepatitis C and E as causes of fulminant or subfulminant hepatic failure in the US and Europe*

Author/country	Number non-A non-B cases examined	Number with HCV markers	Number with HEV markers	Number with HBV DNA
Wright et al. 1991, 1992 – USA	17	0	not tested	7[a]
Feray et al. 1993 – France	23	1	0	1[b]
Liang et al. 1993 – USA	17	2	0	0
Sallie et al. 1993, 1994 – UK	42	0	8	0[c]
Theilmann et al. 1992 – Germany	8	2	0	0
Laskus et al. 1994 Kuwada et al. 1994 – USA	8	0	0	0
Combined	115	5/115 (4.4%)	8/98 (8.2%)	8/115 (7.0%)

[a] Found in explant liver in 6 patients. One additional patient with no explant tissue to examine was found to have posttransplant serum markers of HBV infection as did 4/6 patients with HBV DNA in liver pretransplant.
[b] Only serum samples screened for HBV DNA in this study.
[c] Based on PCR assay for HBV DNA in livers of 45 non-A non-B patients.

hepatic failure have previously been attributed to viral infections because they typically present with the same symptoms, biochemical and histologic manifestations as cases associated with documented hepatitis virus infections (Gimson et al. 1986). However, there is no epidemiologic basis for implicating a virus or other transmissible agent in most cases. Multiple investigators have commented upon the absence of parenteral risk factors in such patients (Laskus et al. 1994; Williams and Wendon 1994; Wright et al. 1991) and no association with epidemics or clusters of hepatitis cases has been reported. The only direct evidence suggesting involvement of infectious agents has derived from several small studies.

The putative non-ABCDE agent was suggested by discovery of Toga virus-like particles on electron microscopic examination of liver biopsies from nine patients with fulminant hepatic failure who presented to the King's College Liver Failure Unit (Fagan et al. 1992). In five of these patients, acute hepatic failure recurred within seven days after liver transplantation. The liver allografts in these patients were characterized by severe hemorrhagic necrosis and presence of similar virus-like particles. However, other transplant centers have yet to report either similar electron microscopic findings or the rapid recurrence of fulminant hepatic failure in patients receiving liver transplants for fulminant non-ABCDE hepatitis. Nevertheless, it should be noted that although HBV and HCV infections frequently recur after liver transplantation, such posttransplant infections rarely manifest unique biochemical or histologic features that clearly distinguish them from allograft rejection or a host of other opportunistic infections.

In 1992, ten patients were described with severe hepatitis characterized histologically by large syncytial hepatocytes containing intracytoplasmic structures thought to be consistent with paramyxoviral nucleocapsids (Phillips et al. 1991). Four of these patients presented with subacute hepatic failure and the other six with a picture consistent with autoimmune chronic active hepatitis. Liver tissue homogenates from one patient were infused into two chimpanzees. Neither animal developed biochemical or histologic evidence of hepatitis but one developed antibodies reactive to two paramyxoviruses (measles and parainfluenza 4) in complement fixation assays. Hemagglutinating antibodies to sheep red blood cells were also found in the convalescent sera from this chimpanzee. In light of the electron microscopic findings in eight of the patients, the presence of autoimmune hemolytic anemia in two human patients and one chimpanzee and the known propensity for giant cell formation in other tissues infected by paramyxoviruses, the authors proposed that this was a new paramyxovirus-mediated form of hepatitis.

Following this report a number of other retrospective analyses were performed on liver biopsy specimens looking for cases of syncytial giant cell hepatitis (Devaney et al. 1992; Lau et al. 1992; Pappo et al. 1994). Most such specimens could not be evaluated by electron microscopy. However, in five cases in which electron microscopy was performed by two different groups of investigators (Devaney et al. 1992; Pappo et al. 1994) no viral particles could be found. Some investigators reported finding "giant cells" in patients with liver disease of defined etiology suggesting that since giant cell formation is a common histologic finding in infants with heterogeneous causes of liver disease, such syncytial giant cell formation in adults, while rare, might merely represent a nonspecific pathologic response.

The recent report from the University of Pittsburgh provides evidence for a transmissible agent in cases of giant cell hepatitis. In this study syncytial giant cells were found in 14 of 3416 native livers removed from patients undergoing allogeneic liver transplantation (Pappo et al. 1994). Giant cell hepatitis developed de novo in only two patients after liver transplantation. However, recurrent syncytial giant cells were observed in post-transplant biopsies in five of fourteen cases. Two of these five patients died and two required repeat transplantation because of recurrent liver failure. One of the latter patients developed giant cell hepatitis again in a second allograft. While these authors could not find viral particles in livers with giant cell hepatitis, they did identify human papilloma virus 6 by PCR analysis in liver tissue from three pretransplant and four posttransplant livers.

Despite ambiguities regarding its etiology, the syndrome of fulminant non-ABCDE hepatitis is characterized by a number of features that tend to distinguish it from other viral or toxic causes of acute liver failure. These characteristics are summarized in Table 2.4. There is a significantly longer mean time interval between onset of either first symptoms or jaundice and development of hepatic encephalopathy and a significantly higher mortality rate than that observed in patients with acute hepatitis A or B (Gimson et al. 1986; O'Grady et al. 1989; Yoshiba et al. 1994). Analysis of the King's College Hospital series of fulminant hepatitis cases has suggested that there is a bimodal distribution in rate of progression to hepatic encephalopathy in cases of severe seronegative hepatitis (Gimson et al. 1986; O'Grady et al. 1993). Patients with onset of hepatic encephalopathy eight to twenty-four weeks after onset of jaundice were older (mean age 44.5 years) than were patients with onset of encephalopathy less than eight weeks after initial jaundice (mean age 25.5 years) and were found to be more likely to develop ascites and renal failure and less likely to develop cerebral edema during their hospital course (Gimson et al. 1986). Both groups had similar acute histologic abnormalities and a high mortality rate.

Cases of aplastic anemia associated with a recent episode of acute hepatitis have been reported over a period of several decades (McNeil et al. 1984; Hibbs et al. 1992). Another rare but striking complication that has been associated with fulminant non-A non-B hepatitis is the development of aplastic anemia often after successful liver transplantation (Tzakis et al. 1988). Most cases have been found not to be associated with markers of HAV or HBV infection. In a survey of liver

Table 2.4. *Distinguishing clinical characteristics of fulminant or subfulminant non-ABCDE hepatitis*

Absence of parenteral or enteric risk factors
Prolonged interval between onset of jaundice and encephalopathy
Multiple transaminase peaks
Higher mortality than fulminant hepatitis A or B
Association with aplastic anemia

transplant centers all cases that occurred after transplantation were found to follow acute non-ABCDE hepatitis. The age range of patients with fulminant non-ABCDE hepatitis and associated aplastic anemia after liver transplantation (5–20 (mean 9) years) and the mean time interval between onset of hepatitis symptoms and transplantation for hepatic coma (less than four weeks in seven of nine patients) is distinctly different from that reported for the majority of patients developing acute liver failure during non-ABCDE hepatitis. Recently, application of anti-HCV and HCV-RNA assays to 28 patients with aplastic anemia and apparent non-ABCDE hepatitis has indicated that HCV markers were absent at time of initial diagnosis prior to initiation of blood product infusions (Hibbs et al. 1992).

In addition to a number of reports directly implicating novel viral agents as causes of fulminant non-ABCDE hepatitis, several new flaviviruses distantly related to HCV have been identified (Simons et al. 1995). The spectrum of human disease mediated by these agents remains to be elucidated. However, these new viruses, like HCV, have been linked to parenteral routes of transmission (Zuckerman 1995). In light of the relatively benign nature of parenterally transmitted non-ABC hepatitis (Alter 1994), it would be surprising if these agents proved to be a major cause of acute liver failure.

Thus, at present, the etiology of a significant fraction of cases of acute liver failure remains an enigma. It remains unclear whether there are multiple distinct etiologic agents responsible for fulminant non-ABCDE hepatitis or if alternatively, the clinical syndromes encompassed by this entity might in part reflect age-related or other individual differences in response to a common, predominant etiologic agent.

REFERENCES

Abzug, M.J. and Levin, M.J. 1991. Neonatal adenovirus infection: four patients and review of the literature. *Pediatrics* 87: 890–3.

Alter, H.J. 1994. Transfusion transmitted hepatitis C and non-A, non-B, non-C. *Vox Sanguinis* 67: 19–24.

Bernuau, J., Rueff, B. and Benhamou, J-P. 1986. Fulminant and subfulminant liver failure: definitions and causes. *Sem Liver Dis* 6: 97–106.

Brechot, C., Bernuau, J., Thiers, V. et al. 1984. Multiplication of hepatitis B virus in fulminant hepatitis B. *BMJ* 288: 270–1.

Chau, K.H., Dawson, G.J., Mushahwar, I.K. et al. 1991. IgM-antibody response to hepatitis C virus antigens in acute and chronic post-transfusion non-A, non-B hepatitis. *J Virol Meth* 35: 343–52.

Chu, C-M., Sheen, I-S. and Liaw, Y-F. 1994. The role of hepatitis C virus in fulminant viral hepatitis in an area with endemic hepatitis A and B. *Gastroenterology* 107: 189–95.

Devaney, K., Goodman, Z.D. and Ishak, K.G. 1992. Postinfantile giant-cell transformation in hepatitis. *Hepatology* 16: 327–33.

Dodson, S.F., Dehara, K. and Iwatsuki, S. 1994. Liver transplantation for fulminant hepatic failure. *ASAIO J* 40: 86–8.

Fagan, E.A., Ellis, D.S., Tovey, G.M. et al. 1992. Toga virus-like particles in acute liver failure attributed to sporadic non-A, non-B hepatitis and recurrence after liver transplantation. *J Med Virol* 38: 71–7.

Fagan, E.A., Yousef, G., Brahm, J. et al. 1990. Persistence of hepatitis A virus in fulminant hepatitis and after liver transplantation. *J Med Virol* 30: 131–6.

Feray, C., Gigou, M., Samuel, D. et al. 1993. Hepatitis C virus RNA and hepatitis B virus DNA in serum and liver of patients with fulminant hepatitis. *Gastroenterology* 104: 549–55.

Forbes, A., Alexander, G.J.M., Smith, H.M., and Williams, R. 1988. Elevation of serum sex hormone-binding globulin in females with fulminant hepatitis B virus infection. *J Med Virol* 26: 93–8.

Gimson, A.E.S., O'Grady, J., Ede, R.J. et al. 1986. Late onset hepatic failure: Clinical, serological and histological features. *Hepatology* 6: 288–94.

Gocke, D.J. 1986. Hepatitis A revisited. *Ann Intern Med* 105: 960–1.

Govindarajan, S., Chin, K.P., Redeker, A.G., Peters, R.L. 1984. Fulminant B viral hepatitis: role of delta agent. *Gastroenterology* 86: 1417–20.

Hibbs, J.R., Frickhofen, N., Rosenfeld, S.J. et al. 1992. Aplastic anemia and viral hepatitis. Non-A, non-B, non-C? *JAMA* 267: 2051–4.

Howard, C.R., Ellis, D.S. and Simpson, D.I.H. 1984. Exotic viruses and the liver. *Sem Liver Dis* 4: 361–74.

Krawczynski, K. 1993. Hepatitis E. *Hepatology* 17: 932–41.

Kuwada, S.K., Patel, V.M., Hollinger, F.B. et al. 1994. Non-A, non-B fulminant hepatitis is also non-E and non-C. *Am J Gastroenterol* 89: 57–61.

Laskus, T., Rakela, J., Weisner, R.H. et al. 1994. Lack of evidence for hepatitis B virus (HBV) infection in fulminant non-A, non-B hepatitis. *Dig Dis Sci* 39: 1677–82.

Lau, J.Y.N., Koukoulis, G., Mieli-Vergani, G. et al. 1992. Syncytial giant-cell hepatitis – a specific disease entity? *J Hepatol* 15: 216–19.

Liang, T.J., Jeffers, L., Reddy, R.K. et al. 1993. Fulminant or subfulminant non-A, non-B viral hepatitis. The role of hepatitis C and E viruses. *Gastroenterology* 104: 556–62.

Liaw, Y.F., Yang, C.Y., Chu, C.M. and Huang, M.J. 1986. Appearance and persistence of hepatitis A IgM antibody in acute clinical hepatitis A observed in an outbreak. *Infection* 14: 156–8.

Mathieson, L.R., Skivoj, P., Nielsen, J.P. et al. 1980. Hepatitis type A, B, and non-A, non-B in fulminant hepatitis. *Gut* 21: 72–7.

McNeil, M., Hoy, J.F., Richards, M.J. et al. 1984. Aetiology of fatal viral hepatitis in Melbourne. A retrospective study. *Med J Aust* 141: 637–40.

Milich, D.R., Jones, J.E., Hughes, J.L. et al. 1994. Is a function of the secreted hepatitis B e antigen to induce immunologic tolerance in utero? *Proc Natl Acad Sci USA* 87: 6599–603.

Mosley, J.W. 1978. Comparison of fulminant type B and non-B hepatitis. *Gastroenterology* 71: 1164.

Myint, H.L.A., Soe, M.M., Khin, T., Myint, T.M. and Tin, K.M. 1985. A clinical and epidemiological study of an epidemic of non-A non-B hepatitis in Rangoon. *Am J Trop Med Hyg* 34: 1183–9.

Nanda, S.K., Yalcinkaya, K., Panigrahi, A.K. et al. 1994. Etiological role of hepatitis E in sporadic fulminant hepatitis. *J Med Virol* 42: 133–7.

O'Grady, J.G., Alexander, G.J.M., Hayllar, K.M. et al. 1989. Early indicators of prognosis in fulminant hepatic failure. *Gastroenterology* 97: 439–45.

O'Grady, J.G., Schalm, S.W. and Williams, R. 1993. Acute liver failure: redefining the syndrome. *Lancet* 342: 273–5.

Papaevangelou, G., Tassopoulos, N., Roumeliotou-Karayannis, A. and Richardson, C. 1984. Etiology of fulminant viral hepatitis in Greece. *Hepatology* 4: 369–72.

Pappo, O., Yunis, E., Jordan, J.A. et al. 1994. Recurrent and de novo giant cell hepatitis after orthotopic liver transplantation. *Am J Surg Pathol* 18: 804–13.

Phillips, M.J., Blendis, L.M., Poucell, S. et al. 1991. Syncytial giant-cell hepatitis. Sporadic hepatitis with distinctive pathological features, a severe clinical course, and paramyxoviral features. *N Engl J Med* 324: 455–60.

Sallie, R., Rayner, A., Naoumov, N. et al. 1993. Occult HBV in NANB fulminant hepatitis. *Lancet* 341: 123.

Sallie, R., Silva, A.E., Purdy, M. et al. 1994. Hepatitis C and E in non-A non-B fulminant hepatic failure: a polymerase chain reaction and serological study. *J Hepatol* 20: 580–8.

Saracco, G., Macagno, S., Rosina, F. et al. 1988. Serologic markers with fulminant hepatitis in persons positive for hepatitis B surface antigen. *Ann Intern Med* 108: 380–3.

Sato, S., Suzuki, K., Akahane, Y. et al. 1995. Hepatitis B virus strains with mutations in the core promoter in patients with fulminant hepatitis. *Ann Intern Med* 122: 241–8.

Seeff, L.B. and Koff, R.S. 1986. Evolving concepts of the clinical and serologic consequences of hepatitis B virus infection. *Sem Liver Dis* 6: 11–22.

Simons, J.N., Pilot-Matias, T.J., Laery, T.P. et al. 1995. Identification of two flavivirus-like genomes in the GB hepatitis agent. *Proc Natl Acad Sci USA* 92: 3401–5.

Sobue, R., Miyazaki, H., Okamato, M. et al. 1991. Fulminant hepatitis in primary human herpesvirus-6 infection. *N Engl J Med* 324: 1290.

Takahashi, Y., Kumada, H. and Shimizu, M. 1994. A multicenter study on the prognosis of fulminant viral hepatitis: early prediction for liver transplantation. *Hepatology* 19: 1065–71.

Takano, S., Omata, M., Ohto, M. and Satomura, Y. 1994. Prospective assessment of incidence of fulminant hepatitis in post-transfusion hepatitis: A study of 504 cases. *Dig Dis Sci* 39: 28–32.

Theilmann, L., Solbach, C., Toex, U. et al. 1992. Role of hepatitis C virus infection in German patients with fulminant and subacute hepatic failure. *Eur J Clin Invest* 22: 569–71.

Tzakis, A.G., Arditi, M., Whitington, P.F. et al. 1988. Aplastic anemia complicating orthotopic liver transplantation for non-A, non-B hepatitis. *N Engl J Med* 319: 393–6.

Williams, R. and Wendon, J. 1994. Indications for orthotopic liver transplantation in fulminant liver failure. *Hepatology* 20: 5S–9S.

Woolf, I.L., El Sheikh, N., Cullens, H. et al. 1976. Enhanced HBsAb production in pathogenesis of fulminant viral hepatitis type B. *BMJ* 2: 669–71.

Wright, T.L., Hsu, H., Donegan, E. et al. 1991. Hepatitis C virus not found in fulminant non-A, non-B hepatitis. *Ann Intern Med* 115: 111–12.

Wright, T.L., Mamish, D., Coombs, C. et al. 1992. Hepatitis B virus and apparent fulminant non-A, non-B hepatitis. *Lancet* 339: 952–5.

Wu, J-C., Chen, C-L., Hou, M-C et al. 1994. Multiple viral infection as the most common cause of fulminant and subfulminant viral hepatitis in an area endemic for hepatitis B: application and limitations of the polymerase chain reaction. *Hepatology* 19: 836–40.

Yoshiba, M., Dehara, K., Inoue, K. et al. 1994. Contribution of hepatitis C virus to non-A, non-B fulminant hepatitis in Japan. *Hepatology* 19: 829–35.

Zhuang, H., Cao, X-Y., Liu, C-B. and Wang, G-M. 1991. Enterically transmitted non-A, non-B hepatitis in China. In *Viral Hepatitis C, D and E*, ed. T. Shikata, R.H. Purcell and T. Uchida, 277–85. Amsterdam: Elsevier Science Publishers B.V.

Zuckerman, A.J. 1995. The new GB hepatitis viruses. *Lancet* 345: 1453–4.

3 Drug hepatotoxicity as a cause of acute liver failure

Gloria Sze and Neil Kaplowitz

INTRODUCTION

Over 800 drugs have been reported to cause liver disease, and the spectrum of disease ranges from asymptomatic reversible transaminase elevations to fatal acute liver failure. Drug-induced liver disease can mimic almost any known liver disorder. Drug hepatotoxicity represents 2 to 3 percent of cases of jaundice, and is responsible for at least 10 to 20 percent of cases of acute liver failure (ALF); since no etiologic virus can be identified in 40–50 percent of cases of ALF, it is conceivable that some additional unknown proportion of these cases are due to drugs, natural toxins or environmental chemicals (Friis and Andreasen 1992; Dossing and Sonne 1993). Precise figures on the incidence of hepatic injury among recipients of most drugs are not available. Most of the information on drug-induced toxicity has come from individual case reports, series of cases, or reviews of the literature.

MECHANISMS OF INJURY

Drug metabolism

The liver is a major site for drug metabolism. The biotransformation of foreign substances into more polar metabolites which are more readily eliminated is classically described to occur in two phases. Phase I reactions are oxidations or reductions of chemicals by cytochrome P450 enzymes. Phase II reactions involve conjugation with glucuronic acid, sulfate, acetic acid or glutathione (GSH) to change the size and solubility of the drug. Phase I reactions may add or expose a functional group, such as hydroxyl, which then can serve as a structural locus for phase II conjugation.

The cytochrome P450 enzymes refer to a superfamily of membrane-bound hemoproteins mostly in the endoplasmic reticulum. More than 40 distinct forms have been isolated from rat liver. In human liver, constitutive expression of CYP1A2, 2C9(19), 2D6, 2E1 and 3A4 are predominant with the latter accounting for 60 percent of total P450 (Watkins 1990; Zimmerman 1982; Murray 1992; Kaplowitz 1996). The P450 system is important in processing foreign substances, but it sometimes gives rise to products more toxic than the parent compound. Some of these products are referred to as electrophiles because they exhibit reactive centers that seek electrons and covalently bind to or alkylate nucleophilic centers, such as sulfhydryl or amino groups, on cellular constituents. Another harmful product of the P450 system is the organic free radical. For example, in either CCl_4 or halothane metabolism, enhanced reduction of substrate occurs in the face of limited oxygen availability, resulting in an electron transfer directly to the drug, producing a free radical metabolite (Williams and Burk 1990). It is also important to realize that some phase II metabolites of drugs are toxic, for example certain ester glucuronide metabolites are unstable due to migration of the ester bond from one hydroxyl group to the next on the glucuronic acid. This can release electrophilic drug intermediates which covalently bind and elicit a hypersensitivity reaction. This is a proposed mechanism for diclofenac hepatotoxicity (Dunk et al. 1982; Helfgott et al. 1990).

One of the most extensively studied examples of a relatively innocuous parent drug that is converted by P450 into a reactive and potentially toxic metabolite is acetaminophen (paracetamol). Acetaminophen, which already contains a hydroxyl group, does not require phase I oxidation in order to undergo phase II conjugation to glucuronide or sulfate. Therefore less than 5 percent of ingested acetaminophen is normally metabolized by P450 (mainly CYP2E1); however, it is this pathway that appears to produce the electrophilic metabolites that are toxic to the hepatocyte (Nelson 1990; Kaplowitz 1996). Hepatotoxicity is usually avoided through the electrophilic metabolite preferentially conjugating to nucleophilic glutathione. However, when a large dose is ingested (>10 g), the increased level of toxic metabolites exhausts the available glutathione stores, resulting in intracellular accumulation of the toxic metabolite and hepatotoxicity. Chronic alcohol ingestion can lead to acetaminophen toxicity with doses of much less than 10 g. One theory is that alcoholic livers are depleted in glutathione, especially in the mitochondria, and have a much reduced capacity to detoxify the reactive metabolite. However, a major factor is that alcoholics actually produce more toxic metabolite at any given dose, secondary to alcohol-induced CYP2E1 levels (Lieber 1994; Whitcomb and Block 1994). Starvation and isoniazid also induce CYP2E1 and increase susceptibility to acetaminophen toxicity. Toxic metabolites may also be produced from acetaminophen by human P450s other than CYP2E1, most notably CYPIA2.

Critical cell targets for toxins

Reactive metabolites of drug metabolism may result in covalent binding, lipid peroxidation and protein–thiol oxidation (Figure 3.1). These chemical reactions do not always correlate with cell injury and their relevance to the pathogenesis of toxicity is uncertain in many cases. A likely theory is that reactive metabolites lead to covalent binding, lipid peroxidation, or protein thiol oxidation of both a large number of noncritical cellular targets and a small number of critical targets. The identification of these critical cell targets that mediate the final pathway to cell death is still controversial. A number of factors probably act in concert, but with varying importance depending on the toxin. One target that has received a great deal of attention in past years is calcium (Reed 1990; Rosser and Gores 1995). Calcium ATPases in the plasma membrane and endoplasmic reticulum pump calcium from the cytosol. A sustained rise in cytosolic calcium can lead to, or contribute to, cell death by activating degradative enzymes such as proteases, phospholipases and endonucleases. Increased cytosolic calcium also can impair mitochondrial function by recycling calcium in and out of mitochondria with the loss of mitochondrial membrane potential. This results in the opening of megachannels (mitochondrial membrane permeability transition), with consequent loss of oxidative phosphorylation and of the availability of ATP needed for cell viability (Nicotera et al. 1992; Zahrebelski et al. 1995). Covalent binding, or oxidation of thiol groups in these calcium pumps can lead to impaired calcium removal. Also, lipid peroxidation can increase plasma and microsomal membrane permeability to calcium, leading to sustained increase in cytosolic calcium. Despite these observations, it is clear that increased calcium levels are not

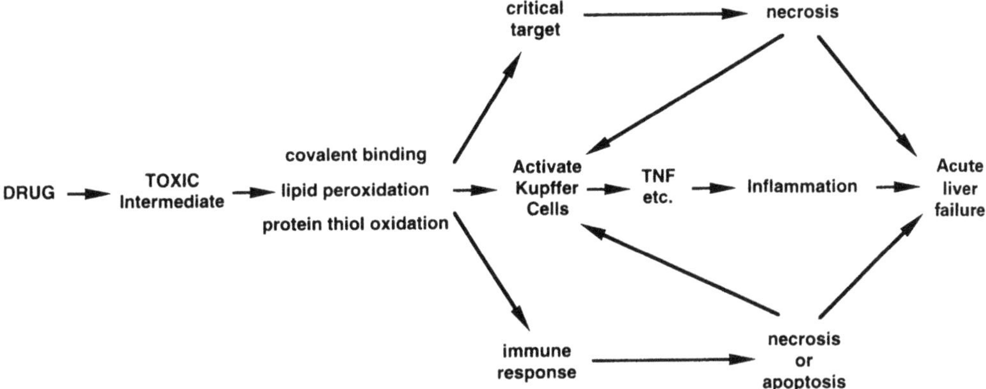

Figure 3.1 Pathogenesis of fulminant hepatic failure from drugs and other toxins. Drugs are converted to toxic intermediates or metabolites which exert specific chemical consequences. As a result, critical targets in the hepatocyte may be disrupted, for example mitochondria, or neoantigens may be generated which elicit an immune response directed at the drug–macromolecular complex or native hepatic proteins. Both processes depend on the generation of toxic metabolites which is influenced by the effects of risk factors listed in Table 3.1 and their impact on the balance of toxification and detoxification. In both, it is likely that the full extent of organ damage and severity of liver disease is determined in part by the participation of Kupffer cells and inflammatory cells and the effect that these cells have on endothelial cells and hepatocytes through the action of cytokines, eicosanoids, reactive oxygen metabolites and proteases.

required for cell necrosis in many instances. Bleb formation and membrane rupture can be observed in the absence of an increased calcium concentration. In fact, removal of calcium from extracellular medium may actually potentiate cell injury through generation of toxic oxygen species by mitochondria.

The integrity of mitochondria and ATP production are critical in cell viability. Recently, much attention has been focused on mitochondria as a critical target leading to necrosis from toxins or anoxia (Imberti et al. 1992; Fujii et al. 1994). Two major modes of cell death have been recognized, apoptosis and lytic necrosis. Intrinsic toxins and anoxia usually kill cells via a lytic process which ultimately involves loss of mitochondrial integrity with opening of a megachannel, that is the mitochondrial membrane permeability transition, with loss of mitochondria membrane potential and matrix constituents and with subsequent cytoskeletal changes, swelling and rupture of cell membrane (lysis) (Zahrebelski et al. 1995). This can be induced by oxidative stress, peroxides, calcium, GSH depletion and can be blocked by cyclosporin A. Toxicants and anoxia may also kill by apoptosis, especially when doses are low or hypoxia is mild. Immune mediated cell death not involving complement, that is cytotoxic T cells, is mainly via apoptosis. This appears as shriveled nuclei with characteristic chromatin condensation and eosinophilic condensation of the whole cell (Councilman body). Lytic necrosis generally elicits a secondary inflammatory reaction whereas apoptosis does not (Searle et al. 1982; Vaux 1993).

Aside from lytic necrosis or apoptosis, certain agents may induce a microvesicular steatosis producing an apparent metabolic poisoning of the liver without collapse. This resembles the histologic findings observed in Reye's syndrome (which also is associated with aspirin) or fatty liver of pregnancy. A similar picture is seen with high dose tetracycline (>2 g, especially intravenous and/or in pregnancy), valproic acid (which also exhibits frank zonal necrosis) and fialuridine (FIAU). The latter impairs mitochondrial DNA synthesis, thereby leading to loss of mitochondrial function resulting in hyperammonia, lactic acidosis and microvesicular steatosis (Sallie et al. 1994).

Certain natural toxins are known to act directly on a specific organelle or function. Thus, the mushroom, *Amanita phalloides*, produces protein synthesis inhibitors, called amatoxins. Cyanobacteria produce microcystins, which irreversibly inhibit protein phosphatases. These natural toxins are cyclical peptides which are targeted to the liver through transport (uptake) by hepatocyte specific multispecific substrate organic anion carriers (Ohta et al. 1994).

Another consideration is the target cell. Although most of the discussion above concerns effects in and on hepatocytes, secondary effects due to activated Kupffer cells or inflammation may contribute to a variable extent. However, some toxins exert a selective effect on endothelial cells of the liver. This may be of importance in veno-occlusive disease. Some of the agents implicated in this form of acute liver failure selectively kill sinusoidal endothelial cells versus hepatocytes in culture. This is determined by unique activation in endothelial cells (e.g. dacarbazine) as well as lower GSH defensive capacity of endothelial cells (e.g. azathioprine and monocrotaline; Yan and Huxtable 1995).

Role of Kupffer cells and inflammation

Inflammatory cells can contribute to liver cell injury in drug hepatotoxicity (Figure 3.1) as well as other types of liver diseases (Laskin 1990). Neutrophils are recruited to areas of injury by cytokines, leukotrienes, and products of oxidative stress by increased expression of adhesion molecules on locally damaged endothelium. Activated neutrophils injure cells by releasing proteases, such as elastase, and oxidants such as H_2O_2 and hypochlorous acid. A recent hypothesis suggests that oxidant generation functions as a permissive factor for protease induced injury (Laskin 1990). Hypochlorous acid and other oxidants from activated neutrophils will inactivate serum and tissue antiproteases. The protease, in the presence of inactivated inhibitors, will subsequently damage cellular membranes, resulting in cell lysis. These effects can be inhibited by antioxidants and antiproteases and the contribution of each of these processes to hepatocyte injury is still under debate.

The Kupffer cells have also been implicated in liver cell injury from drug hepatotoxicity as well as other liver diseases (Thurman et al. 1993). Activated Kupffer cells produce cytokines which may be directly cytotoxic or may recruit additional inflammatory cells (Rosser and Gores 1995). One of these cytokines, tumor necrosis factor, stimulates mitochondrial radical generation and is cytotoxic to some cell lines. Kupffer cells also release proteases, platelet activating factor, toxic oxygen species and eicosanoids. Several studies have suggested a role for Kupffer cells in hepatocyte injury by showing that cell injury can be lessened with inhibition of Kupffer cells either by removal of endotoxin (germ-free) or ablation of Kupffer cells (gadolinium pretreatment) and the injury can be potentiated by activating Kupffer cells (Weiss 1989).

These phenomena are best illustrated by studies showing that Kupffer cells participate in the mechanism of toxicity of carbon tetrachloride, although the participation of similar factors seems likely with virtually all causes of hepatotoxicity (Williams and Burk 1990; Edwards et al. 1993). Carbon tetrachloride increases intracellular calcium, and the release of toxic eicosanoids and cytokines by Kupffer cells is calcium-dependent; alternatively, it is known that carbon tetrachloride activates Kupffer cells also by increasing exposure to endotoxin. The activated Kupffer cells release toxic cytokines and leukotrienes which are chemotactic factors for neutrophils and which up-regulate expression of adhesion molecules. Cellular infiltration of activated neutrophils by release of superoxide anion and other toxic mediators, amplifies the inflammatory response and leads to cell injury and death. Thus, it seems that the action of toxins generated in hepatocytes may be markedly potentiated by factors released from endotoxin activated Kupffer cells either through direct actions on hepatocytes or up-regulation of neutrophil adhesion through actions on sinusoidal endothelial cells. The explanation for enhanced endotoxin activation of Kupffer cells in hepatotoxicity is unknown. Since the ultimate and full extent of liver injury involves these extra-hepatocyte events, targeting therapy or prevention of hepatotoxicity toward blocking tumor necrosis factor (TNF) or leukocyte adhesion appears to be a fruitful area for future clinical investigation.

PREDICTABLE VERSUS UNPREDICTABLE HEPATOTOXICITY

Hepatotoxicity from drugs can be viewed as predictable or unpredictable. Predictable injury is dose-related, usually reproducible in animal models and the liver injury is due to the intrinsic toxicity of a drug or its metabolites. Hepatic necrosis induced by acetaminophen and carbon tetrachloride are typical examples. In clinical practice, unpredictable injury is seen far more commonly than predictable toxicity. These cases, considered examples of idiosyncratic toxicity, represent only a very small proportion of patients who ingest a drug. The incidence of overt drug-induced liver disease among individuals taking a given drug is highly variable, ranging from ~1 percent (isoniazid (INH)) to ~0.1 percent (allopurinol, phenytoin, methyldopa), to 0.01 percent (halothane), to 0.001 percent (NSAIDS) (Dossing and Sonne 1993). With unpredictable toxicity, there seems to be no dose relation, and usually there is no animal model. Reactions often seem to be hypersensitivity mediated, but not infrequently no evidence of hypersensitivity can be found. Rather, the idiosyncrasy may be due to one or more genetically determined or acquired metabolic differences in the biochemical pathways of drug toxification or detoxification (Table 3.1). In most cases of unpredictable hepatotoxicity, the pathogenesis is not clearly known. However, in the future we may be able to predict, from the genetic predisposition of a person to hypersensitivity or from genetically determined differences in pathways of drug metabolism, which persons are at risk for developing significant liver injury from drugs.

Table 3.1. *Risk factors*

Genetic polymorphisms of drug metabolism – acetylator and hydroxylator status
Age
Gender
Nutrition – starvation and obesity
Diseases
Interactions with concomitant drugs and alcohol

Isoniazid is an example of an agent which produces an idiosyncratic drug reaction which usually has no features of hypersensitivity; isoniazid toxicity is not dose-related, and no animal model of isoniazid toxicity is known (Mitchell et al. 1976). Approximately 10–20 percent of isoniazid recipients will have subclinical biochemical evidence of liver injury, and one percent of patients develop overt hepatitis, although the incidence increases with age (Moulding et al. 1989; Snider and Caras 1992; Israel et al. 1992). Studies have noted a relationship between susceptibility to isoniazid hepatotoxicity and metabolism (acetylation) of the drug. Slow acetylators produce more monoacetylhydrazine whereas rapid acetylators produce more diacetylhydrazine. The former is converted by P450 to a toxic intermediate, and P450 activation may be influenced by ethanol. Slow acetylators are also more susceptible to hepatotoxicity due to sulfonamides, dihydralazine and isoniazid (Rieder et al. 1989). But since the frequency of slow acetylator status in Caucasians is 40–50 percent, other factors must be involved to explain low incidence ($\leqslant$ 1 percent) of toxicity. Indeed, it is probably more useful to consider that rapid acetylators are protected by minimizing exposure to the parent drug or monoacetylhydrazine in the case of isoniazid. Other conditions that increase the risk for isoniazid toxicity are alcohol ingestion and simultaneous use of rifampicin, presumably through induction of P450 enzymes (Wu et al. 1990). Isoniazid hepatotoxicity then, occurs when genetic and environmental conditions work together to increase the quantity of toxic metabolites.

In some cases, it is unclear whether unpredictable toxicity is due to hypersensitivity or metabolism. Halothane hepatotoxicity has sometimes been unequivocally immune-mediated; exposure to minuscule ambient halothane can produce a recrudescence of hepatitis in sensitized persons. Circulating antibodies to liver plasma membrane have been found in patients who have recovered from such hepatotoxicity, and in more than 80 percent of these patients, halothane hepatotoxicity occurs after multiple exposures (Benjamin et al. 1985). On the other hand, halothane hepatotoxicity occurs in experimental animals because of conversion of halothane to radical metabolite by inducible cytochrome P450. Although multiple exposures suggest sensitization, the closeness of exposures is a critical factor, with most instances occurring within a one month period. Halothane induces its own metabolism, which may be an alternate explanation for the critical role of multiple exposures. The hepatic biotransformation of a drug can lead to host sensitization to an altered liver macromolecule, perhaps with the drug metabolite serving as a hapten, or it can lead to generation of radical metabolites which mediate toxicity (Pohl 1990). The clinical picture is mostly an allergic reaction with fever and eosinophilia. Halothane is metabolized in two different ways by cytochrome P450. Oxidative metabolism by CYP2E1 in the presence of high oxygen levels produces a trifluoroacetylhalide that can acetylate protein amino groups, and reductive metabolism in the presence of low oxygen leads to a free radical that can induce lipid peroxidation (Kenna et al. 1990). The reductive process can directly cause hepatic injury; however, a most important discovery was the finding that a high proportion of patients with halothane hepatotoxicity contained specific antibodies in their blood that were directed against halothane-altered liver neoantigens. Recent studies have indicated that the halothane-induced antigens comprise a group of halothane metabolite-modified microsomal proteins (trifluoroacetylated proteins) (Satoh et al. 1989; Smith et al. 1993). The generation of trifluoroacetylated microsomal proteins occurs in all anesthetized subjects but overt liver disease is very rare (1:30,000 with single exposure and 1:3,000 with multiple exposures). Multiple different antigens have been identified from the purified microsomal proteins identified by immunoreactivity with patient antisera, including microsomal carboxylesterase, protein disulfide isomerase, and pyruvate dehydrogenase complex–lipoic acid, and these are expressed on the cell surface normally to a small extent (Gut et al. 1992; Martin et al. 1993; Christen et al. 1993; Knight et al. 1994). These proteins appear to become autoantigens since patient antisera can be shown to recognize these proteins. This may be due to some alteration such as trifluoroacetylation leading to autoimmunity to the protein so modified in normal liver, or due to molecular mimicry so that epitopes on unrelated proteins share similarity or cross reactivity with the trifluoroacetylated site (Christen et al. 1993). There is strong evidence to suggest that native epitopes cross-react with trifluoroacetylated protein adducts, that is molecular mimicry. It has been hypothesized that the cross-reacting autoantigen becomes the target of the immune system only in rare individuals who normally express the native protein at very low levels and who therefore have not developed pre-existing tolerance to it (Christen et al. 1993). Antibody-dependent cell-mediated cytotoxicity can be demonstrated using halothane-treated rabbit hepatocytes, patient serum, and normal lymphocytes. However, it is not clearly proven that these immune reactions actually mediate the clinical liver disease, although this seems likely. Therefore, susceptibility factors for halothane may include individual variability in the level of expression of the cytochrome P450 isoenzyme responsible for bioactivation of halothane (probably CYP2E1), the level of expression of the protein targets, the presentation of antigens to the immune system, and/

or the immune response itself. Of note, obesity has been recognized as a risk factor and is associated with increased expression of CYP2E1. Halothane represents an example of the critical importance of drug metabolism as a prerequisite for initiating the hypersensitivity.

Diclofenac hepatotoxicity represents a probable immune reaction to a hapten–protein complex (Scully et al. 1993; Kretz-Rommel and Boelsterli 1993; Kretz-Rommel and Boelsterli 1995). Diclofenac acyl glucuronide metabolites alkylate a 60 kD protein found in microsomes and on the cell surface (Kretz-Rommel and Boelsterli 1993; Kretz-Rommel and Boesterli 1995).

Autoantibodies have also been implicated in other examples of drug-induced hepatotoxicity. In several instances these are anti-LKM antibodies. Some examples in which autoantibodies recognize P450 isoenzymes are tienilic acid hepatitis (CYP2C8, anti-LKM2), dihydralazine induced hepatitis (CYPIA2), and phenytoin, carbamazepine or phenobarbital hepatotoxicity (CYP3A1) (Leeder et al. 1992; Bourdi et al. 1994; Lecoeur et al. 1994). The significance of these autoantibodies in the pathogenesis of disease is still not clear. At the very least, their occurrence may be of diagnostic value.

Phenytoin may cause an allergic reaction in susceptible patients which is associated with fever, rash with exfoliative dermatitis, hepatotoxicity, lymphadenopathy and eosinophilia or a mononucleosis-like picture. The syndrome typically occurs several weeks after therapy is started and can present with a variety of symptoms (Shear and Spielberg 1988). The exact pathogenesis of phenytoin hepatotoxicity has remained obscure. Phenytoin is metabolized by P450 to several products including parahydroxylated, dihydrodiol metabolites, and arene oxides, all of which are reactive, electrophilic compounds. The arene oxides, when generated in vivo, are capable of binding to cellular macromolecules. These drug–macromolecular complexes could lead directly to cytotoxicity, or act as immunogens and initiate allergic responses (Stanley and Fallon-Pellicci 1978; Mullick and Ishak 1979; Spielberg et al. 1981). In patients with the hypersensitivity syndrome to phenytoin, antibodies have been identified that primarily recognized CYP3A1 (Leeder et al. 1992).

RISK FACTORS FOR DRUG HEPATOTOXICITY (Table 3.1)

A number of factors determine whether drug-induced injury will occur in any given situation. New descriptions of the genetic polymorphisms of the expression of P450 (CYP) genes in humans are rapidly emerging (Zimmerman 1993; Kaplowitz 1996; Watkins 1990; Murray 1992). For example, a group of drugs exemplified by debrisoquine are poorly metabolized in about 5–7 percent of Caucasians due to polymorphism of expression of CYP2D6. The role CYP2D6 in the increased susceptibility to hepatotoxicity of certain patients is illustrated by perhexiline maleate, a coronary artery vasodilator. It appears that the parent drug may be responsible for the toxicity in this case, suggesting that poor metabolizers are at greater risk (May 1994). Amineptine and sulfonamide toxicity, in contrast, do not occur in slow hydroxylators indicating that metabolism is required to form the toxic by-product. Acetylator polymorphism has also been implicated as a risk factor for sulfonamide, dihydralazine and isoniazid hepatotoxicity. In slow acetylators, more parent drug is available for P450 activation to a reactive intermediate. Inherited susceptibility to drug toxicity has been suggested to be due to impaired detoxification of P450 generated metabolites of sulfonamides, tricyclics (amineptine), and anticonvulsants (phenytoin, carbamazepine, phenobarbital). Susceptibility of patient or family members' lymphocytes to lethal injury from toxic drug metabolites can be assessed by incubation of the parent drug and human lymphocytes with a fully functional rodent microsomal system (Wolkenstein et al. 1995). Multiple genetic factors may be responsible for creating just the right situation for hepatotoxicity: for example, acetylator status and detoxification status with sulfonamides.

It is important to recognize that these genetic polymorphisms of drug metabolism and detoxification can determine direct toxicity or predispose to hypersensitivity. Thus, in the case of anticonvulsants and sulfonamides discussed above with respect to genetic factors, the clinical syndromes associated with toxicity strongly suggest a hypersensitivity basis. Thus, the extent of exposure to toxic metabolites can determine the likelihood of developing either direct toxicity or hypersensitivity.

Many other factors affect an individual's susceptibility to drug hepatotoxicity. With some medications such as methyldopa, nitrofurantoin, halothane, and benoxaprofen, females appear to be more susceptible to hepatotoxicity. Increasing age also exerts an increased risk for hepatotoxicity due to isoniazid, halothane, and tienilic acid. On the other hand, aspirin-associated liver injury seems to occur more frequently in children under 10 years old. Valproate toxicity also appears to involve patients less than 20 years old (Zimmerman and Ishak 1982; Powell-Jackson et al. 1984). Diet may also play a role in drug hepatotoxicity by inducing increased expression of elements of the cytochrome P450 system: for example, starvation and obesity induce P4502E1 (see below) (Salazar et al. 1994). Theoretically, low intake of sulfur-containing amino acids can lead to glutathione depletion, and low antioxidant intake may also potentiate peroxidative injury. Alcohol ingestion is also an important factor; for example, chronic ethanol exposure induces a form of P450 (CYP2E1) that can oxidize acetaminophen and halothane to an electrophilic product. This probably explains the marked increased susceptibility to the hepatotoxicity of acetaminophen in alcoholics (Lieber 1994). Ethanol also enhances acetaminophen toxicity by glutathione depletion, particularly in hepatic mitochondria, a critical target of toxicity. Alcohol increases susceptibility to toxicity from INH and methotrexate, but the mechanisms are not known. Concurrent medications may also influence hepatotoxicity; for example, specific cytochrome P450 induction by phenobarbital or phenytoin increases susceptibility to toxicity from valproic acid (Zimmerman and Ishak 1982). Other systemic diseases that may increase the risk for drug induced hepatotoxicity are diabetes, thyroid, rheumatic diseases, and AIDS. In advanced liver disease, some phase I metabolic reactions catalyzed by P450 systems are impaired, which may decrease toxic potential, although this is cytochrome P450 specific. For example, CYP2E1 activity seems to be relatively spared in advanced cirrhosis.

CLINICAL MANIFESTATIONS

Acute liver failure has been described with the use of many drugs and natural hepatotoxins. Table 3.2 lists some of the more important agents which have been recognized and emphasizes that the pattern may be that of massive necrosis of hepatocytes, selective metabolic poisoning (as in microvesicular steatosis), or hepatic veno-occlusive disease (Zimmerman 1993; Kaplowitz 1996).

Acute liver failure from drug hepatotoxicity can present in several forms. Acute hepatocellular necrosis usually leads to elevated serum transaminases reflecting the release of enzymes from the cytoplasm of dying cells. Other features are variable and reflect the severity of injury. Serum bilirubin levels and coagulopathy correlate with the severity of damage. Clinically, drug-induced hepatitis may be indistinguishable from necrosis of other causes, such as viral hepatitis and ischemia. Some important features suggesting a drug etiology include recent initiation of therapy with a potentially toxic drug (i.e. temporal association), and other evidences of allergy such as rash and eosinophilia may also be very helpful.

Drug-induced hepatitis associated with overt jaundice tends to be associated with a mortality of at least 10 percent. This emphasizes the severity of the process and is in sharp contrast to the overall mortality of less than one

Table 3.2. *Acute liver failure due to drugs and natural toxins: major reported agents*

Microvesicular steatosis
Tetracycline
NSAIDS, Reye's syndrome
Valproic acid
Fialuridine
Ethanol
Hepatonecrosis
Acetaminophen (paracetamol)
Anesthetics – e.g. halothane
Antiepileptics – e.g. phenytoin, carbamazepine
Antibiotics – e.g. isoniazid, nitrofurantoin, ketoconazole
Dantrolene
Propylthiouracil
Disulfiram
Antihypertensives – e.g. alpha methyldopa, dihydralazine, tienilic acid
NSAIDS – e.g. diclofenac
Phosphorus
Nicotinic acid
Cocaine
Herbal teas – e.g. germander, chaparal, jin bu huan
Mushrooms – *Amanita phalloides* and *Lepiota*
Veno-occlusive disease
6-Thioguanine
Busulfan
Azathioprine
Cyclophosphamide
Dacarbazine
Pyrrolizidine alkaloids – e.g. comfrey, crotolaria (monocrotaline), senecio, heliotropium

percent in viral hepatitis associated with jaundice (Friis and Andreasen 1992; Dossing and Sonne 1993). Possible reasons for the higher mortality with drug-induced hepatitis may include a disproportionate number of older age patients exposed, and the more rapid progression of injury observed with drug-related hepatitis as compared to viral hepatitis. Another general rule is that the longer the patient continues to ingest a drug after onset of drug induced hepatitis symptoms, the more likely it is that the outcome will be fatal. This emphasizes the importance of recognizing the nature of the problem and immediately discontinuing any potentially inciting drug. Latency between start of medication and onset of overt liver disease varies greatly but tends to fall into three patterns. Drugs which produce a hypersensitivity reaction (e.g. phenytoin, allopurinol, etc.) produce injury within the first three months and usually within six to eight weeks. Drugs in which metabolic idiosyncrasy is implicated have a variable latency of weeks to months. Occasionally, the liver injury may follow cessation of the drug by weeks to months (amoxicillin-clavulanate (e.g. Augmentin®) and fialuridine) (Hebbard et al. 1992; Larrey, Vial, Micaleff et al. 1992).

The histologic appearance of the liver is usually not diagnostic for the offending agent or toxin, but is useful in classifying the type of injury (Lee 1995). Certain agents such as acetaminophen and halothane cause a characteristic, sharply demarcated zonal injury in the centrilobular area. Other drugs, such as methyldopa and isoniazid, cause a diffuse or spotty pattern of parenchymal injury similar to that of viral hepatitis. A unique acute injury pattern resembling that in Reye's syndrome or fatty liver of pregnancy, in which there is hepatic failure and infiltration of the liver with microvesicular fat, has been found to occur with high doses of intravenous tetracycline and with valproic acid and fialuridine. However, in most circumstances, liver biopsy specimens will not identify the specific cause and therefore biopsies are not needed. We recommend biopsy only in protracted cases where improvement is slow or there is worsening of the liver disease after at least one month.

Veno-occlusive disease can occur with intensive chemotherapy, with cyclophosphamide, azathioprine, busulfan, dacarbazine, and/or radiation (conditioning for bone marrow transplantation), and some times with ingestion of certain plant extracts such as the Jamaican bush tea (monocrotaline) and other pyrrolizidine alkaloids (comfrey, heliotropium, senecio), which may contaminate food or be used as herbal medicines (Bach et al. 1989; McDonald et al. 1993; Chauvin et al. 1993; Wasserheit et al. 1995). This type of injury presents with rapid onset of tender hepatomegaly, ascites, jaundice, and other features of hepatic failure.

Cocaine abuse is now recognized as a

significant social and medical problem. Hepatotoxicity with periportal necrosis has been reported in patients as a consequence of cocaine abuse. The hepatotoxic metabolite of cocaine is not clearly identified; however, possible factors contributing to liver injury in cocaine intoxicated patients include shock, hypoxia, disseminated intravascular coagulation, and hyperpyrexia. Thus, it is likely that the hepatotoxicity is probably ischemic in nature in many, if not most, cases (Wanless et al. 1990; Mallat and Dhumeaux 1991; Silva et al. 1991). However, true direct hepatotoxicity of cocaine metabolites has been documented in rodents and in a few case reports in humans. Acute liver failure with toxic vasodilatory reaction leading to shock and ischemia has also been described with use of sustained-release niacin (greater than 3 g) (Mullin et al. 1989; Dalton and Berry 1992; Gray et al. 1994).

Natural hepatotoxins also have recently been identified as significant causes of hepatic necrosis. Mushroom poisoning from *Amanita phalloides* leads to hepatotoxicity probably due to ingestions of amatoxins which inhibit RNA polymerase (Fantozzi et al. 1986; Pond et al. 1986; Klein et al. 1989). Acute liver failure after *Lepiota* mushroom ingestion has also been reported (Ramirez et al. 1993). Cyanobacteria (microcystin) poisoning causes hepatotoxicity also through cyclic peptides inhibiting protein phosphatases. Germander is a herbal medicine used to facilitate weight loss and has been reported to cause hepatic injury, probably through transformation (CYP3A?) into toxic metabolites (Larrey, Vial, Pauwels et al. 1992; Loeper et al. 1994). Many other herbal remedies are also being recognized to be hepatotoxic, such as Jin Bu Huan (Stephania and Corydalis), skullcap, valerian, mistletoe, chaparral leaf, senna fruit extract, and the pyrrolizidine alkaloids previously mentioned (MacGregor et al. 1989; Woolf et al. 1994; Kane et al. 1995).

Yellow phosphorus poisoning has become a rare occurrence in the United States; cases are usually the result of accidental ingestion of rat or cockroach poison or the contents of firecrackers (McCarron et al. 1981; Zimmerman 1993). Phosphorus toxicity usually results in severe gastrointestinal symptoms, shock and in some cases, acute liver failure characterized by hepatic steatosis and necrosis. The necrosis is characteristic in its localization to zone 1 (periportal).

ASSESSMENT AND TREATMENT

All forms of acute or chronic hepatobiliary disease are mimicked by drug-induced liver disease, and the possibility of drug-induced hepatotoxicity must be considered in all patients presenting with liver disease, and especially with an acute liver failure picture. A complete drug history, including careful questioning about all nonprescription medications, is essential. Other causes of hepatic necrosis should be excluded by hepatitis serologic testing, and by careful inquiry concerning the clinical setting (travel, transfusions, or evidence of hypotension) preceding the onset of liver injury. Establishing the clinical diagnosis of a drug-induced liver disease is often difficult because the diagnosis is based mainly on circumstantial evidence. The onset of symptoms or laboratory abnormalities occurring within days or weeks of starting therapy with a new medication may provide an initial clue to acute drug toxicity but, as noted above, latency may be prolonged.

With more understanding of the mechanisms of toxicity, methods may be developed to identify people who are biochemically susceptible to toxicity or hypersensitivity from specific drugs. If a drug is implicated as causing either acute or chronic liver disease, the drug should be discontinued immediately and the patient monitored for improvement in hepatic function. After the discontinuation of the offending drug, the activity level of acute or chronic hepatitis will usually respond with rapid improvement over one or two weeks. Indeed, a 50 percent or greater decrease in alanine aminotransferase (ALT) levels in one week is usual. However, certain forms of drug-induced liver disease, such as lesions resembling alcoholic hepatitis and certain cholestatic reactions, will not be alleviated rapidly after stopping the drug. The role of corticosteroids in the treatment of drug induced hepatotoxicity is not clear, but may be considered particularly in patients with features of severe systemic hypersensitivity. Thus, in patients with very severe acute disease with the potential for acute liver failure, especially those with obvious systemic immune hypersensitivity, a short course of corticosteroids in large doses is often used. This approach is reasonable in certain patients, such as those with phenytoin-induced severe hepatic injury, despite its uncertain efficacy.

Rechallenging the patient with the implicated drug and watching for exacerbation of the liver disease provides the most conclusive clinical proof of drug toxicity. Often, patients with drug-induced liver disease may have been rechallenged inadvertently with the drug, and a careful review of the medical record may provide valuable information. Rechallenge in patients with hypersensitivity mediated injury is potentially very dangerous and generally should be avoided. The risk of rechallenging the patient with drug must also be weighed against the potential therapeutic benefits of that drug. If rechallenge is to be done, patients should be tested with a small initial dose and watched closely for any sign of hepatic damage. When an idiosyncratic reaction is due to a minor metabolite of a drug, there may be a long latency between institution of therapy and onset of liver disease. The explanation for the latency is uncertain, but it may reflect the accumulation of a minor but toxic metabolite. In this situation, results of a rechallenge over a short period may be negative. Therefore, a negative response to a rechallenge does not exclude drug-induced liver disease, and it is risky to conclude that chronic reinstitution of the drug is safe.

In conclusion, the use of *N*-acetylcysteine in the emergent treatment of acetaminophen toxicity is the only specific treatment for drug-induced hepatotoxicity; most other therapies are symptomatic and supportive only. Acute liver failure appears with hepatic encephalopathy developing rapidly in cases of drug- or toxin-induced hepatotoxicity. Analysis of sixty cases of acute liver failure referred to University of California at San Francisco (UCSF) from 1989 to 1992 showed that one-third of the cases were drug- or toxin-induced and were associated with a high mortality rate (Hoofnagle et al. 1995). For certain cases in this study, the only successful approach to treatment was emergent liver transplantation. Nevertheless, a more recent study has shown that emergent liver grafting for idiosyncratic drug reactions has a significantly worse outcome than when transplantation is performed for other causes of liver failure (Devlin et al. 1995). Certainly, it is prudent to contact a transplant center when one encounters a patient with overt drug-induced liver disease, in anticipation of the high likelihood of subsequent acute liver failure.

REFERENCES

Bach, N., Thung, S.N. and Schaffner, F. 1989. Comfrey herb tea-induced hepatic veno-occlusive disease. *Am J Med* 87: 97–9.

Benjamin, S.B., Goodman, Z.D., Ishak, K.G., Zimmerman, H.J. and Irey, N.S. 1985. The morphologic spectrum of halothane-induced hepatic injury: Analysis of 77 cases. *Hepatology* 5: 1163–71.

Bourdi, M., Tinel, M., Beaune, P.H. and Pessayre, D. 1994. Interactions of dihydralazine with cytochromes P4501A: a possible explanation for the appearance of anti-cytochrome P4501A2 autoantibodies. *Mol Pharmacol* 45: 1287–95.

Chauvin, P., Dillion, J., Moren, A., Talbak, S. and Barakaev, S. 1993. Heliotrope poisoning in Tadjikistan. *Lancet* 341: 1663–4.

Christen, U., Jeno, P. and Gut, J. 1993. Halothane metabolism: The dihydrolipoamide acetyltransferase subunit of the pyruvate dehydrogenase complex molecularly mimics trifluoroacetyl-protein adducts. *Biochemistry* 32: 1492–9.

Dalton, T.A. and Berry, R.S. 1992. Hepatotoxicity associated with sustained-release niacin. *Am J Med* 93: 102–4.

Devlin, J., Wendon, J., Heaton, N., Tan, K. and Williams, R. 1995. Pretransplantation clinical status and outcome of emergency transplantation for acute liver failure. *Hepatology* 21: 1018–24.

Dossing, M. and Sonne, J. 1993. Drug-induced hepatic disorders. *Drug Safety* 9: 441–9.

Dunk, A.A., Walt, R.P., Jenkins, W.J. and Sherlock, S.S. 1982. Diclofenac hepatitis. *BMJ* 284: 1605–6.

Edwards, M.J., Keller, B.J., Kauffman, F.C. and Thurman, R.G. 1993. The involvement of Kupffer cells in carbon tetrachloride toxicity. *Toxicol Appl Pharmacol* 119: 275–9.

Fantozzi, R., Ledda, F., Caramelli, L., Moroni, F., Blandina, P., Masini, E., Botti, P., Peruzzi, S., Zorn, M. and

Mannaioni, P.F. 1986. Clinical findings and follow-up evaluation of an outbreak of mushroom poisoning – survey of *Amanita phalloides* poisoning. *Klin Wochenschr* 64: 38–43.

Friis, H. and Andreasen, P.B. 1992. Drug-induced hepatic injury: an analysis of 1100 cases reported to The Danish Committee on Adverse Drug Reactions between 1978 and 1987. *J Intern Med* 232: 133–8.

Fujii, Y., Johnson, M.E. and Gores, G.J. 1994. Mitochondrial dysfunction during anoxia/reperfusion injury of sinusoidal endothelial cells. *Hepatology* 20: 177–85.

Gray, D.R., Morgan, T., Chretien, S.D. and Kashyap, M.L. 1994. Efficacy and safety of controlled-release niacin in dyslipoproteinemic veterans. *Ann Intern Med* 121: 252–8.

Gut, J., Christen, U., Huwyler, J., Burgin, M. and Kenna, J.G. 1992. Molecular mimicry of trifluoroacetylated human liver protein adducts by constitutive proteins and immunochemical evidence for its impairment in halothane hepatitis. *Eur J Biochem* 210: 569–76.

Hebbard, G.S., Smith, K.G.C., Gibson, P.R. and Bhathal, P.S. 1992. Augmentin-induced jaundice with a fatal outcome. *Med J Aust* 156: 285–6.

Helfgott, S.M., Sandberg-Cook, J., Zakim, D. and Nestler, J. 1990. Diclofenac-associated hepatotoxicity. *JAMA* 264: 2660–2.

Hoofnagle, J.H., Carithers, R.L., Shapiro, C. and Ascher, N. 1995. Fulminant hepatic failure: summary of a workshop. *Hepatology* 21: 240–52.

Imberti, R., Nieminen, A., Herman, B. and Lemasters, J.J. 1992. Mitochondrial and glycolytic dysfunction in lethal injury to hepatocytes by *t*-butylhydroperoxide: protection by fructose, cyclosporin A and trifluoperazine. *J Pharmacol Exp Ther* 265: 392–400.

Israel, H.L., Gottlieb, J.E. and Maddrey, W.C. 1992. Perspective: preventive isoniazid therapy and the liver. *Chest* 101: 1298–301.

Kane, J.A., Kane, S.P. and Jain, S. 1995. Hepatitis induced by traditional Chinese herbs; possible toxic components. *Gut* 36: 146–7.

Kaplowitz, N. 1996. Drug metabolism and drug-induced liver disease. In *Liver and Biliary Disease*, 2nd edition, ed. N. Kaplowitz, 103–20. Baltimore MD: Williams & Wilkins.

Kenna, J.G., Martin, J.L., Satoh, H. and Pohl, L.R. 1990. Factors affecting the expression of trifluoroacetylated liver microsomal protein neoantigens in rats treated with halothane. *Drug Metab Dispos* 18: 788–93.

Klein, A.S., Hart, J., Brems, J.J., Goldstein, L., Lewin, K. and Busuttil, R.W. 1989. Amanita poisoning: treatment and the role of liver transplantation. *Am J Med* 86: 187–93.

Knight, T.L., Scatchard, K.M., Van Pelt, F.N.A.M. and Kenna, J.G. 1994. Sera from patients with halothane hepatitis contain antibodies to halothane-induced liver antigens which are not detectable by immunoblotting. *J Pharmacol Exp Ther* 270: 1325–33.

Kretz-Rommel, A.K. and Boelsterli, U.A. 1993. Selective protein adducts to membrane proteins in cultured rat hepatocytes exposed to diclofenac: radiochemical and immunochemical analysis. *Mol Pharmacol* 45: 237–44.

Kretz-Rommel, A.K. and Boelsterli, U.A. 1995. Cytotoxic activity of T cells and non-T cells from diclofenac-immunized mice against cultured syngeneic hepatocytes exposed to diclofenac. *Hepatology* 22: 213–22.

Larrey, D., Berson, A., Habersetzer, F., Tinel, M., Castot, A., Babany, G., Letteron, P., Freneaux, E., Loeper, J., Dansette, P. and Pessayre, D. 1989. Genetic predisposition to drug hepatotoxicity: role in hepatitis caused by amineptine, a tricyclic antidepressant. *Hepatology* 10: 168–73.

Larrey, D., Vial, T., Micaleff, G.B., Morichau-Beauchant, M., Michel, H. and Benhamou, J.P. 1992. Hepatitis associated with amoxycillin-clavulanic acid combination report of 15 cases. *Gut* 33: 368–71.

Larrey, D., Vial, T., Pauwels, A., Castot, A., Biour, M., David, M. and Michel, H. 1992. Hepatitis after germander (*Teucrium chamaedrys*) administration: another instance of herbal medicine hepatotoxicity. *Ann Intern Med* 117: 129–32.

Laskin, D.L. 1990. Nonparenchymal cells and hepatotoxicity. *Sem Liver Dis* 10: 293.

Lecoeur, S., Bonierbale, Challine, D., Gautier, J., Valadon, P., Dansette, P.M., Catinot, R., Ballet, F., Mansuy, D. and Beaune, P.H. 1994. Specificity of in vitro covalent binding of tienilic acid metabolites to human liver microsomes in relationship to the type of hepatotoxicity: comparison with two directly hepatotoxic drugs. *Chem Res Toxicol* 7: 434–42.

Lee, W.M. 1995. Medical review. Drug-induced hepatotoxicity. *N Engl J Med.*

Leeder, J.S., Riley, R.J., Cook, V.A. and Spielberg, S.P. 1992. Human anti-cytochrome P450 antibodies in aromatic anticonvulsant-induced hypersensitivity reactions. *J Pharmacol Exp Ther* 263: 360–7.

Lieber, C.S. 1994. Mechanisms of ethanol-drug-nutrition interactions. *Clin Toxicol* 32: 631–81.

Loeper, J., Descatoire, V., Letteron, P., Moulis, C., Degott, C., Dansette, P., Fau, D. and Pessayre, D. 1994. Hepatotoxicity of germander in mice. *Gastroenterology* 106: 464–72.

MacGregor, F.B., Abernethy, V.E., Dahabra, S., Cobden, I. and Hayes, P.C. 1989. Hepatotoxicity of herbal remedies. *BMJ* 299: 1156–7.

Mallat, A. and Dhumeaux, D. 1991. Cocaine and the liver. *J Hepatol* 12: 275–8.

Martin, J.L., Kenna, J.G., Martin, B.M., Thomassen, D., Reed, G.F. and Pohl, L.R. 1993. Halothane hepatitis patients have serum antibodies that react with protein disulfide isomerase. *Hepatology* 18: 858–63.

May, D.G. 1994. Genetic differences in drug disposition. *J Clin Pharmacol* 34: 881–97.

McCarron, M.M., Gaddie, G.P. and Trotter, A.T. 1981. Acute yellow phosphorus poisoning from pesticide pastes. *Clin Toxicol* 18: 693.

McDonald, G.B., Hinds, M.S., Fisher, L.D., Schoch, H.G., Wolford, J.L., Banaji, M., Hardin, B.J., Shulman, H.M. and Clift, R. 1993. Veno-occlusive disease of the liver and multiorgan failure after bone marrow transplantation: a cohort study of 355 patients. *Ann Intern Med* 118: 255–67.

Mitchell, J.R., Zimmerman, H.J., Ishak, K.G., Thorgeirsson, U.P., Timbrell, J.A., Snodgrass, W.R. and Nelson, S.D. 1976. Isoniazid liver injury: clinical spectrum, pathology, and probable pathogenesis. *Ann Intern Med* 84: 181–92.

Moulding, T.S., Redeker, A.G. and Kanel, G.C. 1989. Twenty isoniazid-associated deaths in one state. *Am Rev Respir Dis* 140: 700–5.

Mullick, F.G. and Ishak, K.G. 1979. Hepatic injury associated with diphenylhydantoin therapy. *Am J Clin Pathol* 74: 442–52.

Mullin, G.E., Greenson, J.K. and Mitchell, M.C. 1989. Fulminant hepatic failure after ingestion of sustained-release nicotinic acid. *Ann Intern Med* 111: 253–5.

Murray, M. 1992. P450 Enzymes, inhibition mechanisms, genetic regulation and effects of liver disease. *Clin Pharmacokinet* 23: 132–46.

Nelson, S.D. 1990. Molecular mechanisms of the hepatotoxicity caused by acetaminophen. *Sem Liver Dis* 10: 267.

Nicotera, P., Bellomo, G. and Orrenius, S. 1992. Calcium-mediated mechanisms in chemically induced cell death. *Ann Rev Pharmacol Toxicol* 32: 449–70.

Ohta, T., Sueoka, E., Iida, N., Komori, A., Suganuma, M., Nishiwaki, R., Tatematsu, M., Kim, S., Carmichael, W.W. and Fujiki, H. 1994. Nodularin, a potent inhibitor of protein phosphatases 1 and 2A, is a new environmental carcinogen in male F344 rat liver. *Cancer Res* 54: 6402–6.

Pohl, L.R. 1990. Drug-induced allergic hepatitis. *Sem Liver Dis* 10: 305–15.

Pond, S.M., Olson, K.R., Woo, O.F., Osterloh, J.D., Ward, R.E., Kaufman, D.A. and Moody, R.R. 1986. Amatoxin poisoning in Northern California, 1982–1983. *West J Med* 145: 204–9.

Powell-Jackson, P.R., Tredger, J.M. and Williams, R. 1984. Hepatotoxicity to sodium valproate: a review. *Gut* 25: 673–81.

Ramirez, P., Parrilla, P., Bueno, F.S., Robles, R., Pons, J.A., Bixquert, V., Nicolas, S., Nunez, R., Alegria, S., Miras, M. and Rodriguez, J.M. 1993. Fulminant hepatic failure after *Lepiota* mushroom poisoning. *J Hepatol* 19: 51–4.

Reed, D.J. 1990. Status of calcium and thiols in hepatocellular injury by oxidative stress. *Sem Liver Dis* 10: 285.

Rieder, M.J., Uetrecht, J., Shear, N.H., Cannon, M., Miller, M. and Spielberg, S.P. 1989. Diagnosis of sulfonamide hypersensitivity. *Ann Intern Med* 110: 286–9.

Rosser, B.G. and Gores, G.J. 1995. Liver cell necrosis: cellular mechanisms and clinical implications. *Gastroenterology* 108: 252–75.

Salazar, D.E., Sorge, C.L., Jordan, S.W. and Corcoran, G.B. 1994. Obesity decreases hepatic glutathione concentrations and markedly potentiaties allyl alcohol-induced periportal necrosis in the overfed rat. *Int J Obesity* 18: 25–33.

Sallie, R., Kleiner, D., Richardson, F., Conjeevaram, H., Zullo, S., Mutimer, D., Hoover, S., Fox, C. and Hoofnagle, J.H. 1994. Mechanisms of FIAU induced hepatotoxicity. *Hepatology* 20 (Suppl. (2)): A209.

Satoh, H., Martin, B.M., Schulick, A.H., Christ, D.D., Kenna, J.G. and Pohl, L.R. 1989. Human anti-endoplasmic reticulum antibodies in sera of patients with halothane-induced hepatitis are directed against a trifluoroacetylated carboxylesterase. *Proc Natl Acad Sci USA* 86: 322–6.

Scully, L.J., Clarke, D. and Barr, R.J. 1993. Diclofenac induced hepatitis. *Dig Dis Sci* 38: 744–51.

Searle, J., Kerr, J.F.R. and Bishop, C.J. 1982. Necrosis and apoptosis: distinct modes of cell death with fundamentally different significance. *Pathol Ann* 17: 229–59.

Shear, N.H., Spielberg, S.P., Grant, D.M., Tang, B.K. and Kalow, W. 1986. Differences in metabolism of sulfonamides predisposing to idiosyncratic toxicity. *Ann Intern Med* 105: 179–84.

Shear, N.H. and Spielberg, S.P. 1988. Anticonvulsant hypersensitivity syndrome *J Clin Invest* 82: 1826–32.

Silva, M.O., Roth, D., Reddy, K.R., Fernandez, J.A., Albores-Saavedra, J. and Schiff, E.R. 1991. Hepatic dysfunction accompanying acute cocaine intoxication. *J Hepatol* 12: 312–15.

Smith, G.C., Kenna, J.G., Harrison, D.J., Tew, D. and Wolf, C.R. 1993. Autoantibodies to hepatic microsomal carboxylesterase in halothane hepatitis. *Lancet* 342: 963–4.

Snider, D.E. and Caras, G.J. 1992. Isoniazid-associated hepatitis deaths: a review of available information. *Am Rev Respir Dis* 145: 494–7.

Spielberg, S.P., Gordon, G.B., Blake, D.A., Goldstein, D.A. and Herlong, H.F. 1981. Predisposition to phenytoin hepatotoxicity assessed in vitro. *N Engl J Med* 305: 722–7.

Stanley, J. and Fallon-Pellicci, V. 1978. Phenytoin hypersensitivity reaction. *Arch Dermatol* 114: 1350–3.

Thurman, R.G., Bunzendahl, H. and Lemasters, J.J. 1993. Role of sinusoidal lining cells in hepatic reperfusion injury following cold storage and transplantation. *Sem Liver Dis* 13: 93–100.

Vaux, D.L. 1993. Toward an understanding of the molecular mechanisms of physiological cell death. *Proc Natl Acad Sci USA* 90: 786–9.

Wanless, I.R., Dore, S., Gopinath, N., Tan, J., Cameron, R., Heathcote, E.J., Blendis, L.M. and Levy, G. 1990. Histopathology of cocaine hepatotoxicity. *Gastroenterology* 98: 497–501.

Wasserheit, C., Acaba, L. and Gulati, S. 1995. Abnormal liver function in patients undergoing autologous bone marrow transplantation for hematological malignancies. *Cancer Invest* 13: 347–54.

Watkins, P.B. 1990. Role of cytochromes P450 in drug metabolism and hepatotoxicity. *Sem Liver Dis* 10: 235–50.

Weiss, S.J. 1989. Tissue destruction by neutrophils. *N Engl J Med* 320: 365–76.

Whitcomb, D.C. and Block, G.D. 1994. Association of acetaminophen hepatotoxicity with fasting and ethanol use. *JAMA* 272: 1845–50.

Williams, A.T. and Burk, R.F. 1990. Carbon tetrachloride hepatotoxicity: an example of a free radical mediated injury. *Sem Liver Dis* 10: 279.

Wolkenstein, P., Charue, D., Laurent, P., Revuz, J., Roujeau, J. and Bagot, M. 1995. Metabolic predisposition to cutaneous adverse drug reactions. *Arch Dermatol* 131: 544–51.

Woolf, G.M., Petrovic, L.M., Rojter, S.E., Wainwright, S., Villamil, F.G., Katkov, W.N., Michieletti, P., Wanless, I.R., Stermitz, F.R., Beck, J.J. and Vierling, J.M. 1994. Acute hepatitis associated with the Chinese herbal product Jin Bu Huan. *Ann Intern Med* 121: 729–35.

Wu, J., Lee, S., Yeh, P., Chan, C., Wang, Y., Huang, Y., Tsai, Y., Lee, P., Ting, L. and Lo, K. 1990. Isoniazid-rifampin-induced hepatitis in hepatitis B carriers. *Gastroenterology* 98: 502–4.

Yan, C.C. and Huxtable, R.J. 1995. Relationship between glutathione concentration and metabolism of the pyrrolizidine alkaloid, monocrotaline, in the isolated, perfused liver. *Toxicol Appl Pharmacol* 130: 132–9.

Zahrebelski, G., Nieminen, A., Al-Ghoul, K., Qian, T., Herman, B. and Lemasters, J.J. 1995. Progression of subcellular changes during chemical hypoxia to cultured rat hepatocytes: a laser scanning confocal microscopic study. *Hepatology* 21: 1361–72.

Zimmerman, H.J. 1993. Hepatotoxicity. *Dis Mon* 39: 677–787.

Zimmerman, H.J. and Ishak, K.G. 1982. Valproate-induced hepatic injury: analyses of 23 fatal cases. *Hepatology* 2: 591–7.

4 Acetaminophen-induced acute liver failure

Alistair J. Makin and Roger Williams

INTRODUCTION

Acetaminophen (paracetamol; *N*-acetyl-*p*-aminophenol), a para-aminophenol derivative, is an active metabolite of both acetanilide and phenacetin. Acetanilide, the parent compound, was first introduced as an antipyretic and analgesic in 1886 but its use was limited by its toxicity. Consequently other para-aminophenol derivatives were tested which led to the introduction of phenacetin in 1887 followed by acetaminophen in 1893, which was first used in medicine by von Mering (Insel 1990). In the USA, acetaminophen has been available since 1952 and in the UK it has steadily gained in popularity as an analgesic from 1956 onwards. It is available without prescription and, when used at the recommended dosage, has few side effects and is considered safer than aspirin (*Lancet* 1981). Currently, in the UK and USA, there are more than one hundred proprietary preparations of acetaminophen, and more than two hundred proprietary multi-ingredient acetaminophen preparations.

The hepatotoxic effects of acetaminophen were first reported by Eder in 1964, during long-term toxicity studies in cats (Eder 1964), and two years later extensive centrilobular necrosis was observed in rats given high doses of acetaminophen (Boyd and Bereczky 1966). The first cases of severe and fatal liver damage in man following acetaminophen overdose were reported in the UK in the same year (Davidson and Eastham 1966; Thomson and Prescott 1966).

INCIDENCE

Acetaminophen overdose, with deliberate suicidal intent, is increasing in most Western countries. In the USA during 1987 there were 60,000 calls to Poison Control Centers concerning acetaminophen overdoses (Smilkstein et al. 1988) and in 1993 over 90,000 were recorded, although in the same year only 92 deaths were directly related to overdose of acetaminophen (Litovitz et al. 1994). In the UK, the most recent available figures indicate that acetaminophen overdose caused about 150 deaths in England and Wales in 1992 (Office of Population Censuses and Surveys, 1994). Acetaminophen-induced hepatotoxicity remains the commonest cause of acute liver failure (ALF) accounting for between 50 and 60 percent of the cases seen (O'Grady et al. 1989). According to previous statistics from England and Wales there were over 500 deaths in 1990, suggesting that the incidence is decreasing (Office of Population Censuses and Surveys 1991) but a detailed investigation of autopsy and coroner's reports from that year revealed that in only 150 of these 500 cases was there any evidence of hepatic damage (Spooner and Harvey 1993), the primary cause of death from acetaminophen toxicity. The additional deaths were likely to have been the result of respiratory depression caused by the dextropropoxyphene component of the mixed drug formulation coproxamol (Spooner and Harvey 1993). These data suggest that there has been little change in the annual number of deaths from acetaminophen-induced hepatotoxicity in recent years.

In the rest of Europe, death from acetaminophen overdose taken with suicidal intent is uncommon. In France it accounts for only 2 percent of the cases of ALF and is implicated in less than ten deaths annually (Benhamou 1991; Garnier and Bismuth 1993). In Denmark the death rate from acetaminophen poisoning is ten times lower than in the UK for unclear reasons (Ott et al. 1990). Nevertheless, instances of hepatotoxicity due to acetaminophen overdose occur world-wide with reports from South Africa (Monteagudo and Folb 1987), Israel (Oren and Levy 1992), Australia (Brotodihardjo et al. 1992) and Hong Kong (Chan et al. 1993), but both the mortality and severe poisoning rates appear to be much lower than in the UK.

MECHANISMS OF TOXICITY

In therapeutic doses, acetaminophen is metabolized predominantly in the liver where over 90 percent of the dose undergoes glucuronidation or sulfation, producing nontoxic metabolites that are excreted in the urine. Approximately 5 percent of the dose is excreted unchanged in the urine and the remainder is metabolized by the hepatic cytochrome P450 (mixed function oxidase) system to *N*-acetyl-*p*-benzoquinone imine (NAPQI), a highly reactive arylating metabolite, which is preferentially conjugated with reduced glutathione and excreted as mercapturic acid and cysteine conjugates (Figure 4.1).

After an overdose, the half-life of acetaminophen is prolonged as a result of the saturation of both glucuronidation and sulfate conjugation (Prescott and Wright 1973; Prescott 1983). Consequently, increasing quantities of NAPQI are produced which overwhelm glutathione synthesis, with manifestations of toxicity appearing when glutathione levels fall below 30 percent of normal (Mitchell, Jollow, Potter, Gillette and Brodie 1973).

NAPQI is capable of both arylation and oxidation, but arylation, particularly to protein thiol groups, appears to be the most important event (Mitchell, Jollow, Potter, Gillette and Brodie 1973; Streeter et al. 1984). Following covalent binding the exact series of events that produce cell death are not fully understood but a number of possible mechanisms have been implicated. NAPQI disrupts Ca^{2+} homeostasis by its oxidation of thiol groups in the key calcium-regulating proteins Ca^{2+}/Mg^{2+}-ATPase of the plasma membrane (Tsokos-Kuhn et al. 1987), the ATP-dependent Ca^{2+}-sequestering system of the endoplasmic reticulum and NAD(P)H-dehydrogenase of the mitochondrion (Moore et al. 1985). Damage to these proteins produces an intracellular accumulation of Ca^{2+} which mediates cell death either by DNA fragmentation (Shen et al. 1991; Ray et al. 1993) or by damage to the cell cytoskeletal elements (Glenney et al. 1981). Inhibition of mitochondrial respiration may be the key event in the development of acetaminophen-induced hepatotoxicity (Meyers et al. 1988; Donnelly et al. 1994) as changes in mitochondrial morphology are one of the earliest histological changes seen (Placke et al. 1987) and NAPQI binds covalently to mitochondria (Jollow et al. 1973). Lipid peroxidation has also been implicated but it is unclear at what stage this occurs (Nelson 1990).

HEPATOTOXIC DOSE OF ACETAMINOPHEN

Severe hepatotoxicity is an uncommon consequence of an acetaminophen overdose

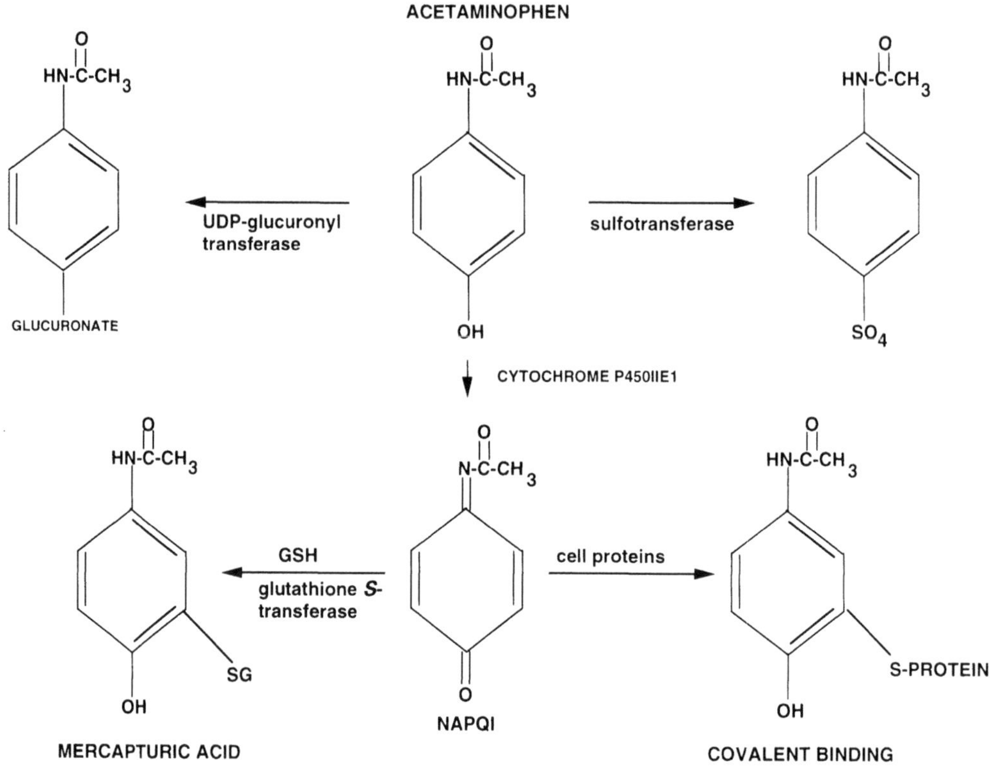

ACETAMINOPHEN

HN-C-CH$_3$ / O / OH

UDP-glucuronyl transferase → GLUCURONATE

sulfotransferase → SO_4

CYTOCHROME P450IIE1

NAPQI

GSH glutathione S-transferase → MERCAPTURIC ACID (SG, OH)

cell proteins → COVALENT BINDING (S-PROTEIN, OH)

Figure 4.1 Metabolic pathway of acetaminophen. Acetaminophen primarily undergoes sulfation and glucuronidation (phase 2 reactions) but is metabolized by cytochrome P450 2E1 (in a phase 1 reaction) to *N*-acetyl-*p*-benzoquinoneimine (NAPQI) if the capacity of the phase 2 reactions is exceeded or if cytochrome P450 2E1 synthesis is induced. Glutathione-*S*-transferase is capable of detoxifying NAPQI to yield mercapturic acid and its derivatives, if glutathione is available. In the absence of glutathione substrate, covalent binding to cell proteins occurs. *N*-acetylcysteine is an excellent source of glutathione substrate. UDP denotes uridine diphosphate, and GSH reduced glutathione.

because the majority of patients do not absorb more than 125 mg/kg of the drug which is thought to be the minimum dose that can produce hepatic damage. Doses above 250 mg/kg (15 g, or 30 standard 500 mg tablets in a 60 kg individual) often produce hepatotoxicity whereas those in excess of 350 mg/kg invariably result in severe liver damage (aspartate aminotransferase (AST) >1000 units/l).

The most reliable method of assessing the potential risk of an overdose is to use the standard semilogarithmic plot, produced from the original work by Prescott (Prescott et al. 1971), which relates plasma acetaminophen concentration to time after ingestion. Those patients with a plasma concentration above a line joining values of 200 g/ml (1.32 mmol/l) at 4 h and 30 μg/ml (0.19 mmol/l) at 15 h are considered to have taken a major overdose with a 60 percent chance of developing liver damage. Above a parallel line joining 300 μg/ml (1.98 mmol/l) at 4 h to 45 μg/ml (0.28 mmol/l) at 15 h, patients have a 90 percent chance of developing severe hepatic damage (Prescott 1983) (Figure 4.2). Levels that fall between these two lines result in severe liver damage in only 25–30 percent of cases.

In a study of 560 consecutive admissions to the Liver Failure Unit at King's College Hospital with severe acetaminophen-induced hepatotoxicity, we found no correlation between the dose taken and outcome. Of these patients, 90 percent had taken more than 12 g (24 tablets) and 71 percent more than 24 g.

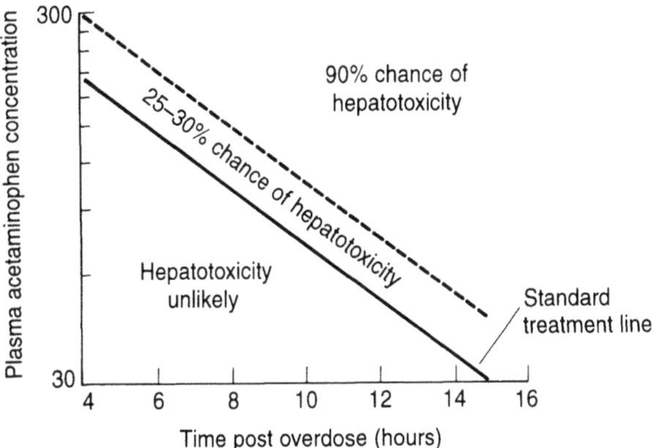

Figure 4.2 Relationship between plasma acetaminophen concentration and the relative risk of developing hepatotoxicity.

This suggests that once the minimum threshold dose of acetaminophen has been exceeded, the ensuing hepatic damage and outcome are not dose related.

HIGH RISK GROUPS

There have been a number of cases where the occurrence of severe hepatotoxicity after ingestion of therapeutic or near therapeutic doses of acetaminophen has been reported in chronic alcoholics or in patients taking hepatic enzyme-inducing medication (Seeff et al. 1986; McClain et al. 1988; Wootton and Lee 1990). The main enzyme-inducing drugs implicated have been anticonvulsants (phenytoin, carbamazepine, primadone and phenobarbital) and antituberculous drugs (rifampicin and isoniazid). Animal studies have demonstrated that both chronic alcohol intake (Sato et al. 1989) and treatment with enzyme-inducing drugs (Mitchell, Jollow, Potter, Davis, Gillette and Brodie 1973) can increase the hepatotoxic effect of acetaminophen by induction of the cytochrome P-450 system. Enhanced toxicity of acetaminophen might be expected to occur in such groups of patients as a result of increased NAPQI production and more rapid glutathione depletion. In addition, the low levels of hepatic glutathione associated with the malnutrition so common in alcoholics could further increase susceptibility (Lauterburg and Velez 1988; Whitcomb and Block 1994) and may also account, at least in part, for the increased suspectibility of HIV-positive individuals (Henry 1990). It has also been suggested that individuals with genetically determined defects of glucuronidation, such as Gilbert's syndrome, may have an increased susceptibility to the toxic effects of acetaminophen (De Morais et al. 1992) although no clinical evidence to support this has been reported.

The clinical data with respect to these high-risk groups are not so clear-cut. An increased susceptibility to a normal or near-normal dose is not a necessary prerequisite to the development of hepatotoxicity as, in fact, in the majority of cases a major overdose has been taken (Seeff et al. 1986; Bray et al. 1991, 1992). Prescott, in a detailed review of the early literature reached a similar conclusion, namely that although some individuals may have a true increased susceptibility to acetaminophen the majority of cases of severe hepatotoxicity in alcoholics are the direct result of the size of the overdose taken (Prescott 1986). Therefore, although one cannot be certain about an individual's susceptibility, the practice in the UK is to recommend that any patient thought to come from a high-risk group should be given *N*-acetylcysteine at half the serum acetaminophen concentration levels of the standard plot. In the USA the standard treatment guidelines are followed for both alcoholics and patients on enzyme-inducing drugs (Ferner 1993; Anker and Smilkstein 1994) but the line for treatment used in that country is 25 percent below the plot used in the UK (Rumack et al. 1981). In practice, *N*-acetylcysteine should be used whenever there is any doubt concerning the timing, dose ingested, or plasma concentration, since the use of the antidote is much less hazardous than the consequences of withholding it (Figure 4.3).

One often-overlooked group of patients who are particularly at risk of developing hepatotoxicity are those who have either taken alcohol or sedating drugs at the same time or who are psychiatrically ill. These patients cannot be relied upon to give an accurate history which renders the standard treatment plot of serum acetaminophen concentration to time after overdose uninterpretable. Measurement of the serum acetaminophen concentration in patients who have taken sequential overdoses over a number of hours or days is also meaningless because of the variable absorption. As a result, *N*-acetylcysteine treatment may be inadvertently or inappropriately withheld in these patients, thus increasing the risk of hepatotoxicity and serious complications. This group appears to be more common in series from the USA than from the UK, and recent reports emphasize the greater severity and higher mortality associated with "therapeutic misadventures" (Zimmerman and Maddrey 1995; Rochling et al. 1995).

EARLY MANIFESTATIONS OF HEPATOTOXICITY

The majority of patients do not develop any symptoms or signs after acetaminophen overdosage, and may not even feel unwell. If the dose is sufficient to produce hepatotoxicity, nausea and vomiting can occur within the first few hours, followed by abdominal pain and hepatic tenderness which are often the reason for presentation to hospital. Hepatic enzymes become elevated within 12–24 h of the overdose with the maximum derangement occurring by day 3, when AST levels can exceed 10,000 units/l. Jaundice may become apparent from 24 h after the overdose and deepens rapidly in patients with severe hepatic damage who may remain jaundiced for a number of weeks. Most importantly, the prothrombin time becomes prolonged as a result of decreased synthesis of clotting factors. This may be detected within a few hours of overdose in severe cases and usually peaks by day 3.

Renal failure, oliguric (urine output <300 ml/24 h and serum creatinine >300 μmol/l) or non-oliguric, occurs in 1–2 percent of all overdoses and in 11 percent of severely

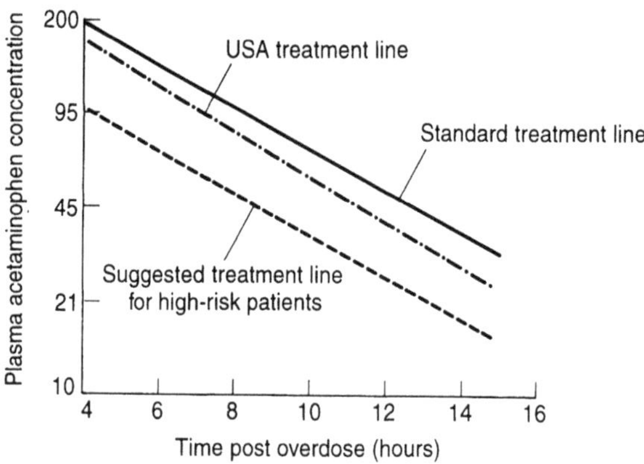

Figure 4.3 Treatment guidelines used for high-risk patients.

poisoned patients (AST >1000 units/l) (Prescott 1979). Acetaminophen is concentrated 5–7-fold in the renal medulla where it is also metabolized to NAPQI and cellular damage occurs when renal glutathione is depleted (Kincaid-Smith 1986). Renal failure becomes evident 24–72 h after overdose and can occur in cases which do not progress to ALF (Davenport and Finn 1988). Exceptionally, it may develop without any clinical or biochemical evidence of severe liver damage (Prescott et al. 1982). Once ALF has developed, renal failure occurs in about 70 percent of cases (O'Grady et al. 1988).

Hypophosphatemia is a common finding and may occur early after a major overdose, although it is not invariably associated with the development of ALF (Davenport and Will 1988). The degree of hypophosphatemia correlates with the severity of the hepatic damage and is thought to be due to renal loss of phosphate (Jones et al. 1989) although intracellular redistribution is more important when there is associated renal failure. Other metabolic disturbances are seen only with severe cases of hepatotoxicity. Hypoglycemia, often marked, can occur within the first 24 h after overdose and should be looked for in all major overdoses, particularly if the level of consciousness is impaired. It is the consequence of impaired gluconeogenesis, an inability to mobilize hepatic glycogen stores, and elevated levels of circulating insulin. Metabolic acidosis, another well recognized complication, can occur at two distinct time periods after overdose in all but minor cases (Gray et al. 1987). An initial transient metabolic acidosis (compensated in half of the cases) appears within 15 h of ingestion and is due to the direct effect of the acetaminophen overdose on hepatic lactic acid uptake and metabolism (Gray et al. 1987). Hypovolemia as a result of vomiting produces poor tissue perfusion and anaerobic tissue respiration which may exacerbate this initial acidosis and is rapidly improved by colloid infusions. Metabolic acidosis occurring later than 15 h after overdose is invariably the consequence of deteriorating hepatic function and is then the result of decreased hepatic lactic acid clearance (Gray et al. 1987) and increased peripheral lactic acid production by anaerobic metabolism resulting from profound tissue hypoxia (Bihari et al. 1985). Acidosis that either fails to respond to adequate fluid resuscitation or that develops with deteriorating hepatic function carries a very poor prognosis.

N-ACETYLCYSTEINE TREATMENT

Cysteamine was the first drug shown to be an effective antidote for acetaminophen-induced hepatotoxicity and subsequently both methionine and *N*-acetylcysteine (NAC) were found to have similar properties. NAC has emerged as the treatment of choice (Prescott et al. 1979; Smilkstein et al. 1988); cysteamine proved to have unpleasant central nervous and gastrointestinal side-effects, and methionine is less effective than NAC and unreliably absorbed in the presence of vomiting. The action of NAC as an antidote to acetaminophen is via several mechanisms (Figure 4.1). As a source of cysteine its main action is to increase hepatic glutathione production, which allows increased conjugation of NAPQI (Lauterburg et al. 1983). In addition, NAC has the capacity to act as a direct substitute for glutathione in the reduction of NAPQI (Huggett and Blair 1983). By its action as a sulfur donor it increases the nontoxic sulfation of acetaminophen and directly reduces NAPQI back to acetaminophen (Lauterburg et al. 1983) although the contribution of these pathways is relatively minor. Additional antioxidant properties of NAC may prevent the inflammatory response initiated by oxidative damage and it may improve microcirculatory blood flow by restoring normal vascular responsiveness to endothelial-derived relaxing factor.

As an antidote, NAC is most effective when administered within 8 h of the overdose (Smilkstein et al. 1988). In the early studies, NAC was considered to be ineffective after 15 h (Prescott et al. 1979), but more recent data suggest that NAC administration is both safe and effective when administered more than 15 h after overdose even if hepatic damage is already developing (Parker et al. 1990). In a large trial in the USA, NAC decreased the incidence of hepatotoxicity when administered up to 24 h after overdose (Smilkstein et al. 1988), and NAC given up to 72 h after overdose not only decreases the occurrence of grade III/IV encephalopathy and hypotension requiring inotropic support but also decreases mortality when compared to untreated control patients (Harrison, Keays et al. 1990; Keays et al. 1991).

A recent analysis of cases of severe hepatotoxicity admitted to King's College Hospital, UK in 1987–1993 demonstrated that survival was very closely correlated with the use of NAC (Makin, Wendon and Williams 1995). Patients given NAC within 12 h and those administered it between 12 and 24 h after overdose had overall survival rates of 80.1 percent and 79.6 percent respectively. Patients not receiving NAC until after 24 h had a significantly poorer outcome of 72 percent and the worst survival of 48.4 percent was in the group of patients in whom the administration of NAC had, for various reasons, been delayed until the stage of established hepatic failure (Figure 4.4).

EARLY MANAGEMENT

Acetaminophen is rapidly absorbed over the first 4 h after ingestion. Gastric lavage is therefore worthwhile up to this time, but this also means that a true measurement of the plasma acetaminophen concentration cannot be obtained until at least 4 h after overdose when absorption is complete. As the efficacy of NAC as an antidote decreases after 8 h (Smilkstein et al. 1988), its administration should be commenced immediately once the patient has been found to have ingested a potentially toxic dose of acetaminophen (>150 mg/kg or 12 g) or a lesser dose if a high risk setting is apparent (alcohol, fasting, other drugs involved). Treatment may be stopped if the serum acetaminophen concentration, when obtained, is well below the treatment line. In this way, although more cases are given therapy than may be necessary, potentially fatal delays are averted (Meredith et al. 1986). Patients should be discharged from observation only if the plasma concentration is known to be below the treatment line and if they are not from a potentially high-risk group.

Patients requiring treatment may be discharged from the observation ward (where

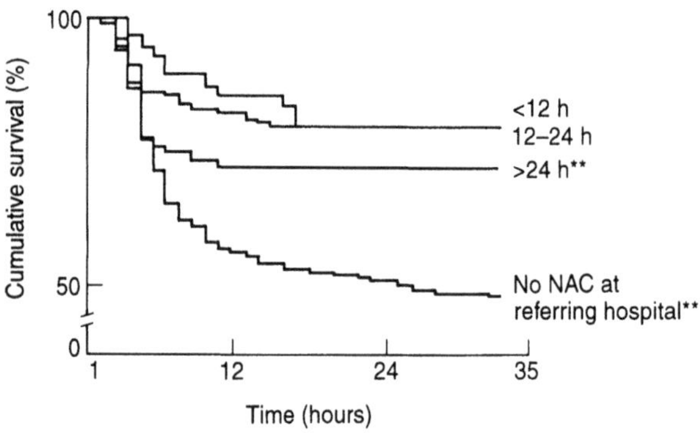

Figure 4.4 Survival related to time of acetylcysteine treatment: $^{**}P<0.0001$.

they have usually been treated) on completion of the appropriate NAC regime, provided there is no clinical or biochemical evidence of hepatoxicity or nephrotoxicity. All patients should be advised to return to hospital if they develop abdominal pain, vomiting or any other untoward symptoms whether they have received treatment or not.

The route of administration, duration and the dosing protocol for NAC is not standard worldwide. In Europe and Canada administration is intravenous with a 150 mg/kg loading dose given over 15–30 min followed by 50 mg/kg over 4 h, and then 100 mg/kg over 16 h (total of 300 mg/kg over 20 h) (Prescott et al. 1979; Vale and Proudfoot 1995). In the USA, oral administration only is approved in a loading dose of 140 mg/kg followed by 70 mg/kg every 4 h for 17 doses (total of 18 doses of 1330 mg/kg over 68 h) (Rumack et al. 1981). Because of the potential benefits of late and continued NAC treatment already referred to, the 100 mg/kg dose should be continued over 16 h for all patients where there is evidence of worsening hepatic damage, indicated by increasing aminotransferases or prothrombin time after the initial 20 h course of treatment.

MANAGEMENT OF SEVERE POISONING

All patients found to have developed a coagulopathy or elevated serum creatinine should be detained in hospital for further daily measurements of the international normalized ratio (INR) and serum creatinine. Since urea production is impaired by hepatic damage, plasma urea should not be used as an index of renal function. NAC therapy should be continued at a dose of 150 mg/kg every 24 h until the INR has fallen below 2. The patient must be kept adequately hydrated, preferably intravenously. With the development of renal failure, acidosis or a progressive coagulopathy the central venous pressure should be maintained at +6–10 cmH_2O with 4.5 percent human albumin solution. Renal dose dopamine (2–3 μg/kg/min) can be started if urine output fails to respond to colloid infusion. Once the INR has risen above 2, both antibiotics and gastric prophylaxis (either sucralfate or H_2 antagonists) need to be commenced because of the increased risk of infection and gastrointestinal bleeding in these patients.

Patients with a progressive coagulopathy where the INR is >2 at 24 h, >4 at 48 h or >6 at 72 h are the group most likely to develop ALF. Encephalopathy usually develops 3–4 days after overdose but can occur much earlier in the most severe cases. Rapid deterioration from minimal encephalopathy to a highly agitated state and then deep coma, with the development of cerebral edema, can occur with extraordinary rapidity over 24 h in cases with the most severe hepatic damage.

Transient polymorphonuclear leukocytosis is common and profound thrombocytopenia (Thornton and Losowsky 1990; Fischereder and Jaffe 1994) may occur on the second or third day after overdose in up to 3 percent of cases. The thrombocytopenia correlates with the degree of hepatic damage and appears to be a transient direct toxic effect of acetaminophen on platelets or megakaryocytes (Fischereder and Jaffe 1994).

Instances of pancreatitis have been reported following acetaminophen overdose but in most cases chronic or acute ingestion of alcohol was also implicated (Mofenson et al. 1991). In a series of autopsies of 96 patients with acute liver failure, evidence of pancreatitis was found in nine cases (four of which occurred after acetaminophen overdose) and some degree of pancreatic damage may be more prevalent than previously thought (Gazzard et al. 1975).

Cardiotoxicity has also been reported following large acetaminophen overdoses but this has been in association with the development of severe hepatic failure. Cardiovascular disturbances can occur in all etiologies of ALF, suggesting that they are not the result of the direct action of acetaminophen on the heart.

Small varices are known to develop in ALF from other causes (Lebrec et al. 1980) and there has been one case reported of varices that developed and bled shortly after an acetaminophen overdose (Thornton and Losowsky 1989).

THE ROLE OF TRANSPLANTATION

A previously unsalvageable group of patients are now surviving as a result of improved intensive care medicine along with the use of liver transplantation as a treatment for ALF. This group of patients must be recognized and transferred to a specialized liver center to enable appropriate assessment and treatment to be undertaken as early as possible. In selecting those patients with the poorest prognosis, who need to be considered for transplantation, a number of sets of laboratory and clinical criteria have been proposed (Table 4.1). An arterial pH <7.3 that fails to correct with colloid infusion is one of the best prognostic indicators, these patients having a survival rate of <10 percent (O'Grady et al. 1989).

Table 4.1. *Indications for transplantation in acetaminophen-induced hepatotoxicity used by the Liver Unit at King's College Hospital, London, UK*

Used routinely
Arterial pH <7.3 (that fails to correct with adequate colloid infusion)
Normal arterial pH but all three of the following concomitantly
prothrombin time >100 s
creatinine >300 µmol/l
grade III encephalopathy
Not used routinely
Prothrombin time increase from day 3 to day 4 post overdose
Admission Factor V level <10 percent of normal with factor VIII/V ratio >30 percent

In patients with a normal pH, the coexistence of a prothrombin time of >100 s, serum creatinine >300 µmol/l, and grade 3 encephalopathy is indicative of a survival rate of <20 percent (O'Grady et al. 1989). Other poor risk criteria that have been proposed include a peak prothrombin time of >180 s (Harrison, O'Grady et al. 1990), a prothrombin time rising on day 4 after overdose (Harrison, O'Grady et al. 1990) and an admission factor V value <10 percent of normal (Pereira et al. 1992) but these are not used routinely. In France, factor V levels below 20 percent of the normal range with hepatic encephalopathy constitute the principal selection criteria for transplantation (Bernuau et al. 1986).

FACTORS AFFECTING OUTCOME

In a recent analysis from our unit of 560 cases of severe acetaminophen-induced hepatotoxicity, we found a number of factors indicative of an improved outcome (Makin et al. 1995). Those patients who presented within 24 h of the overdose had significantly better survival rates than those presenting later. Survival was also closely correlated to NAC administration as untreated patients had a worse outcome than treated cases, even those who had not received NAC within 24 h of their overdose. The level of encephalopathy also correlated closely with outcome. Patients with grade I or II encephalopathy had survival rates in excess of 95 percent whereas with grade IV encephalopathy and cerebral edema the survival rate was reduced to only 22 percent. The improvement in overall survival following severe acetaminophen-induced hepatotoxicity from 50 percent in 1987 to 78 percent in 1993 was the result of both the increasing availability and success of transplantation and the improved survival rates of the medically managed patients.

REFERENCES

Anker, A.L. and Smilkstein, M.J. 1994. Acetaminophen. Concepts and controversies (Review). *Emer Med Clin North Am* 12: 335–49.

Benhamou, J-P. 1991. Fulminant and subfulminant liver failure: definitions and causes. In *Acute Liver Failure. Improved understanding and better therapy*, eds. R. Williams and R.D. Hughes, 6–10. London: Mitre Press.

Bernuau, J., Goudeau, A., Poynard, T., Dubois, F., Lesage, G., Yvonnet, B., Degott, C., Bejeaud, A., Rueff, B. and Benhamou, J-P. 1986. Multivariate analysis of

prognostic factors in fulminant hepatitis B. *Hepatology* 6: 648–51.
Bihari, D., Gimson, A.E.S., Waterson, M. and Williams, R. 1985. Tissue hypoxia during fulminant hepatic failure. *Crit Care Med* 13: 1034–9.
Boyd, E.M. and Bereczky, G.M. 1966. Liver necrosis from paracetamol. *Br J Pharmacol* 26: 606–14.
Bray, G.P., Mowat, C., Muir, D.F., Tredger, M. and Williams, R. 1991. The effect of chronic alcohol intake on prognosis and outcome in paracetamol overdose. *Hum Exp Toxicol* 10: 435–8.
Bray, G.P., Harrison, P.M., O'Grady, J.G., Tredger, M. and Williams, R. 1992. Long-term anticonvulsant therapy worsens outcome on paracetamol-induced fulminant hepatic failure. *Hum Exp Toxicol* 11: 265–70.
Brotodihardjo, A.E., Batey, R.G., Farrell, G.C. and Byth, K. 1992. Hepatotoxicity from paracetamol self-poisoning in western Sydney: a continuing challenge. *Med J Aust* 157: 382–5.
Chan, T.Y.K., Chan, A.Y.W. and Critchley, J.A.J.H. 1993. Paracetamol poisoning and hepatotoxicity in Chinese – the Prince of Wales Hospital (Hong Kong) experience. *Singapore Med J* 34: 299–302.
Davenport, A. and Finn, R. 1988. Paracetamol (acetaminophen) poisoning resulting in acute renal failure without hepatic coma. *Nephron* 50: 55–6.
Davenport, A. and Will, E.J. 1988. Hypophosphatemia in acute liver failure. *BMJ* 296: 131.
Davidson, D.G. and Eastham, W.N. 1966. Acute liver necrosis following overdose of paracetamol. *BMJ* 2: 497–9.
De Morais, S.M.F., Uetrecht, J.P. and Wells, P.G. 1992. Decreased glucuronidation and increased bioactivation of acetaminophen in Gilbert's Syndrome. *Gastroenterology* 102: 577–86.
Donnelly, P.J., Walker, R.M. and Racz, W.J. 1994. Inhibition of mitochondrial respiration in vivo is an early event in acetaminophen-induced hepatotoxicity. *Arch Toxicol* 68: 110–18.
Eder, H. 1964. Chronic toxicity studies on phenacetin, *N*-acetyl-*p*-aminophenol (NAPA) and acetylasalicylic acid on cats. *Acta Pharmacol Toxicol* 21: 197–204.
Ferner, R. 1993. Paracetamol poisoning – an update. *Prescriber's J* 33: 45–50.
Fischereder, M. and Jaffe, J.P. 1994. Thrombocytopenia following acute acetaminophen overdose. *Am J Hematol* 45: 258–9.
Garnier, R. and Bismuth, C. 1993. Liver failure induced by paracetamol. *BMJ* 306: 718.
Gazzard, B.G., Portmann, B., Murray-Lyon, I. and Williams, R. 1975. Causes of death in fulminant hepatic failure and the relationship to quantitative histological assessment of parenchymal damage. *Quart J Med* 44: 615–26.
Glenney Jr, J.R., Kaulfus, P. and Weber, K.F. 1981. Actin assembly modulated by villin: Ca^{2+}-dependent nucleation and capping of the barbed end. *Cell* 24: 471–80.
Gray, T.A., Buckley, B.M. and Vale, J.A. 1987. Hyperlactataemia and metabolic acidosis following paracetamol overdose. *Quart J Med* 65: 811–21.
Harrison, P.M., Keays, R., Bray, G.P., Alexander, G.J.M. and Williams, R. 1990. Improved outcome of paracetamol-induced fulminant hepatic failure by late administration of acetylcysteine. *Lancet* 335: 1572–3.
Harrison, P.M., O'Grady, J.G., Keays, R.T., Alexander, G.J.M. and Williams, R. 1990. Serial prothrombin time as prognostic indicator in paracetamol induced fulminant hepatic failure. *BMJ* 301: 964–6.
Henry, J.A. 1990. Glutathione and HIV infection. *Lancet* 335: 235–6.
Huggett, A. and Blair, I. 1983. The mechanism of paracetamol-induced hepatotoxicity: implications of therapy. *Hum Toxicol* 2: 399–405.
Insel, P.A. 1990. Analgesics: antipyretics and anti-inflammatory agents; drugs employed in the treatment of rheumatoid arthritis and gout. In *Goodman and Gilman's The Pharmacological Basis of Therapeutics*, eds. A.G. Gilman, T.W. Rall, A.S. Nies and P. Taylor, 656–9. New York: Pergamon Press.
Jollow, D.J., Mitchell, J.R., Davis, D.C., Gillette, J.R. and Brodie, B.B. 1973. Acetaminophen-induced hepatic necrosis. II. Role of covalent binding in vivo. *J Pharmacol Exp Ther* 187: 195–202.
Jones, A.F., Harvey, J.M. and Vale, J.A. 1989. Hypophosphatemia and phosphaturia in paracetamol poisoning. *Lancet* 2: 607–9.
Keays, R., Harrison, P.M., Wendon, J., Forbes, A., Gove, C., Alexander, G.J.M. and Williams, R. 1991. Intravenous acetylcysteine in paracetamol-induced fulminant hepatic failure: a prospective controlled trial. *BMJ* 303: 1026–9.
Kincaid-Smith, P. 1986. Effects of non-narcotic analgesics on the kidney. *Drugs* 32: 109–28.
Lancet. 1981. Editorial. Aspirin or paracetamol? 2: 287–9.
Lauterburg, B.H., Corcoran, G.B. and Mitchell, J.R. 1983. Mechanism of action of *N*-acetylcysteine in the protection against the hepatotoxicity of acetaminophen in rats in vivo. *J Clin Invest* 71: 980–91.
Lauterburg, B.H. and Velez, M.E. 1988. Glutathione deficiency in alcoholics: risk factor for paracetamol hepatotoxicity. *Gut* 29: 1153–7.
Lebrec, D., Nouel, O., Bernuau, J., Rueff, B. and Benhamou, J. 1980. Portal hypertension in fulminant viral hepatitis. *Gut* 21: 541–51.
Litovitz, T.L., Clark, L.R. and Soloway, R.A. 1994. 1993 Annual Report of the American Association of Poison Control Centers Toxic Exposure Surveillance System. *Am J Emer Med* 12: 546–84.
Makin, A.J., Wendon, J., Williams, R. 1995. A 7-year experience of severe acetaminophen-induced hepatotoxicity (1987–1993). *Gastroenterology* 109: 1907–16.
McClain, C.J., Holtzman, J., Allen, J., Kromhout, J. and Shedlofsky, S. 1988. Clinical features of acetaminophen toxicity. *J Clin Gastroenterol* 101: 76–80.
Meredith, T.J., Prescott, L.F. and Vale, J.A. 1986. Why do patients still die from paracetamol poisoning? *BMJ* 293: 345–6.
Meyers, L.L., Beierschmitt, W.P., Khairallah, E.A. and Cohen, S.D. 1988. Acetaminophen-induced inhibition of hepatic mitochondrial respiration in mice. *Toxicol Appl Pharmacol* 93: 378–87.
Mitchell, J.R., Jollow, D.J., Potter, W.Z., Davis, D.C., Gillette, J.R. and Brodie, B.B. 1973. Acetaminophen-induced hepatic necrosis. I. Role of drug metabolism. *J Pharmacol Exp Ther* 187: 185–94.
Mitchell, J.R., Jollow, D.J., Potter, W.Z., Gillette, J.R. and Brodie, B.B. 1973. Acetaminophen-induced hepatic necrosis IV: Protective role of glutathione. *J Pharmacol Exp Ther* 187: 211–17.
Mofenson, H.C., Caraccio, T.R., Nawaz, H. and Steckler, G. 1991. Acetaminophen induced pancreatitis. *Clin Toxicol* 29: 223–30.

Monteagudo, F.S. and Folb, P.I. 1987. Paracetamol poisoning at Groote Schuur Hospital. *South Afr Med J* 72: 773–6.

Moore, M., Thor, H., Moore, G., Nelson, S., Moldeus, P. and Orrenius, S. 1985. The toxicity of acetaminophen and *N*-acetyl-*p*-benzoquinone imine in isolated hepatocytes is associated with thiol depletion and increased cytosolic Ca^{2+}. *J Biol Chem* 260: 13035–40.

Nelson, S.D. 1990. Molecular mechanisms of the hepatotoxicity caused by acetaminophen. *Sem Liver Dis* 10: 267–78.

Office of Population Censuses and Surveys. 1991. *Mortality statistics: injury and poisoning 1990*. London: Her Majesty's Stationery Office.

Office of Population Censuses and Surveys. 1994. *Mortality statistics: injury and poisoning 1992*. London: Her Majesty's Stationery Office.

O'Grady, J.G., Gimson, A.E.S., O'Brien, C.J., Pucknell, A., Hughes, R.D. and Williams, R. 1988. Controlled trials of charcoal hemoperfusion and prognostic factors in fulminant hepatic failure. *Gastroenterology* 94: 1186–92.

O'Grady, J.G., Alexander, G.J.M., Hayllar, K.M. and Williams, R. 1989. Early indicators of prognosis in fulminant hepatic failure. *Gastroenterology* 97: 439–45.

Oren, R. and Levy, M. 1992. Paracetamol overdosage in Jerusalem, 1984–89. *Israel J Med Sci* 28: 795–6.

Ott, P., Dalhoff, K., Hansen, P.B., Loft, S. and Poulsen, H.E. 1990. Consumption, overdose and death from analgesics during a period of over-the-counter availability of paracetamol in Denmark. *J Intern Med* 227: 423–8.

Parker, D., White, J.P., Paton, D. and Routledge, P.A. 1990. Safety of late acetylcysteine treatment in paracetamol poisoning. *Hum Exp Toxicol* 9: 25–7.

Pereira, L.M., Langley, P.G., Hayllar, K.M., Tredger, J.M. and Williams, R. 1992. Coagulation factor V and VIII/V ratio as predictors of outcome in paracetamol induced fulminant hepatic failure: relation to other prognostic indicators. *Gut* 33: 98–102.

Placke, M.E., Ginsberg, G.L., Wyand, D.S. and Cohen, S.D. 1987. Ultrastructural changes during acute acetaminophen-induced hepatotoxicity in the mouse. A time and dose study. *Toxicol Pathol* 15: 431–8.

Prescott, L.F., Wright, N., Roscoe, P. and Brown, S.S. 1971. Plasma paracetamol half-life and hepatic necrosis in patients with paracetamol overdosage. *Lancet* **i**: 519–22.

Prescott, L.F. and Wright, N. 1973. The effects of hepatic and renal damage on paracetamol metabolism and excretion following overdosage. A pharmacokinetic study. *Br J Pharmacol* 43: 603–13.

Prescott, L.F., Illingworth, R.N., Critchley, J.A., Stewart, M.J., Adam, R.D. and Proudfoot, A.T. 1979. Intravenous *N*-acetylcysteine: the treatment of choice for paracetamol poisoning. *BMJ* 2: 1097–100.

Prescott, L.F. 1979. The nephrotoxicity and hepatotoxicity of antipyretic analgesics. *J Clin Pharmacol* 7: 453–62.

Prescott, L.F., Proudfoot, A.T. and Cregreen, R.J. 1982. Paracetamol-induced acute renal failure in the absence of fulminant liver damage. *BMJ* 284: 421–2.

Prescott, L.F. 1983. Paracetamol overdosage. Pharmacological considerations and clinical management. *Drugs* 25: 290–314.

Prescott, L.F. 1986. Effects of non-narcotic analgesics on the liver. *Drugs* 32: 129–47.

Ray, S.D., Kamendulis, L.M., Gurule, M.W., Yorkin, R.D. and Corcoran, G.B. 1993. Ca^{2+} antagonists inhibit DNA fragmentation and toxic cell death induced by acetaminophen. *FASEB J* 7: 453–63.

Rochling, F.A., Casey, D.L., Weiss, R., Lee, W.M. 1995. Incidence of acetaminophen overdose and hepatotoxicity in an urban U.S. hospital. *Hepatology* 22: 379A.

Rumack, B.H., Peterson, R.C., Koch, G.G. and Amarai, A.I. 1981. Acetaminophen overdose. 662 cases with evaluation of oral acetylcysteine treatment. *Arch Intern Med* 141: 380–5.

Sato, C., Matsuda, Y. and Lieber, C.S. 1989. Increased hepatotoxicity of acetaminophen after chronic ethanol consumption in the rat. *Gastroenterology* 80: 140–8.

Seeff, L.B., Cuccherini, B.A., Zimmerman, H.J., Adler, E. and Benjamin, S.B. 1986. Acetaminophen hepatotoxicity in alcoholics; a therapeutic misadventure. *Ann Intern Med* 104: 399–404.

Shen, W., Kamendulis, L.M., Ray, S.D. and Corcoran, G.B. 1991. Acetaminophen-induced cytotoxicity in cultured mouse hepatocytes: correlation of nuclear Ca^{2+} accumulation and early DNA fragmentation with cell death. *Toxicol Appl Pharmacol* 111: 242–54.

Smilkstein, M.J., Knapp, H.L., Kulig, K.W. and Rumack, B.H. 1988. Efficacy of oral *N*-acetylcysteine in the treatment of acetaminophen overdose. *N Engl J Med* 319: 1557–62.

Spooner, J.B. and Harvey, J.G. 1993. Paracetamol overdose – facts not misconceptions. *Pharmaceut J* 252: 706–7.

Streeter, A.J., Dahlin, D.C., Nelson, S.D. and Baillie, T.A. 1984. The covalent binding of acetaminophen to protein. Evidence for cysteine residues as major sites of arylation *in vitro*. *Chem-Biol Interact* 48: 349–66.

Thomson, J.S. and Prescott, L.F. 1966. Liver damage and impaired glucose tolerance after paracetamol overdosage. *BMJ* 2: 506–7.

Thornton, J.R. and Losowsky, M.S. 1989. Fatal variceal hemorrhage after paracetamol overdose. *Gut* 30: 1424–5.

Thornton, J.R. and Losowsky, M.S. 1990. Severe thrombocytopenia after paracetamol overdose. *Gut* 31: 1159–60.

Tsokos-Kuhn, J.O., Todd, E.L., McMillin-Wood, J.B. and Mitchell, J.R. 1987. ATP-dependent calcium uptake by rat liver plasma membrane vesicles. Effect of alkylating toxins in vivo. *Mol Pharmacol* 28: 56–61.

Vale, J.A. and Proudfoot, A.T. 1995. Paracetamol (acetaminophen) poisoning. *Lancet* 346: 547–52.

Whitcomb, D.C. and Block, G.D. 1994. Association of acetaminophen hepatotoxicity with fasting and alcohol use. *JAMA* 272: 1845–50.

Wootton, F.T. and Lee, W.M. 1990. Acetaminophen hepatotoxicity in the alcoholic. *South Med J* 83: 1047–9.

Zimmerman, H.J. and Maddrey, W.C. 1995. Acetaminophen (paracetamol) hepatotoxicity with regular intake of alcohol: analysis of instances of therapeutic misadventure. *Hepatology* 22: 767–73.

5 Unusual causes of acute liver failure

Mark D. Uhl and Caroline A. Riely

INTRODUCTION

Viral hepatitis, hepatotoxic drugs, and toxins make up the common causes of acute liver failure. Using a thorough case history, in combination with liver function studies and serological data, the diagnosis is usually very straightforward. However, less common etiologies must be investigated when the initial evaluation is not conclusive. In this chapter, some of the more unusual causes of acute liver failure will be discussed, along with the specific features of their presentation, and distinctive aspects of their management.

BUDD–CHIARI SYNDROME

Budd–Chiari syndrome is defined as obstruction to outflow in the major hepatic veins. Most commonly, the underlying pathology is thrombosis in these vessels. Many patients have an underlying coagulopathy or tendency to thrombosis, such as a myeloproliferative disorder, malignancy, polycythemia rubra vera, paroxysmal nocturnal hemoglobinuria, or deficiencies in protein C, protein S, or antithrombin III. The use of oral contraceptives has also been implicated in Budd–Chiari syndrome. Although not common in Western society, anatomical anomalies such as membranous webs of the inferior vena cava (IVC) can also impede the flow of blood from the liver. Whatever the underlying etiology, the high pressures which are transmitted to the liver result in progressive hepatocyte death, portal hypertension, and liver failure (Mitchell et al. 1982; Gupta et al. 1986).

Most patients with Budd–Chiari syndrome present with a subacute illness of less than three months' duration, characterized by ascites, abdominal pain, and hepatomegaly. Bleeding from esophageal varices is a less common initial complication of this disease. Some patients may even have a fulminant presentation, with accompanying encephalopathy and hepatorenal syndrome. In acute cases, the clinical picture may resemble a surgical abdominal emergency. Without aggressive treatment, acute liver failure from Budd–Chiari syndrome is uniformly fatal (Sandle et al. 1980; Powell-Jackson et al. 1986; Langnas and Sorrell 1993).

The diagnosis of Budd–Chiari syndrome can usually be made with combined clinical and radiographic information. A significant coagulopathy associated with massive ascites will preclude a percutaneous liver biopsy in many cases. However, if one of the hepatic veins can be catheterized via the transjugular approach, liver biopsy may be feasible. Liver histology in the acute presentation of Budd–Chiari syndrome demonstrates centrilobular congestion, hemorrhage, necrosis, and sinusoidal dilatation. Indeed, most of the hepatic parenchyma may be replaced by blood. Persistent congestion and hemorrhage may lead to fibrosis and even cirrhosis in cases of weeks' or months' duration. Analysis of the ascitic fluid reveals portal hypertensive ascites, with a serum-to-ascites albumin gradient of greater than 1.1 g/dl.

Without measures to decompress the liver, there will be continued deterioration of hepatic function. Surgical shunting procedures such as a portocaval shunt can be performed to reduce hepatic congestion by converting the portal vein to an outflow tract. If there is compression of the IVC by a hypertrophied caudate lobe, elevated pressures are transmitted to the vena cava inferior to the liver. A portocaval shunt will not be effective in this situation, and a mesoatrial shunt provides a viable surgical alternative, by bypassing the narrowed (or thrombosed) IVC. Recent reports indicate that a transjugular intrahepatic portosystemic shunt (TIPS) may provide at least some short-term benefit in patients with Budd–Chiari syndrome. This metal mesh stent is placed radiographically and connects the hepatic venous system with the portal system through the hepatic parenchyma, thus creating a side-to-side portosystemic shunt. The long-term risks and benefits of TIPS in treating Budd–Chiari syndrome are still unknown. Many patients with Budd–Chiari syndrome may eventually require liver transplantation. Systemic anticoagulation after the procedure may be necessary to prevent recurrence of thrombosis (Bismuth and Sherlock 1991; Ochs et al. 1993).

VENO-OCCLUSIVE DISEASE

Veno-occlusive disease (VOD) of the liver refers to nonthrombotic hepatic vascular obstruction resulting from fibrous obliteration of terminal hepatic venules and small sublobular veins. VOD was first diagnosed in Jamaican children who had ingested a herbal tea known as "bush tea", which contains toxic pyrrolizidine alkaloids. Today, acute VOD most commonly occurs after combination chemotherapy and high-dose irradiation, usually administered before bone marrow transplantation. These treatments are probably toxic to both hepatocytes and hepatic venular endothelial cells. After the injury, the hepatic congestion due to obstruction results in increased pressure and ischemia, which then leads to more extensive hepatocyte necrosis, which is most severe in the centrilobular zone. Up to 21 percent of patients undergoing bone marrow transplantation will develop this complication (McDonald et al. 1984). Acute fatal VOD has also been seen after high-dose chemotherapy without irradiation, however (McIntyre et al. 1981). Veno-occlusive disease is a separate process from graft-versus-host disease of the liver, which occurs later (4–6 weeks) after bone marrow transplantation and has not been associated with acute liver failure (McDonald et al. 1986).

The development of jaundice, ascites, weight gain, hepatomegaly, abdominal pain, and encephalopathy in patients who have recently undergone bone marrow transplantation is characteristic of VOD. These symptoms usually occur within two weeks of transplantation, and are more likely to develop in patients with pre-existing hepatitis. Severe cases are characterized by deeper jaundice, greater amount of ascites and weight gain, and higher levels of transaminases. Patients who experience acute liver failure or a more severe form of VOD are likely to have a fatal outcome, but patients with milder disease often go on to complete hepatic recovery (Woods et al. 1980).

In the acute stage of VOD, massive centrilobular hemorrhage and hepatocellular necrosis, which obscures the terminal hepatic venules, dominate the histologic picture (Shulman et al. 1980). These findings resemble those seen in right-sided heart failure. Liver biopsy in later stages reveals concentric subendothelial thickening and luminal narrowing of the hepatic venules.

Treatment for this condition consists of managing fluid and electrolyte status, diuretic therapy for ascites, aggressive treatment of encephalopathy, and minimizing the use of drugs which require hepatic metabolism. Surgical intervention such as a shunting procedure is rarely performed, as these procedures are unlikely to alter the outcome and carry a high risk in these critically ill patients.

WILSON'S DISEASE

Wilson's disease is a treatable autosomal recessive disorder of copper metabolism. Deposition of excess copper in the liver and central nervous system results in the hepatic and neuropsychiatric manifestations of this disease. Hepatic manifestations include chronic asymptomatic hepatitis, cirrhosis with portal hypertension, and acute liver failure. Patients frequently present during adolescence and rarely after age 40 years. Kayser–Fleischer rings are associated with, but not pathognomonic for, Wilson's disease. These appear as greenish-brown areas of discoloration of Descemet's membrane in the peripheral cornea, which result from the deposition of copper granules.

When acute liver failure develops due to Wilson's disease, the typical presentation resembles other forms of acute liver failure, with rapid onset of altered mental status and coagulopathy. Unique features may include a history of previous psychiatric disorder, movement disorder with choreiform movements, or previous treatment for chronic active hepatitis (misdiagnosed because of the histologic and clinical similarity). The diagnosis of Wilson's disease may not have been made previously, or the patient may have been treated successfully previously but discontinued treatment. The diagnosis is based on a high index of suspicion, coupled with low serum ceruloplasmin levels. Up to 15 percent of patients, however, may have normal or only borderline ceruloplasmin levels (Berman et al. 1991). Typically, a very high serum bilirubin concentration, out of proportion to the other hepatic tests, is present. There is often marked elevation of serum and urinary copper. The presence of a high concentration of serum bilirubin, with only modest elevation of transaminases and normal to low levels of alkaline phosphatase, may help to differentiate acute liver failure secondary to Wilson's disease from other causes (McCullough et al. 1983; Berman et al. 1991). An additional finding which may be of help is an unusually low serum uric acid level, the result of the renal tubular defect caused by copper accumulation. The elevated bilirubin level (often in excess of 25 or 35 mg/dl), provides evidence of liver disease in combination with intravascular hemolysis, the latter the result of the oxidative effect of elevated serum copper on red blood cells (Roche-Sicot and Benhamou 1977; Hartleb et al. 1987). Histologic evaluation in the acute setting reveals massive hepatocyte necrosis, chronic active hepatitis, cirrhosis with nodular regeneration, Mallory-hyaline bodies, and positive staining for hepatic copper.

Debate exists as to whether this condition qualifies as a cause of acute liver failure, since cirrhosis is invariably present on biopsy at the time of presentation. Nevertheless, many patients have not been diagnosed as having Wilson's disease before this acute, and often catastrophic, presentation. In this sense, the timing of clinical illness is less than six or eight weeks, at least meeting the temporal definition for acute disease. The definitive diagnostic test for Wilson's disease is increased quantitative hepatic copper, but tissue may not be obtainable if severe coagulopathy is present. Recognition of acute liver failure secondary to Wilson's disease is critical, as mortality is virtually 100 percent without transplantation. Treatment with D-penicillamine which is usually effective for chronic disease is of no help in the acute hemolytic crisis, and transfer to a transplant facility should be accomplished as soon as it is feasible. Transplantation resolves the genetic disease, so that patients generally live normal life expectancies, with no further requirement of D-penicillamine treatment. Central nervous system disease often improves dramatically after transplantation. Family members of the index case must also be screened, since there are frequently other affected siblings with subclinical disease.

HEATSTROKE

Heatstroke is characterized by extreme (>41°C) rectal temperatures, anhidrosis, diffuse tissue injury, and neuropsychiatric manifestations. Coma and shock are common in fatal cases (Rubel 1984; Feller and Wilson 1994). The elderly, those with chronic illnesses, alcoholics, and people who are not acclimatized to the environment or to physically strenuous exercise are at highest risk for heatstroke. Outbreaks of heatstroke are often seen in situations involving vigorous training exercise for young, healthy adults, such as conditioning programs for police and military recruits. Use of certain medications such as diuretics and anticholinergics also increases the risk of heatstroke.

The overall mortality in heatstroke is as high as 25 percent, due to multiorgan involvement (Hassanein et al. 1992). Severe lactic acidosis and rhabdomyolysis with renal failure are often present. Patients are frequently unconscious at the time of presentation, and early mortality is usually due to central nervous system damage. If patients survive the first few days, however, death may still result from systemic complications such as liver failure, renal failure, or sepsis.

Evidence of liver damage is seen in most patients with heatstroke, usually within 24–36 h of presentation (Kew et al. 1970). Hepatic injury ranges from mild abnormalities in hepatocellular enzymes to acute liver failure. Hepatocyte necrosis likely results from hypoxia and direct thermal injury. Profound ischemia and hypoxia result from systemic hypotension and circulatory collapse, increased oxygenation requirements in the febrile state, and disseminated intravascular coagulation (DIC). Thermal damage to the sinusoids may trigger DIC which may result in microthrombi in the hepatic sinusoids, causing infarction and hemorrhage (Hassanein et al. 1992).

Liver biopsy in heatstroke reveals massive centrilobular zonal necrosis, congestion, prominent cholestasis, and proliferation of intralobular bile ductules. Cholangioles may be dilated, with invasion by neutrophils (Bianchi et al. 1972). Serial liver biopsies will show resolution of the histologic changes if the patient recovers (Bianchi et al. 1972). In contrast to chronic viral hepatitis or alcohol-induced liver disease, a single event leads to hepatic necrosis in heatstroke. Therefore, minimal reticulin collapse is seen, and subsequent fibrosis usually does not occur.

Heatstroke results from failure of the normal physiological dissipation of heat. Therefore, early and aggressive external cooling is the mainstay of treatment. Therapy directed toward management of shock and sepsis is also necessary. Some patients may require dialysis until renal function returns. Patients surviving the initial few days may have progressive liver failure with worsening coagulopathy and encephalopathy. Liver transplantation is an option for some patients who show continued deterioration of hepatic function, but transplantation should only be performed when it is accomplished early enough to avoid irreversible central nervous system damage (Hassanein et al. 1991).

LIVER FAILURE ASSOCIATED WITH PREGNANCY

Liver failure is a rare but well recognized complication of pregnancy. There are three main situations which may result in hepatic failure in pregnancy. These are: the syndrome of hemolysis, elevated liver tests, and low platelet count (HELLP syndrome) (Weinstein 1982), hepatic rupture, and acute fatty liver of pregnancy (AFLP). HELLP syndrome and hepatic rupture are most often associated with pre-eclampsia or eclampsia. Pre-eclampsia is a multisystem disorder of unclear pathogenesis associated with hypertension, proteinuria, and generalized edema during pregnancy. Eclampsia refers to the previous findings with accompanying seizures.

HELLP syndrome

The liver may be involved in 5–10 percent of patients with pre-eclampsia, often as part of HELLP syndrome (Weinstein 1982). Approximately 12 percent of patients with pre-eclampsia or eclampsia fulfill the criteria for the HELLP syndrome (MacKenna et al. 1983). Patients with HELLP syndrome present late in pregnancy with nonspecific symptoms, such as malaise, nausea with or without vomiting, epigastric pain, and right upper quadrant tenderness. These nonspecific symptoms, however, are also frequently seen in pre-eclamptic patients without liver involvement. Transaminases are elevated, but do not accurately reflect the degree of hepatic necrosis. Hyperbilirubinemia is secondary to liver dysfunction and hemolysis. While liver biopsies are often normal in patients with pre-eclampsia, specific histologic changes have been described in the liver specimens of patients with HELLP syndrome. These include periportal parenchymal necrosis with deposition of fibrin-like material in the sinusoids and fibrin microthrombi (Arias and Mancilla-Jimenez 1976; Barton et al. 1992). Macrovesicular and microvesicular steatosis may be noted.

Liver failure associated with the HELLP syndrome may be manifested by ascites and elevation of the prothrombin time. Concurrent renal dysfunction is also usually present. Maternal mortality is low (3.5 percent), but fetal morbidity and mortality is high (44–60 percent) (Weinstein 1985). The disease tends to be progressive, and conservative treatment increases maternal and fetal morbidity, along with the risk of spontaneous rupture of a liver hematoma. Therefore, prompt delivery is usually recommended. Some infants born to patients with HELLP syndrome may manifest thrombocytopenia. Following delivery, hepatic necrosis in the mother usually heals quickly without subsequent fibrosis.

Spontaneous rupture of the liver

Spontaneous rupture of the liver usually occurs in the setting of pre-eclampsia, and is a life threatening complication of pregnancy (Henny et al. 1983). This condition is more common in older multiparous women (Aziz et al. 1983). Overall maternal and fetal mortality rates are as high as 59 percent and 62 percent, respectively (Gonzalez et al. 1984). This diagnosis should be considered in a pregnant woman presenting late in pregnancy with sudden onset of right upper quadrant pain, especially with evidence of hypovolemia or impending shock.

Spontaneous hepatic rupture may be part of the HELLP syndrome, where a periportal hemorrhage may occur close to the capsule, which then subsequently coalesces. The hemorrhage usually involves the right lobe of the liver, and may be managed conservatively if bleeding is contained in a subcapsular hematoma. However, when frank rupture occurs, aggressive intervention is required, including immediate delivery of the fetus, fluid and blood replacement, and control of hemorrhage. Survival rates with hepatic hematoma evacuation and packing have been reported to be higher than with hepatic lobectomy (Hunter et al. 1995). Other treatment modalities have included ligation of the appropriate branch of the hepatic artery to control hemorrhage, hepatic artery embolization, percutaneous angiographic embolization, topical hemostatic agents, and oversewing the liver (Gonzalez et al. 1984; Loevinger et al. 1985). Liver transplantation has also been successful in treating this complication, in a patient who was anhepatic for 13 h (Hunter et al. 1995).

Acute fatty liver of pregnancy

A rare but potentially fatal hepatic complication of pregnancy, occurring almost exclusively in the third trimester, is acute fatty liver of pregnancy (AFLP). There is a wide clinical spectrum of presentation, but severe cases can result in acute liver failure. Maternal mortality rates were once as high as 85 percent and even with earlier recognition and treatment, mortality rates remain 10–33 percent (Ockner et al. 1990; Schoeman et al. 1991). Fetal mortality rates are also high, ranging from 25 to 66 percent. The pathogenesis, at least in some patients, is probably secondary to a defect in fatty acid oxidation, with resultant accumulation of toxic free fatty acids in cells and tissues (Treem et al. 1994)

Patients may initially present with a number of nonspecific symptoms, such as nausea, vomiting, malaise, and abdominal discomfort. Over the next one to two weeks, these symptoms may progress to jaundice and change in mental status. Indeed, evidence of portosystemic encephalopathy is seen in over half of the patients with AFLP (Rolfes and Ishak 1985). Signs of pre-eclampsia or eclampsia are present in at least one third of patients (Rolfes and Ishak 1985; Riely et al. 1987). Laboratory evaluation reveals prolongation of the prothrombin time and elevation of serum bilirubin levels. Serum transaminases are elevated, but not to the degree seen in viral hepatitis or hepatic failure from other causes. Transaminase levels are usually less than 500 units. Other abnormalities include increased serum uric acid levels and nucleated red blood cells in the circulation. Worsening coagulopathy and encephalopathy, and the development of extrahepatic complications, such as renal failure, DIC, hypoglycemia requiring intravenous dextrose, pancreatitis, and gastrointestinal bleeding indicate a poor prognosis.

Early diagnosis is the key to increased survival for the mother and fetus, and AFLP should be considered in all pregnant patients with evidence of hepatic dysfunction late in pregnancy. Ruling out acute viral hepatitis is critical, since early delivery is not usually indicated for patients with viral hepatitis. Liver biopsy may be required if the diagnosis is in question. Biopsy specimens from patients with AFLP reveal microvesicular steatosis, more prominent in zone 3, similar in appearance to damage from valproic acid, tetracycline, alcoholic foamy degeneration, and Reye's syndrome (Partin 1975). Special stains for fat should be performed on the frozen sections, because on routine stains, the biopsy may mimic acute viral hepatitis with ballooning degeneration of hepatocytes.

The only treatment of AFLP is prompt delivery of the fetus and supportive care. After delivery, most patients improve over the next two to three days. In these patients, the liver heals completely, and there is no hepatic fibrosis. However, some patients may experience a steady downhill course, with persistent coagulopathy and worsening encephalopathy. These patients should receive maximal support in an intensive care setting, and have been reported to require liver transplantation (Ockner et al. 1990; Usta et al. 1994). Recurrence of AFLP is rare but has been reported (Schoeman et al. 1991).

GRAFT FAILURE AFTER LIVER TRANSPLANTATION

Acute liver failure can also be seen after liver transplantation. The incidence of primary graft failure is 10–20 percent, and these failures often occur in the first month after transplantation (Quiroga et al. 1991). The main causes of liver graft failure are primary nonfunction of the graft, severe ischemic injury, hyperacute or severe acute rejection, and vascular complications (Quiroga et al. 1991). As the name implies, primary nonfunction of the graft refers to absent or diminished initial hepatic function after transplantation. Laboratory and clinical assessment reveals signs of hepatic failure, including massive elevations of transaminases, severe persistent uncorrectable coagulopathy, daily rises in serum bilirubin, advanced encephalopathy, worsening renal failure, acidosis, and hemodynamic instability (Shaw et al. 1985). This dreaded complication is usually fatal without urgent retransplantation. Significant fatty infiltration in the donor organ may predispose to primary nonfunction (D'Alessandro et al. 1991; Ploeg et al. 1993). Some liver transplant patients may recover from initial dysfunction of the graft, only to develop liver failure after a few days. Such a course is probably secondary to prolonged cold ischemia, preservation injury, warm ischemia before revascularization, moderate steatosis, or donor age greater than 50 years (Ploeg et al. 1993; Strasberg et al. 1994). Hyperacute or severe acute rejection may also result in early graft failure. This damage may be humorally mediated, as evidenced by linear deposition of immunoglobulin and complement along hepatic vessels (Quiroga et al. 1991). Finally, hepatic artery thrombosis can result in acute liver failure due to massive hepatic necrosis and gangrene. This devastating complication usually occurs within the first two months after transplantation (Shaw et al. 1985; Tzakis et al. 1985), and requires retransplantation.

Any of the above complications should be considered in the early postoperative liver transplant patient who develops hepatic deterioration. While survival rates for retransplantation are less than with primary grafting, this is often the only available treatment option (Shaw et al. 1985).

SEPSIS, CIRCULATORY FAILURE, METASTASES, SICKLE CELL DISEASE

Clinical jaundice is present in about 14 percent of patients with pneumococcal lobar pneumonia (Zimmerman and Thomas 1950). Jaundice is also common in patients with extrahepatic bacterial sepsis, especially when secondary to Gram-negative organisms. In septic shock, clinical and laboratory parameters may resemble those seen in acute liver failure, including fever, leukocytosis, thrombocytopenia, severe prolongation of the prothrombin time, renal failure, and hypoglycemia (Dirix et al. 1989). However, in contrast to hepatic failure from other etiologies, there is a disproportionate elevation of bilirubin compared with the elevations observed in transaminase and alkaline phosphatase levels.

A well-described hepatic histologic finding seen with marked hyperbilirubinemia in the face of sepsis and multi-system organ failure is bile ductular (cholangiolar) cholestasis (Lefkowitch 1982; Riely et al. 1989). Here, inspissated bile is seen in the dilated and proliferated ductules at the margin of the portal tracts. This finding is histologically distinct from the centrilobular cholestasis with polymorphonuclear leukocyte infiltrates seen in extrahepatic biliary obstruction. The diagnosis of cholangiolar cholestasis usually indicates the terminal stages of sepsis, and aggressive medical management is warranted.

Massive hepatocyte necrosis and liver failure can also result from cardiovascular and hemodynamic instability unrelated to sepsis. This clinical picture is most likely to develop in a patient over fifty, with chronic congestive heart failure, who has a documented episode of circulatory collapse (Nouel et al. 1980). In patients with compensated chronic congestive heart failure, congestive hepatopathy may be manifested by hepatomegaly, mild abnormalities of the transaminases, bilirubin, and prothrombin time, and even ascites. If these patients sustain an episode of circulatory collapse, acute liver failure may result over the next two to three days, even if the hemodynamic instability is corrected. The usual sequelae of massive hepatocyte necrosis, including marked elevation of transaminases and prothrombin time, encephalopathy, jaundice, renal failure, and hypoglycemia will be present. Biopsy or necropsy specimens reveal massive centrilobular necrosis. Chronic severe congestive heart failure may also result in acute liver failure even when a definite hypotensive episode is not documented (Kisloff and Schaffer 1976; Cohen and Kaplan 1978; Kaymakcalan et al. 1978). Some cases of acute liver failure have been discovered before the diagnosis of cardiac failure, particularly in obese patients with occult cardiomyopathy (Hoffman et al. 1990).

Elevated bilirubin, transaminases, and alka-

Table 5.1. *Unusual causes of acute liver failure*

Budd–Chiari syndrome
Veno-occlusive disease
Wilson's disease
Heatstroke
Pregnancy-associated complications
HELLP syndrome
Spontaneous rupture of the liver
Acute fatty liver of pregnancy
Graft failure after liver transplantation
Sepsis
Circulatory failure
Metastatic malignancy
Sickle cell crisis

line phosphatase are common when tumors metastasize to the liver. Some patients with extensive metastases present with rapidly worsening liver tests, and may progress to hepatic coma from hepatic failure. Liver failure in this situation results from ischemia secondary to tumor emboli, massive hepatocyte necrosis secondary to tumor infiltration and infarction, and pressure atrophy from massive infiltration (Krauss et al. 1979; Zafrani et al. 1983; Sawabe et al. 1990; Karl 1991). The most common tumors implicated are breast, lymphoma (Woolf et al. 1994), melanoma and oat cell tumors of the lung. Hepatomegaly of massive proportions should be the tip-off to this diagnosis, and liver biopsy is often of value to confirm the specific etiology. Rapid clarification of the diagnosis is important, since palliative treatment may be an option. A specific diagnosis of tumor will preclude consideration of transplantation and yet allows a reasonable prognosis to be made. Without treatment, life expectancy is measured in days, and this condition is uniformly fatal.

Sickle cell disease patients are frequently jaundiced and the etiology is multifactorial, with many developing cirrhosis and hepatic failure in their later years. However, the occasional patient may develop acute sickle crisis featuring primarily hepatic necrosis. This may occur after a period of anoxia such as a seizure, and is seldom seen in a setting in which the liver is the only organ injured (Hassell et al. 1994).

SUMMARY

While severe hepatic injury from hepatitis viruses and drugs account for the majority of cases of acute liver failure, other etiologies exist (Table 5.1) and may present a diagnostic challenge. Therefore, clinicians caring for patients with acute liver failure must be aware of less common etiologies, and pursue the appropriate clinical investigations so that optimal treatment can be delivered to each patient.

REFERENCES

Arias, F. and Mancilla-Jimenez, R. 1976. Hepatic fibrinogen deposits in pre-eclampsia: immunofluorescent evidence. *N Engl J Med* 295: 578–82.

Aziz, S., Merrell, R.C. and Collins, J.A. 1983. Spontaneous hepatic hemorrhage during pregnancy. *Am J Surg* 146: 680–2.

Barton, J.R., Riely, C.A., Adamec, T.A., Shanklin, D.R., Khoury, A.D. and Sibai, B.M. 1992. Hepatic histopathologic condition does not correlate with laboratory abnormalities in HELLP syndrome (hemolysis, elevated liver enzymes, and low platelet count). *Am J Obstet Gynecol* 167: 1538–43.

Berman, D.H., Leventhal, R.I., Gavaler, J.S., Cadoff, E.M. and VanThiel, D.H. 1991. Clinical differentiation of fulminant Wilsonian hepatitis from other causes of hepatic failure. *Gastroenterology* 100: 1129–34.

Bianchi, L., Ohnacker, H., Beck, K. and Zimmerli-Ning, M. 1972. Liver damage in heatstroke and its regression. A biopsy study. *Hum Pathol* 3: 237.

Bismuth, H. and Sherlock, D.J. 1991. Portosystemic shunting versus liver transplantation for the Budd–Chiari syndrome. *Ann Surg* 214: 581–9.

Cohen, J.A. and Kaplan, M.M. 1978. Left-sided heart failure presenting as hepatitis. *Gastroenterology* 74: 583–7.

D'Alessandro, A.M., Kalayoglu, M., Sollinger, H.W., Hoffmann, R.M., Reed, A., Knechtle, S.J., Pirsch, J.D., Hafez, G.R., Lorentzen, D. and Belzer, F.O. 1991. The predictive value of donor liver biopsies on the development of primary nonfunction after orthotopic liver transplantation. *Transpl Proc* 23: 1536–7.

Dirix, L., Polson, R.J., Richardson, A. and Williams, R. 1989. Primary sepsis presenting as fulminant hepatic failure. *Quart J Med* 73: 1037–43.

Feller, R.B. and Wilson, J.S. 1994. Hepatic failure in fatal exertional heatstroke. *Aust NZ J Med* 24: 69.

Gonzalez, G.D., Rubel, H.R., Giep, N.N. and Bottsford, J.E. 1984. Spontaneous hepatic rupture in pregnancy: management with hepatic artery ligation. *South Med J* 77: 242–5.

Gupta, N., Blumgart, L.H. and Hodgson, H.J.F. 1986. Budd–Chiari syndrome: long-term survival and factors affecting mortality. *Quart J Med Ser* 60: 781–91.

Hartleb, M., Zahorska-Markiewicz, B. and Ciesielski, A. 1987. Wilson's disease presenting in sisters as fulminant hepatitis with hemolytic episodes. *Am J Gastroenterol* 82: 549–51.

Hassanein, T., Perper, J.A., Tepperman, L., Starzl, T.E. and Van Thiel, D.H. 1991. Liver failure occurring as a component of exertional heatstroke. *Gastroenterology* 100: 1442–7.

Hassanein, T., Razack, A., Gavaler, J.S. and Van Thiel, D.H. 1992. Heatstroke: its clinical and pathological presentation, with particular attention to the liver. *Am J Gastroenterol* 87: 1392–98.

Hassell, K.L., Eckman, J.R. and Lane, P.R. 1994. Acute multiorgan failure syndrome; a potentially catastrophic complication of severe sickle cell pain episodes. *Am J Med* 96: 155–62.

Henny, C.P., Lim, A.E., Brummelkamp, W.H., Buller, H.R. and Ten Cate, J.W. 1983. A review of the importance of acute multidisciplinary treatment following spontaneous rupture of the liver capsule during pregnancy. *Surg Gynecol Obstet* 156: 593–8.

Hoffman, B.J., Pate, M.B., Marsh, W.H. and Lee, W.M. 1990. Cardiomyopathy unrecognized as a cause of hepatic failure. *J Clin Gastroenterol* 12: 306–9.

Hunter, S.K., Martin, M., Benda, J. and Zlatnik, F.J. 1995. Liver transplant after massive spontaneous hepatic rupture in pregnancy complicated by preeclampsia. *Obstet Gynecol* 85: 819–22.

Karl, M.M. 1991. Hepatic encephalopathy in a 40 yr old woman. Clinicopathologic conference. *Am J Med* 90: 374–80.

Kaymakcalan, H., Dourdourekas, D., Szanto, P.B. and Steigmann, F. 1978. Congestive heart failure as cause of fulminant hepatic failure. *Am J Med* 65: 384–8.

Kew, M., Bersohn, I., Seftel, H. and Kent, G. 1970. Liver damage in heatstroke. *Am J Med* 49: 192–202.

Kisloff, B. and Schaffer, G. 1976. Fulminant hepatic failure secondary to congestive heart failure. *Dig Dis Sci* 21: 895–900.

Krauss, E.A., Ludwig, P.W. and Sumner, H.W. 1979. Metastatic carcinoma presenting as fulminant hepatic failure. *Am J Gastroenterol* 72: 651–4.

Langnas, A.N. and Sorrell, M.F. 1993. The Budd–Chiari syndrome: a therapeutic Gordian knot? *Sem Liver Dis* 13: 352–9.

Lefkowitch, J.H. 1982. Bile ductular cholestasis: an ominous histopathologic sign related to sepsis and "cholangitis lenta". *Hum Pathol* 13: 19–24.

Loevinger, E.H., Vujic, I., Lee, W.M. and Anderson, M.C. 1985. Hepatic rupture associated with pregnancy: treatment with transcatheter embolotherapy. *Obstet Gynecol* 65: 281–4.

MacKenna, J., Dover, N.L. and Brame, R.G. 1983. Preeclampsia associated with hemolysis, elevated liver enzymes, and low platelets – an obstetric emergency. *Obstet Gynecol* 62: 751–4.

McCullough, A.J., Fleming, C.R., Thistle, J.L., Baldus, W.P., Ludwig, J., McCall, J.T. and Dickson, E.R. 1983. Diagnosis of Wilson's disease presenting as fulminant hepatic failure. *Gastroenterology* 84: 161–7.

McDonald, G.B., Sharma, P., Matthews, D.E., Shulman, H.M. and Thomas, E.D. 1984. Venocclusive disease of the liver after bone marrow transplantation: diagnosis, incidence and predisposing factors. *Hepatology* 4: 116–22.

McDonald, G.B., Shulman, H.M., Sullivan, K.M. and Spencer, G.D. 1986. Intestinal and hepatic complications of human bone marrow transplantation. Part 1. *Gastroenterology* 90: 460–77.

McIntyre, R.E., Magidson, J.G., Austin, G.E. and Gale, R.P. 1981. Fatal veno-occlusive disease of the liver following high-dose 1,3-(2-chloroethyl)-1 nitrosourea (BCNU) and autologous bone marrow transplantation. *Am J Clin Pathol* 75: 614–17.

Mitchell, M.C., Boitnott, J.K., Kaufman, S., Cameron, J.L. and Maddrey, W.C. 1982. Budd–Chiari syndrome: etiology, diagnosis and management. *Medicine* 61: 199–218.

Nouel, O., Henrion, J., Bernuau, J., Degott, C., Rueff, F. and Benhamou, J.P. 1980. Fulminant hepatic failure due to transient circulatory failure in patients with chronic heart disease. *Dig Dis Sci* 25: 49–52.

Ochs, A., Sellinger, M., Haag, K., Noldge, G., Herbst, E.W., Walter, E., Gerok, W. and Rossle, M. 1993. Transjugular intrahepatic portosystemic stent-shunt (TIPS) in the treatment of Budd–Chiari syndrome. *J Hepatol* 18: 217–25.

Ockner, S.A., Brunt, E.M., Cohn, S.M., Krul, E.S., Hanto, D.W. and Peters, M.G. 1990. Fulminant hepatic failure caused by acute fatty liver of pregnancy treated by orthotopic liver transplantation. *Hepatology* 11: 59–64.

Partin, J.C. 1975. Reye's syndrome (encephalopathy and fatty liver). Diagnosis and treatment. *Gastroenterology* 69: 511–18.

Ploeg, R.J., D'Alessandro, A.M., Knechtle, S.J., Stegall, M.D., Pirsch, J.D., Hoffmann, R.M., Sasaki, T., Sollinger, H.W., Belzer, F.O. and Kalayogul, M. 1993. Risk factors for primary dysfunction after liver transplantation – a multivariate analysis. *Transplantation* 55: 807–13.

Powell-Jackson, P.R., Ede, R.J. and Williams, R. 1986. Budd–Chiari syndrome presenting as fulminant hepatic failure. *Gut* 27: 1101–5.

Quiroga, J., Colina, I., Demetrius, A.J., Starzl, T.E. and Van Thiel, D.H. 1991. Cause and timing of first allograft failure in orthotopic liver transplantation: a study of 177 consecutive patients. *Hepatology* 14: 1054–62.

Riely, C.A., Dean, P.J., Park, A.L. and Levinson, M.J. 1989. A distinct syndrome of liver disease with multisystem organ failure associated with bile ductular cholestasis. *Hepatology* 10: 73A.

Riely, C.A., Latham, P.S., Romero, R. and Duffy, T.P. 1987. Acute fatty liver of pregnancy. A reassessment based on observations in nine patients. *Ann Intern Med* 106: 703–6.

Roche-Sicot, J. and Benhamou, J.P. 1977. Acute intravascular hemolysis and acute liver failure associated as a first manifestation of Wilson's disease. *Ann Intern Med* 86: 301–3.

Rolfes, D.B. and Ishak, K.G. 1985. Acute fatty liver of pregnancy: a clinicopathologic study of 35 cases. *Hepatology* 5: 1149–58.

Rubel, L.R. 1984. Hepatic injury associated with heatstroke. *Ann Clin Lab Sci* 14: 130–6.

Sandle, G.I., Layton, W., Record, C.O. and Cowan, W.K. 1980. Fulminant hepatic failure due to Budd–Chiari syndrome. *Lancet* **i**: 1199.

Sawabe, M., Kato, Y., Ohashi, I. and Kitagawa, T. 1990. Diffuse intrasinusoidal metastases of gastric carcinoma to the liver leading to fulminant hepatic failure. *Cancer* 65: 169–73.

Schoeman, M.N., Batey, R.G and Wilcken, B. 1991. Recurrent acute fatty liver of pregnancy associated with a fatty-acid oxidation defect in the offspring. *Gastroenterology* 100: 544–8.

Shaw, B.W., Jr., Gordon, R.D., Iwatsuki, S. and Starzl, T.E. 1985. Hepatic retransplantation. *Transpl Proc* 17: 264–71.

Shulman, H.M., McDonald, G.B., Matthews, D., Doney, K.C., Kopecky, K.J., Gauvreau, J.M. and Thomas, E.D. 1980. An analysis of hepatic venocclusive disease and centrilobular hepatic degeneration following bone marrow transplantation. *Gastroenterology* 79: 1178–91.

Strasberg, S.M., Howard, T.K., Molmenti, E.P. and Hertl, M. 1994. Selecting the donor liver: risk factors for poor function after orthotopic liver transplantation. *Hepatology* 20: 829–38.

Treem, W.R., Rinaldo, P., Hale, D.E., Stanley, C.A., Millington, D.S., Hyams, J.S., Jackson, S. and Turnbull, D.M. 1994. Acute fatty liver of pregnancy and long-chain 3 hydroxyacyl-coenzyme A dehydrogenase deficiency. *Hepatology* 19: 339–45.

Tzakis, A.G., Gordon, R.D., Shaw, B.W., Jr., Iwatsuki, S. and Starzl, T.E. 1985. Clinical presentation of hepatic artery thrombosis after liver transplantation in the cyclosporine era. *Transplantation* 40: 667–71.

Usta, I.M., Barton, J.R., Amon, E.A., Gonzalez, A. and Sibai, B.M. 1994. Acute fatty liver of pregnancy: an experience in the diagnosis and management of fourteen cases. *Am J Obstet Gynecol* 171: 1342–7.

Weinstein, L. 1982. Syndrome of hemolysis, elevated liver enzymes, and low platelet count: a severe consequence of hypertension in pregnancy. *Am J Obstet Gynecol* 142: 159–67.

Weinstein, L. 1985. Preeclampsia/eclampsia with hemolysis, elevated liver enzymes, and thrombocytopenia. *Obstet Gynecol* 66: 657–60.

Woods, W.G., Dehner, L.P., Nesbit, M.E., Krivit, W., Coccia, P.F., Ramsay, N.K.C., Kim, T.H. and Kersey, J.H. 1980. Fatal veno-occlusive disease of the liver following high dose chemotherapy, irradiation and bone marrow transplantation. *Am J Med* 68: 285–90.

Woolf, G.M., Petrovic, L.M., Rojter, S.E. et al. 1994. Acute liver failure due to lymphoma. A diagnostic concern when considering liver transplantation. *Dig Dis Sci* 39: 1351–8.

Zafrani, E.S., Leclerq, B., Vernant, J.P., Pinaudeau, V.Y., Chomette, G. and Dhuemot, D. 1983. Massive blastic infiltration of the liver: a cause of fulminant hepatic failure. *Hepatology* 3: 428–32.

Zimmerman, H.J. and Thomas, L.J. 1950. The liver in pneumococcal pneumonia: observations in 94 cases on liver function and jaundice in pneumonia. *J Lab Clin Med* 35: 556–67.

6 Pediatric aspects of acute liver failure

Ian D. D'Agata and William F. Balistreri

INTRODUCTION

The consequences of acute liver failure (ALF) have presented formidable challenges to both pediatricians and general physicians. Several important differences are observed in ALF when it occurs in different age groups. For example, hepatic encephalopathy is considered a cardinal component of the definition of ALF in adults, but in children encephalopathy need not be present to make the diagnosis of acute liver failure. Although ALF in children exhibits similarities to ALF in adults, there exist age-related differences in etiology and liver metabolism which demand an approach tailored specifically for the pediatric patient. The objective of this chapter is to discuss the unique aspects of ALF in children.

DEFINITION

The term acute liver failure is best employed to describe all forms of hepatic failure occurring de novo in a given time frame. The terms fulminant hepatic failure (FHF) and subacute and late-onset hepatic failure have been used to distinguish between clinical patterns of disease in adults (Trey and Davidson 1970). However, strict application of these definitions to ALF in children is problematic. In children, ALF is most often fulminant in nature (Sokol 1990; Balistreri 1994). Likewise, the lack of pre-existing liver disease is an essential part of the definition of FHF in adults, but in children, FHF is often the presenting feature of a chronic liver disorder (such as Wilson's disease or autoimmune hepatitis) which may have remained quiescent for months or years. Since ALF in neonates is most often the result of inborn errors of metabolism or in utero infections, the liver, in one sense, was never truly disease-free in these patients. As previously mentioned, severe FHF without encephalopathy can occur in pediatric patients, most notably in infants. The evaluation of encephalopathy, especially its earliest stages, is extremely difficult in neonates and infants. Although changes in mental status are always followed closely, in pediatrics greater importance is given to failing liver functions and biopsy results. Finally, a number of pediatric disorders present with signs and symptoms compatible with ALF (urea cycle defects, Reye's syndrome); however, in these cases either "true" liver dysfunction does not occur, or the observed encephalopathy may not be secondary to liver disease.

INCIDENCE

The relative rarity of pediatric ALF explains the paucity of published literature addressing the subject or defining the incidence. As a consequence, most recommendations regarding management of these patients are based on the experience accumulated by pediatric hepatologists and the extrapolation of data acquired from studies of adult patients. Mortality remains high and supportive medical management and orthotopic liver transplantation are the cornerstones of treatment in pediatric ALF. Nonetheless, recent scientific advances have improved the outlook for pediatric patients affected by ALF. The development of sensitive molecular biology techniques to establish the specific causes of ALF has reduced the number of cases in which the etiology remains unknown and in which a poor prognosis is typically observed. Medical management now offers the possibility of reversing conditions associated with ALF such as neonatal hemochromatosis, tyrosinemia, inborn errors of bile acid biosynthesis, and galactosemia. Furthermore, certain metabolic disorders may soon be treated through molecular manipulation techniques such as gene therapy and targeted enzyme replacement, thereby affording a possible alternative to orthotopic liver transplantation in affected patients (Balistreri 1994).

ETIOLOGY

Acute viral hepatitis is the most common presumed cause of pediatric ALF in all age groups. However, a distinct age dependency exists with regards to etiology in pediatric ALF, as age at presentation is a characteristic of certain disorders (Sokol 1990). Table 6.1 details the causes of ALF by age group. As previously noted, the most common causes of ALF in neonates are congenital infections and inherited metabolic disorders. Many viruses that do not usually cause ALF in older children and adolescents may lead to ALF in neonates. Because of the relative immaturity of the neonatal immune system, which is unequipped to confront overwhelming viral infections,

Table 6.1. *Etiologies of acute liver failure in pediatric patients*

Neonates	
Infectious	HSV, ECHO, coxsackie, adenovirus, EBV, HBV, CMV, parvovirus, non-A, non-B, non-C, sepsis
Metabolic	Tyrosinemia, galactosemia, fructose intolerance, respiratory enzyme chain defects, Zellweger syndrome, neonatal hemochromatosis, alpha-1 antitrypsin deficiency, inborn errors of bile acid biosynthesis
Vascular	Congenital heart disease, asphyxia, epilepsy, myocarditis, Budd–Chiari syndrome
Other	Leukemia, neuroblastoma, hepatoblastoma, hemophagocytic lymphohistiocytosis
Infants and older children	
Infectious	HAV, HBV, HCV, HDV, EBV, CMV, HSV, non-A, non-B, non-C, leptospirosis, Togavirus, bacterial sepsis
Drugs	Valproic acid, acetaminophen (paracetamol), isoniazid, salicylates
Toxins	*Amanita phalloides*, carbon tetrachloride, iron overload
Metabolic DNA	Hereditary fructose intolerance, Wilson's disease, mitochondrial DNA depletion, Alper's disease
Vascular	Shock, myocarditis, sequelae of cardiac surgery, sickle cell anemia
Other	Leukemia, TPN-associated, erythropoietic protoporphyria, autoimmune hepatitis, neuroblastoma, choledochal cyst
Adolescents	
Infectious	HAV, HBV, HCV, HDV, EBV, CMV, HSV, non-A, non-B, non-C, leptospirosis, bacterial sepsis, treponemal infection
Drugs and toxins	Acetaminophen (paracetamol), glue sniffing, cocaine
Metabolic	Wilson's disease, fatty liver of pregnancy
Neoplastic	Lymphoma, leukemia, hepatocellular carcinoma

neonates may succumb to congenital infections with multisystem organ failure. Congenital infections manifest with the typical signs of cardiovascular instability, petechiae and exanthems, and myelosuppression. Inborn errors of metabolism are characterized by impairment of hepatic synthetic function, with often only mild elevation of transaminases and subtle findings such as elevated lactate levels and unexplained metabolic acidosis. In older children, the most common causes of ALF are the known (and the unknown) hepatitis viruses as well as drugs and toxins (Table 6.2). In adolescents, voluntary ingestion of medication with suicidal intent as well as drug abuse become more prominent causes of ALF. Although ALF associated with Wilson's disease usually manifests in children over age ten years, there have been reports of this presentation in younger children (Walia et al. 1992).

Hepatitis viruses

The risk of developing ALF in pediatric patients with symptomatic hepatitis A virus (HAV) is low, estimated to be 0.1–0.4 percent of affected patients (Fagan 1994). The prevalence is higher for intravenous drug abusers (Akrividias and Redeker 1989); this may be of concern in the adolescent age group. In a review of patients undergoing liver transplantation because of ALF, HAV was more common in children than adults (10.3 percent versus 6.6 percent) (Hoofnagle et al. 1995). Two large pediatric series, from Saudi Arabia and Hong Kong, have confirmed the low incidence of ALF consequent to HAV infection (Chow et al. 1989; Yohannan and Rannia, 1990). Hepatitis B virus (HBV) remains a common cause of ALF, although it is less common in the pediatric age group than it is in adults (Psacharopoulos et al. 1980). It is an especially rare cause of ALF in North America and Western Europe. In one series from Great Britain, not one of 31 children with ALF had documented HBV infection (Chang et al. 1986). This is, of course, in striking contrast to reports from other parts of the world where the virus is endemic. Chang and colleagues reported that, of 16 children with viral-induced ALF, 11 were positive for anti-HBc IgM as evidence of acute HBV infection (Chang et al. 1986). Overall, it is estimated that only 1 percent of all HBV infections are associated with ALF, although rarely overwhelming HBV infections are capable of causing ALF in the absence of positive HBV serological markers (Whitington 1994). Infants born to HBsAg and anti-HBe positive mothers who are negative for HBeAg (but who are HBV-DNA positive) constitute a particularly high risk group. These infections, due to mutant HBV strains which are unable to code for HBeAg, are believed to be rare in the Western hemisphere. Although this serological profile is associated with a smaller risk of vertical transmission of HBV, it does substantially increase the risk of ALF (Ewing and Davidson 1985). Hepatitis C virus (HCV) is

Table 6.2. *Drugs and toxins causing acute liver failure in children*

Frequent	Infrequent	Rare
Acetaminophen (paracetamol)	Valproic acid	Carbamazepine
	Fluorinated and chlorinated hydrocarbons	VP-16
	Halothane	Ketoconazole
	Sulfa-containing antibiotics	Imipramine
	Diphenylhydantoin	Ciprofloxacin
	Amanita toxin	Tetracycline
	Salicylate overdose	
	Ferrous sulfate overdose	
	Solvents	
	Propylthiouracil	

generally regarded as an extremely rare cause of ALF; there are no reports of HCV-induced ALF in children (Nowicki and Balistreri 1995). However, HCV may be capable of producing severe liver damage in patients with a concomitant HBV infection (Feray et al. 1993). Hepatitis delta virus (HDV), acquired either as a co-infection with HBV or as a superinfection in patients previously infected with HBV, is known to increase the likelihood of developing ALF (Hsu et al. 1988): data in pediatric patients is limited. Hepatitis E virus (HEV) is an important cause of ALF in pregnant women, but nothing is known regarding the role of this virus leading to ALF in children. Viruses may trigger liver failure in patients with underlying chronic liver disease. A recent report has described the association between HEV and Wilson's disease in a 6-year-old girl (Sallie et al. 1994).

Other viruses and infectious agents

"Unknown viral" or "non-alphabet" virus induced ALF is still the most common cause of presumed infectious ALF in the pediatric age group; this form carries the poorest prognosis. In three large series of pediatric patients, 25–75 percent of patients with ALF were diagnosed as having so-called non-A non-B non-C hepatitis (Psacharopoulos et al. 1980; Devictor et al. 1992; Tan et al. 1979). Interestingly, in a number of these patients with "non-alphabet" virus-associated ALF there was simultaneous or subsequent development of aplastic anemia, indicating that at least some of these as yet unidentified viruses are capable of myelosuppression (Cattral et al. 1994). ALF associated with other known viruses is most commonly seen in neonates (Halfon and Spector 1981; Gillam et al. 1986). The members of the herpes virus family have all been implicated in ALF, especially in immunocompromised patients (Benador et al. 1990; Shaw and Evans 1988). Recently, togavirus-like particles have been reported to cause ALF; three of the reported patients were children aged between 3 and 16 years of age (Fagan et al. 1992). Similar virus particles had been described in patients from Thailand (Mitarnum 1990) and in a patient from Nepal who had HEV co-infection (Shavrina-Asher et al. 1990). Finally, in rare instances, other infectious agents such as *entamoeba, leptospira, plasmodia,* and *coxiella* have been associated with ALF. Bacterial sepsis due to Gram-negative organisms can also present with signs and symptoms of ALF. It is important to recognize these infections since specific therapy is available.

Drugs and toxins

Exposure to toxic agents represent the second most common cause of ALF in children. Mitchell and associates reported that 2 percent of all pediatric hospital admissions are for drug-related illnesses, although drug-induced liver failure is relatively rare in children (Mitchell et al. 1988). These disparate statistics may result from under-diagnosis, faster or alternate metabolism of the drugs by the developing liver, and the relative infrequency of prescription or illicit drug use in the pediatric age population (Schmuckler and Wong 1980). In general, idiosyncratic reactions to medications appear to be less common in pediatrics.

In evaluating a patient with ALF, obtaining a thorough history is essential, with particular care given to eliciting information regarding "over the counter" medications, use of illicit drugs or solvent sniffing in teenagers, mushroom ingestions, and use and doses of anticonvulsants. Acetaminophen (paracetamol) is the single most common cause of ALF in the UK (Vale and Proudfoot 1995), and is the most commonly implicated drug in causing ALF in the USA (Lee 1993), accounting for 2 percent of ALF cases in children and 5 percent in adults (Hoofnagle et al. 1995). The hepatotoxic effect of acetaminophen is greatly heightened by the concomitant ingestion of alcohol; teenagers bent on suicide and binge drinkers receiving therapeutic doses are at greatest risk. The prompt use of *N*-acetylcysteine in the setting of acetaminophen ingestion, either suicidal or unintentional, can be lifesaving. Table 6.2 lists drugs that are most often associated with ALF in children.

Inborn errors of metabolism

The major causes of ALF in this group are galactosemia, tyrosinemia, and hereditary fructose intolerance. Symptoms of galactosemia and hereditary fructose intolerance begin when the offending carbohydrate is first introduced into the diet. Tyrosinemia is manifest shortly after birth. Neonatal iron storage disease is a rare cause of ALF in neonates (Rand et al. 1992). Defects in bile acid synthesis, such as delta-3-oxosteroid-5-beta-reductase deficiency, can cause a particularly severe form of ALF (Balistreri 1995). Diagnosis requires examination of the urine by fast atom bombardment mass spectroscopy; in this disorder bile acid replacement therapy has proven life-saving. Wilson's disease is the most common metabolic disorder to cause ALF in older children; liver transplantation is the current standard of therapy for Wilsonian ALF (Schilsky et al. 1994; and see Chapter 5). Other hereditary causes of ALF include mitochondrial DNA depletion (Mazziotta et al. 1992) and defects in oxidative phosphorylation (Bioulac-Sage et al. 1993).

PATHOLOGY

The pathologic lesions present in ALF in children are, for the most part, similar to those observed in adults (see Chapter 8). One classification is that of Jones and Schafer (1990). Type I lesions are the result of viral infections, most toxin associated liver injuries, ischemia, and a few metabolic diseases such as Wilson's disease and neonatal iron storage disease. Type II lesions are characterized by microvesicular steatosis and special lipid stains may be necessary to identify the presence of fat. The macrovesicular pattern of fatty infiltration is classified as a Type III lesion.

In mitochondrial cytopathies in which fatal acute liver failure is the major clinical and biochemical feature, the histopathologic appearance consists of significant steatosis (mostly microvesicular), with widespread hepatocytic, canalicular, and bile duct cholestasis with bile thrombi and cholangiolar proliferation. Fibrosis may be perisinusoidal, periportal or even precirrhotic. Mitochondria, either densely or loosely packed, are abnormal, appearing pleiomorphic with few or altogether absent cristae and a fluffy, granular matrix (Mazziotta et al. 1992). The histopathologic picture seen in valproate-induced liver failure is also unusual. The lesion is a hybrid one, characterized by mixed cholestatic/toxic hepatitis with diffuse hepatocellular injury, terminating in centrilobular microvesicular fatty change and submassive necrosis (Suchy et al. 1979).

PATHOGENESIS

The complex and incompletely understood pathogenesis of ALF is discussed in detail elsewhere in this volume. Therefore, in this chapter we will highlight certain aspects that are pertinent to the pathogenesis of this condition in pediatrics.

As observed in adults, the reasons for certain individuals being at greater risk than others to develop ALF are poorly understood. In general, increased age is associated with increased vulnerability to drug and toxin-mediated hepatic damage. For example, the incidence of isoniazid-induced hepatitis is increased with advanced age (Black 1975), and the same is true of acetaminophen and halothane. By contrast, children appear to be particularly susceptible to aspirin and sodium valproate-induced hepatic injury (Zimmerman 1981; Zimmerman and Ishak 1982).

Age-related developmental changes in the metabolic capabilities of the liver are important. Studies of acetaminophen pharmacokinetics and metabolism have elucidated the biochemical basis for the greater resistance of children to acetaminophen toxicity. Although the elmination half-life of acetaminophen is essentially the same in children and adults (but somewhat longer in neonates), the profile of metabolite production differs in early childhood from that present in adolescents and adults. In young children, sulfation, rather than glucuronidation, is the primary detoxification pathway; the switch to the adult pattern occurs at approximately 12 years of age (Miller et al. 1976).

Anti-epileptic medications also induce cytochrome enzyme systems and can thereby generate highly reactive oxygen species during periods of ischemia and reperfusion. This may enhance hepatic injury during periods of hypoxia (Decell 1994). Hepatic damage appears to be most severe when multiple anti-convulsants are employed simultaneously. In one series, 16.6 percent of pediatric patients required liver transplantation for carbamazepine-induced ALF (Devictor et al. 1992).

Valproate hepatotoxicity occurs commonly and almost exclusively in pediatric patients. The typical picture is that of mildly elevated transaminases being observed in the absence of symptoms; the transaminases typically return to normal when valproate dosage is reduced (Coulter 1991). However, valproate has been associated with ALF and death in children (Dreifuss et al. 1989). The risk appears to be highest in children under 2 years old who are receiving multiple anticonvulsants. A combination of vomiting, nausea, and anorexia occur in 82 percent of patients with valproate-induced ALF, while lethargy and drowsiness occur in 40 percent. Vomiting is the most frequent reported initial symptom in fatal cases (Gerber et al. 1979). Increasing seizure activity in the presence of concomitant febrile infections is also common. Hyperammonemia may be present whether valproate-induced ALF is to resolve or have a terminal outcome. Consequently, this test is of little or no value as a screening tool. Similarly, the clinical presentation has no prognostic value in determining which patients will have a fatal outcome and which will not (Willmore et al. 1991; Konig et al. 1994), but children older than 10 years are more likely to survive. In view of the serious consequences of valproate administration in some children, it is recommended that all children (and for that matter, adults as well) being treated with valproate who have vomiting, lethargy, or increased seizures, undergo a careful clinical evaluation and appropriately detailed metabolic assessment (Willmore et al. 1991).

The explanation for valproate hepatotoxicity remains unclear but it is hypothesized that it is due to valproate-induced carnitine deficiency. This hypothesis stems from experiments in which exposure of rat hepatocytes to valproate in tissue culture resulted in increased cellular leakage of aminotransferases and lactic dehydrogenase into the culture medium. The leakage was prevented by the addition of carnitine to the medium (Coulter 1991). At the biochemical level, valproate inhibits mitochondrial beta-oxidation of long-chain fatty acids by two mechanisms. One is through the formation of valproyl Co-A with sequestration of free Co-A so that less is available for fatty acid metabolism. A second, more potent and long-lasting mechanism, involves the inhibition of enzymes involved in beta oxidation by valproate metabolites, especially 4-en-valproate. The protective effect of L-carnitine supplementation might be due to the formation of carnitine esters with these metabolites, which then allows for transport of the toxins out of the mitochondrion. Despite these theoretical benefits, results of carnitine supplementation have been disappointing. L-carnitine therapy (up to 100 mg/kg/day) has failed consistently to reverse ALF in pediatric patients. Interestingly, several children with fatal reactions to valproate were subsequently found to have underlying, previously undiagnosed metabolic abnormalities including urea cycle defects and a sub-type of Alper's disease (an infantile diffuse cerebral degeneration) with associated hepatic disease (Blackwood et al. 1963). It may be that in some instances, but not all, use of valproate further aggravated a latent carnitine deficiency due to the underlying metabolic disorder. It should be noted that ALF is not always the result of hepatocellular necrosis; in most cases of inborn errors of metabolism, hepatocyte organelle dysfunction is responsible. For example, in tyrosinemia, hereditary fructose intolerance and in some of the disorders of fatty acid metabolism, functional hepatic failure exists in a setting of minimal liver parenchymal necrosis.

CLINICAL FEATURES

ALF in children usually presents following a mild bout of hepatitis characterized by the typical prodrome of malaise, nausea, myalgias, vomiting, diarrhea, and anorexia. At times, there may be a brief period of improvement, following which clinical deterioration recurs. In other cases, there is a progressive, increasingly severe jaundice that may quickly lead to hepatic decompensation. Asterixis and flapping tremors are not commonly elicited in children; rather, short myoclonic jerks and even seizures may be present, especially in infants. Fetor hepaticus is often not present in infants and young children. Laboratory evaluation reflects these diverse presentations: at times there may be only slightly elevated aminotransferase values. Observation and supportive measures are all that is recommended. Often, however, there are ominous signs at presentation such as greatly elevated aminotransferase and bilirubin values, increased prothrombin times, and low serum albumin values. Electrolyte abnormalities and acidosis are present and blood ammonia levels may be high. Blood urea nitrogen and serum creatinine are often elevated, and hypoglycemia is usually present. Either leukocytosis (stress related) or leukopenia (myelosuppression) may be present, usually accompanied by thrombocytopenia. Bleeding may be evident due to deficiencies of clotting factors and consumptive coagulopathy. A prothrombin time that does not correct following parenteral vitamin K administration is a clear sign of failure of hepatocyte regeneration. Mortality without transplantation is 90 percent if the international normalized prothrombin ratio (INR) is greater than 4, rising to 100 percent if over 6 (Chiyende and Mowat 1992). It is recommended that any child with apparent acute liver disease and encephalopathy, or having an INR of greater than 1.6 (which is not corrected by intravenous vitamin K) represents a clear indication for transplantation. These patients should be admitted to hospital immediately and placed under close observation. It is at this point in time that a rapid and precise decision must be made regarding transfer of the patient to an intensive care setting in a center prepared to perform liver transplantation. This is a critical point in guaranteeing optimal management of pediatric patients in ALF. Although hepatic encephalopathy may develop insidiously in pediatric patients over the course of two weeks, it may appear as early as 24 h after onset of illness, as late as 50 days after onset or not at all. However, progression of ALF in pediatric patients is usually very rapid, and it is not justifiable to delay transfer to specialized centers or intensive care units once the diagnosis of ALF has been made. In one series of pediatric patients, the average interval between onset of encephalopathy and death was approximately four days (Devictor et al. 1993).

Another important question facing the pediatric hepatologist is whom (and when) to biopsy. In cases of serologically diagnosed acute viral hepatitis, liver biopsy is not indicated; but in protracted cases in which chronic hepatitis may be evolving, biopsy may prove helpful in decision-making. In the case of autoimmune hepatitis, biopsy helps establish the underlying chronic hepatitis. Postponement of liver biopsy in this setting usually leads to a delay in institution of corticosteroids which generally prove to be very effective therapy.

COMPLICATIONS

A number of complications observed in children are similar to those seen in adults. These include coagulopathy, metabolic changes, renal dysfunction, and infectious complications. These are covered in detail elsewhere in this volume. Those listed here represent not a complete list but those worth comment as having particular relevance to children.

Encephalopathy

While encephalopathy always occurs in adult patients, this is not true of children. The earliest signs are behavioral and psychological modifications that are difficult to diagnose in neonates and infants. Parents usually report inappropriate behaviors such as excessive yawning, hiccuping, and sucking. They may also describe excessive drowsiness and confusion, as well as loss of previously achieved motor and verbal milestones. Older children may be quite agitated and have day–night reversal of sleep. Regressive behavior, as well as unexplained hostility towards the parents and/or siblings, with use of uncharacteristic (for the patient) foul language is not uncommon. As coma progresses, confusion and combative behavior intensify and agitated delirium may appear, an eventuality that appears to be more common in children than in adults (Colon 1990). A staging system describing the clinical grades of hepatic encephalopathy used routinely in adults is of little use in pediatrics; an age-dependent grading scale is needed. A modified pediatric Glasgow Coma Scale in which cry is taken as a normal verbal response (as opposed to the "incomprehensible sounds" of the adult scale) may be helpful in assessing pediatric patients. Another classification of grades of hepatic encephalopathy as adapted to infants and children is shown in Table 6.3 (Mullen 1992).

Table 6.3. *Classification of hepatic encephalopathy adapted to infants and children*

Grade 1	Infant/child is confused and has mood changes
Grade 2	Infant/child is drowsy and displays inappropriate behavior
Grade 3	Infant/child is stuporous but obeys simple commands or is sleeping but arousable
Grade 4A	Infant/child is comatose but arousable with painful stimuli
Grade 4B	Infant/child is in deep coma and not arousable with any stimuli

Cerebral edema

Increased intracranial pressure (ICP) is more common in children than adults (Mullen 1992; Waranabe et al. 1992). Although it may occur within 24 h of coma onset, increased ICP usually evolves over two or three days and is heralded by changes in the neurological examination such as abnormally reactive or unequal pupils, mild clonus and focal seizures, and loss of brain stem reflexes. When intracranial pressure is being monitored, cerebral edema is anticipated to occur when the ICP consistently exceeds 30 mmHg. In any case, prognosis for ALF is poor in the setting of cerebral edema. In one series of pediatric patients, ten of 22 patients with ALF developed irreversible brain damage and died before or after surgery (Devictor et al. 1992). Furthermore, four of the six patients in this series who died after transplantation had severe encephalopathy on admission that did not improve after transplantation. Tan and colleagues recommend (in case of signs of cerebral edema) the insertion of an extradural intracranial pressure monitor and state that monitoring of ICP is the best guide for the management of episodes of cerebral edema (Tan et al. 1979). Such episodes may be successfully treated by hyperventilation combined with mannitol and thiopental infusions. However, to date, there has been resistance to ICP monitoring in the setting of ALF in pediatric patients. Reasons given by some centers for failing to monitor ICP are that placement of the ICP monitor may precipitate intracranial bleeding, or may serve as a site of infection, and that placement requires correction of a coagulation disorder that leads to the loss of an important prognostic factor, namely, coagulation studies. Use of total hepatectomy as treatment for cerebral edema and shock has been performed rarely in children, with mixed results (Rozga et al. 1993).

Cardiovascular and pulmonary abnormalities

Although cardiac arrhythmias are seen in pediatric patients with ALF, these are less common than in adults. Sinus tachycardia and sinus bradycardia, ectopic beats, heart block, atrial and ventricular fibrillation may all be induced by hypoxia, hypocapnia, hyperkalemia or increased intracranial pressure. Hypoxia, even in the absence of overt pulmonary symptoms, may be due to neurogenic pulmonary edema, fluid overload from hyperaldosteronism and increased anti-diuretic hormone (ADH) activity, or intra-pulmonary shunting due to ventilation–perfusion mismatch. Hypoxia is seen in 40–60 percent of patients with ALF, and the development of intrapulmonary shunts with or without pulmonary hypertension can result in respiratory failure, complicating OLT (Mews et al. 1990). Pulmonary edema in children is much rarer that in adults and, when present, is usually mild and responsive to albumin and diuretic therapy.

DIAGNOSIS

The diagnosis of ALF is not a difficult one, especially when confronted with a classical, catastrophic presentation. At presentation, a careful history is required to eliminate possible metabolic or iatrogenic causes of ALF, which may require specific diagnostic tests and therapy.

THERAPY

In view of the possible rapid evolution of ALF in pediatric patients, it is particularly important to intervene quickly. One must anticipate the onset and minimize the eventual impact of complications, which almost invariably alter the prognosis. Currently, the only definitive therapy for ALF is liver transplantation, along with specific medical therapies employed in the setting of disorders such as defects of bile acid biosynthesis or tyrosinemia. However, for many disorders, medical therapy is not yet available. Therefore, the goal of management in ALF is to improve the overall clinical condition of the child such that if spontaneous hepatic recovery is not possible, the patient is at least a better candidate for transplantation.

General supportive measures

In any patient with ALF, admission to the intensive care unit is mandatory. Universal blood and body fluid precautions must be enforced. Blood and body secretions should be considered infectious until proven otherwise. Intravenous, radial and central venous catheters are necessary for monitoring of continuous arterial and central venous pressures. Vascular access is also imperative for the administration of fluids, medications, blood products and, if needed, plasmapheresis. Pulse oximeters and cardiorespiratory monitoring are essential. Frequent vital signs, fluid input and output measurements, along with daily or twice daily weights, are of paramount importance, as ascites develop quickly in pediatric patients with ALF. A urinary tract catheter allows for exact quantification of urinary output. Nasogastric intubation, which is helpful in detecting gastrointestinal bleeding, can also be used as an accessory route for administration of medication; this is recommended only for patients who are intubated. Intravenous fluid administration should consist of 10 percent dextrose in 0.25 N saline at 75–100 percent maintenance requirements; the fluid type and rate of administration are based upon calculations of overall fluid and electrolyte status and ongoing losses. Total daily sodium intake of 1 mEq/kg/day is sufficient, as indiscriminate administration of both sodium and fluid can precipitate ascites. In the face of massive ascites and hyponatremia, vigorous fluid restriction is important. Provision of sodium only aggravates water retention in this setting. Large potassium requirements

(3–6 mEq/kg/day) are the rule in these patients. Hypophosphatemia may be treated by administering part of the daily potassium supplementation as a phosphate salt. Care must be exercised with potassium supplementation in general, but especially so if potassium-sparing diuretics such as spironolactone are being used.

Respiratory alkalosis is managed by mechanical ventilation. Metabolic acidosis may require sodium bicarbonate administration. Anemia needs to be corrected in order to allow for maximum oxygen carrying capacity and delivery to the tissues. Therapy of coagulopathy hinges upon fresh frozen plasma and platelets as needed. It is virtually impossible to normalize coagulation parameters. In general, only marked coagulopathy or active bleeding requires active intervention with platelets or fresh frozen plasma. If plasma is given, the usual dose is 10 ml/kg every 6 h. It is essential to remember that all administered blood products have to be included in the daily fluid input and output calculations. Plasmapheresis may be indicated in case of severe coagulopathy, hemorrhage, or encephalopathy. H_2 blockers may be administered to diminish the likelihood of bleeding due to stress-induced gastropathy or ulcers. Antacids may also be used to augment gastric pH to levels above five, although nasogastric administration of antacids may lead to tube occlusion and the necessity of frequent tube replacement. ICP monitoring should be performed in pediatric patients with stage III and IV coma in order to control cerebral edema, which remains the most common cause of death in these patients (Psacharopoulos et al. 1980). Lactulose or neomycin administration may be used to diminish ammonia production; lactulose has the disadvantage of causing an osmotic diarrhea, further complicating fluid management in these patients. Protein intake needs to be restricted to 1 g/kg/day. Enteral feeding, if possible, or total parenteral nutrition allow for exact quantification of a daily adequate caloric and volume intake. Daily neurological assessment is necessary and all drugs that may impair mental status examination are to be avoided. Elective intubation may be necessary when progression into deeper stages of hepatic encephalopathy has occurred, and risk of aspiration and pneumonia are high. Prophylactic use of antibiotics is discouraged. All fevers need to be investigated thoroughly, and paracentesis considered when no source can be found. Twice weekly surveillance cultures of blood and urine are recommended.

Transplantation

The availability of liver transplantation has greatly improved the success of therapy of ALF in children (Whitington 1994). With supportive measures alone, the mortality in ALF is 70–90 percent; with transplantation survival is >60%. The advantages of transplantation are that it not only replaces the damaged organ, but also corrects the phenotype if a metabolic disease is present. Currently, ALF accounts for approximately 7 percent of all liver transplants performed in the USA (Hoofnagle et al. 1995). ALF is a more frequent indication in children (11–13 percent). Patients with ALF undergoing transplant are more likely to be receiving life support than those undergoing transplant for other indications, and the waiting period is shorter (7.5 days versus 106.1 days). In contrast to adults, children with ALF are less likely to receive organs from donors with similar characteristics, and it is more likely that they will receive organs from older donors. Also, children in ALF are more likely to receive ABO-incompatible grafts (17.7 percent in children versus 5.7 percent in adults). In a recent review of emergency liver transplantation for ALF in children from France, 22 were placed on a waiting list and 19 underwent the operation (three died awaiting transplant) (Devictor et al. 1992). Of these 19 patients, 13 (62.8 percent) are alive without significant sequelae after six months to four years of follow-up. In a similar study from Great Britain, 12 children with ALF underwent transplantation and eight (66 percent) are living after a follow-up period of 18 months (Tan et al. 1979). Results from the French study also highlight the absolute necessity of rapid transfer of patients in ALF to transplant centers, as 4/19 patients undergoing the operative procedure suffered irreversible brain damage and died.

Organ availability remains a major problem for emergency treatment of children with ALF. The recent use of size-reduced, split segment, and living related donor grafts may help to overcome this predicament at least in part (Bismuth and Houssin 1984; Strong et al. 1990; Whitington and Balistreri 1991). Interestingly, ten of the twelve children in the British study cited above (Tan et al. 1979) received reduced-size transplants and survival was comparable to other pediatric series (Devictor et al. 1992). Auxiliary liver transplantation has also been performed with encouraging results (Broelsch et al. 1990). This technique is of particular interest for it allows regeneration of the native liver, when possible, after which the implanted liver may be removed (see Chapter 17).

Even though transplantation has proven invaluable in the management of pediatric patients in ALF, certain questions need to be asked when evaluating a child in ALF for transplantation. Is spontaneous recovery likely? Clearly, in most cases of acetaminophen toxicity medical management is as effective as transplantation. If recovery is not likely, is transplantation feasible? It is generally accepted that transplantation should not be performed in patients who have suffered irreversible brain damage or have signs of severe cerebral edema. Although transplantation has proven to be remarkably successful in improving outcome in pediatric ALF, it involves a major operation and the commitment to a lifetime of immunosuppression, with all the attendant consequences which this entails.

Nontransplant options

Nontransplant options are especially important for the treatment of metabolic liver diseases. Of 5180 liver transplants performed in the USA, 5.3 percent were carried out for metabolic liver disease (Kilpe et al. 1993). The paucity of organs available and the ensuing long waiting periods render the development of novel medical therapeutic modalities an absolute necessity in order to improve the prognosis for children with ALF. Flumazenil, a benzodiazepine antagonist, has been reported to improve encephalopathy in some uncontrolled reports in adult patients (Gyr and Meier 1991). However, the therapeutic value of flumazenil in children with ALF remains open to question. In a small series of nine pediatric patients in ALF and awaiting transplant, administration of flumazenil transiently improved EEG abnormalities in one child and increased arousal in another child who moved from grade III to grade II coma. Encephalopathy worsened in all other children despite the continuous administration of flumazenil (Devictor et al. 1995).

Recent advances in medical therapy for some inborn errors of metabolism have met with phenomenal success. The oral administration of bile acids has proven to be life-saving for neonates with genetic defects in bile acid biosynthesis (Daugherty et al. 1993). Tyrosinemia type I responds well to NTBC therapy (Linstedt et al. 1992). The success of these treatments rests on the fact that correction of the underlying problem should diminish the likelihood of development of ALF, and thereby reduce the need for transplantation. Recently, an aggressive chelation and antioxidant therapy has been proposed for ALF associated with neonatal iron storage disease (Shamieh et al. 1993). This "designer cocktail" provides a trio of antioxidants (vitamin E, *N*-acetylcysteine, and selenium) along with desferroxamine and prostaglandin E1. The goal is to chelate iron while modifying oxygen radical production capable of damaging hepatocellular membranes. It can be hypothesized that a similar approach may be beneficial in patients with Wilson's disease-induced ALF (Balistreri 1994), in whom, at present, transplantation represents the only viable treatment option. By addressing oxidant injury to hepatic mitochondria, an aggressive chelation/antioxidant therapy might convert the rapidly progressive Wilsonian ALF picture to one of chronic liver disease, which carries a considerably better prognosis. The advent of artificial hepatic support systems is eagerly awaited by pediatric and adult hepatologists (Sussman et al. 1992; and see Chapters 20 and 21).

PROGNOSIS

For adult and pediatric patients, clinical variables relative to the final outcome in patients with ALF can be divided into static and dynamic. Static variables are present at time of admission and do not vary with time, and include the age, race, and sex of the patient and the cause of disease. Dynamic variables change over the course of the illness (degree of encephalopathy, prothrombin time). Static variables which correlate with survival are patient age and etiology. Outcome is best for patients between 10 and 40 years of age, while it is poorer for those below 10 and over 40 years of age (less than 10 percent survival) (Hoofnagle et al. 1995). Etiology is important since ALF due to HAV infection has a better prognosis than ALF due to HBV, and better still than unidentified infectious etiologic agents. Amongst the dynamic variables, the degree of encephalopathy is most correlated to outcome. In one large pediatric series, all the patients presenting in stage I and II coma recovered completely after transplantation as opposed to those in grade III and IV coma, in which group only 21 percent recovered and 54 percent died (Devictor et al. 1992). The same series showed that the reduction in factor V levels was much greater in patients who died or needed transplant, suggesting that factor V may serve as a useful predictive criterion. Finally, prognosis in pediatrics has to also take into account long term effects on growth and cognitive development. Height and weight percentiles improve in children who have undergone successful liver transplantation, as does cognitive development (Urbach et al. 1987; Stewart et al. 1989; Stewart et al. 1991; Hobbs and Sexson 1993).

SUMMARY

ALF in pediatric patients remains a serious condition characterized by a high mortality. For any reasonable measure of success, management of these patients mandates a rapid transfer to a center with intensive care facilities, and which specializes in liver transplantation. The advent of liver transplantation and the development of specific medical therapies aimed at correcting and underlying metabolic disorder have improved outcomes in ALF. Management of these patients would be helped by an effective/age-controlled prognostic scale which would provide quicker and better identification of those patients at greatest risk for the development of irreversible ALF, and for determination of which patients will progress most rapidly. Development of prognostic scoring for decison-making in pediatric ALF is a matter of paramount importance and ought to be one aim of future multicenter trials.

REFERENCES

Akrividias, E.A. and Redeker, A.G. 1989. Fulminant hepatitis A in intravenous drug abusers with chronic liver disease. *Ann Intern Med* 110: 838.

Balistreri, W.F. 1994. Nontransplant options for the treatment of metabolic liver disease: saving livers while saving lives. *Hepatology* 19: 782–7.

Balistreri, W.F. 1995. Inborn errors of bile acid biosynthesis: Clinical and therapeutic aspects. In *Bile Acids in Gastroenterology: Basic and Clinical Advances*, eds. A.F. Hofmann, G. Paumgartner and A. Stiehl, 333–53. London: Kluwer Academic Publishers.

Benador, N., Mannhardt, W., Shranz, D. et al. 1990. Three cases of neonatal herpes simplex virus infection presenting as fulminant hepatitis. *Eur J Pediatr* 149: 555.

Bioulac-Sage, P., Parrot-Roulaud, F., Mazat, J.P. et al. 1993. Fatal neonatal liver failure with mitochondrial cytopathy: a light and electron microscopic study of the liver. *Hepatology* 18: 839–46.

Bismuth, H. and Houssin, D. 1984. Reduced size orthotopic liver grafts in hepatic transplantation in children. *Surgery* 95: 367–70.

Black, M. 1975. Isoniazid associated hepatitis in 114 patients. *Gastroenterology* 69: 289.

Blackwood, W., Buxton, P.H., Cummings, J.N. et al. 1963. Diffuse cerebral dysfunction in children (Alper's disease). *Arch Dis Child* 33: 193.

Broelsch, C.E., Emond, J.C., Whitington, P.F., Thistlewaite, J.R., Baker, A. and Lichtor, J.L. 1990. Application of reduced size liver transplantation as split graft auxiliary orthotopic grafts and living related segment transplantation. *Ann Surg* 212: 358–67.

Cattral, M.S., Langnas, A.N., Markin, R.S. et al. 1994. Aplastic anemia post orthotopic liver transplantation for fulminant hepatic failure. *Hepatology* 20: 813–18.

Chang, M.H., Lee, C.Y., Chen, D.S. et al. 1986. Fulminant hepatitis in children in Taiwan: important role of HBV. *J Pediatr* 3: 74–8.

Chiyende, J. and Mowat, A.P. 1992. Liver transplantation. *Arch Dis Child* 67: 1124–7.

Chow, L.B., Law, T.T.Y., Leung, N.K. et al. 1989. Acute viral hepatitis: aetiology and evolution. *Arch Dis Child* 64: 211–13.

Colon, A.R. 1990. Hepatic encephalopathy. In *Textbook of Pediatric Hepatology, 2nd edn.*, ed. A.R. Colon, 233–44. Yearbook Publishers.

Coulter, D.L. 1991. Carnitine, valproate and toxicity. *J Child Neurol* 6: 7–14.

Daugherty, C.C., Setchell, K.D.R., Heubi, J.E. and Balistrieri, W.F. 1993. Resolution of liver biopsy alterations in three siblings with bile acid treatment of an inborn error of metabolism (delta-3-oxosteroid 5 beta reductase deficiency). *Hepatology* 18: 1096–101.

Decell, M.K., Gordon, J.B., Silver, K. and Meagher-Villemure, K. 1994. Fulminant hepatic failure associated with status epilepticus in children: three cases and a review of potential mechanisms. *Intens Care Med* 20: 375–8.

Devictor, D., Desplanques, L., Debray, D. et al. 1992. Emergency liver transplantation for fulminant liver failure in infants and children. *Hepatology* 16: 1156–62.

Devictor, D., Tahiri, C., Lanchier, C., Navelet, Y., Durand, P. and Rousset, A. 1995. Flumazenil in the treatment of hepatic encephalopathy in children with fulminant liver failure. *Intens Care Med* 21: 253–6.

Devictor, D., Tahiri, C., Rousset, A., Massenavette, B., Russo, M. and Huault, G. 1993. Management of fulminant hepatic failure in children. An analysis of 56 cases. *Crit Care Med* 21: S348–9.

Dreifuss, F.E., Langer, D.H., Moline, K.A. et al. 1989. Valproic acid hepatic fatalities. II. US experience since 1984. *Neurology* 39: 201–7.

Ewing, C.L. and Davidson, D.C. 1985. Fatal hepatitis B in infant born to HBsAg carrier with HBe Ab. *Arch Dis Child* 60: 265–7.

Fagan, E.A., Ellis, D.S., Tovey, G.M. et al. 1992. Togavirus-like particles in acute liver failure attributed to sporadic NANB hepatitis and recurrence after liver transplantation. *J Med Virol* 38: 71–7.

Fagan, E.A. 1994. Acute liver failure of unknown pathogenesis: the hidden agenda. *Hepatology* 19: 1307–12.

Feray, C., Gigou, M., Samuel, D. et al. 1993. Hepatitis C virus and hepatitis B virus DNA in serum and liver of patients with fulminant hepatitis. *Gastroenterology* 104: 549–55.

Gerber, N., Dickinson, G., Harland, R.C. et al. 1979. Reye-like syndrome associated with valproic acid therapy. *J Pediatr* 95: 142–4.

Gillam, G.L., Stokes, K.B., McLellan, J. et al. 1986. Fulminant hepatic failure with intractable ascites due to Echovirus 11 infection successfully managed with a peritoneovenous shunt. *J Pediatr Gastroenterol Nutr* 5: 476–80.

Gyr, K. and Meier, R. 1991. Flumazenil in the treatment of portal systemic encephalopathy. *Intens Care Med* 17: S39–42.

Halfon, N.S. and Spector, S.A. 1981. Fatal Echovirus type II infections. *AJDC* 35: 1017–19.

Hobbs, S.A. and Sexson, S.B. 1993. Cognitive development and learning in the pediatric organ transplant recipient. *J Learn Disab* 26: 104–13.

Hoofnagle, J.H., Carithers, R.L., Shapiro, C. and Ascher, N. 1995. Fulminant hepatic failure: summary of a workshop. *Hepatology* 21: 240–52.

Hsu, H.Y., Chey, M.H., Chen, D.S. et al. 1988. Hepatitis D virus in children with active or chronic HBV infection in Taiwan. *J Pediatr* 12: 888–92.

Jones, E.A. and Schafer, D.F. 1990. Fulminant hepatic failure. In *Hepatitis*, eds. D. Zakim and T.D. Boyer, 460–92. Philadelphia: W. Saunders.

Kilpe, V.E., Krakauer, H. and Wren, R.E. 1993. An analysis of the liver transplantation experience from 37 transplantation centers as reported to medicare. *Transplantation* 56: 554–61.

Konig, S.A., Seimes, H., Blaker, F. et al. 1994. Severe hepatotoxicity during valproate therapy: an update and report of eight new fatalities. *Epilepsia* 35: 1005–15.

Lee, W.M. 1993. Medical progress: Acute liver failure. *N Engl J Med* 329: 1862–72.

Linstedt, S., Holme, E., Lock, E.A., Hjalmarson, O. and Strandvik, B. 1992. Therapy of hereditary tyrosinemia type I by inhibition of 4-hydroxyphenylpyruvate-dioxygenase. *Lancet* 340: 813–17.

Mazziotta, M.R., Ricci, E., Bertini, E. et al. 1992. Fatal infantile liver failure associated with mitochondrial DNA depletion. *J Pediatr* 121: 896–901.

Mews, C.F., Dorney, S.F., Sheil, A.G., Forbes, D.A. and Hill, R.E. 1990. Failure of liver transplantation in Wilson's disease with pulmonary arteriovenous shunts. *J Pediatr Gastroenterol Nutr* 10: 230–3.

Miller, R.P., Roberts, R.J. and Fisher, L.F. 1976. Acetaminophen elimination kinetics in neonates, children, adolescents. *Clin Pharmacol Ther* 19: 284–94.

Mitarnum, W. 1990. Fulminant hepatitis, possible viral origin: a report of 17 cases in southern Thailand. *J Med Assoc Thai* 73: 674–82.

Mitchell, A.A., Lacouture, P.G., Sheehan, J.E. et al. 1988. Adverse drug reactions in children leading to hospital admission. *Pediatrics* 82: 24.

Mullen, K.D. 1992. Hepatic encephalopathy. In *Complications of Chronic Liver Disease*, ed. W.G. Rector, 127–60. St. Louis: Mosby-Yearbook.

Nowicki, M.J. and Balistreri, W.F. 1995. The hepatitis C virus: identification, epidemiology, and clinical controversies. *J Pediatr Gastroenterol Nutr* 20: 248–74.

Psacharopoulos, H.T., Mowat, A.P., Davies, M. et al. 1980. Fulminant hepatic failure in children: an analysis of 31 cases. *Arch Dis Child* 55: 252–8.

Rand, E.B., McClenathan, D. T. and Whitington, P.F. 1992. Neonatal hemochromatosis: report of successful orthotopic liver transplantation. *J Pediatr Gastroenterol Nutr* 15: 325–9.

Rozga, J., Podesta, L., LePage, E., et al. 1993. Control of cerebral edema by total hepatectomy and extracorporeal liver support in fulminant hepatic failure. *Lancet* 342: 898–9.

Sallie, R., Chiyende, J., Tan, K.C. et al. 1994. Fulminant hepatic failure resulting from coexisting Wilson's disease and hepatitis E virus. *Gut* 35: 849–53.

Schilsky, M.L., Scheinberg, I.H. and Sternlieb, I. 1994. Hepatic transplantation for Wilson's disease: indications and outcome. *Hepatology* 19: 583–7.

Schmucker, D.L. and Wong, R.K. 1980. Age-related changes in liver drug metabolism: structure as function. *Proc Soc Exp Biol Med* 165: 178–87.

Shamieh, I., Kibort, P.K., Suchy, F.J. and Freese, D.K. 1993. Antioxidant therapy for neonatal iron storage disease (abstract). *Pediatr Res* 33: 109A.

Shavrina-Asher, L.V., Innis, B.L., Shresta, M.P., Ticehurst, J. and Base, W.B. 1990. Virus like particles in the liver of a patient with fulminant hepatitis and antibodies to hepatitis E virus. *J Med Virol* 31: 229–33.

Shaw, N.J. and Evans, J.H.C. 1988. Liver failure and Epstein–Barr infection. *Arch Dis Child* 63: 432–45.

Sokol, R.J. 1990. Fulminant hepatic failure. In *Pediatric Hepatology*, eds. W.F. Balistreri and J.T. Stocker, 355–62. New York: Horn Publishing.

Stewart, S.M., Hiltebeitel, C., Nici, J., Waller, D.A., Uauy, R. and Andrews, W.S. 1991. Neuropsychological outcome of pediatric liver transplantation. *Pediatrics* 87: 367–76.

Stewart, S.M., Uauy, R., Waller, D.A., Kennard, B.D., Benser, M. and Andrews, W.S. 1989. Mental and motor development, social competence, and growth one year after successful pediatric liver transplantation. *J Pediatr* 114: 574–81.

Strong, R.W., Lynch, S.V., Ong, T.H., Matsumani, H., Koide, Y. and Balderson, G. 1990. Successful liver transplantation from a live donor to her son. *N Engl J Med* 322: 1505–7.

Suchy, F.J., Balistreri, W.F., Buchino, J.J. et al. 1979. Acute hepatic failure associated with the use of sodium valproate. *N Engl J Med* 300: 962–6.

Sussman, N.L., Chang, M.G., Koussaye, T. et al. 1992. Reversibility of fulminant hepatic failure using an extracorporeal liver assist device. *Hepatology* 16: 60–5.

Tan, K.C., Mondragon, R.S., Vougas, V. et al. 1979. Liver transplantation for fulminant hepatic failure and late onset hepatic failure in children. *Br J Surg* 11:1182–92.

Trey, C. and Davidson, L.S. 1970. The management of fulminant hepatic failure. In *Progress in Liver Disease*, eds. H. Popper and F. Schaffner, 282–98. New York: Grune and Stratton.

Urbach, A.H., Gartner, J.C. Jr., Malatack, J.J. et al. 1987. Linear growth following pediatric liver transplantation. *AJDC* 141: 547–9.

Vale, J.A. and Proudfoot, A.T., 1995. Paracetamol (acetaminophen) poisoning. *Lancet* 346: 547–52.

Walia, B.N., Singh, S., Marwaha, R.K., Bhusnurmath, S.R. and Dilawari, J.B. 1992. Fulminant hepatic failure and acute intravascular hemolysis as presenting manifestations of Wilson's disease in young children. *J Gastroenterol Hepatol* 7: 370–3.

Waranabe, A., Shista, A. and Tsuji, T. 1992. Cerebral edema during hepatic encephalopathy in fulminant hepatic failure. *J Med* 23: 29–38.

Whitington, P.F. and Balistreri, W.F. 1991. Liver transplantation in pediatrics: indications, contraindications, and pretransplant management. *J Pediatr* 118: 169–77.

Whitington, P.F. 1994. Fulminant hepatic failure in children. In *Liver Disease in Children*, ed. F.J. Suchy, 180–213. St. Louis: Mosby Yearbook.

Willmore, L.J., Triggs, W.J. and Pellock, J.M. 1991. Valproate toxicity: risk-screening strategies. *J Child Neurol* 6: 3–6.

Yohannan, A.M. and Rannia, S. 1990. Aetiology of icteric hepatitis with fulminant hepatic failure in children and the possibility of predisposition to hepatic failure by sickle cell disease. *Acta Paediatr Scand* 79: 201–5.

Zimmerman, H.J. and Ishak, K.G. 1982. Valproate induced hepatic injury: analysis of 23 fatal cases. *Hepatology* 2: 591–7.

Zimmerman, H.J. 1981. Effect of aspirin/acetaminophen on the liver. *Arch Intern Med* 141: 333–42.

PART TWO Mechanisms of Disease and Multisystem Involvement

7 Role of cytokines and immune mechanisms in acute liver failure

Kevork M. Peltekian and Gary A. Levy

INTRODUCTION

Acute liver failure (ALF) is a syndrome which results from a large number of inciting agents including viruses and toxins, whose common endpoint is massive hepatic necrosis (Lee 1993). Although the inciting agent may directly damage hepatocytes, recent evidence has suggested that inflammatory cells and their products contribute to the hepatic necrosis (Andus et al. 1991; Winwood and Arthur 1993; Izumi et al. 1994; Rosser and Gores 1995). Furthermore, in patients with liver failure, endotoxemia occurs which contributes to the pathogenesis of this disorder (Verhoef and Mattsson 1995). Recent interest has focused on the intermediate pathways activated during the initial injury that lead to progressive and rapid hepatocyte destruction. A number of studies have implicated the resident cell population of the liver, especially Kupffer and endothelial cells, in combination with elements of the immune system as key participants in the destructive process which ultimately leads to liver failure (Winwood and Arthur 1993). Kupffer cells have been implicated in liver necrosis during hepatotoxicity, endotoxemia, and viral-induced liver disease. Several studies have suggested this destructive role by showing amelioration of injury with inhibition of Kupffer cell function and potentiation of injury by activating these cells. Of particular interest is the rapidly increasing body of evidence identifying biological modifiers such as cytokines which are thought to play a major role in the pathogenesis of liver injury. Cytokines have numerous effects including increasing the expression of adhesion molecules, production of nitric oxide and activation of the immune coagulation system all of which have been implicated in the pathogenesis of liver injury (Halloran et al. 1993; O'Garra and Murphy 1994; Essani et al. 1995).

In spite of the presence of a large number of cytokines at foci of inflammation, and the complex interactions which may appear uncoordinated, the cytokine network has a rigorous internal organization. The complexity of the cytokine network is illustrated by cytokines such as interleukin 1 (IL-1) and tumor necrosis factor (TNF) that not only contribute to hepatocyte destruction, but also have potent antiviral activity, stimulate synthesis of acute phase proteins in liver cells and mediate hepatocyte regeneration. The potential role of cytokines in the pathogenesis of liver injury has been established primarily in a number of animal models of acute or fulminant liver failure in which levels of cytokines are markedly elevated, correlating with the extent of hepatic injury (Sekiyama et al.

1994). In this chapter, we will describe the intricacies of the cytokine system and its involvement in the initiation and progression of cellular injury and death as it pertains to the pathogenesis of acute liver failure.

THE CYTOKINE NETWORK

Cytokines are regulatory proteins that function as messengers for cell to cell communication to modify cellular growth, differentiation and function (Table 7.1). They are glycoproteins or simple polypeptides, of molecular weight 15 to 30 kDa, many of which are highly conserved among species. Constitutively, the production of cytokines is usually low or absent. Following stimulation, cytokine activity is often transient and its action radius short suggesting that cytokines act in an autocrine or paracrine fashion and less likely in an endocrine fashion (Halloran et al. 1993). Most cytokine actions can be attributed to an altered pattern of gene expression in target cells leading to either an increase or decrease in the rate of cell proliferation or change in cell differentiation. Various stimuli including antigens, adhesion molecules, as well as other cytokines induce both cytokines and cytokine receptors.

Cytokines produce their actions by binding to high affinity cell surface receptors. With the exception of the α/β homologues of IL-1, TNF and interferon (IFN) each cytokine binds to a unique receptor and does not compete for binding with other cytokine receptors. However, these receptors are inducible and may be modulated by their own or other ligands. The signalling systems associated with cytokine receptors include tyrosine kinases, threonine kinases and G proteins. The receptor engagement signal is transmitted to intracellular enzymes and often involves the transcription of cytokine genes with common features. These genes tend to be relatively small with four or five exons including a leader sequence, usually without a membrane anchor. The 3′ untranslated region often is rich in AT sequences, which seems to confer a very short half-life on the mRNA. The polypeptide produced often has 100–200 amino acids and variable numbers of carbohydrate groups, which may enhance stability and solubility of the molecule. The major control of the cytokine production tends to be mainly at the level of transcription, but in certain cytokines, such as TNF-α and transforming growth factor-β (TGF-β), this control occurs during translation. Thus, the regulation of the cytokine response may occur at multiple levels including cytokine production, receptor expression and receptor signal transduction. The regulation may be built into some

Table 7.1. *Cytokines in immunity, inflammation and disease states*

Inflammation	B and T cell stimulation	Immuno-suppression	Tissue remodeling	Antiviral	Antitumor
IL-1α, IL-1β	IL-1α, IL-1β	IFN-α	FGF	IFN-α	IFN-α
IL-6	IL-2	IL-10	IL-1α, IL-1β	IFN-β	IFN-β
IL-8	IL-4	TGF-β	IL-6	IFN-γ (weak)	IFN-γ
TNF-α	IL-5 (mice)		TNF-α	TNF-α	IL-1α, IL-1β
GM-CSF	IL-6		TGF-β	TNF-β	IL-2
G-CSF	IL-12				IL-4
M-CSF	IL-13				IL-6
	IFN-α				TNF-α
	IFN-β				TNF-β
	TNF-α				
	TNF-β				

IL = interleukin; CSF = colony stimulating factor; FGF = fibroblast growth factor; GM = granulocyte-macrophage; TNF = tumor necrosis factor; TGF = transforming growth factor; IFN = interferon.

cytokine genes so that bursts of transcription are followed by repression due to negative feedback. In many disorders, there are circulating soluble receptors which may play regulatory role by binding to their ligands.

The importance of cytokines and cytokine receptors in the immune system is further highlighted by observations of infectious agents adopting features from the cytokine system to manipulate the host defense responses. For example, Epstein–Barr virus (EBV), has a gene sequence homologous with the interleukin-10 (IL-10) gene. It has been suggested that EBV uses the anti-inflammatory and immunosuppressive capabilities of IL-10 to suppress host defense. The pox virus has been shown to have a truncated IFN-γ receptor-like molecule, which may antagonize the IFN-γ-mediated genes in host defenses. The human immunodeficiency virus (HIV) uses cytokines in a number of ways to promote viral replication. *T. brucei* can induce CD8$^+$T-cells into releasing IFN-γ promoting the growth of the organism. Thus, organisms have developed mechanisms for both triggering production of cytokines and using cytokines for their growth.

At present, the best classification system for cytokines is based on the nature of the cytokine receptors (Halloran et al. 1993). Cytokines may be subdivided into several classes: chemokines, hematopoietins, immunoglobulin superfamily members, interferons and TNF-related molecules. Another classification is based on cytokine production by mouse CD4$^+$ T-cell clones. TH1 T cells produce IL-2, IL-12, IFN-γ and TNF-α, whereas TH2 T cells produce IL-4, IL-5, IL-6, IL-10 and IL-13 (Figure 7.1). This classification has allowed the grouping of cytokines in a larger cross-regulating organization.

Although members of each of the cytokine class affect the liver (Table 7.2) and play regulatory roles in the immune response, in this chapter only those cytokines that have been implicated directly with the pathogenesis of acute liver failure will be discussed.

Experimental ALF

In a number of animal models of liver injury, including those that are caused by carbon tetrachloride, endotoxin, galactosamine, acetaminophen (paracetamol) and

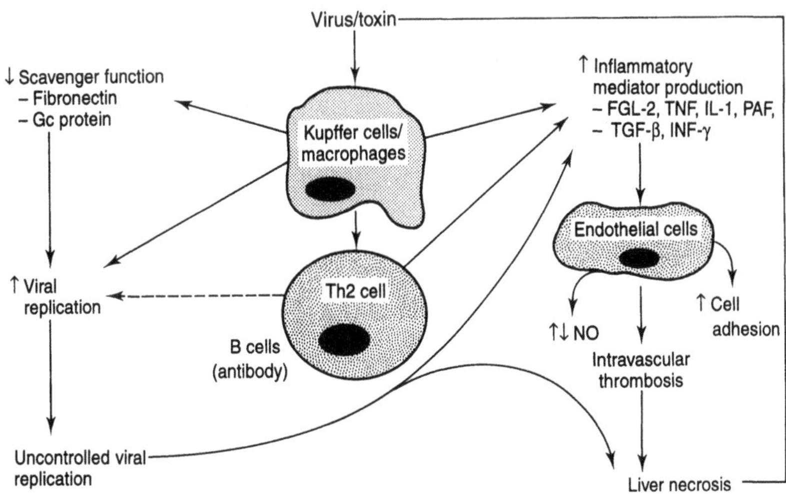

Figure 7.1 Proposed mechanisms for the pathogenesis of fulminant hepatic failure: TNF, tumor necrosis factor; IL-1, interleukin-1; TGF-β, transforming growth factor beta; PAF, platelet activating factor; FGL2, procoagulant activity; IFN-γ, interferon gamma; and NO, nitric oxide.

Table 7.2. *Cytokines affecting the liver*

Cytokine	Cellular source
Interleukin-1α, 1β	Monocytes-macrophages, smooth muscle cells, endothelial cells
Interleukin-2	Lymphocytes (Th0, Th1)
Interleukin-4	Lymphocytes (Th2) mast cells
Interleukin-6	Monocytes-macrophages, endothelial cells, lymphocytes, neoplastic cells
Interferon-α/β	Leukocytes, virus-infected cells
Interferon-γ	Lymphocytes (Th0, Th1), smooth muscle cells, endothelial cells
Tumor necrosis factor-α	Monocytes-macrophages
Tumor necrosis factor-β	Lymphocytes (Th1)
Transforming growth factor-β	Monocytes-macrophages, platelets, lymphocytes, placenta, kidney, endothelial cells, smooth muscle cells
Fibroblast growth factor	Endothelial cells, smooth muscle cells
Platelet-derived growth factor	Platelets, endothelial cells, smooth muscle cells
Insulin-like growth factor-I, II	Hepatocytes, tumor cells
Hepatocyte growth factor	Monocytes-macrophages, endothelial cells

murine hepatitis virus strain-3 (MHV-3), the hepatic injury observed is associated with fibrin deposition, sinusoidal thrombosis and accumulation of inflammatory cells (Pope et al. 1995). In the hepatocellular necrosis associated with these pathologic processes, resident macrophages within the liver (Kupffer cells) exhibit morphologic features of activation and release a number of inflammatory mediators including TNF, IL-1, proteolytic enzymes, eicosanoids as well as superoxide anions and nitric oxide (Laskin 1990). In the liver necrosis induced by *Corynebacterium parvum* and endotoxin, a correlation has been demonstrated between the amount of liver injury and serum levels of lipid peroxidation products (Arthur et al. 1988), while pretreatment with superoxide dismutase reduced the extent of the liver damage and mortality (Arthur et al. 1985). Furthermore, liver injury associated with alcohol and endotoxin correlated with macrophage production of eicosanoids and TNF-α (McClain and Cohen 1989). Associated with cytokine release endotoxin (LPS) induces the activation of polymorphonuclear cells (PMN) and macrophages resulting in the release of toxic oxygen species leading to tissue damage. At the same time, membrane associated phospholipases are activated and products of the arachidonic acid cascade are released (Verhoef and Mattsson 1995). In addition platelet activating factor (PAF) is generated and in combination these products generate a generalized inflammatory state involving the influx of PMNs, a capillary leak syndrome, thrombosis, and myocardial suppression.

We have shown recently that following infection with MHV-3, macrophages from susceptible animals showed a rapid increase in the production of IL-1, TNF, TGF-β, leukotriene (LTB_4). A unique procoagulant, mouse fibrinogen-like protein (musfiblp) which cleaves prothombin directly to thrombin also was increased in this setting. By contrast, macrophages from resistant mice either did not produce these mediators or produced them in lesser amounts or for a shorter duration. Furthermore, evaluation of mRNA transcripts indicated that the levels of these inflammatory mediators paralleled the expression of the functional proteins (Parr et al. 1995).

A role for TNF-α in liver injury has also been suggested in the fulminant hepatitis induced by *Propionobacterium acnes* and galactosamine (Nakagawa et al. 1991). Both TNF and IL-1 are known to activate endothelial cells to produce activators of the coagulation system and thus, may contribute to the sinusoidal thrombosis which is a characteristic feature of these models of fulminant hepatic failure. Furthermore, LTB_4 may also contribute to the development of hepatic necrosis by causing changes in vascular permeability, or by directly damaging hepatocytes as has been described following infection with frog virus 3.

One possible mechanism underlying the differential susceptibility to infection and differential induction of macrophage inflammatory products might be the production of transforming growth factor-β (TGF-β). During MHV-3 infection, TGF-β, a known immunosuppressive cytokine, was found to be produced by macrophages from susceptible, but not resistant mice. Although the exact role for TGF-β in MHV-3 infection was not defined, it is known that TGF-β primes macrophages to express increased amounts of procoagulants and inhibits production of interleukins contributing to the immunosuppressed state of susceptible animals.

The evidence that inflammatory cytokines play a central role in the virulence of hepatitis B virus infection comes from studies of transgenic mice whose hepatocytes produce the hepatitis B virus large envelope polypeptide and retain hepatitis B surface antigen (HBsAg) within the endoplasmic reticulum (Ando et al. 1993). In these mice, bacterial endotoxin inducing inflammatory cytokines causes severe acute liver disease. In contrast, no liver cell injury was detected in nontransgenic litter-mate controls or in transgenic mice whose hepatocytes secrete HBsAg rather than retain it. In this model, the hepatocellular injury appeared to be mediated by IFN-γ and TNF, since the inflammation was significantly reduced by prior administration of neutralizing antibody to IFN-γ and TNF.

As early as 1978, Ferluga and Allison (1978) reported that soluble factors released by infiltrating mononuclear cells in the liver were responsible for necrosis of hepatocytes in lethal hepatitis. They suggested that the cells responsible for the secretion of these factors were mononuclear phagocytes (macrophages) and it is likely that the soluble factors were interleukin 1 and tumor necrosis factor. Recent studies have demonstrated increased levels of TNF and IL-1 in patients with ALF (Muto et al. 1988). Additional studies in patients with ALF showed an increase in acute phase response protein gene expression such as C reactive protein and interleukin 6 (IL-6). Although the mechanism for the increased production of these mediators is not known, both endotoxemia and sepsis, which are common in ALF, may contribute to their production. It has been suggested that production of these mediators may account for the massive liver necrosis, high mortality and many of the clinical characteristics and histological changes which resemble those of experimental animals with endotoxin and TNF induced liver injury.

INTERCELLULAR ADHESION MOLECULES

Cells at inflammation foci are chemotactic for neutrophils and macrophages. Neutrophils are involved in phagocytosis, particularly of pathogens that have been opsonized by antibody and complement. They can be recruited to the liver by inflammatory mediators such as TNF-α, activated complement factors, and Kupffer cell-induced oxidant stress and injury (Halloran et al. 1993). Neutrophils reach sites of inflammation by specific adherence to the endothelium, mediated by surface receptors that interact with cognate molecules expressed on vascular endothelium under stimulus by locally released cytokines. The expression of adhesion molecules P and E selectins on endothelial cells initiates neutrophil rolling (Essani et al. 1995). The rolling enhances contact between endothelial cells and neutrophils via the interaction of integrins and intercellular adhesion molecules. The transendothelial migration of neutrophils is dependent on the β_2 integrins LFA-1 and Mac-1 on neutrophils as well as the intercellular adhesion molecule-1 (ICAM-1) receptor on endothelial cells. The cells migrate through the vessel wall by diapedesis toward the area of maximum inflammation. After adherence to opsonized pathogens, phagocytosis takes place which activates the intracellular killing mechanism involving the generation of free radicals, superoxide, and halide. This process is energy dependent and involves the cytochrome system.

Mononuclear phagocytes (circulating monocytes and tissue macrophages including Kupffer cells) have similar capabilities and also express specific receptors for adherence, chemotaxis, and phagocytosis. They have additional function in the processing of phagocytosed antigens and their presentation to T and B cells in the context of major histocompatibility (MHC) antigens to stimulate specific immune responses. These cells also play an important role in cytokine release such as IL-1 and TNF-β that are involved in the systemic manifestations of infection such as fever, cachexia, and acute phase response.

Viral infections and drug metabolites can induce local or systemic neutrophil activation, which may be involved in liver dysfunction. Neutrophils accumulate initially in the sinusoids and hepatic venules and have been shown to cause liver injury in experimental models of endotoxic shock through the production of oxygen free radicals (Jaeschke et al. 1991). Previous studies have shown the protective effects of anti-Mac 1 antibodies in endotoxin-induced liver injury (Sekiyama et al. 1994). Immunohistochemical analysis identified ICAM-1 expression on parenchymal cells during hepatic injury (Volpes et al. 1990), as well as in human liver cells during various inflammatory states (Steinhoff et al. 1990; Kvale and Brandtzaeg 1993). In vitro studies using isolated murine hepatocytes and a human hepatocyte cell line showed that ICAM-1 expression after stimulation with cytokines such as TNF-α, IL-1, and IFN-γ (Morita et al. 1994). Further studies have shown that TNF-α and IL-1 are the main mediators responsible for upregulation of ICAM-1 mRNA in the liver during endotoxemia. The upregulation of both adhesion molecules, ICAM-1 and Mac-1, is necessary for a neutrophil-induced liver injury to occur. Blocking ICAM-1 or interfering with ICAM-1 induction attenuated liver injury in the endotoxin-induced murine model of acute liver failure (Essani et al. 1995).

At early stages, the accumulation of neutrophils and blood monocytes at sites of inflammation in the liver may explain the initial focal hepatitis seen in the MHV model of murine hepatitis. Once there, these cells become activated in response to cytokines produced by local tissue cells such as endothelial cells or Kupffer cells. Host mechanisms become amplified, and when cellular processes are overstimulated by the continuous production of mediators at high levels, further liver damage and destruction results. The pathogenic stimuli may be of such intensity that massive production of inflammatory mediators occurs, their spillage into the circulation can cause acute-phase responses and fever as well as detrimental changes such as endotoxic shock, which threaten the well-being of the host. The acute phase response represents an additional non-specific response to infections and inflammatory stimuli. It is mediated by a number of "acute-phase proteins" synthesized in the liver. Control of the acute-phase response is integrated with the immune system through interleukin-6 (IL-6), formally known as hepatocyte stimulatory factor, as the major stimulus to hepatic synthesis. As well as increasing serum concentrations of complement components, transport proteins such as α-2 macroglobulin, and protease inhibitors, IL-6 stimulates the synthesis of the C-reactive protein, which binds to DNA as well as to bacterial substances and promotes phagocytosis.

In addition to neutralizing pathogenic microorganisms, activated macrophages, and neutrophils remove the pathogenic stimuli by phagocytosis and digestion. Subsequently, they may present the processed foreign antigens in combination with MHC molecules to T-lymphocytes to initiate immune responses. This leads to the activation of T-helper cells and subsequent release of cytokines such as IFN-γ, IL-3, and IL-6, which in turn stimulates B-cell proliferation, secretion of antibodies, the growth and differentiation of hemopoietic precursors, and the activation of cytotoxic T-lymphocytes, macrophages and granulocytes. By a combination of humoral and cell-mediated processes, pathogenic stimuli are then eliminated. Furthermore, cytokines produced by T-lymphocytes and macrophages may stimulate tissue repair and hepatic regeneration. If, however, the immunogenic stimulus persists, then this may lead to overproduction of cytokines and other inflammatory mediators resulting in cell mediated delayed hypersensitivity responses and chronic inflammatory disease in some cases.

NITRIC OXIDE

Nitric oxide has now been established to be an important endogenous messenger molecule in mammals and has been implicated in a wide range of biological processes, such as regulation of vasomotor tone, neurotransmission and host defenses against intracellular pathogens (Nathan 1992). It is synthesized from L-arginine by a family of complex enzymes known as nitric oxide synthases, which includes at least three different isoforms: the neuronal (nNOS, NOS1), inducible (iNOS, NOS2) and endothelial constitutive (ecNOS, NOS3), originally purified from neurons, cytokine-activated macrophages and endothelium respectively. The three NOS isoforms are expressed in a wide range of cell types and tissues. A cell may even express two NOS isoforms. NOS are cytochrome P-450-like hemoproteins which catalyze the NADPH-dependent, five-electron oxidation of L-arginine to generate NO and L-citrulline. The nNOS and ecNOS isoforms are constitutively expressed, and are activated through stimulation of the Ca^{2+}-independent, high-output enzyme whose expression can be stimulated by cytokines or lipopolysaccharide in almost every murine tissue and cell type over a period of hours. Although, for reasons as yet unclear, human cells express less iNOS mRNA in response to cytokines than rodent cells, sepsis and "septic-like" states in humans have been associated with increased urinary excretion of nitrite, suggesting that in vivo activation of the L-arginine–NO pathway does occur in humans (Hibbs et al. 1992). Functional characterization of the murine iNOS promoter has demonstrated a proximal region which interacts with the Nfkβ trans-acting factor and which is critical for lipopolysaccharide (LPS)-induced transcription of iNOS, as well as a more distal region involved in IFN-γ-stimulated changes in transcription. IFN-γ and LPS also exert their stimulatory effects on NO synthesis by stabilizing iNOS mRNA transcripts.

The induction of an antiviral state by interferons is an early response to viral infection that is essential for host survival. IFN-γ-induced nitric oxide production by macrophages has been implicated in resistance to intracellular pathogens, such as parasites, fungi, mycobacteria, and more recently viruses, including ectromelia, vaccinia and herpes simplex type 1 (Karupiah et al. 1993). In biological systems, NO reacts with oxygen (O_2), superoxide (O_3), and transition metals, leading to the formation of reactive products that support additional nitrosative reactions at thiol groups. Iron sulfur clusters and heme proteins which are now known to be regulated by NO include membrane, cytosolic, and nuclear proteins involved in signal transduction. Although the exact mechanism by which NO exerts its antiviral action remains unknown, the multiplicity of its host target enzymes makes it probable that multiple alterations in host cell proteins are involved. In vaccinia virus infection of RAW 264.7 cells, NO has been known to inhibit viral DNA synthesis, late protein synthesis and virus particle formation. We have recently shown that resistance to MHV-3 infection is dependent on NO production. Macrophages from resistant mice produced a five-fold higher level of NO and higher levels of mRNA transcripts of iNOS in response to interferon gamma than macrophages from susceptible mice. In sepsis, however, overproduction of NO by both Kupffer cells and hepatocytes may contribute to the systemic vasodilatation and shock-like syndrome that is observed. Thus, NO has been shown to be an important antiviral and vasoproductive molecule, but its overproduction in prolonged or severe sepsis may contribute to the hepatocellular dysfunction seen in organ failure states.

ACTIVATION OF THE IMMUNE COAGULATION SYSTEM IN ACUTE LIVER FAILURE

About 50 percent of cases of ALF are associated with a moderate to severe consumption coagulopathy, or disseminated intravascular coagulation (DIC) (Sinclair et al. 1990). Histopathological studies in man have revealed severe and extensive hepatic cell necrosis as the most conspicuous and common abnormality seen in the liver. This morphologically resembles hepatic necrosis produced experimentally in the rabbit by a Schwartzman reaction using *Escherichia coli* endotoxin (Mori et al. 1981). This has led to the hypothesis that the acute, severe and extensive hepatic cell necrosis which is seen in these cases is probably the result of an anoxic state caused in most instances by intrahepatic circulatory disturbances (Mori et al. 1986). Thrombus formation has been noted in and around the necrotic areas in a significant number of cases of ALF in humans. Further experimental evidence to support a role for activation of the immune coagulation system was seen in a murine model of viral hepatitis (MHV-3) as well as virus infection in which production of a macrophage serine protease [procoagulant activity (PCA)] precedes and is genetically linked to the evolution of ALF (Dindzans et al. 1986). Abrogation of production of PCA either by heparin and/or prostaglandins prevented ALF although it did not prolong survival. Macrophages stimulated with endotoxin can be induced to express monokines such as IL-1 and TNF. These have been shown to be capable of initiating induction of procoagulants by endothelial cells. Activated endothelial cells also produce an adhesion molecule (endothelial-leukocyte adhesion molecule 1, ELAM-1) which promotes adhesion of lymphocytes, endothelial cells and produces vascular stasis. The normal function of endothelium is to inhibit thrombosis, therefore nonstimulated endothelial cells have very little surface procoagulant activity and normally augment the anticoagulant function of activated protein C. However, following stimulation of endothelial cells, the balance is tipped in favor of thrombosis. The promotion of coagulation as a result of interaction of monocytes and endothelial cells may be beneficial in limiting the spread of the infectious agent and this may act as a natural defense mechanism. On the other hand, the same tendency to coagulation may lead to disseminated intravascular coagulation as has been seen in certain infections and malignancies and this may be detrimental to the host.

SCAVENGER MOLECULES

The liver is a principal clearance organ of circulatory cytokines (Andus et al. 1991). The rapid clearance of cytokines may be an important mechanism limiting both the local and systemic effects of cytokines. Lack of hepatic clearance may account for the disturbances in the immune system and microcirculation in patients with ALF.

Fibronectin

The circulating soluble form of fibronectin has important properties (Almasio et al. 1986). It acts as an opsonin for fibrin and bacteria and is involved in hemostasis. Severe deficiency of fibronectin has now been reported in patients with ALF which may contribute to deposition of particulate debris in capillary beds as well as to impaired Kupffer cell function with decreased clearance of bacterial endotoxins and impaired phagocytosis which will result in an increased incidence of infection and septicemia all of which will contribute to multiorgan failure.

Serum Gc protein

Plasma Gc protein, an alpha-2-globulin is a component of the extracellular actin-scavenger system (Lee and Galbraith 1992; Lee et al. 1995) and is produced by the liver. It has been shown to be greatly reduced both in an animal model of ALF (Lee et al. 1987) and low levels are productive of a poor outcome in patients with ALF (Lee et al. 1995). In addition in the setting of ALF, the percentage of circulating Gc complexed with actin released from damaged hepatocytes is markedly increased. Depletion of Gc protein and increased formation of Gc-actin complexes could result in deposits of actin and actin-Gc complexes in hepatic sinusoids and in the peripheral circulation which could contribute to the microcirculatory disturbances which are a hallmark of ALF.

LIVER CELL DEATH OR REGENERATION

Liver cell injury may ultimately result in an irreversible process by either necrosis or apoptosis (Alison and Sarraf 1994). Necrosis refers to the morphology of cellular death following a severe and sudden injury, such as ischemia, sustained hyperthermia, physical trauma, or hepatotoxic drugs. This is sometimes referred to as accidental cell death. In necrosis, there are early changes in mitochondrial shape and function disrupting cellular homeostasis. The plasma membrane loses ability to regulate osmotic pressure, the cell swells with vacuolization and blebbing, and ruptures. Its contents are spilled into the surrounding tissue space and provoke an inflammatory response. The final irreversible changes are heralded by the cellular coagulation, shrinkage and karyolysis. Since this type of cell injury is often extensive, the inflammatory response is often desirable, so that debris may be efficiently cleared and the process of repair started.

On the other hand, apoptosis is a form of cell death in which the process is more subtle and the plasma membrane integrity is preserved. There is shrinkage of cells with pyknosis, followed by budding and karyorrhexis. The final irreversible process is the breakup of these cells into a cluster of apoptotic bodies which are phagocytosed by macrophages, resident Kupffer cells, or nearby hepatocytes. This last step in apoptosis results in the formation of Councilman bodies in the liver. In contrast to cell necrosis, which occurs as a result of an injurious environment, in apoptosis, the cell commits suicide by the purposeful activation of a specific program of events. There are many stimuli that induce apoptosis, including: stimulation of T and B cells via the antigen receptor, withdrawal of growth factor, exposure to cytokines such as TGF-β and TNF, ionizing irradiation, thermal shock and synthetic inducers or inhibitors of signal-transduction pathways. However, a distinction between necrosis and apoptosis as a response to injury is not so clear. Toxins, for example CCl_4 or acetaminophen (paracetamol), generally, but not exclusively produce injury by necrosis. Histologically the picture is one of large "lakes" of centrilobular necrosis. Some drugs such as phenytoin and chlorpromazine invoke an immunologically mediated damage through an apoptotic process. Viruses may produce injury either by necrosis or apoptosis directly or by an immunologic process. Electron microscopy can be utilized to distinguish between necrosis and apoptosis. Cell blebbing and organelle disruption are features of necrotic cells whereas cell condensation and fragmentation results in membrane-bound cryptotic bodies containing well-preserved organelles. More recently the task of identifying isolated apoptotic cells has been made easier by in situ end labeling of DNA strand breaks.

TREATMENT STRATEGIES

Based on our understanding of the role of inflammatory mediators leading to vasoconstriction, thrombosis, and necrosis, newer forms of treatment have been directed at modifying the early inflammatory events or at preserving blood flow in the liver.

Pharmacologic

Prostaglandins

Prostaglandins may be beneficial in patients with critical illness and ALF by virtue of their vasodilatory action, ability to inhibit cytokines and beneficial effects on the microcirculation, by improving blood flow and inhibiting aggregation of platelets and adherence of white blood cells (Peltekian et al. 1995).

Infusion of prostacyclin (PGI_2) to patients with ALF resulted in increased oxygen delivery and consumption (Bihari et al. 1985).

Interest in prostaglandin analogues led to a clinical trial in 1989 with promising positive results (Sinclair et al. 1989). However, a recent randomized controlled double-blind trial, involving 41 consecutive patients with ALF who were treated with either intravenous PGE_1 (prostin VR) or placebo, failed to show an overall benefit for PGE_1 therapy. Whether this agent is of use in the setting of ALF awaits further studies.

N-acetyl cysteine

N-acetyl cysteine is an established antidote following acetaminophen overdose if given up to 10 h after overdose (see Chapter 4). Recently, it has been suggested that even late administration of acetylcysteine may result in an improved outcome of acetaminophen-induced ALF (Harrison et al. 1991). The improvement in survival after acetylcysteine was attributed to improvement in hemodynamics and oxygen transport by enhancing tissue oxygen delivery and consumption. However, the beneficial effect may also be related to the inhibition of the production of proinflammatory cytokines including leukotrienes, TNF and oxygen free radicals. Furthermore, the benefit achieved might be secondary to enhanced production of nitric oxide with inhibition of aggregation and adhesion of platelets.

Molecular

Charcoal hemoperfusion and adsorbent columns

Charcoal is an effective adsorbent for a wide range of potentially toxic substances. Additionally, adsorbent columns have a role in the removal of a variety of cytokines. Although the circulating levels of toxic substances significantly decreased in patients treated by charcoal hemoperfusion (Gimson et al. 1982), in a subsequent controlled trial, an improvement in survival over conventional care was not noted (O'Grady et al. 1988). Recent work has suggested that a variety of circulating cytokines and endotoxin could be effectively removed using a variety of adsorbent columns (Nagaki et al. 1991) and thus, this form of therapy could be important in combination with other modalities.

Antibodies

With the development of new methods to neutralize cytokines, it is now possible to alter the outcome of a number of inflammatory diseases by specifically blocking the effects of a particular cytokine (Pugh-Humphreys and Thomson 1994; Czaja et al. 1995). Recently, it has been demonstrated that carbon-tetrachloride-induced liver injury could be prevented by treatment with a soluble tumor necrosis factor receptor antibody which neutralized the effects of TNF. The lethality of MHV-3 induced ALF can be prevented by the administration of a monoclonal antibody to the MHV-3 induced prothrombinase musfiblp (Li et al. 1992). These data provide direct evidence for a role of cytokines in induced ALF and demonstrate a role for antibodies to the cytokine or receptor in treatment of these disorders.

Hepatocyte columns

A potentially promising approach is the development of the "bioartificial" liver: in essence, a hollow-fiber dialysis cartridge that contains living hepatocytes (Cattral and Levy 1994). Two such devices are now being evaluated clinically: one that contains hepatocytes derived from a well-differentiated human hepatoblastoma cell line and is perfused with the patient's whole blood treated with heparin (Sussman et al. 1992), and one that uses pig hepatocytes and is perfused with plasma in a technique similar to plasmapheresis (Rozga et al. 1994). Whether these devices can provide sufficient liver function to support a patient with acute liver failure has not yet been determined. The devices currently used contain only about 200 g of hepatocytes, as compared with 1200 g in the typical adult human liver. In addition, there are no accessory cells, such as bile-duct epithelial cells, Kupffer cells, or endothelial cells which contribute substantially to overall hepatic functions.

SUMMARY AND CONCLUSIONS

Although the pathogenesis of ALF is not completely known, data is now emerging to support the hypothesis that irrespective of the etiology of ALF (toxic versus viral), the host's immune response including production of cytokines and inflammatory mediators contributes to microcirculatory disturbances which results in hypoxic injury and cell death (Figure 7.1). Impairment of scavenger function of the reticuloendothelial cell system further contributes to reduced hepatic blood flow and ischemic necrosis.

In this chapter, we have highlighted recent advances in our understanding of the molecular mechanisms contributing to hepatic necrosis in ALF. We have defined the importance of cytokines in the pathogenesis of ALF and some key points at which the production and action of cytokines might be controlled and might thereby modulate the immune response and the evolution of acute liver failure. This increased knowledge has allowed for new avenues of therapy both in experimental and human ALF. Given the complexity, the challenge is to provide a rational basis for the management of patients with acute liver failure with enhancement or suppression of the immune responsiveness by manipulation of endogenous cytokine synthesis or by cytokine administration.

REFERENCES

Alison, M.R. and Sarraf, C.E. 1994. Liver cell death: patterns and mechanisms. *Gut* 35: 577–81.

Almasio, P.L., Hughes, R.D. and Williams, R. 1986. Characterization of the molecular forms of fibronectin in fulminant hepatic failure. *Hepatology* 6: 1340–5.

Ando, K., Moriyama, T., Guidotti, L.G. et al. 1993. Mechanisms of class 1 restricted immunopathology. A transgenic mouse model of fulminant hepatitis. *J Exp Med* 178: 1541–54.

Andus, T., Bauer, J. and Gerok, W. 1991. Effects of cytokines on the liver. *Hepatology* 13: 364–75.

Arthur, M.P.J., Bentley, I. and Kowalski-Saunders, P. 1985. Oxygen-derived free radicals promote hepatic injury in the rat. *Gastroenterology* 89: 1114–22.

Arthur, M.P.J., Kowalski-Saunders, P. and Wright, R. 1988. Effect of endotoxin on release of reactive oxygen intermediates by rat hepatic macrophages. *Gastroenterology* 95: 1588–94.

Bihari, D., Gimson, A.E., Waterson, M. and Williams, R. 1985. Tissue hypoxia during fulminant hepatic failure. *Crit Care Med* 13: 1034–9.

Cattral, M. and Levy, G.A. 1994. Artificial liver support – pipe dream or reality? *N Engl J Med* 331: 268–9.

Czaja, M.J., Xu, J. and Alt, E. 1995. Prevention of carbon tetrachloride-induced rat liver injury by soluble tumor necrosis factor receptor. *Gastroenterology* 108: 1849–54.

Dindzans, V.J., Skamene, E. and Levy, G.A. 1986. Susceptibility/resistance to mouse hepatitis virus strain 3 and macrophage procoagulant activity are genetically linked and controlled by two non-H-2-linked genes. *J Immunol* 137: 2355–9.

Essani, N.A., Fisher, M.A., Farhood, A. et al. 1995. Cytokine-induced upregulation of hepatic intercellular adhesion molecule-1 messenger RNA expression and its role in the pathophysiology of murine endotoxin shock and acute liver failure. *Hepatology* 21: 1632–9.

Ferluga, J. and Allison, A.C. 1978. Role of mononuclear infiltrating cells in pathogenesis of hepatitis. *Lancet* i: 610–11.

Gimson, A., Braude, S., Mellon, P. et al. 1982. Earlier charcoal hemoperfusion in fulminant hepatic failure. *Lancet* 2: 681–3.

Halloran, P., Batiuk, T. and Goes, N. 1993. An overview of the cytokines in transplantation. *Transpl Sci* 3: 69–76.
Harrison, P.M., Wendon, J.A., Gimson, A.E.S. et al. 1991. Improvement of acetylcysteine of hemodynamics and oxygen transport in fulminant hepatic failure. *N Engl J Med* 324: 1852–7.
Hibbs, J.J., Westenfelder, C., Taintor, R. et al. 1992. Evidence for cytokine-inducible nitric oxide synthase from L-arginine in patients receiving interleukin-2 (IL-2) therapy. *J Clin Invest* 89: 867–77.
Izumi, S., Hughes, R.D., Langley, P.G., Pernambuco, J.R.B. and Williams, R. 1994. Extent of the acute phase response in fulminant hepatic failure. *Gut* 35: 982–6.
Jaeschke, H., Farhood, A. and Smith, C.W. 1991. Neutrophil-induced liver cell injury in endotoxin shock is a CD11b/CD18-dependent mechanism. *Am J Physiol* 261: G1051–6.
Karupiah, G., Xie, Q., Buller, M.L. et al. 1993. Inhibition of viral replication by interferon-gamma-induced nitric oxide synthase. *Science* 261: 1445–8.
Kvale, D. and Brandtzaeg, P. 1993. Immune modulation of adhesion molecules ICAM-1 (CD54) and LF-3 (CD58) in human hepatocytic cell lines. *J Hepatol* 17: 347–52.
Laskin, D.L. 1990. Nonparenchymal cells and hepatotoxicity. *Sem Liver Dis* 10: 293–304.
Lee, W.M. 1993. Acute liver failure. *N Engl J Med* 329: 1862–72.
Lee, W.M., Emerson, D.L., Young, W.O. et al. 1987. Diminished serum Gc (Vitamin D-binding protein) levels and increased Gc:G-Actin complexes in a hamster model of fulminant hepatic necrosis. *Hepatology* 7: 825–30.
Lee, W.M. and Galbraith, R. 1992. The extracellular actin-scavenger system and actin toxicity. *N Engl J Med* 326: 1335–41.
Lee, W.M., Galbraith, R.M., Watt, G.H. et al. 1995. Predicting survival in fulminant hepatic failure using serum Gc protein concentrations. *Hepatology* 21: 101–5.
Li, C., Fung, L.S., Crow, A. et al. 1992. Monoclonal anti-prothrombinase (3D4.3) prevents mortality from murine hepatitis virus infection (MHV-3). *J Exp Med* 176: 689–97.
McClain, C.J. and Cohen, D.A. 1989. Increased tumor necrosis factor production by monocytes in alcoholic hepatitis. *Hepatology* 9: 349–51.
Mori, W., Naoto, A. and Shiga, J. 1981. Acute hepatic cell necrosis experimentally produced by viral agents in rabbits. *Am J Pathol* 103: 31–5.
Mori, W., Shiga, J. and Irie, H. 1986. Schwartzman reaction as a pathogenetic mechanism in fulminant hepatitis. *Sem Liver Dis* 6: 267–9.
Morita, M., Watanabe, Y. and Akaike, T. 1994. Inflammatory cytokines upregulate intercellular adhesion molecule-1 expression on primary cultured mouse hepatocytes and T-lymphocyte adhesion. *Hepatology* 19: 426–31.
Muto, Y., Nouri-Aria, K.T., Meager, A. et al. 1988. Enhanced tumour necrosis factor and interleukin-1 in fulminant hepatic failure. *Lancet* 2: 72–4.
Nagaki, N., Hughes, R.D., Lau, J.Y.N. and Williams, R. 1991. Removal of endotoxin and cytokines by absorbents and the effect of plasma protein binding. *Int J Artif Org* 14: 43–50.
Nakagawa, J., Hishinuma, I., Hirota, K. et al. 1991. Involvement of tumor necrosis factor alpha in pathogenesis of activated-macrophage mediated hepatitis. *Gastroenterology* 100: 1153–4.
Nathan, C. 1992. Nitric oxide as a secretory product of mammalian cells. *FASEB J* 6: 3051–64.
O'Garra, A. and Murphy, K. 1994. Role of cytokines in determining T-lymphocyte function. *Curr Opin Immunol* 6: 458–66.
O'Grady, J.G., Gimson, A.E., O'Brien, C.J. et al. 1988. Controlled trials of charcoal hemoperfusion and prognostic factors in fulminant hepatic failure. *Gastroenterology* 94: 1186–92.
Parr, R.L., Fung, L.S., Reneker, J., Myers-Mason, N. et al. 1995. Association of mouse fibrinogen-like protein with murine hepatitis virus-induced prothrombinase activity. *J Virol* 69: 5033–8.
Peltekian, K., Makowka, L., Williams, R., Blendis, L., Levy, G., Prostaglandins in Liver Transplantation Research Group. 1996. Prostaglandins in Liver Failure and Transplantation: Regeneration, Immunomodulation, and Cytoprotection. *Liver Transpl Surg* 2: 171–84.
Pope, M., Rotstein, O., Cole, E. et al. 1995. Pattern of disease following murine hepatitis virus strain 3 (MHV-3) infection correlates with macrophage activation and not viral replication. *J Virol* 69: 5252–600.
Pugh-Humphreys, R.G.P. and Thomson, A.W. 1994. Cytokines and their receptors as potential therapeutic targets. In *The Cytokine Handbook*, 2nd edn., Chapter 26, 525–63. London: Academic Press.
Rosser, B.G. and Gores, G.J. 1995. Liver cell necrosis: Cellular mechanisms and clinical implications. *Gastroenterology* 108: 252–75.
Rozga, J., Podesta, L., Lepage, E. et al. 1994. A bioartificial liver to treat severe acute liver failure. *Ann Surg* 219: 538–46.
Sekiyama, K.D., Yoshiba, M. and Thomson, A.W. 1994. Circulating proinflammatory cytokines (IL-1β, TNF-α, and IL-6) and IL-1 receptor antagonist (IL-1Ra) in fulminant hepatic failure and acute hepatitis. *Clin Exp Immunol* 98: 71–7.
Sinclair, S.B., Greig, P.D., Blendis, L.M. et al. 1989. Biochemical and clinical response of fulminant viral hepatitis to administration of prostaglandin E: A preliminary report. *J Clin Invest* 84: 1063–9.
Sinclair, S.B., Wakefield, A.J. and Levy, G.A. 1990. Fulminant hepatitis. *Springer Seminars in Immunopathology* 12: 1–13.
Steinhoff, G., Behrend, M. and Pichlmayr, R. 1990. Induction of ICAM-1 on hepatocyte membranes during liver allograft rejection and infection. *Transpl. Proc.* 22: 2308–9.
Sussman, N.L., Chong, M.G., Koussayer, T. et al. 1992. Reversal of fulminant hepatic failure using an extracorporeal liver assist device. *Hepatology* 16: 60–5.
Verhoef, J. and Mattsson, E. 1995. The role of cytokines in Gram-positive bacterial shock. *Trends Microbiol* 3: 136–40.
Volpes, R., Van Den Oord, J.J. and Desmet, V.J. 1990. Immunohistochemical study of adhesion molecules in liver inflammation. *Hepatology* 12: 59–65.
Winwood, P.J. and Arthur, M.J.P. 1993. Kupffer cells: Their activation and role in animal models of liver injury and human liver disease. *Sem Liver Dis* 13: 50–9.

8 Pathology of acute liver failure

Bernard Portmann and Romil Saxena

INTRODUCTION

Confluent necrosis and loss of liver parenchyma in either zonal or nonzonal distribution is the commonest pathology underlying acute liver failure. More rarely microvesicular fatty change in the absence of significant parenchymal loss, or another pathology may dominate the histologic picture and indicate the likely etiology. When confluent necrosis does occur, there is usually a lack of specificity of pathologic features. However, different patterns of damage may reflect different etiology and/or disease duration and prognosis and at times influence management and likelihood of recovery.

In this chapter, the terminology and main patterns of liver necrosis are reviewed and then related to the various causes of liver failure. The morphologic changes associated with some rarer causes, in particular Wilson's disease, Budd–Chiari syndrome, malignant infiltration, as well as those of liver failure following orthotopic liver transplantation and in the immunocompromised host are discussed separately. The section ends with some considerations on liver regeneration as observed in human liver after severe necrosis, with the experimental aspects of regeneration being treated in the next chapter.

CONFLUENT PARENCHYMAL NECROSIS

Forms of confluent liver necrosis

Necrosis and/or loss of confluent areas of parenchyma show a variety of patterns which depend on: their distribution in relation to both the acinar architecture and the liver as a whole; whether or not cell dropout has taken place; and the degree and distribution of the regeneration process.

Macroscopic examination

Previously, information about the gross appearances of the liver in acute hepatitis were obtained from laparoscopic views in nonfatal cases and at autopsy in cases of fulminant failure. With transplantation as a regular therapeutic option for acute liver failure, the pathologist has the unique opportunity to study in detail the explanted liver. Three main patterns are recognized:

- A diffuse, more or less uniform involvement of the whole organ without evidence of nodular regeneration. The liver is variably reduced in size, or may be slightly enlarged and swollen, its capsular surface being accordingly wrinkled or smooth. The cut surface is homogeneous yellow or red, depending largely on the degree of cell dropout; in a number of cases, a red mottling on a yellowish background indicates perivenular confluent cell loss and congestion with a substantial sparing of periportal hepatocytes (Figure 8.1a, Plate I).

- A diffuse pattern with micronodular regeneration. The liver shows diffuse collapse, but the cut surface displays a seeding of minute yellow or greenish nodules of regeneration which are just discernible with the naked eye (Figure 8.1b, Plate I).
- A "map-like" or geographic pattern where broad areas of multiacinar parenchymal collapse alternate with large nodules of apparently spared and regenerating parenchyma (Figure 8.2a, Plate II). The collapsed areas are darkly colored, sunken and rubbery in consistency. They contrast sharply with the large nodules which are yellow or green in color, soft in consistency and often protrude from the capsular or cut surface (Figure 8.2b, Plate II).

Histologic findings

The changes vary according to both mechanisms and the time of observation after onset of the tissue damage.

Eosinophilic (coagulative) necrosis

This is usually observed in cases with a short disease duration (hyperacute liver failure) and more often in relation to toxic than to viral injury (O'Grady et al. 1993). The necrosis is zonal, affecting predominantly acinar zones 3 and 2, but in severe cases acinar zone 1 becomes partially or totally engrossed in the necrotic process (submassive or panacinar necrosis) (Figure 8.3a, Plate II). Throughout the necrotic areas, coagulated hepatocytes are shrunken, rounded, separated from each other by clear spaces and have lost their nuclei by pyknosis or karyorrhexis. Infiltration by inflammatory cells is minimal and consists of a few polymorphonuclear cells located in portal areas and/or at the periphery of the necrotic areas. However, considerable numbers of activated sinusoidal lining cells are observed, especially in cases where cell dropout has started in the perivenular regions. These cells include perisinusoidal cells (Ito cells) reactive with α-smooth muscle actin antibodies (Enzan et al. 1995) and CD68-positive activated macrophages (Mathew et al. 1994). Usually, the areas of necrosis remain sharply demarcated from the periportal surviving parenchyma which comprises enlarged, pale staining hepatocytes arranged in two or more cell-thick plates. The intervening sinusoids are attenuated (Figure 8.3b, Plate II). In places where the necrosis has reached portal boundaries, small elongated cells, closely resembling the "oval cells" described in animal studies, are observed seemingly sprouting from the portal margin into the necrotic parenchyma (Koukoulis et al. 1992) (Figure 8.4, Plate II).

Confluent cell dropout

Confluent cell dropout, as opposed to actually visible necrosis, is more commonly seen, particularly in livers removed at transplantation or in those with a long disease duration. Cell dropout follows coagulative and/or lytic necrosis and is characterized by a complete loss of hepatocytes with collapse of the reticulin framework, variable sinusoidal congestion and a generally more intense mixed inflammatory cell infiltration throughout the post-necrotic areas (Figure 8.5a, Plate III). Material released from the necrotic cells appears as ceroid pigment within macrophages which stain positively with periodic acid Schiff (PAS) after diastase digestion. Sparse lymphocytes, plasma cells, neutrophils and eosinophils are also present in various combinations which may reflect different etiology and/or disease duration. In a number of cases, hepatic venules show a picture of endotheliitis or venulitis resembling that seen in the acutely rejected liver allograft (Figure 8.5b, Plate III). The inflammatory cell infiltrate is also reinforced within the enlarged portal tracts where lymphocytes often predominate. Confluent cell dropout may be zonal, leaving a significant mantle of surviving parenchyma around the portal tracts, panacinar with nearly complete hepatocyte loss affecting the whole liver or multiacinar, as in the collapsed areas of the map-like pattern of necrosis. In this situation the approximated portal tracts are surrounded by exuberant ductular structures which express biliary epithelium cytokeratin 19 (Figure 8.6a and b, Plate III) or a combination of hepatocytic plates and ductules. These include structures of mixed phenotype referred to as neocholangioles (Phillips and Poucell 1981). In the map-like pattern, these collapsed areas are sharply demarcated from macronodules of regeneration which show lesser degrees of damage, an increased pleomorphism of large hepatocytes arranged in thickened plates, and an apparent paucity of portal areas with few, if any proliferated ductules. Active hepatocyte proliferation in these areas is demonstrated by an intensive nuclear staining for proliferative markers such as proliferating cell nuclear antigen (PCNA) (Figure 8.3b, Plate II) or Ki67.

A third pattern, confluent focal cell necrosis/dropout with cell sparing, is an intermediate form between a classical lobular hepatitis of extreme severity and submassive confluent necrosis. Foci of confluent cell dropout, best appreciated on the reticulin preparation, are widely distributed throughout the liver acini and are intermingled with spared single liver cells or groups of liver cells throughout (Figure 8.6c, Plate III). The islands of surviving parenchyma show a marked cell pleomorphism due to a mixture of ballooned, eosinophilic degenerated, or smaller and slightly basophilic hepatocytes, together with ductal plate structures having acquired a bile duct phenotype. This pattern is observed in cases due to virus or drug hepatitis or of undetermined cause, but not with direct toxins.

Cholestasis

Cholestasis is absent in areas with coagulative necrosis and/or complete cell dropout; restricted to areas of surviving parenchyma, its severity parallels that of clinical cholestasis and reflects the degree of surviving parenchyma rather than necrosis and is not necessarily a sign of bad prognosis. Histologic cholestasis includes intracellular bile pigments, canalicular bile plugs and, in the majority of cases presenting a severe cholestatic syndrome clinically, cholangiolar or extravasated bile casts which are often surrounded by neutrophils. These deposits disposed at the portal periphery or along the interface between collapsed and regenerating parenchyma, resemble those described in association with sepsis (Lefkowitch 1982) (Figure 8.7, Plate IV). When observed after severe liver necrosis, it is not certain whether the inspissated bile results from altered bile secretion due to the parenchymal damage or from septic complications that often develop in these patients. This type of cholestasis is commonly seen from ten days or so after the onset of liver damage irrespective of the cause. In extreme cases, bile lakes or infarcts may form surrounded by a foreign-body-type giant cell reaction. In general, the prominent parenchymal collapse assists in distinguishing the changes from those of large duct obstruction.

Pattern of necrosis related to etiology

Acetaminophen (paracetamol) toxicity

The liver damage is the prototype of a direct and predictable hepatotoxin that causes severe but time-limited injury to the liver. Owing to the number of cases observed at various stages after the toxic insult, an orderly sequence of changes has been described after acetaminophen overdose (Portmann et al. 1975), which roughly corresponds to that seen in animal models, yet in a different time-scale (Dixon et al. 1971). Although rarely observed in man, early changes prior to significant clinical symptoms are characterized by extensive cell swelling with cytoplasmic microvacuolation resembling that of acute fatty liver of pregnancy. This early phase is followed by zonal eosinophilic coagulative necrosis affecting acinar zones 3 and 2, and in more severe cases, zone 1 (Figures 8.3a and 8.4a, Plate II). This is associated with high serum aminotransferase levels and is mainly observed in toxic injury or ischemic liver injury due to circulatory failure. Between days six and seven, the necrotic cells have disappeared, leaving areas of reticulin collapse and an infiltrate which comprises predominantly activated sinusoidal lining cells and pigmented macrophages. By day ten after overdose, the postnecrotic areas have shrunk further, often taking the form of bridging collapse with a "star-fish" pattern, highlighting the boundaries of acinar zones 3. Bile ductules are present in periportal areas and areas adjacent to postnecrotic collapse. These neocholangioles show atypical epithelial lining and inspissated bile concretions are often present in their lumens. As a rule, the longer the interval between overdose and tissue examination, the denser the inflammatory cell infiltrate, to the extent that after 12 days the picture becomes indistinguishable from that of fulminant viral hepatitis (Figure 8.5b, Plate III). Early features of regeneration are discussed later in this chapter. Subsequent developments have been documented in the past on the basis of a few sequential liver biopsies from patients who survived (Portmann et al. 1975), and, recently, in native livers of patients who have received auxiliary orthotopic grafts (unpublished data). Even in areas of complete necrosis, there is indirect evidence of periportal "oval cell" proliferation which might later replenish hepatocytic plates, but the extent to which this happens is still a matter of speculation. When necrosis has spared a periportal cuff of hepatocytes, regeneration is explosive and nodules of thickened plates composed of large, pale staining, and actively dividing hepatocytes are identified as early as two weeks after injury. Long term follow up specimens taken from patients who had survived grade 4 coma have shown a remarkable restoration of the liver architecture with only fine irregular scarring (Figure 8.8a and b, Plate IV). Clinically, signs of chronic liver disease or portal hypertension have not been observed after a single overdose.

Other toxic agents

Carbon tetrachloride (CCl_4), a rare cause of accidental human poisoning occurring especially in alcoholics, produces changes similar to those induced by acetaminophen. In both acetaminophen and CCl_4 toxicity, large fatty vacuoles within both necrotic and surviving parenchyma reflect previous alcohol intake. Pre-existing perivenular fibrosis may also be observed. Experimentally, CCl_4 is widely used to study toxic hepatic necrosis. It is still a favored model of cirrhosis which regularly develops after repeated injections of CCl_4 (Sokal et al. 1990), but it is worth mentioning that surprising reversal of the process often occurs in animals kept for long periods of time after the last injection (personal observation).

Poisoning by mushrooms (most frequently *Amanita phalloides*) is characterized by centrizonal coagulative necrosis with panacinar fatty infiltration in small or medium-sized vacuoles (Figure 8.9, Plate IV). The main toxin, α-amanitin is a potent inhibitor of RNA polymerase, which even at very low concentrations inhibits m-RNA synthesis and leads to loss of synthesis of enzymes, structural proteins and apoproteins with subsequent fat accumulation and necrosis of hepatocytes (Scheurlen et al. 1994).

A characteristically periportal coagulative necrosis (acinar zone 1) has been attributed to toxins such as phosphorus, poisonous doses of ferrous sulfate, allyl alcohol and its esters, and the endotoxin of *Proteus vulgaris* (Zimmerman and Ishak 1994).

Ischemic hepatitis

Acute liver failure may follow an acute episode of circulatory failure, or more often when there is acute-on-chronic cardiac failure (Nouel et al. 1980). The liver shows coagulative necrosis affecting acinar zones 3 and 2, but in some instances, there may be a preservation of perivenular hepatocytes producing an acinar zone 2 or midzonal necrosis (Figure 8.10, Plate V) (de la Monte et al. 1984). Dystrophic calcification may later develop (Shibuya et al. 1985).

Fulminant viral hepatitis

Whereas toxic insults to the liver are generally

(a)

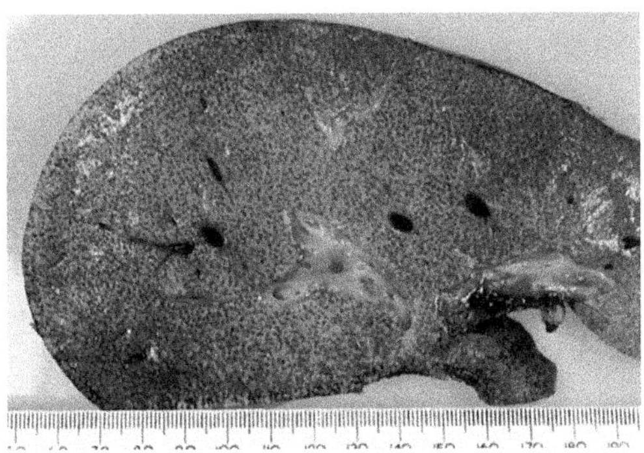

(b)

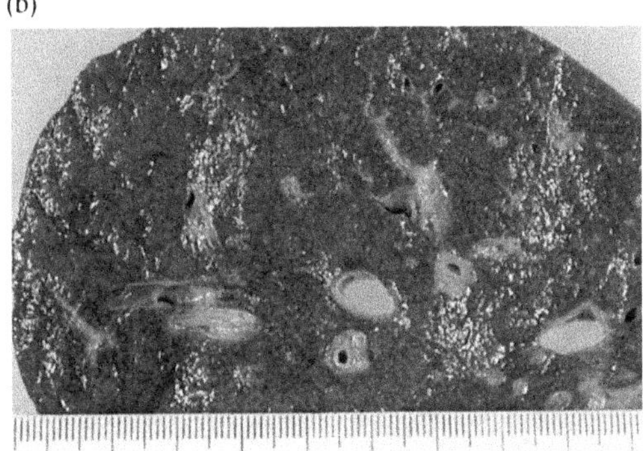

Figure 8.1 Gross appearance of bisected livers removed at transplantation: (a) day 5 after a massive acetaminophen overdose; red mottling indicating confluent centrilobular necrosis and absence of nodular regeneration and (b) micronodular regeneration just seen with the naked eye in fulminant hepatitis B of 10 days' duration.

(a)

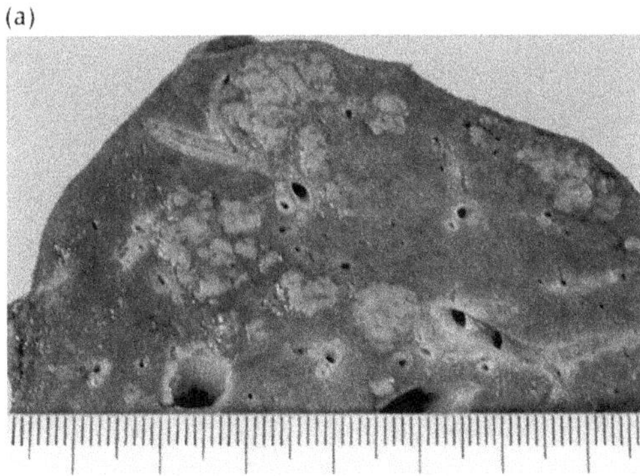

(b)

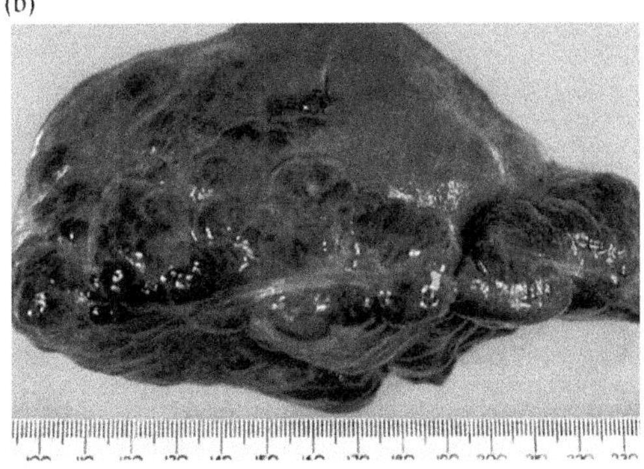

Figure 8.2 Subacute liver failure of undetermined etiology: (a) liver cut surface showing extensive areas of multiacinar collapse (brown) and scattered regenerative nodules (yellow); and (b) external view showing cholestatic nodules protruding on the anterior margins of both left and right lobes.

(a)

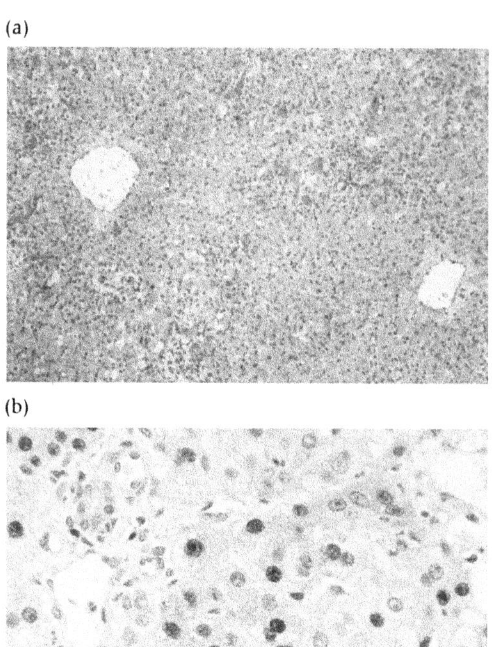

(b)

Figure 8.3 Acetaminophen toxicity: (a) a submassive eosinophilic necrosis on day 4 with only few islands of "viable" cells in periportal areas (seen at higher magnification in Figure 8.4); (b) periportal regenerating parenchyma with enlarged, pale staining hepatocytes of which most nuclei are stained positively for proliferating cell nuclear antigen (PCNA), immunoperoxidase using MAB clone PC10.

(a)

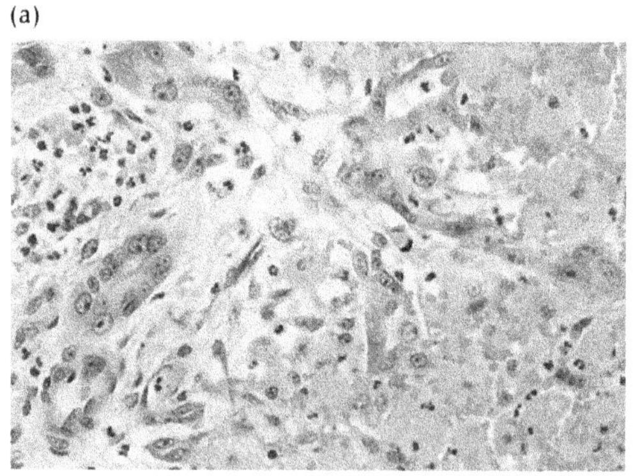

(b)

(c)

Figure 8.4 Submassive eosinophilic necrosis due to acetaminophen toxicity. "Oval" cells expressing biliary epithelium cytokeratin appear sprouting from the portal margin into the necrotic parenchyma: (a) H&E; (b) cytokeratin 19 and (c) PCNA clone PC10 immunoperoxidase.

PLATE II

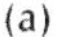

(a)

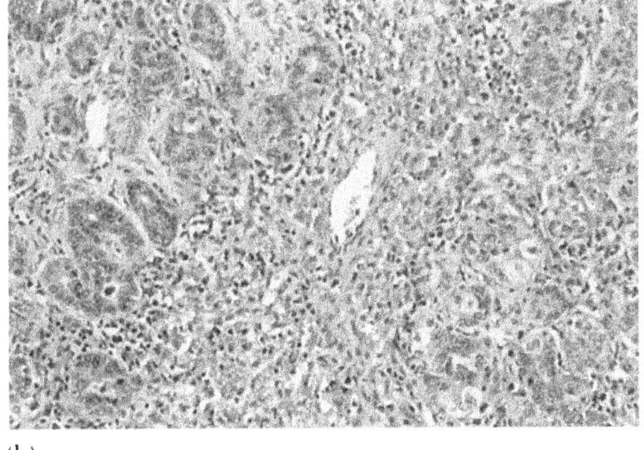

(b)

Figure 8.5 (a) Acute liver failure due to hepatitis B. There is confluent hepatocyte dropout with sparse mixed inflammatory cells and predominantly ductular structures around portal tracts. (b) Acinar zone 2 and 3 confluent cell dropout with zone 1 regeneration, mixed inflammatory cell infiltrate including pigmented macrophages and prominent hepatic venulitis on day 12 after an acetaminophen overdose.

(a)

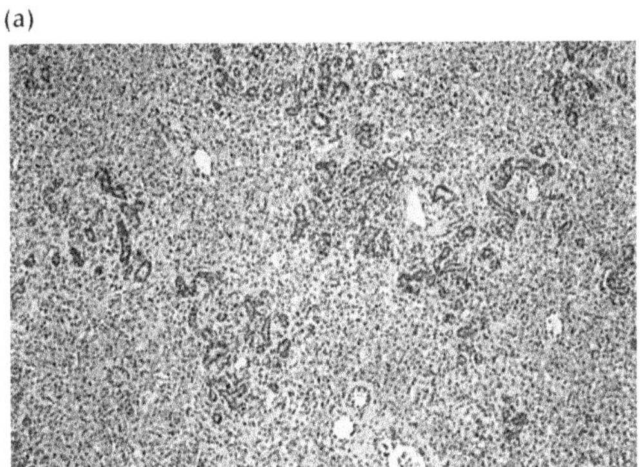

(b)

(c)

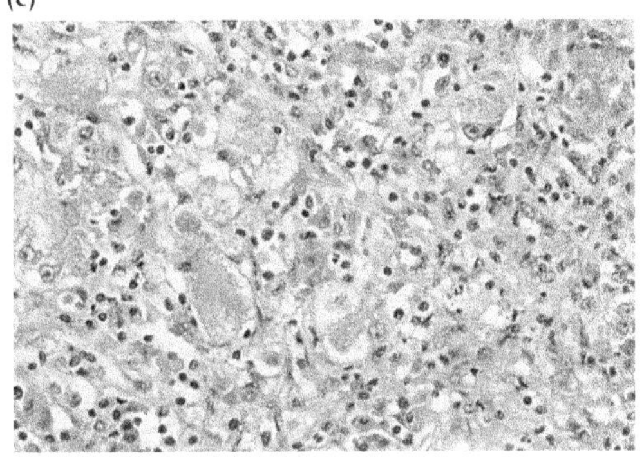

Figure 8.6 (a) Multiacinar parenchymal collapse of undetermined cause with approximated portal areas surrounded by neoductules; (b) PCNA positive staining of a high proportion of ductular nuclei support their proliferative state; and (c) widespread foci of cell dropout and inflammatory cell infiltrates intermingled with pleomorphic surviving hepatocytes in sulfonamide-related acute liver failure. (a) and (c) H&E; (b) PCNA clone PC10 immunostaining.

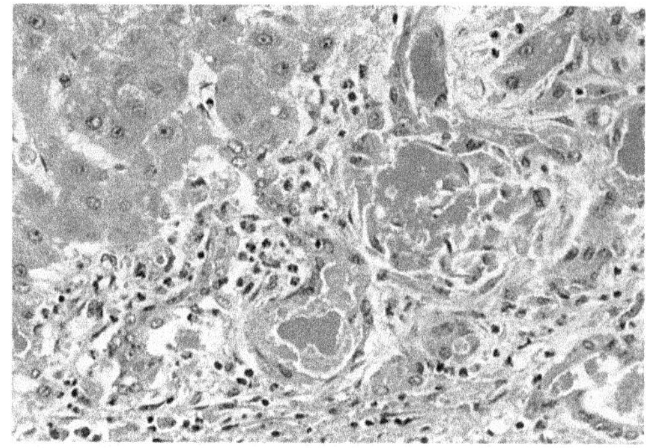

Figure 8.7 Severe cholestasis after subacute liver failure associated with ketoconazole exposure. Histology shows cholangiolar and extravasated bile casts at the portal periphery, a feature suggestive of septic complications.

(a)

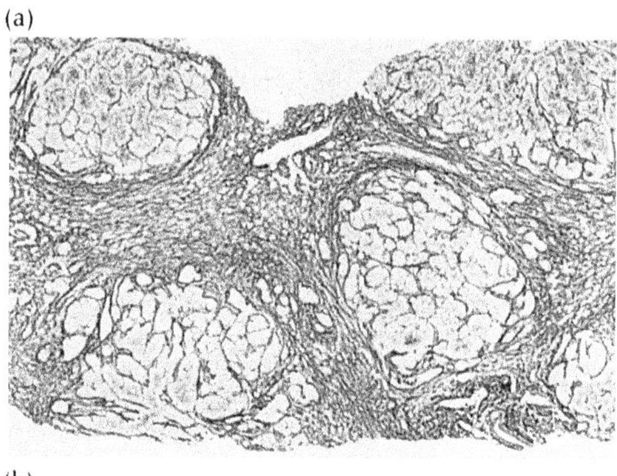

(b)

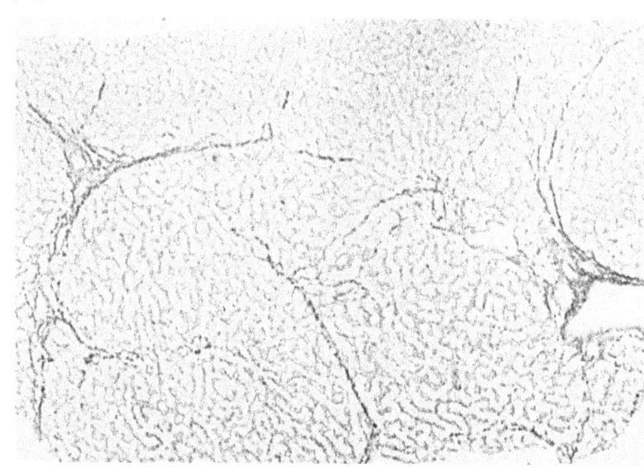

Figure 8.8 Reticulin preparation of liver biopsy specimens taken after recovery from grade IV encephalopathy due to acetaminophen toxicity: (a) extensive parenchymal bridging collapse with micronodule formation at two months; (b) remarkable restoration of the parenchyma with only thin postnecrotic scarring at one year. Silver for reticulin.

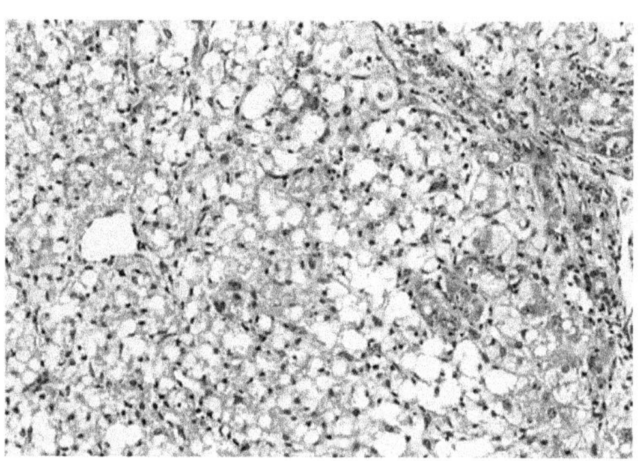

Figure 8.9 Panacinar hepatocyte necrosis with fatty infiltration in acute liver failure due to *Amanita phalloides* poisoning.

PLATE IV

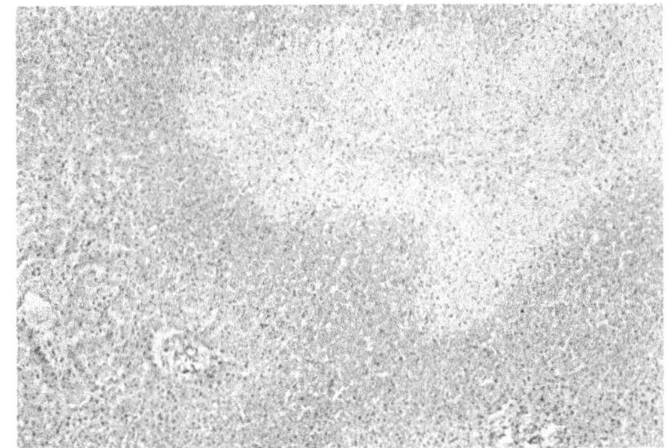

Figure 8.10 Predominantly acinar zone 2 confluent necrosis in acute liver failure due to circulatory failure.

(a)

(b)

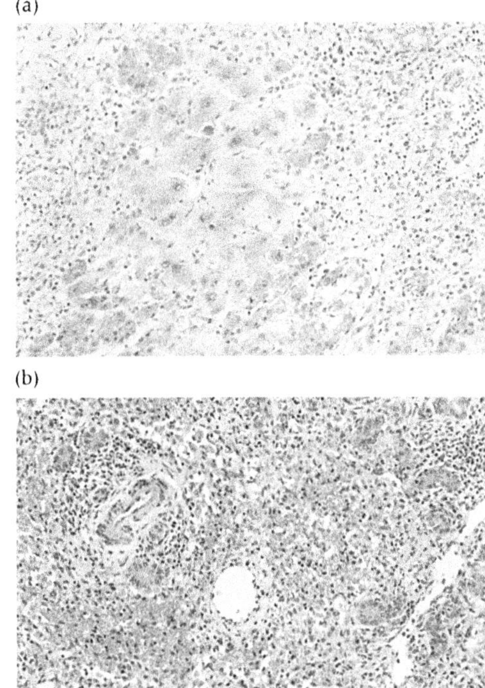

Figure 8.11 (a) Sparing of perivenular hepatocytes (center of the field) and acinar zone 1 and 2 necrosis characteristic of fulminant hepatitis A; (b) panacinar cell dropout due to fulminant hepatitis B in a baby born to mother carrying the precore mutant.

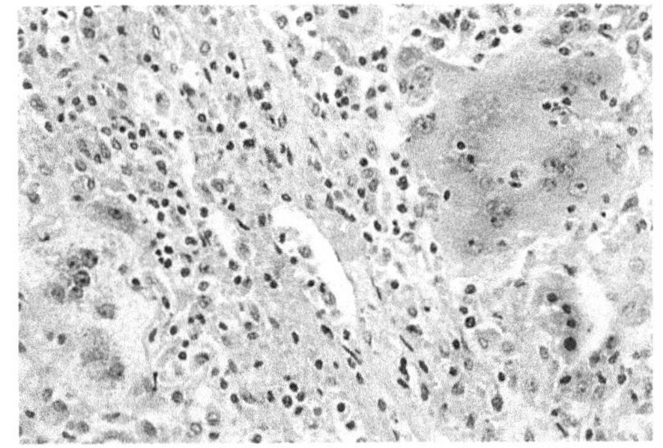

Figure 8.12 Multinucleated syncytial hepatocytes lining areas of parenchymal collapse in a case of acute liver failure of undetermined cause.

These plates are available for download in colour from www.cambridge.org/9780521188944

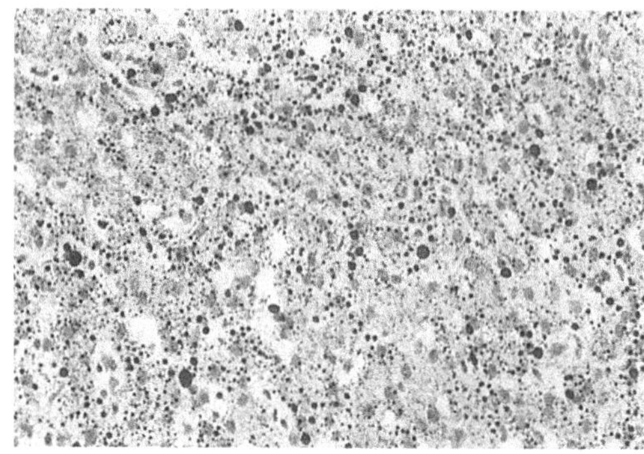

Figure 8.13 Reye's syndrome. There is widespread, microvesicular fatty infiltration in otherwise preserved liver parenchyma. Frozen section stained with Oil red O.

(a)

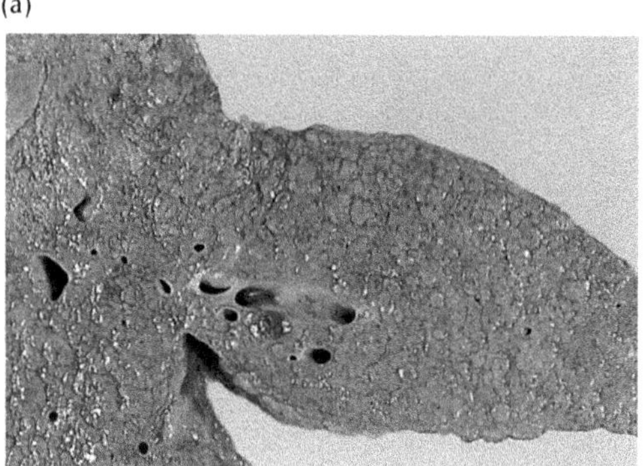

(b)

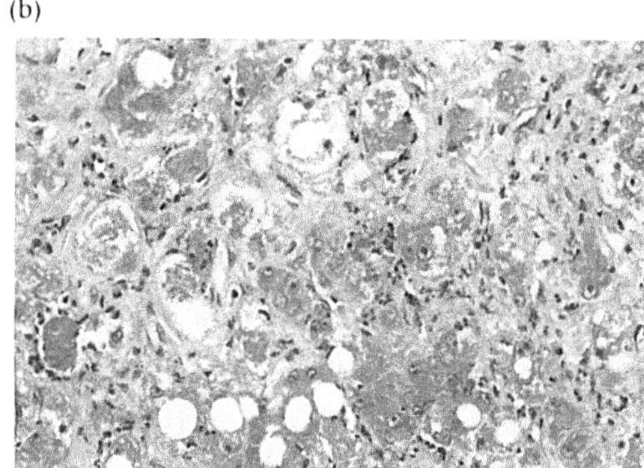

(c)

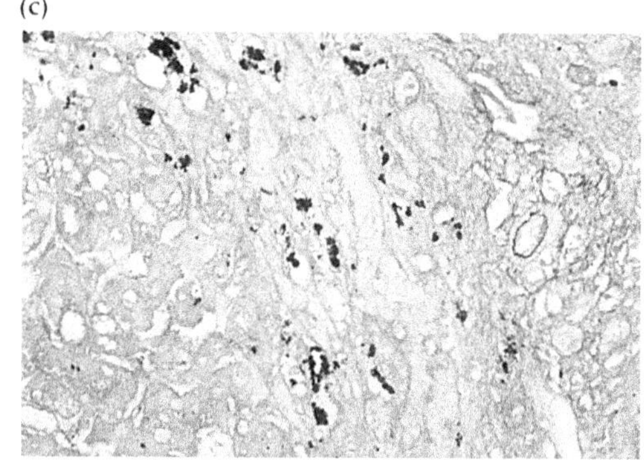

Figure 8.14 Wilson's disease presenting as acute liver failure. (a) Cut section of liver removed at transplantation showing cirrhosis with yellow, fat-loaded parenchymal nodules of variable size; (b) histologically, there is severe hepatocyte damage with ballooning, fatty infiltration and Mallory bodies; and (c) coarse granules of copper associated protein are present in Kupffer cells and porto-septal macrophages. (b) H&E; (c) orcein staining.

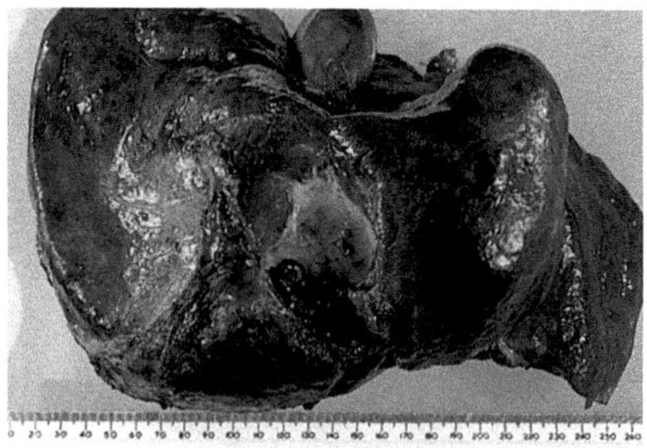

Figure 8.15 Acute liver failure secondary to the Budd–Chiari syndrome. Posteroinferior view of autopsy liver with the vena cava cut open to show a recent thrombus obliterating its lumen. There are small organized thrombi occluding outlets of accessory hepatic veins.

PLATE VI

(a)

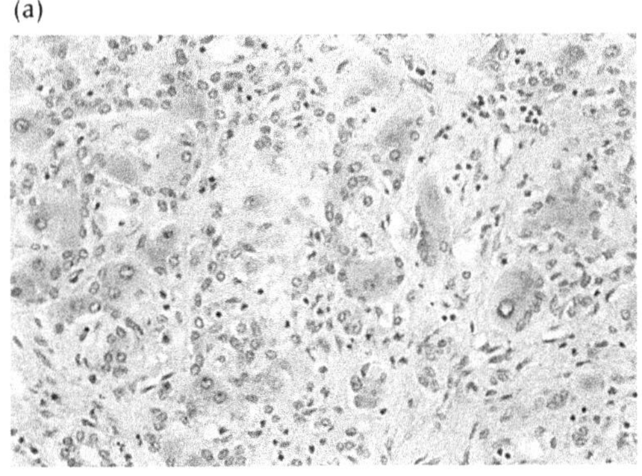

(b)

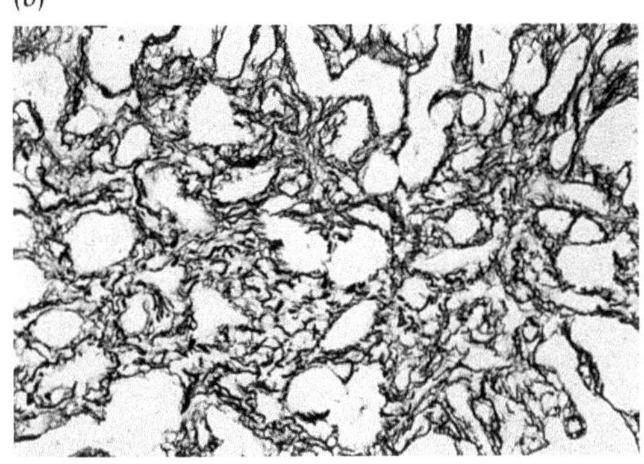

(c)

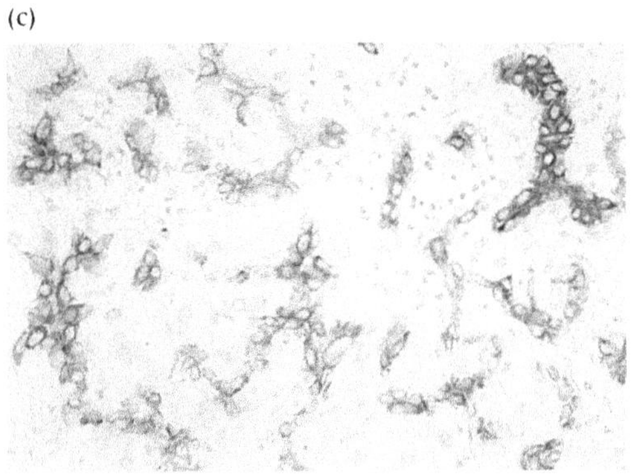

(d)

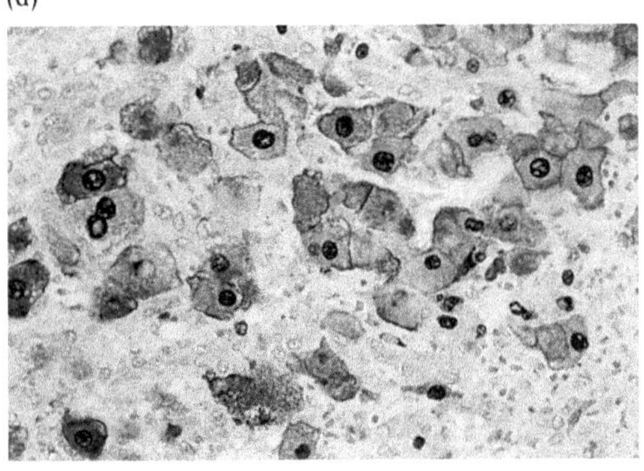

Figure 8.16 Liver failure due to recurrent HBV infection in the liver allograft, pattern of fibrosing cholestatic hepatitis: (a) enlarged hepatocytes intermingled with ductal plates and dissociated by diffuse pericellular fibrosis; (b) fibrosis is better shown on the reticulin preparation and (c) ductal plates by cytokeratin immunostaining; (d) massive nuclear and cytoplasmic HB_cAg deposition is observed. (a) H&E, (b) reticulin silver stain; immunoperoxidase staining for cytokeratin 19 (c) and HB_cAg (d).

(a)

(b)

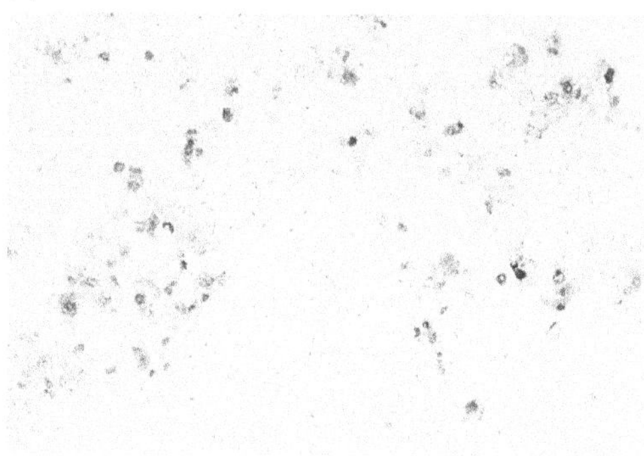

Figure 8.17 Liver allograft removed for acute failure due to adenovirus hepatitis in a 3.5-year-old boy at 3 weeks after transplantation. (a) Necrotic areas with little inflammation are bordered by hepatocytes containing prominent viral inclusions; (b) positive nuclear immunostaining with an adenovirus-group antibody (MAB805 Chemicon).

(a)

(b)

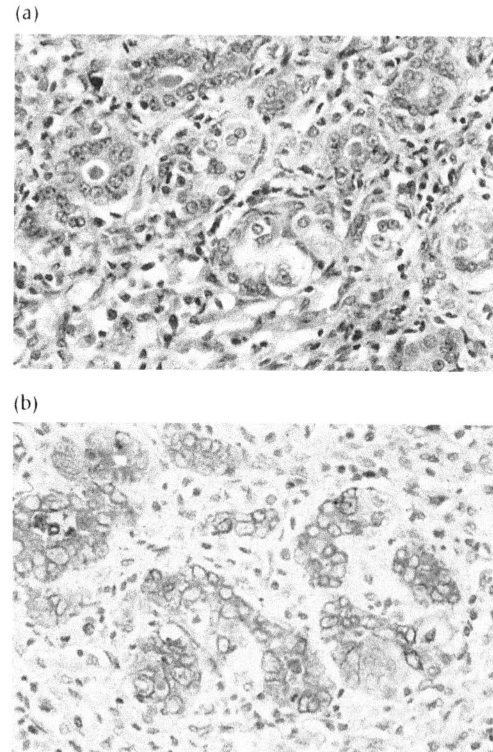

Figure 8.18 Submassive necrosis related to isoniazid treatment. Periportal neoductules include mixed structures showing both biliary and hepatocellular components. (a) H&E; (b) immunoperoxidase for cytokeratin 19.

PLATE VIII

short-lived and their precise time of occurrence is known, viral induced liver damage generally results from a complex and prolonged interplay between virus replication and host defense. The exact time of onset is difficult to determine and acute liver failure may in fact represent the culmination of a process of long duration. As a consequence, liver histology in fulminant viral hepatitis is more likely to show zonal or submassive cell dropout with varying degrees of cell sparing and regeneration, rather than coagulative necrosis.

Hepatitis A

Hepatitis A virus, a rare cause of acute liver failure, may present with a particularly short history and submassive eosinophilic necrosis in the liver. However, in most instances submassive cell dropout is already present and in many instances there is a distinctive preservation of hepatocytes adjacent to hepatic venules (Figure 8.11a, Plate V). This pattern is in keeping with the prominent periportal distribution of the necro-inflammatory activity observed in milder forms of the disease. The portal inflammatory cell infiltrate is rich in plasma cells. Microvesicular change attributed to finely divided fat vacuoles in surviving hepatocytes may be striking, similar to that reported in delta hepatitis in the Venezuelan Indians (Buitrago et al. 1986).

Hepatitis B

The most common change encountered in fulminant hepatitis B is submassive cell dropout with variable and random hepatocyte sparing. Pleomorphic cells with ballooning and eosinophilic shrinkage are reminiscent of a classical lobular hepatitis, but with more extensive cell loss. Viral markers in the tissue are generally negative on immunohistochemical preparations and the overall changes do not substantially differ from those of other viral forms. Rarely, HB_c antigen is demonstrated in an occasional hepatocyte nucleus. A positive immunostaining for HB_s antigen in hepatocyte cytoplasm points toward either acute HB_e antigen–antibody seroconversion or acute delta or another hepatotropic virus infection superimposed on a chronic HBV carrier state. In such a situation evidence of pre-existing liver damage is present in the form of portal and/or parenchymal scarring. Delta co-infection (Smedile et al. 1982) and HBV mutations in the precore (Omata et al. 1991; Liang et al. 1991) or core promoter regions (Sato et al. 1995) which respectively affect translation or transcription of the HB_e coding region have been associated with a higher rate of fulminant hepatitis. Cases occurring in infants born to mothers carrying the pre-core mutant are well documented (Hawkins et al. 1994) (Figure 8.11b, Plate V).

Hepatitis C

Few reports of detailed histology in fulminant hepatitis C are available since the incidence is decidedly rare. However, when compared with seven cases of B-related acute hepatitis, type C cases and most of the non-A non-B non-C cases were characterized as having slower and less severe, but more persistent hepatocyte destruction (Yoshiba et al. 1994). We are not aware that features classically described in chronic forms of hepatitis C infection (Lefkowitch et al. 1993), namely lymphoid aggregates/follicles and bile duct damage have been observed in fulminant cases ascribed to HCV.

Hepatitis E

The changes closely resemble other fulminant viral hepatitis, but appear to most closely resemble hepatitis A, with extensive parenchymal necrosis and collapse, swollen and foamy appearances of surviving hepatocytes and prominent ductular proliferation and cholestatic rosettes (Asher et al. 1990).

Yellow fever

The viral hemorrhagic fevers (Yellow fever, Dengue, Lassa fever, Ebola and Marburg fevers) share several epidemiologic and clinicopathologic features, in particular small vessel damage and overlapping changes in the liver (Ishak et al. 1982). Much attention has been paid to the hepatic pathology, but death from liver failure is exceedingly rare, except in yellow fever. At autopsy, the liver is yellow and soft, with occasional patches of hemorrhagic necrosis present under the capsule. Microscopically, there is confluent focal necrosis with a predominantly midzonal distribution and striking acidophilic degeneration forming the classic, but non-specific, Councilman bodies. Fatty change may be prominent.

Hepatitis of undetermined cause

In 17 percent of cases of acute liver failure in the UK (O'Grady et al. 1993) the cause remains undetected. These cases were presumed to be of viral etiology, and were allocated to the category non-A non-B hepatitis, and more recently non-A non-B non-C hepatitis following exclusion of HCV as a cause. In other centers, clinically comparable cases are still referred to as indeterminate. The majority of patients with acute or subacute liver failure of undetermined etiology have had at least two weeks' duration of jaundice before the development of encephalopathy. The pathology of the liver removed at transplantation falls almost invariably into the map-like category with areas of multiacinar parenchymal collapse which alternate with large macronodules of regenerative parenchyma in a random distribution (Figure 8.2a and b, Plate I). The reason for such a patchy distribution is not known. Vascular occlusion is usually not found, although intrahepatic microthrombi were detected on sections stained with phosphotungstic acid hematoxylin (trichrome) (Mori et al. 1984). In extreme situations, one lobe may show near total collapse whereas the other lobe is spared, or swollen with features of regeneration. Good preservation of the caudate lobe is commonly observed.

Unpredictable drug reactions

An injury pattern which in every way recapitulates the changes described above for viral hepatitis, has been observed with idiosyncratic reactions to a number of drugs, irrespective of dosage and length of administration (Davies and Portmann 1994). Most prominent in the list of drugs associated with confluent parenchymal necrosis are halothane, the antituberculous agents isoniazid/rifampicin, disulfiram, ketoconazole, sulfonamide, and some nonsteroidal anti-inflammatory drugs (see Chapter 3). In most instances histologic differentiation between drug- and viral-induced acute hepatitis is not possible. A sharply demarcated zonal parenchymal loss with prominent accumulation of pigmented macrophages may be more marked in drug-induced damage, such as halothane or isoniazid hepatitis. An eosinophil rich and/or granulomatous inflammatory cell infiltrate, or a particularly severe cholestasis may point to a drug as a possible cause. In that respect large cholangiolar casts of inspissated bile, which closely resemble those described in benoxaprofen-induced cholestasis (Goudie et al. 1982), may suggest drug-induced damage. However, as alluded to above, these cholestatic features are commonly found following confluent parenchymal necrosis, whether of viral, drug, or undetermined causes.

Features of uncertain significance

Multinucleated giant hepatocytes are occasionally observed in adult liver at the margin of areas of confluent necrosis, most often, but not invariably in cases of undetermined etiology (Figure 8.12, Plate V). Paramyxoviral features have been found in a few such cases by electron microscopy (Phillips et al. 1991), but the finding has not been confirmed by others, nor has it been serologically substantiated; there is insufficient evidence to incriminate a specific virus at the present time. Giant cell transformation and confluent necrosis are more commonly seen in livers of neonates, whether liver failure is idiopathic, associated with severe tissue iron load (perinatal hemochromatosis) or with an autoimmune hemolytic anemia (see Chapter 6). In the latter condition, recent parenchymal necrosis including many neutrophils has been emphasized (Bernard et al. 1981) and the disease has been shown to recur after transplantation.

Toga-like virus particles have been demonstrated by thorough electron microscopic screening in livers removed at transplantation for acute liver failure of undetermined cause, and occasionally in cases attributed to a drug reaction. These cases had no distinctive histologic features, and serologic markers against representative panels of arboviruses, which the ultrastructural features resembled to, have remained negative (Fagan et al. 1992).

PATHOLOGIC CHANGES OTHER THAN NECROSIS

Microvesicular fatty change

There is a heterogeneous group of well defined conditions and syndromes, all of which have in common acute liver failure, a high mortality and microvesicular fatty change on histology. Necrosis is seen to a variable extent in some of these conditions but is never the prominent or predominant feature. The most important members of the group are discussed below.

Reye's syndrome

Reye's syndrome is now rare due to increasing awareness of its association with salicylates and the cessation of salicylate use in young children (Waldman et al. 1982). In the liver, there is panacinar microvesicular steatosis. The hepatocytes are slightly enlarged and packed with small lipid droplets that do not displace the nucleus. The lipid droplets have been observed to be smaller in acinar zone 3 than in zones 2 and 1. The lipid infiltration is not evident by light microscopy in the first 24 h after the onset of encephalopathy, although abundant fat can be detected on frozen sections stained for neutral fat by oil red O (Figure 8.13, Plate VI) or Sudan black B (Bove et al. 1975). Actual necrosis of hepatocytes, portal inflammation and cholestasis are rare. Glycogen depletion correlates with the severity of the disease process and with hypoglycemia. Electron microscopy reveals distinctive abnormalities of the mitochondria which are enlarged, misshapen with reduced number and size of cristae. Some of these changes have been correlated with the stage of encephalopathy (Partin et al. 1971).

Valproic acid toxicity

Microvesicular steatosis is also observed in patients on the anticonvulsant valproic acid. In the majority of cases, the drug causes minor elevations of the serum transaminases which return to normal on decreasing the dose of the drug (Powell-Jackson et al. 1984), but death from acute liver failure is well recorded (Zimmerman and Ishak 1982), especially in children and particularly males. The reaction suggests an idiosyncratic metabolic aberration with direct interference of metabolites with mitochondrial function and fatty acid oxidation. Histologically, there is panacinar microvesicular steatosis, and in half the cases conspicuous confluent necrosis which affects predominantly acinar zone 3. It is not certain whether the necrosis is due to valproic acid itself, as up to 85 percent of children also received other anticonvulsants (Zafrani and Berthelot 1982). A few fatal cases showed cirrhosis (Zimmerman and Ishak 1982).

Tetracycline toxicity

Histology of the liver shows finely-divided lipid droplets that do not displace the nucleus; initially the fat is confined to acinar zone 3 but soon becomes panacinar in distribution. There is little, if any cholestasis and no significant necrosis. Tetracycline is known to bind tRNA with inhibition of protein synthesis including lipoproteins; in addition, an increase of both uptake of fatty acids and formation of triglycerides, and an impairment of mitochondrial fatty acid oxidation seem to contribute to the severe intrahepatocytic lipid retention (Breen et al. 1975).

Acute fatty liver of pregnancy

Histologically, the liver shows microvesicular fatty change which begins in perivenular hepatocytes and then extends to acinar zones 3 and 2, a rim of periportal hepatocytes often remaining unaffected. Cholestasis and cholangiolitis have been described in some cases (Rolfes and Ishak 1985). Although cell necrosis is not appreciated on routine hematoxylin and eosin staining, the reticulin stain shows focal areas of collapse. Necrotic debris are present in Kupffer cells on staining with PAS after diastase digestion. In the survivors, biopsy specimens obtained during the phase of recovery show patchy residual fatty change which is maximal in the perivenular areas; cholestasis and inflammation are more marked and the picture may at times be difficult to distinguish from that of a resolving hepatitis, but the extent of parenchymal collapse is invariably much less than that observed in the liver of patients recovering from a severe hepatitis having led to encephalopathy. There is no evidence of progression to chronic liver impairment in women who survive.

The pathogenesis of acute fatty liver of pregnancy is not known, but a close resemblance to Reye's syndrome which is attributed to a mitochondrial functional defect, provides ample grounds for speculation. In that respect it is of interest that acute fatty liver developed in two successive pregnancies in a patient whose offspring were subsequently shown to have an inherited defect in fatty acid oxidation (Schoeman et al. 1991).

Acute liver failure in Wilson's disease

Although Wilson's disease is accepted as a cause of acute liver failure, all 20 livers examined at autopsy or removed at transplantation in our center up to July 1992 have been cirrhotic (Davies, Williams and Portmann 1989; Rela et al. 1993); the one exception was the liver from the youngest (6 year old) patient, which was shrunken with a map-like pattern of recent parenchymal necrosis and nodular regeneration due to coexistent fulminant hepatitis E (Sallie et al. 1994). Cirrhosis is predominantly of micronodular or mixed type with yellowish nodules 0.3–1.0 cm in diameter, contrasting sharply on a red background (Figure 8.14a, Plate VI). Histologically, portoseptal and parenchymal inflammation is moderate, a few cases showing a pattern of severe chronic hepatitis, closely resembling an autoimmune hepatitis. There is evidence of recent parenchymal necrosis and/or collapse and scattered spotty necrosis with or without clusters of neutrophils. Severe hepatocyte ballooning with moderate fatty infiltration is frequent, and extensive Mallory bodies are found in approximately half the cases (Figure 8.14b, Plate VI). Florid ductular proliferation with cholestasis is common. A distinctive feature is the presence of orcein-positive granules in a patchy distribution within hepatocytes, Kupffer cells and portoseptal macrophages. Their weaker reaction for copper by the rhodanine method is presumably due to leaching of copper during tissue fixation (Figure 8.14c, Plate VI). Copper and copper-associated protein deposits predominate in periseptal areas, but the overall distribution is markedly uneven with parenchymal nodules being either diffusely loaded, or totally lacking copper. The uneven distribution of both copper and copper-free connective tissue may account for the marked variation in values of tissue copper estimation performed on small needle biopsy samples.

Budd–Chiari syndrome

The rare cases of Budd–Chiari syndrome presenting clinically as acute liver failure may reflect a very rapid onset and severe extent of the hepatic venous occlusion. Some cases follow incidental exploratory surgery without portal decompression (Powell-Jackson et al. 1986). The liver at autopsy or transplantation shows complete occlusion of the main hepatic veins with often an extension of the thrombotic process into the lumen of the inferior vena cava (Figure 8.15, Plate VI). Histologically, features of venous outflow block with extreme sinusoidal dilatation and congestion are present with particularly severe hepatocyte loss. Coagulative necrosis may be seen in this situation, probably secondary to the associated circulatory failure and shock.

Malignant infiltration

Malignant liver infiltration accounts for less than 2 percent of cases presenting with acute liver failure. Hodgkin's (Lefkowitch et al. 1985), and non-Hodgkin's lymphomas (Braude et al. 1982; Colby and La Brecque 1982), acute blastic transformation in chronic leukemia (Zafrani et al. 1983) and metastatic melanoma (Bouloux et al. 1986) and carcinomas (Schneider and Cohen 1984) have been most often incriminated. Tissue is necessary to secure the diagnosis and a liver biopsy in this situation may be rewarding especially if the infiltration is lymphomatous. In our experience, nodular or sinusoidal tumor infiltration is particularly extensive; features of venous outflow block and parenchymal necrosis are often present, but in a number of cases the extent of tumor infiltration or associated liver damage does not differ from that seen in cases without significant functional liver impairment.

ACUTE LIVER FAILURE EARLY AFTER LIVER TRANSPLANTATION

Acute allograft failure in the early post-transplant period includes primary nonfunction and hemorrhagic necrosis due to hyperacute rejection, hepatic artery thrombosis or of undetectable cause.

Primary nonfunction

Primary graft nonfunction (PGN) with no identifiable cause has been variably reported from different centers PGN is probably due to preservation injury (Chazouillères et al. 1993) and has a very high mortality unless urgent re-transplantation is performed. The explanted graft shows variable amounts of coagulative necrosis with neutrophilic infiltration and is sometimes intensely hemorrhagic. PGN cannot be predicted from changes seen in reperfusion specimens, except for the finding of severe macrovesicular fatty change for which association with PGN has been previously recognized (Portmann and Wight 1987). Large fat vacuoles are thought to interfere with the perfusion procedure and intracellular lipids may activate phospholipases with free radical formation and exacerbation of reperfusion injury (Todo et al. 1989). The explanted graft in this situation shows an oily cut surface which on histologic examination shows the formation of large sinusoidal spaces (lipopeliosis) presumably from rupture of fatty microcysts.

Hemorrhagic necrosis

In a small proportion of recipients, initial graft function is followed by sudden deterioration progessing to acute liver failure within 3 to 15 days of transplantation. In early series, such cases were ascribed to kinking of the hepatic artery and called septic hepatic gangrene because of the frequent contamination of the necrotic tissue by Gram-negative organisms. More recently, the nonspecific terminology of massive hemorrhagic necrosis was used to acknowledge the frequently hemorrhagic appearance of the graft in this situation (Hübscher et al. 1989) and the uncertainty as to the actual cause.

Hyperacute rejection

There is now good evidence that a number of cases of hemorrhagic necrosis are examples of antibody-mediated rejection or hyperacute rejection (Starzl et al. 1989). Morphologically, the major vessels are patent, the graft is swollen with a dark red congested appearance. Histology shows hemorrhagic necrosis affecting both parenchyma and portal tracts, fibrin thrombi are present in vessels, and immunohistochemistry will demonstrate bound IgG, Clq and C3. The diagnosis should be confirmed by the demonstration of donor-specific antibodies in an eluate from the failed graft (Demetris et al. 1992). Hyperacute rejection is usually, but not always, associated with a known presensitized state of the recipient, in particular ABO incompatibility (Gugenheim et al. 1990). The condition is much rarer (and the speed of onset is also slower) after liver than after kidney transplantation. This immunologic privilege of the liver has been attributed to its dual blood supply and sinusoidal architecture which makes vascular occlusion less likely. Other proposed factors include the vast number of Kupffer cells which are available for phagocytosis of any fibrin or immune complexes formed, and the release by the liver of HLA class I antigens to bind to and remove damaging antibodies (Davies, Pollard and Calne 1989).

Arterial thrombosis

Arterial thrombosis is commonest in the first few weeks after transplantation but may develop after several months. The results are often catastrophic with massive or submassive infarction of the graft. Macroscopically, the liver shows geographic areas of infarction that variously appear yellow to dark brown in color. They are softer in consistency than the adjacent parenchyma, sharply demarcated and may show a red or greenish rim at the interface with the adjacent parenchyma. After two or three weeks, severe bile duct destruction due to ischemic cholangitis often occurs producing a perihilar crescentic area of necrosis which is deeply bile stained presumably due to leakage of bile from necrotic bile ducts. There is frequent breakdown of necrotic tissue with cavity formation which may simulate an abscess on ultrasonography. This ischemic necrosis of the duct reflects the essentially arterial blood supply of the peribiliary vascular plexus.

Undetermined cause

Rarely, a similar pattern of hemorrhagic necrosis is observed within ten days of transplantation without evidence of arterial thrombosis or hyperacute rejection. A delayed preservation injury (Chazouillères et al. 1993) may be responsible in some cases, possibly aggravated by hypovolemic injury to which the denervated liver seems to be more susceptible (Henderson et al. 1992). In our center similar hemorrhagic necrosis leading to acute liver failure seven days after transplantation occurred in five patients grafted for acute liver failure of presumed viral cause, but non-A non-B non-C. In all five cases, Toga-like viral particles had been identified by electron microscopy both in the native livers and in even greater number in the hemorrhagic necrotic grafts, suggesting that hemorrhagic necrosis may also result from graft viral re-infection, possibly a single organ Shwarztman reaction (Fagan et al. 1992).

ACUTE LIVER FAILURE IN THE IMMUNOCOMPROMISED HOST

Allograft reinfection with HBV or HCV

Allograft reinfection with hepatitis B or C virus may rarely present with acute liver failure. An acute lesion with bridging and multiacinar necrosis, unlike that observed in naturally occurring HCV infection, appears exceptional (Paradis et al. 1995); superimposed on chronic changes it may lead to seemingly acute graft failure (Martin et al. 1991). The same pattern is occasionally observed in HBV recurrence and in allografts of patients who remain HBV and HCV negative. In addition, HBV recurrence may show the unique histologic pattern of fibrosing cholestatic hepatitis (FCH) (Davies et al. 1991; Benner et al. 1992) which in approximately 25 percent of cases rapidly progresses to graft failure. Once established, the lesion appears refractory to therapeutic measures. However, re-transplantation has resulted in an accelerated pace of disease recurrence and progression (O'Grady et al. 1992). Histologically, the lesion is characterized by severe parenchymal damage with hepatocyte ballooning, cytoplasmic vacuolation and glassy transformation (Figure 8.16a, Plate VII), massive accumulation of both HBV genome, and HBsAg and HBcAg products (Figure 8.16d, Plate VII). Ductal plates extend from the periportal areas into the acinus, being focally present in acinar zone 3 (Figure 8.16a and c, Plate VII). There is an extensive perisinusoidal fibrosis (Figure 8.16b) and both cellular and canalicular cholestasis is often severe. Phillips et al. (1992) have described a distinct form with particularly extensive fatty infiltration (steatoviral hepatitis B) and suggest that the cholestatic component may reflect associated sepsis. Besides the immunosuppressive therapy, the lack of identity between graft and recipient immune system and amino-acid substitutions in the HBV core gene might contribute to the unprecedented viral replication, the viral burden having been estimated at 10^{18} core particles in one liver with FCH (Phillips et al. 1992). This is bound to interfere with cell function with consequent hepatocyte injury as shown in vitro (Roingeard et al. 1991), and in HBV transgenic mice. Inhibition of normal hepatocyte regeneration is shown by a reduction in proliferative nuclear antigen (PCNA) nuclear staining, whereas the widespread occurrence of ductular plates suggests activation of an alternative cell compartment.

The lesion has become rarer due to patient selection (nonreplicators) and the use of anti-HBs immunoglobulins. FCH has been occasionally reported in HBV infection after renal transplantation (Chen et al. 1994) and in HCV recurrence after liver transplantation (Paradis et al. 1995).

Opportunistic viral infection

Adenovirus, herpes simplex virus and, to a lesser extent varicella zoster virus rarely cause acute liver failure in immunocompromised hosts (Lucas 1994). A number of fatal cases have been reported, particularly in liver transplant children who had required additional immunosuppression (Cames et al. 1992; Michaels et al. 1992). Histologically, initial changes show focal necrosis with neutrophilic collections resembling the microabscesses seen in uncomplicated cytomegalovirus infection. Viral material can be demonstrated by immunohistochemistry before typical viral inclusions can be detected by routine histologic examination (Saxena et al. 1996). These areas later develop into extensive regions of confluent necrosis. Numerous purple nuclear inclusions with a clear surrounding halo are present within viable hepatocytes at the edge of the necrotic areas (Figure 8.17a and b, Plate VIII). The specific viral agent can be demonstrated by immunostaining using corresponding antibodies or by electron microscopy.

LIVER REGENERATION AFTER CONFLUENT NECROSIS IN MAN

Liver regeneration after severe necrosis has been the subject of intense investigation, particularly in experimental animals (see Chapter 9). In man, contrary to previous belief, there is evidence that significant regeneration does occur in acute liver failure (Milandri et al. 1980). However, the regenerative process does not seem to be sufficient to sustain adequate function suggesting that the positive forces of regeneration cannot keep pace with those that cause cell necrosis. Morphologic studies in man have been somewhat hampered by the difficulty of obtaining adequate tissue, the difficulty in interpreting the complex picture produced by variably damaged or regenerating hepatocytes intermingled with mixed inflammatory cells and activated sinusoidal cells, and indeed the impossibility to make sequential observations. The first two impediments have been improved by transplantation as a unique source of better preserved liver tissue with a range of well defined patterns of damage seen at different stages of development.

After zonal necrosis or multiacinar collapse,

the spared parenchyma respectively in periportal areas or in nodules of the map-like pattern are composed of large hepatocytes with a pale staining, often microvesicular cytoplasm arranged in two-or-more cell thick plates. The sinusoids appear slit-like, mitoses are observed and over half the hepatocyte nuclei exhibit positive staining for PCNA (Koukoulis et al. 1992), indicating cell proliferation (Wolf and Michalopoulos 1992). The overall changes closely resemble those observed in the regenerating parenchyma after partial hepatectomy, with extensive confluent necrosis producing a comparable stimulus to that of partial liver resection. In cases with subtotal necrosis, as exemplified by massive coagulative necrosis after a recent acetaminophen overdose, a different type of regeneration seems to set in. In areas where necrosis reaches the portal boundaries, foci of small elongated cells with scanty, basophilic cytoplasm seem to sprout from the portal margin into the necrotic parenchyma (Figure 8.4a, Plate II) (Koukoulis et al. 1992). The cells strongly express biliary cytokeratin 19 and the majority of their oval nuclei stain for PCNA (Figure 8.4b and c, Plate II). They are morphologically identical to the oval cells described experimentally after partial hepatectomy when hepatocyte proliferation is chemically inhibited (Fausto 1994). This pattern suggests an activation of a stem cell compartment, supposedly located in the smallest units of the biliary tree (the so-called canals of Hering) into a multipotent progenitor cell which eventually differentiates. The fate of proliferating oval cells in man is unknown, but their ultimate differentiation into bile ducts or hepatocytes undoubtedly involves a delicate interplay of growth promoting factors, growth inhibiting factors and cell–matrix interactions (Sell 1990; Michalopoulos 1992; Travis 1993). In liver where total cell dropout has occurred, the periportal areas show predominantly ductular structures whose nuclei are often positive for PCNA (Figure 8.6b, Plate III). Overall, livers with complete cell dropout have had a longer disease duration and the location and proliferative state of these neoductules suggests that they may in part have originated from the "oval cells" observed earlier. A biliary modulation of residual hepatocytes seems less likely in this situation, but may also contribute to the formation of these structures. Occasional rosettes of hepatocytes which appear to be budding at the extremity of these neoductules (Figure 8.18a and b, Plate VIII) provide some support for the idea that they differentiate into hepatocytes. The factors that trigger such a differentiation may hold the key to therapy in acute liver failure.

REFERENCES

Asher, L.V.S., Innis, B.L., Shrestha, M.P., Ticehurst, J. and Baze, W.B. 1990. Virus-like particles in the liver of a patient with fulminant hepatitis and antibody to hepatitis E virus. *J Med Virol* 31: 229–33.

Benner, K.G., Lee, R.G., Keeffe, E.B. et al. 1992. Fibrosing cytolytic liver failure secondary to recurrent hepatitis B after liver transplantation. *Gastroenterology* 103: 1307–12.

Bernard, O., Hadchouel, M., Scotto, J., Odièvre, M. and Alagille, D. 1981. Severe giant cell hepatitis with autoimmune hemolytic anema in early childhood. *J Pediatr* 99: 704–11.

Bouloux, P.G.M., Goligher, J.E., Scott, R.J. and Kindell, C. 1986. Fulminant hepatic failure secondary to diffuse liver infiltration by melanoma. *J Roy Soc Med* 79: 302–3.

Bove, K.E., McAdams, A.J., Partin, J.C., Partin, J.S., Hug, G. and Schubert, W.K. 1975. The hepatic lesion in Reye's syndrome. *Gastroenterology* 69: 605–97.

Braude, S., Gimson, A.E.S., Portmann, B. and Williams, R. 1982. Fulminant hepatic failure in non-Hodgkin's lymphoma. *Postgrad Med J* 58: 301–4.

Breen, K.J., Schenker, S. and Heimberg, M. 1975. Fatty liver induced by tetracycline in the rat. Dose–response relationships and effects of sex. *Gastroenterology* 69: 714–23.

Buitrago, B., Popper, H., Hadler, S.C., Thung, S.N., Gerber, M.A., Purcell, R.H. and Maynard, J.E. 1986. Specific histological features of Santa Maria hepatitis: a severe form of hepatitis D-virus in Northern South America. *Hepatology* 6: 1285–91.

Cames, B., Rahier, J., Burtomboy, G., de Ville de Goyetet, J., Reding, R., Lamy, M., Otte, J.B. and Sokal, E.M. 1992. Acute adenovirus hepatitis in liver transplant recipients. *J Pediatr* 120: 33–7.

Chazouillères, O., Calmus, Y., Vaubourdolle, M. and Ballet, F. 1993. Preservation-induced liver injury. Clinical aspects, mechanisms and therapeutic approaches. *J Hepatol* 18: 123–34.

Chen, C.-H., Chen, P.-J., Chu, J.-S., Yeh, K.-H., Lai, M.-Y. and Chen, D.-S. 1994. Fibrosing cholestatic hepatitis in a hepatitis B surface antigen carrier after renal transplantation. *Gastroenterology* 107: 1514–18.

Colby, T.V. and La Brecque, D.R. 1982. Lymphoreticular malignancy presenting as fulminant hepatic disease. *Gastroenterology* 82: 339–45.

Davies, H.S., Pollard, S.G. and Calne, R.Y. 1989. Soluble HLA antigens in the circulation of liver graft recipients. *Transplantation* 47: 524–7.

Davies, S.E., Williams, R. and Portmann, B. 1989. Hepatic morphology and histochemistry of Wilson's disease presenting as fulminant hepatic failure: a study of 11 cases. *Histopathology* 15: 385–94.

Davies, S.E., Portmann, B.C., O'Grady, J.G. et al. 1991. Hepatic histological findings after liver transplantation for chronic hepatitis B virus infection, including a unique pattern of fibrosing cholestatic hepatitis. *Hepatology* 13: 150–7.

Davies, S.E. and Portmann, B.C. 1994. Drugs and toxins. In *Systemic Pathology, 3rd edn. Vol 11, Liver biliary Tract and Exocrine Pancreas*, eds. D.G.D. Wight and W.St.C. Symmers, 201–36. Edinburgh: Churchill Livingstone.

de la Monte, S.M., Arcide, J.M., Moore, G.W. and Hutchins, G.M. 1984. Midzonal necrosis as a pattern of hepatocellular injury after shock. *Gastroenterology* 86: 627–31.

Demetris, A.J., Nakamura, K., Yagihashi, A., Iwaki, Y., Takaya, S., Hartman, G.C., Murase, N., Bronsther, O., Manez, R., Fung, J.J., Iwatsuki, S. and Starzl, T.E. 1992. A clinicopathological study of human liver allograft recipents harboring preformed IgG lymphocytoxic antibodies. *Hepatology* 16: 671–82.

Dixon, M.F., Nimmo, J. and Prescott, L.F. 1971. Experimental paracetamol-induced hepatic necrosis: a histopathological study. *J Pathol* 103: 225–9.

Enzan, H., Himeno, H., Iwamura, S., Saibara, T., Onishi, S., Yamamoto, Y., Miyazaki, E. and Hara, H. 1995. Sequential changes in human Ito cells and their relation to postnecrotic liver fibrosis in massive and submassive hepatic necrosis. *Virchows Archiv* 426: 95–101.

Fagan, E.A., David, E.S., Tovey, G.M., Lloyd, G., Smith, H.M., Portmann, B., Tan, K-C., Zuckerman, A.J. and Williams, R. 1992. Toga virus-like particles in acute liver failure attributed to sporadic non-A, non-B hepatitis and recurrence after liver transplantation. *J Med Virol* 38: 71–7.

Fausto, N. 1994. Liver stem cells. In *The Liver: Biology and Pathobiology*, 3rd edn., eds. I.M. Arias, J.L. Boyer, N. Fausto, W.B. Jakoby, D.A. Schachter and D.A. Shafritz, 1501–18. New York: Raven Press.

Goudie, B.M., Birnie, G.F., Watkinson, G., MacSween, R.N.M., Kissen, L.H. and Cunningham, N.E. 1982. Jaundice associated with the use of benoxaprofen. *Lancet* i: 959.

Gugenheim, J., Samuel, D., Reynès, M. and Bismuth, H. 1990. Liver transplantation across ABO blood group barriers. *Lancet* 336: 519–23.

Hawkins, A.E., Gilson, R.J., Beath, S.V., Boxall, E.H., Kelly, D.A., Tedder, R.S. and Weller, I.V. 1994. Novel application of a point mutation assay: evidence for transmission of hepatitis B viruses with precore mutations and their detection in infants fulminant hepatitis. *Br J Med Virol* 44: 13–21.

Henderson, J.M., Mackay, G.J., Lumsden, A.B., Atta, H.M., Brouillard, R. and Kutner, M.H. 1992. The effect of liver denervation on hepatic haemodynamics during hypovolaemic shock in swine. *Hepatology* 15: 130–3.

Hübscher, S.G., Adams, D.H., Buckles, J.A.C., McMaster, J.A., Neuberger, J. and Elias, E. 1989. Massive haemorrhagic necrosis of the liver after liver transplantation. *J Clin Pathol* 42: 360–70.

Ishak, K.G., Walker, D.H., Coetzer, J.A.W., Gardner, J.J. and Gorelkin, L. 1982. Viral hemorrhagic fevers with hepatic involvement: pathologic aspects with clinical correlations. In *Progress in Liver Diseases*, vol VII, eds. H. Popper and F. Schaffner, 495–515. New York: Grune & Stratton.

Koukoulis, G., Rayner, A., Tan, K.C., Williams, R. and Portmann, B. 1992. Immunolocalization of regenerating cells after submassive liver necrosis using PCNA staining. *J Pathol* 166: 359–68.

Lefkowitch, J.H. 1982. Bile ductular cholestasis: an ominous histopathologic sign related to sepsis and "cholangitis lenta". *Hum Pathol* 13: 19–24.

Lefkowitch, J.H., Falkow, S. and Whitlock, R.T. 1985. Hepatic Hodgkin's disease simulating cholestatic hepatitis with liver failure. *Arch Pathol Lab Med* 109: 424–6.

Lefkowitch, J.H., Schiff, E.R., Davis, G.L., Perrillo, R.P., Lindsay, K., Bodenheimer, H.C. Jr., Balart, L.A., Ortego, T.J., Payne, J., Dienstag, J.L., Gibas, A., Jacobson, I.M., Tamburro, C.H., Carey, W., O'Brien, C., Sampliner, R., Van Thiel, D.H., Feit, D., Albrecht, J., Maschievitz, C., Sanghavi, B. and Vaughan, R.D. 1993. Pathological diagnosis of chronic hepatitis C: a multicenter comparative study with chronic hepatitis B. *Gastroenterology* 104: 595–603.

Liang, T.J., Hasegawa, K., Rimon, N., Wands, J.R. and Ben-Porath, E. 1991. A hepatitis B virus mutant associated with an epidemic of fulminant hepatitis. *N Engl J Med* 324: 1705–9.

Lucas, S.B. 1994. Other viral and infectious diseases and HIV-related liver disease. In *Pathology of the Liver*, 3rd edn., eds. R.N.M. MacSween, P.P. Anthony, P.J. Scheuer, A.D. Burt and B.C. Portmann, 269–315. Edinburgh: Churchill Livingstone.

Martin, P., Munoz, S.J., Di Bisceglie, A.M., Rubin, R., Waggoner, J.G., Armenti, V.T., Moritz, M.J., Jarrell, B.E. and Maddrey, W.C. 1991. Recurrence of hepatitis C virus infection after orthotopic liver transplantation. *Hepatology* 13: 719–21.

Mathew, J., Hines, J.E., James, O.F.W. and Burt, A.D. 1994. Non-parenchymal cell response in paracetamol (acetaminophen)-induced liver injury. *J Hepatol* 20: 537–41.

Michaels, M.G., Green, M., Wald., E.R. and Starzl, T.E. 1992. Adenovirus infection in pediatric liver transplant recipients. *J Infect Dis* 165: 170–4.

Michalopoulos, G. 1992. Liver regeneration and growth factors: Old puzzles and new perspectives. *Lab Invest* 67: 413–15.

Milandri, M., Gaub, J. and Ranek, L. 1980. Evidence for liver cell proliferation during fatal hepatic failure. *Gut* 21: 423–7.

Mori, W., Machinami, R., Shiga, J., Taguchi, T., Tanaka, K., Fukusato, T., Hasegawa, A., Aoki, N., Narita, T., Kikuchi, F., Kodama, T., Irie, H., Oka, T., Yoshimura, A. and Aoyama, H. 1984. A pathological study of fulminant liver disease. *Acta Pathol Jpn* 34: 727–42.

Nouel, O., Herrion, J. and Degott, C. 1980. Fulminant hepatic failure due to transient circulatory failure in patients with chronic heart disease. *Dig Dis Sci* 25: 49–52.

O'Grady, J.G., Smith, H.M., Davies, S.E., Daniels, H.M., Doanaldson, P.T., Tan, K.C., Portmann, B., Alexander, G.J.M. and Williams, R. 1992. Hepatitis B reinfection after orthotopic liver transplantation. Serological and clinical implication. *J Hepatol* 14: 104–11.

O'Grady, J.G., Portmann, B. and Williams, R. 1993. Fulminant hepatic failure. In *Diseases of the Liver*, 7th edn., Vol. 2, eds. L. Schiff and E.R. Schiff, 1077–90. Philadelphia: JB Lippincott.

Omata, M., Ehata, T., Yokosuka, O., Hosoda, M. and Ohta, M. 1991. Mutations in the pre-core region of hepatitis B virus DNA in patients with fulminant and severe hepatitis. *N Engl J Med* 324: 1699–704.

Paradis, V., Sebagh, M., Fétay, C., Samuel, D. and Bismuth, H. 1995. Unusual and severe evolution of liver transplant recipients reinfected by hepatitis C virus. *Path Res Pract* 191–748 (Abstract).

Partin, J.C., Schubert, W.K. and Partin, J.S. 1971. Mitochondrial ultrastructure in Reye's syndrome (encephalopathy and fatty degeneration of the viscera). *N Engl J Med* 285: 1339–43.

Phillips, M.J., Blendis, L.M., Poucell, S., Patterson, J., Petrie, M., Roberts, E., Levy, G.A. et al. 1991. Syncitial giant-cell hepatitis: sporadic hepatitis with distinctive pathological features, a severe clinical course, and paramyxoviral features. *N Engl J Med* 324: 455–60.

Phillips, M.J. and Poucell, S. 1981. Modern aspects of the morphology of viral hepatitis. *Hum Pathol* 12: 1060–84.

Phillips, M.J., Cameron, R., Flowers, M.A., Blendis, L.M., Greig, P.D., Wanless, I., Sherman, M., Superina, R., Langer, B. and Levy, G.A. 1992. Post-transplant recurrent hepatitis B viral disease: Viral-burden, steatoviral, and fibroviral hepatitis B. *Am J Pathol* 140: 1295–308.

Portmann, B. and Wight, D.G.D. 1987. Pathology of liver transplantation (excluding rejection). In *Liver Transplantation*, ed. R.Y. Calne, 2nd edn., 437–70. London: Grune & Stratton.

Portmann, B., Talbot, I.C., Day, D.W., Davidson, A.R., Murray-Lyon, I.M. and Williams, R. 1975. Histopathological changes in the liver following a paracetamol overdose: correlation with clinical and biochemical parameters. *J Pathol* 117: 169–81.

Powell-Jackson, P.R., Tredger, J.M. and Williams, R. 1984. Hepatotoxicity to sodium valproate: a review. *Gut* 25: 673–81.

Powell-Jackson, P.R., Ede, R.J. and Williams, R. 1986. Budd–Chiari syndrome presenting as fulminant hepatic failure. *Gut* 27: 1101–5.

Rela, M., Heaton, N.D., Vougas, V., McEntee, G., Gane, E., Fahrat, B., Chiyende, J., Mieli-Vergani, G., Mowat, A.P., Portmann, B. and Williams, R. 1993. Orthotopic liver transplantation for hepatic complications of Wilson's disease. *Br J Surg* 80: 909–11.

Roingeard, P., Romet-Lemonne, J-L. and Essex, M. 1991. Correlation between cytoplasmic HBcAg and HBV replication in HepG2 transfected cloned cells and cytopathic effect associated with nuclear HBcAg accumulation in an HBV nonproducer clone. In *Viral Hepatitis and Liver Disease*, eds. F.B. Hollinger, S.M. Lemon, H.S. Margolis, 308–13. Baltimore: Williams & Wilkins.

Rolfes, D.B. and Ishak, K.G. 1985. Acute fatty liver of pregnancy: a clinicopathologic study of 35 cases. *Hepatology* 5: 1149–58.

Sallie, R., Silva, A.E., Purdy, M., Smith, H., McCaustland, K., Tibbs, C., Portmann, B., Eddleston, A., Bradley, D. and Williams, R. 1994. Hepatitis C and E in non-A non-B fulminant hepatic failure: polymerase chain reaction and serological study. *J Hepatol* 20: 580–8.

Sato, S., Susuki, K., Akahane, Y., Akamatsu, K., Akiyama, K., Unomura, K., Tsuda, F., Tanaka, T., Okamoto, H., Miyakawa, Y. and Mayumi, M. 1995. Hepatitis B virus strains with mutations in the core promoter in patients with fulminant hepatitis. *Ann Intern Med* 122: 241–8.

Saxena, R., Tovey, D.G., Dhawan, A., Ellis, D.S. and Portmann, B.C. 1996. Acute liver failure due to adenoviral hepatitis in a pediatric liver transplant. *Int J Surg Pathol* 3: 189–94.

Scheurlen, C., Spannbrucker, N., Spengler, U., Zachoval, R., Schulte-Witte, H., Brensing, K.-A. and Sauerbruch, T. 1994. *Amanita phalloides* intoxications in a family of Russian immigrants. Case report and review of the literature with a focus on orthotopic liver transplantation. *Z Gastroenterol* 32: 399–404.

Schneider, R. and Cohen, A. 1984. Fulminant hepatic failure complicating metastatic breast carcinoma. *South Med J* 77: 84–6.

Schoeman, M.N., Batey, R.G. and Wilcken, B. 1991. Recurrent acute fatty liver of pregnancy associated with a fatty-acid oxidation defect in the offspring. *Gastroenterology* 100: 544–8.

Sell, S. 1990. Is there a liver stem cell? *Cancer Res* 50: 3811–15.

Shibuya, A., Unuma, T., Sugimoto, T., Yamakado, M., Tagawa, H., Tagawa, K., Tanaka, S. and Takanashi, R. 1985. Diffuse hepatic calcification as a sequela to shock liver. *Gastroenterology* 89: 196–201.

Smedile, A., Farci, P., Verme, G., Caredda, F., Cagnel, A., Caporaso, N., Dentico, P., Trepo, C., Opolon, P., Gimson, A., Vergani, D. and Williams, R. 1982. Influence of delta infection on severity of hepatitis B. *Lancet* ii: 945–7.

Sokal, E.M., Trivedi, P., Portmann, B. and Mowat, A.P. 1990. Adaptive changes of metabolic zonation during the development of cirrhosis in the growing rats. *Gastroenterology* 99: 785–92.

Starzl, T.E., Demetris, A.J., Todo, S., Kang, Y., Tzakis, A., Duquesnoy, R., Makowka, L., Banner, B., Concepcion, W. and Porter, K.A. 1989. Evidence for hyperacute rejection of human liver grafts: The case of the canary kidneys. *Clin Transpl* 3: 37–48.

Todo, S., Demetris, A.J., Makowaka, L., Teperman, L., Podesta, L., Shaver, T., Tzakis, A. and Starzl, T.E. 1989. Primary nonfunction of hepatic allografts with preexisting fatty infiltration. *Transplantation* 47: 903–5.

Travis, J. 1993. The search for liver stem cells picks up. *Science* 259: 1829.

Waldman, R.J., Hall, W.N., McGee, H. and Amburg, G.V. 1982. Aspirin as a risk factor in Reye's syndrome. *JAMA* 247: 3089–94.

Wolf, H.K. and Michalopoulos, G.K. 1992. Hepatocyte regeneration in acute fulminant and nonfulminant hepatitis: A study of proliferating cell nuclear antigen expression. *Hepatology* 15: 707–13.

Yoshiba, M., Dehara, K., Inoue, K., Okamoto, H. and Mayumi, M. 1994. Contribution of hepatitis C virus to non-A, non-B fulminant hepatitis in Japan. *Hepatology* 19: 829–35.

Zafrani, E.S. and Berthelot, P. 1982. Sodium valproate in the induction of unusual hepatotoxicity. *Hepatology* 2: 648–9.

Zafrani, E.S., Leclercq, B., Vernan, J.-P., Pinaudeau, Y., Chomette, G. and Dhumeaux, D. 1983. Massive blastic infiltrations of the liver: a cause of fulminant hepatic failure. *Hepatology* 3: 428–32.

Zimmerman, H.J. and Ishak, K.G. 1982. Valproate-induced hepatic injury: analysis of 23 fatal cases. *Hepatology* 2: 591–7.

Zimmerman, H.J. and Ishak, K.G. 1994. Hepatic injury due to drugs and toxins. In *Pathology of the Liver*, 3rd edn., eds. R.N.M. MacSween, P.P. Anthony, P.J. Scheuer, A.D. Burt and B.C. Portmann, 563–633. Edinburgh: Churchill Livingstone.

9 Hepatocyte replication and liver regeneration

Nelson Fausto

INTRODUCTION

Hepatocytes are highly differentiated cells which have little proliferative activity in adult livers of humans or animals. Nevertheless, the proliferative capacity of hepatocytes is not lost and is rapidly activated in response to decreases in functional hepatic mass caused by tissue resection or cell death (Bucher and Malt 1971; Fausto and Webber 1994). During the last few years much new information has become available on the role of transcription factors, proto-oncogenes and growth factors as mediators of the process by which quiescent hepatocytes enter the cell cycle and replicate. Most of this knowledge has been obtained from studies of liver regeneration after partial hepatectomy (PH) in rodents and from work with cultured hepatocytes. In liver regeneration induced by partial hepatectomy, hepatocyte replication occurs in the absence of concomitant cell death and fibrogenesis. Thus, the system is most suitable for the analysis of the molecular mechanisms of hepatocyte replication and growth factor effects. Moreover the results of these studies are applicable to the understanding of growth regulation in human livers. However, hepatocyte replication in humans often takes place in diseased livers in which the tissue architecture is grossly altered, or, in the case of acute hepatic failure, in an organ with massive cell death and impaired function.

It is not known whether the molecular mechanisms of hepatic replication after partial hepatectomy of a normal organ differ from those which regulate hepatocyte proliferation after severe injury. It appears that once hepatocytes enter the cell cycle, the progressive steps traversed by these cells is the same, regardless of the nature of the inducing event. There are, however, some identifiable differences between regeneration after PH and hepatocyte replication in response to cell death.

1. After PH, practically all hepatocytes replicate and there is no evidence for the activation of a stem cell compartment. In contrast, in regeneration after injury and specifically in acute hepatic failure there is involvement of a stem cell compartment (Fausto and Webber 1994; Fausto 1994).
2. Although the cell cycle progression steps taken by hepatocytes may be the same in any type of liver growth, the mediators responsible for initiating the process and making the cells move from quiescence into the cycle (priming or competence step) may differ depending on the cause of the regenerative process.
3. Hepatocyte replication taking place in an organ with intact extracellular matrix scaffolding results in complete restoration of liver structure. This is the case after PH and even in situations such as experimental acute toxic liver injury and in livers of patients who recover from acute

failure in which widespread destruction of hepatocytes has occurred. In contrast, hepatocyte proliferation in cirrhotic livers or in experimentally induced chronic liver injury leads to distorted tissue architecture and nodule formation (Figure 9.1).

GENERAL PRINCIPLES OF LIVER GROWTH REGULATION

The liver has the capacity to regulate its growth and size. This property is unique to hepatic tissue and is quite remarkable when one considers the multitude of stimuli and factors both systemic and intrahepatic, that influence liver growth. Hepatocyte replication can be controlled by growth factors and cytokines produced by hepatocytes themselves (autocrine regulation), or by liver nonparenchymal cells (paracrine regulation). Growth factors, cytokines, and hormones which have effects on hepatocyte DNA synthesis can also be produced in extrahepatic sites and be released in the circulation (endocrine regulation). Finally, within the liver, growth regulation may take place through the effects of growth factors or cytokines which are anchored in the cell membrane as part of large precursor molecules. Such molecules can serve to promote both growth and cell adhesion by linking the cell containing membrane-bound ligands with adjacent cells that have the specific receptors for the ligands (juxtacrine regulation). Regardless of their site of production and mode of action many growth factors induce hepatocyte replication (see below). However, transforming growth factor beta (TGF-β), activin and the FAS antigen/ligand system inhibit DNA synthesis and cause apoptosis (Braun et al. 1988; Yasuda et al. 1993; Schwall et al. 1993; Schulte-Hermann et al. 1993).

The simplest way to understand the mechanisms of liver growth regulation is to assume that they involve an appropriate balance between positive and negative stimuli. Although in a general sense this is a valid concept, certain experimental observations do not entirely support this assumption. For instance, if a balance between positive and negative effectors determines hepatocyte replication, it would be expected that expression of inhibitor molecules would be high in normal livers, and would decrease during growth processes. Yet, expression of the inhibitor molecules TGF-β and activin is very low in normal livers but increases during liver regeneration, a pattérn of change that is the opposite of that predicted (Yasuda et al. 1993; Schwall et al. 1993; Jakowlew et al. 1991). Moreover, these factors not only inhibit hepatocyte DNA synthesis but also cause apoptosis. This is demonstrated by increased expression of TFG-β, activin and FAS (Oberhammer et al. 1992) in conditions in which there is either a reduction in the number of hepatocytes (during starvation or the withdrawal of growth stimuli) or an increase in hepatocyte turnover (hepatocarcinogenesis). In particular, the FAS system appears to play a major role in massive hepatocyte death occurring in acute hepatic failure (Ogasawara et al. 1994). Although expression of inhibitors or inducers of apoptosis would be expected to occur in physiologic and pathologic conditions that involve cell death, it is still a puzzle why TGF-β and activin expression increase during liver regeneration after PH. Perhaps the simultaneous activation of factors that promote and inhibit DNA replication during liver regeneration is a hallmark of regulated growth processes in the liver, that is, processes which have a defined end point. The simultaneous activity of positive and negative regulatory loops in the regenerating may be the key feature that makes the liver capable of regulating its own growth. It follows that the disruption of either one or both of these circuits can lead to uncontrolled growth and eventually, carcinogenesis.

The set point which determines the appropriate liver size is the ratio between hepatic functional mass and body mass. This ratio is relatively constant in adult human and animals and is rapidly corrected whenever its optimal level is exceeded or decreased. Decrease of the functional liver mass/body

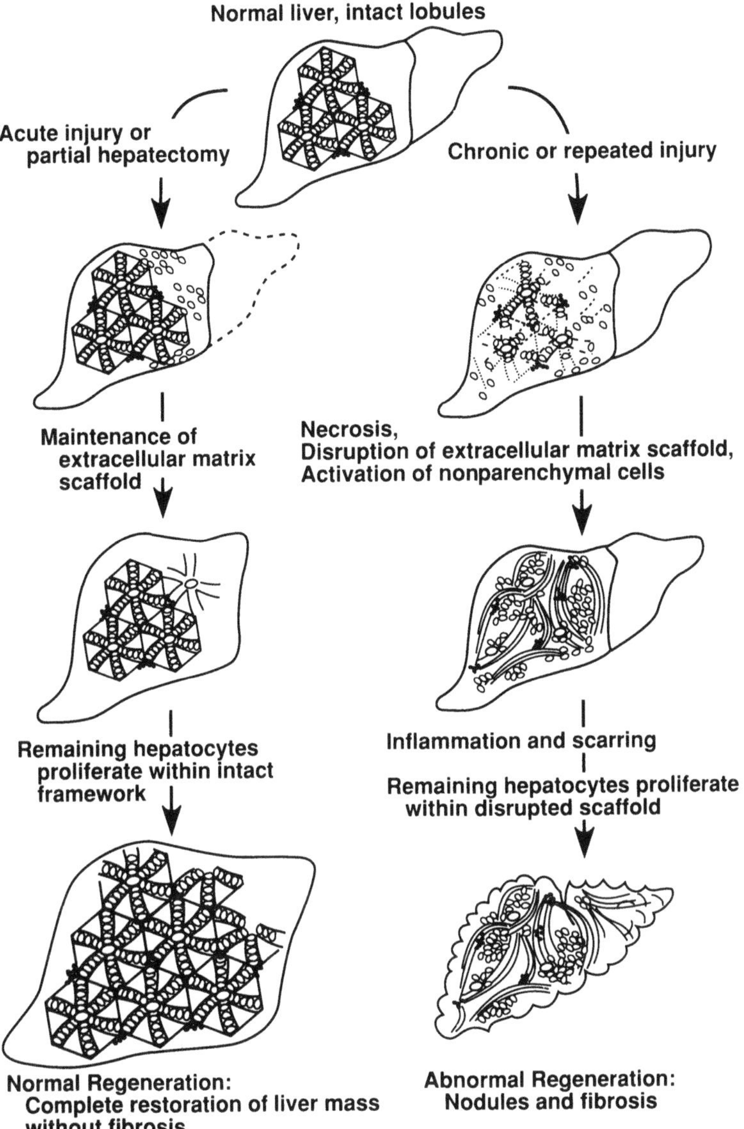

Figure 9.1 Diagram of normal and abnormal liver regeneration. The left side of the figure illustrates complete restoration of liver mass after acute injury, partial hepatectomy and acute hepatic failure without pre-existing chronic liver disease. The right side illustrates hepatocyte replication occurring in chronic or repeated acute injury in which despite hepatocyte proliferation, the liver architecture is abnormal with scar formation and cirrhosis.

mass ratio occurs in conditions such as partial hepatectomy, acute liver failure and "small for size" transplants. In contrast, where there is excess functional hepatic tissue in relationship to body demands the liver mass/body mass ratio increases, as in drug or hormonally induced liver hyperplasia and "large for size" transplants. Decreases in the ratio initiate a growth response in the liver while its increase triggers apoptosis. These general rules are best demonstrated by examining the patterns of growth and apoptosis which occur after liver transplantation in animals and humans. A "small for size" transplant will grow until the transplanted liver reaches the appropriate size for that particular host, at which point growth terminates (Francavilla et al. 1994). In contrast, a "large for size" transplant will not grow and may diminish in size presumably by apoptosis (Kam et al. 1987). The understanding of these properties of hepatic tissue have led to the successful development of split transplant procedures as well as liver transplantation from living donors. A further example of a similar type of growth regulation is provided by cases of heterotopic liver transplantation in which, for unknown reasons, the natural liver recovered its function after transplantation of the new liver (Willemse et al. 1992). Under these conditions the heterotopically transplanted liver became atrophic, indicating that at any one time after transplantation the functional equivalent of only a single liver (either the natural organ or the transplant) was operative.

How does the liver "know" when to start and stop growing? On the basis of experimental and clinical data one can postulate that there may be a coordinate regulation of hepatocyte proliferation and apoptosis. A transgenic mouse model in which the animals overexpress transforming growth factor alpha (TGF-α) provides an interesting example of a linkage between proliferation and apoptosis in the liver (Webber, Wu et al. 1994). Because TGF-α is a strong hepatic mitogen, young TGF-α transgenic mice have hyperplastic livers which are 25–40 percent larger than normal. However, by six months of age, livers of the transgenic mice have similar weights as those of nontransgenic animals the same age, despite enhanced hepatocyte proliferation (Sandgren et al. 1990; Webber, Wu et al. 1994). In the transgenic mouse livers of six-month-old animals, high levels of hepatocyte proliferation are compensated by fast cell turnover and apoptosis, which restore the normal ratio between hepatic functional mass and body weight. Eventually, the balance between proliferation and apoptosis breaks down and liver tumors develop in most of the transgenic mice after 12 months of age. These studies suggest that excessive (non-neoplastic) hepatocyte proliferation may by itself trigger an apoptotic response. The understanding of the interactions between hepatocyte proliferation and apoptosis is of fundamental importance and requires the detailed knowledge of each of these processes. This chapter deals with only one of these processes and focuses on the molecular mechanisms of cell proliferation.

MOLECULAR MECHANISMS OF LIVER REGENERATION

Studies of liver regeneration after partial hepatectomy have shown that replication of hepatocytes in the regenerating liver involves a series of steps (Fausto and Mead 1989; Michalopoulos 1990). We have proposed that the events can be broadly divided into two phases: priming or competence, corresponding to the G_0 to G_1 transition; and progression, in which hepatocytes progress through the cell cycle and replicate. After PH in rats, the priming phase roughly corresponds to the first 2–4 h of the process while DNA synthesis (S phase) starts at 12–14 h and reaches a maximum 24 h later. The process is well synchronized and is followed by a wave of mitosis between 24 and 32 h. During liver regeneration after PH about 95 percent of hepatocytes divide at least once while a smaller proportion of hepatocytes divides twice (Bucher and Malt 1971; Grisham 1962). The regenerative process consists of the growth of a liver remnant corresponding to 30–32 percent of the original liver into an organ which weighs approximately the same as the original liver before resection. In rodents, regeneration after PH takes approximately 7–10 days to complete. In humans, complete regeneration after PH may take 2–3 months but the rate of growth depends on the extent of the resection and the integrity of the liver tissue (Yamanaka et al. 1993). In rodents there is a threshold value for the extent of resection below which no growth response is elicited (Bucher 1963). In adult animals, removal of less than one third of the liver (the standard operation is a 68 percent hepatectomy) does not induce growth. Both in humans and animals the hepatic lobes or segments excised at surgery do not regrow. Instead, the growth process consists of the expansion of the remaining parts of the organ to compensate for the loss of tissue. Thus, "regeneration" of the liver is actually a process of compensatory hyperplasia that does not involve the restitution of lost parts.

Many of the studies on hepatocyte replication after PH have sought to establish links between the events which occur in the first 2–4 h after the operation and the wave of DNA synthesis which starts at 12 h and reaches a maximum at 24 h. Analysis of the role of transcription factors, growth factors, protooncogenes and cyclins have received particular emphasis in these studies. A possible sequence of events for liver regeneration after PH which includes all of these agents is presented in Figure 9.2. The sequential gene activation events occurring during liver regeneration can be placed into three categories: transcription factor activation; primary or "immediate early" gene response; and secondary gene response. These responses are outlined in Figure 9.3 and discussed below.

Transcription factor activation after partial hepatectomy

Transcription factors: Tissue specificity and relationship with gene activation

Transcription factors are proteins that bind to specific recognition sequences in DNA and cause transcription of the genes to which they bind (Zaret 1994). Some years ago it was assumed that each transcription factor would specifically bind only a single gene. It is now known that binding sequences for the same transcription factor are found in many different genes and that individual genes have a multitude of sites capable of binding many different transcription factors. Genes for proteins that are preferentially expressed in the liver are regulated by families of transcription factors which are enriched in hepatic tissue (Zaret 1994). For instance, the transcriptional activity of liver "specific" genes such as those for albumin, alphafetoprotein, fibrinogens and alpha-1-antitrypsin is regulated by at least four families of transcription factors which include the hepatocyte nuclear factors 1, 3, and 4 (HNF-1, HNF-3 and HNF-4) and CAAT/enhancer binding protein (C/EBP). Genes not associated with proteins which are preferentially expressed in the liver are regulated by different sets of transcriptional factors. Most importantly, the expression of genes involved in mitogenic and stress responses is regulated by transcription factors found in most cell types and not preferentially restricted to the liver. These ubiquitous factors control transcription of sets of genes required for these responses in whatever tissue they may occur. At least three of these non-tissue specific transcription factors namely NF-κB, AP1 and STAT3 (Table 9.1) are of major interest for liver regeneration because they are activated and bind to DNA within the first 30 min after PH

Table 9.1. *Transcription factor families*

Liver enriched transcription factor families	
Factor	*Family*
HNF1 (Hepatocyte nuclear factor 1)	"POU – homeodomain protein family"
HNF3 (Hepatocyte nuclear factor 3)	"Forkhead family"
HNF4 (Hepatocyte nuclear factor 4)	"Nuclear receptor family"
C/EBP (CAAT enhancer binding protein)	"Leucine zipper family"
Non-tissue-enriched transcription factors involved in liver proliferative responses	
NF-κB	(Nuclear factor for kappa gene enhancer of B cells)
AP1	(Complex formed by jun homodimers or jun/fos heterodimers)
STAT3	(Signal transducers and activators of transcription also known as APRF, acute-phase response factor)

(FitzGerald et al. 1995; Tewari et al. 1992; Diehl et al. 1994; Cressman et al. 1994; Cressman et al. 1995). NF-κB responds to a variety of extracellular stimuli and activates genes involved in many different types of responses (see below and Figure 9.4). AP1 is induced in cell cultures by mitogenic stimuli and is constituted by c-jun/c-fos heterodimers or jun homodimers. API regulates the transcription of genes that respond to mitogens and initiate a proliferative cascade, although the same genes may also be involved in

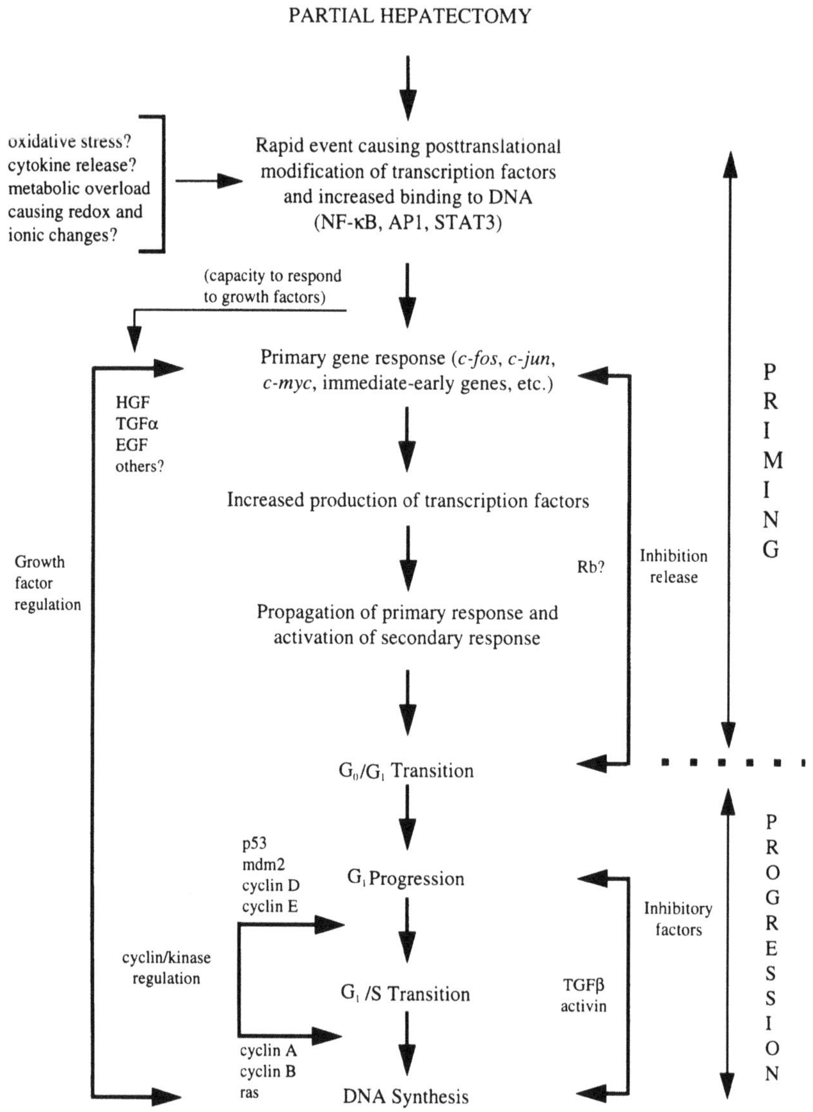

PARTIAL HEPATECTOMY
oxidative stress?
cytokine release?
metabolic overload
causing redox and
ionic changes?
Rapid event causing posttranslational modification of transcription factors and increased binding to DNA (NF-κB, AP1, STAT3)
(capacity to respond to growth factors)
Primary gene response (*c-fos*, *c-jun*, *c-myc*, immediate-early genes, etc.)
HGF
TGFα
EGF
others?
Increased production of transcription factors
Growth factor regulation
Rb?
Inhibition release
Propagation of primary response and activation of secondary response
G_0/G_1 Transition
PRIMING
p53
mdm2
cyclin D
cyclin E
G_1 Progression
cyclin/kinase regulation
G_1 /S Transition
TGFβ
activin
Inhibitory factors
cyclin A
cyclin B
ras
DNA Synthesis
PROGRESSION

Figure 9.2 Overview of major events in hepatocyte replication after partial hepatectomy. The events are divided into two major phases, priming and progression. Priming involves the transit of quiescent hepatocytes into the G_1 phase of the cell cycle and include two major steps: (a) a rapid phase of transcription factor activation (NF-κB, AP1 and STAT3) and (b) the primary ("immediate-early") gene response. Several potential initiators of liver regeneration are listed. The diagram indicates that transcription factor activation may make hepatocytes fully respond to growth factors which regulate the primary gene response. The progression phase involves a secondary gene response in which cyclins and cell cycle progression genes are expressed.

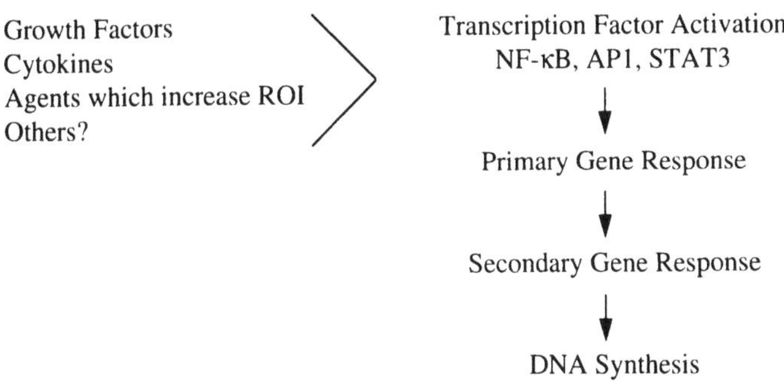

Figure 9.3 Summary of the major phases of liver regeneration (see Figure 9.2 for details).

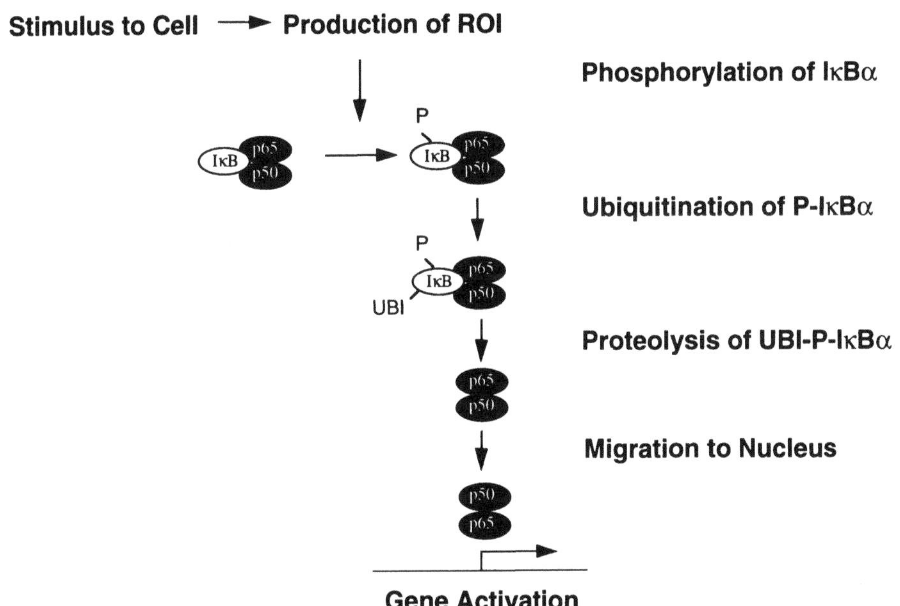

Figure 9.4 Activation of the transcription factor NF-κB at the start of liver regeneration. The factor is present in the cytoplasm in an inactive complex in which its heterodimer components p65 and p50 are bound to the inhibitor molecule IκB. Activation of NF-κB depends on the removal of IκB from the complex which takes place in several steps. It is believed that the initiation stimulus involves the production of reactive oxygen intermediates (ROI) by either metabolic overload or the action of a cytokine such as TNF. It is not known whether liver growth factors such as EGF, TGF-α and HGF can also generate ROI to activate the system. Degradation of IκB requires three steps shown on the right side of the figure. The active NF-κB complex migrates to the nucleus and turns on transcription of target genes which contain a NF-κB recognition sequence.

nonproliferative responses. STAT3 belongs to the category of factors known as signal transducers and activators of transcription, that is proteins that shuttle from the cell membrane into the nucleus where they bind to DNA target sequences (Figure 9.5). In cultured cells STAT3 can be activated by growth factors (EGF) and cytokines (IL-6). In this chapter we confine the analysis of transcription factor activation after PH to NF-κB activity. A listing of various transcription factors and their abbreviations is shown in Table 9.1.

NF-κB activation after partial hepatectomy

NF-κB comprises a family of proteins related to the rel oncogene and the *Drosophila* gene dorsal that can form homo- and heterodimers (Grilli et al. 1993). In most cells the major

STAT 3 Signal Transduction and Gene Activation

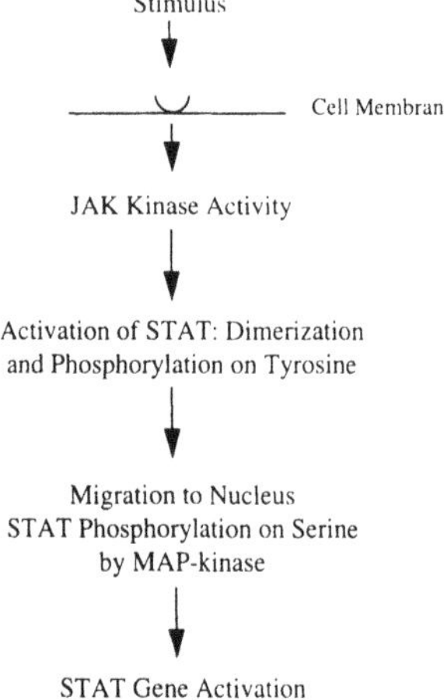

Figure 9.5 STAT3 activation and Signal Transduction Mechanisms. STAT3 is a transcription factor which belongs to the STAT (signal transduction and activation of transcription) family. It is also known as APRF (acute phase response factor) because it can be activated by cytokines such as IL-6 in acute phase response. It is also activated by EGF. STAT3 receives an extracellular stimulus, becomes activated and migrates into the nucleus where it binds and turns on transcription in genes that have a STAT3 recognition sequence. STAT3 activation involves: (a) dimerization and phosphorylation of a tyrosine residue which is accomplished by an enzyme named JAK kinase and (b) a second phosphorylation event in which a serine residue is phosphorylated by an enzyme named MAP-kinase.

NF-κB form is a heterodimer formed by two subunits referred to as p50 and p65 (Figure 9.4). The heterodimer containing the two subunits forms a complex with a protein named IκB (inhibitor of κB). The complex is inactive and its activation degradation of IκB (Beg and Baldwin 1993). Freed from the inhibitor, the heterodimer migrates into the cell nucleus and binds to a specific recognition sequence contained in many genes (target genes). Originally described in lymphocytes, NF-κB proteins have been detected in many different cell types and found to participate in diverse cellular responses that include gene activation associated with injury, inflammation, vascular reactions, viral replication, and cell proliferation (Liou and Baltimore 1993). NF-κB activation is a rapid process that involves post-translation modification of proteins triggered by many different types of stimuli such as endotoxins (LPS), TNF, IL-1, IL-2, ultraviolet light, and oxidants. Its target genes include surface immunoglobulins, adhesion molecules, cytokines, acute phase response genes, the c-myc proto-oncogene and viruses such as HIV (Grilli et al. 1993; Liou and Baltimore 1993). The activation pathway for NF-κB induced by most if not all agents, converges into an intracellular step that involves oxidant molecules. Anderson et al. (1994) suggested that the common pathway of NF-κB activation involves the generation of mitochondrial oxidants followed by protein phosphorylation and degradation of IκB (Figure 9.4). Recent data demonstrate that degradation of IκB involves two steps: phosphorylation by an oxidant sensitive kinase; and digestion of the phosphorylated form of proteases contained in proteasomes, which are large multiprotease cytoplasmic particles (Palombella et al. 1994).

Analysis by electrophoretic shift mobility assays (ESMA) showed that NF-κB (p50/p65 heterodimer), is activated in the liver very shortly after PH (Cressman et al. 1994; Fitz-Gerald et al. 1995). In addition, there is also increased binding of p50 homodimers as well as binding of a smaller component of lower molecular weight that corresponds to the partial hepatectomy factor (PHF) described by Tewarí et al. (1992). NF-κB activation reaches a maximum at approximately 1 h after PH and returns to normal values by 2–3 h. Little, if any, activation of NF-κB as assessed by its binding to DNA occurs after sham operation. In addition to analyses done with whole liver preparations, increased NF-κB binding was detected in nuclear extracts of hepatocytes isolated 30 min after PH (FitzGerald et al. 1995). In addition to NF-κB hepatocyte nuclei also contained p50 homodimers and a minor band corresponding to PHF. The three complexes (p50/p65; p50/p50 and PHF) were also present in nuclear extracts of normal liver nonparenchymal cells but no increase in NF-κB binding (p50/p65 heterodimer) was detected in these cells after PH. These experiments demonstrate that immediately after PH, there is activation of NF-κB in hepatocytes with a dramatic increase in NF-κB DNA binding. The binding may transactivate sets of target genes that contain the NF-κB motifs (for instance c-myc) and initiate the primary gene response after PH (see below). Increased NF-κB binding to DNA was also detected 1–2 h after 30 percent hepatectomy, a procedure which is below the tissue deficit threshold needed to elicit regeneration. However, animals with 30 percent hepatectomy go through the initial stages of liver regeneration and acquire the capacity to respond to growth factors but do not undergo DNA synthesis (Webber, Godowski and Fausto 1994; FitzGerald 1995). Thus NF-κB activation may be required for the initiation of liver regeneration, but is not sufficient by itself to cause DNA synthesis.

NF-κB activity is required for liver development

Mice lacking the p65 component of NF-κB die at 15–16 days of embryonic development with widespread hepatic apoptosis (Beg et al. 1995). Embryos of p65 knockout mice are normal up to 14 days after conception but one day after show massive destruction of hepatocytes which causes embryonic death. Neither hepatic hemopoietic cells nor any other tissue display morphological abnormalities. Experiments done with fibroblasts from 13-day embryos demonstrated that p65 deficiency interferes with inducible but not basal levels of NF-κB activity (Beg et al. 1995). The studies done with p65 knockout mice indicate that p65 is essential for liver development and acts at a time in embryonic development in which cell proliferation is probably rapidly enhanced. It is of interest that knockout mice which lack p50 (the other component of the NF-κB heterodimer) have completely normal development and postnatal growth. Lack of lethality from p50 deficiency most likely occurs because p65 activity compensates for the loss of the p50 component.

Primary gene response during liver regeneration

When cells are stimulated to proliferate in culture by serum or growth factors, there is rapid and almost immediate gene activation. This event is referred to as a primary gene response or immediate early gene response. The original genes to be identified as participants in this response after PH were the protooncogenes c-fos, c-jun and c-myc (Fausto and Mead 1989). Through the work of Taub and her colleagues, it is now known that the immediate early genes expressed after PH include as many as 70 genes (Haber et al. 1993). A major challenge for the future is to characterize these genes and identify those which may be required for hepatocyte proliferation. In addition to protooncogenes, the immediate early response after PH includes genes coding for phosphatases, growth factor receptors, proteases, growth factor binding factors and many others which remain to be identified. The primary response after PH takes place even when protein synthesis is inhibited and the activation of this set of genes is actually stimulated by protein synthesis inhibition. This observation suggests that in addition to synthesis, degradative processes and inhibitors play a role in controlling the levels of transcripts for these genes. Indeed, the mechanisms which regulate the expression of some of these genes are multiple and quite complex. For instance, c-myc regulation after PH involves both transcriptional and post-transcriptional mechanisms (Morello, FitzGerald et al. 1990; Morello, Lavenu and Babinet 1990). Transcriptional control of c-myc expression takes place both at the initiation of transcription and the elongation of transcripts. The post-transcriptional mechanisms may involve lowering the rate of degradation of newly synthesized transcripts and increasing the stability of cytoplasmic mRNA. Some of the immediate early genes such as c-jun and c-fos are themselves transcription activators (components of the API complex). Thus, the increased expression of these genes shortly after PH leads to propagation of the primary response by stimulating the transcription of other sets of genes (secondary response). Post-transcriptional mechanisms that control mRNA stability also contribute to the establishment of the secondary gene response.

Secondary gene response during liver regeneration

The secondary gene response corresponds to the progression of hepatocytes through the G_1 phase of the cell cycle culminating in cell replication. Genes which are expressed during the period of time (approximately between 6 and 24 h after PH) have received less attention than immediate early genes. Nevertheless, secondary response genes are likely to be directly involved in the machinery necessary for cell cycle progression. Among them are p53, mdm2 and cyclins D and E. p53 has been studied in other systems mostly in its role as a tumor suppression gene (Albrecht et al. 1993; Lu et al. 1992; Loyer et al. 1994). Yet, during physiologic hepatocyte replication after PH, it functions as a cell cycle gene. Both its mRNA and protein increase between 8 and 18 h after partial hepatectomy, a few hours before the maximal period of DNA synthesis (Fausto and Mead 1989). Increased p53 expression is followed by the increased expression of mdm2, one of the p53 target genes which can bind to other components of the cell cycle machinery and promote cell cycle progression. Another p53 target gene, waf1 (also known as Cip1, sd1 or p21) is also transiently expressed during liver regeneration. Although it has not been directly determined whether p53 or mdm2 actions are indispensable for hepatocyte DNA synthesis, transfection of cultured differentiated hepatocytes of the AML-12 line with p53 mutants prevents mdm2 increase in late G_1 and causes a delay in DNA synthesis when synchronized cells are released from a block in the G_1/S boundary during the cell cycle (Yamada and Fausto, unpublished). Expression of cyclin D1 and of the cyclin dependent kinase p34 cdc2 are important correlates of DNA replication in hepatocytes.

ROLE OF GROWTH FACTORS AND CYTOKINES IN HEPATOCYTE REPLICATION

The primary and secondary gene responses described above are regulated by growth factors and cytokines. A relatively large number of growth factors can stimulate DNA synthesis in cultured hepatocytes. Among these are, EGF, TFG-α, HGF, aFGF, HB-EGF and KGF (see Table 9.2 for complete names). In addition, ALR, HSS, insulin, glucagon, and norepinephrine (Table 9.2), which on their own have little effect on DNA synthesis, can augment the effect of growth factors on hepatocyte replication (Fausto and Webber 1994; Michalopoulos 1990). The factors which have been better studied are EGF, TFG-α, HGF but recent work demonstrated that aFGF, KGF, and HB-EGF are also complete hepatocyte mitogens (Tanahashi et al. 1994; Housley et al. 1994; Ito et al. 1994). In addition to factors which stimulate DNA replication, others such as TGF-β and activin have an opposite effect, that is, they inhibit DNA synthesis (Table 9.2). Moreover, TGF-β,

Table 9.2. *Main growth factors with effects on hepatocyte replication*

Hepatocyte mitogens
Epidermal growth factor (EGF)
Transforming growth factor alpha (TGF-α)
Hepatocyte growth factor (HGF)
Acidic fibroblast growth factor (aFGF or FGF2)
Heparin binding EGF-like growth factor (HG-EGF)
Keratinocyte growth factor (KGF)
Adjuvant agents for hepatocyte replication
Augmenter of liver regeneration (ALR)
Hepatic stimulating substance (HSS)
Insulin, glucagon, norepinephrine
Inhibitors of hepatocyte replication and/or apoptosis inducers
Transforming growth factor beta (TGF-β)
Activin
FAS antigen/ligand system (apoptosis)

activin and the FAS receptor/ligand system promote apoptosis. Recent work also suggests that cytokines such as TNF and IL-6 may be involved in the initiation steps of liver regeneration (Akerman et al. 1992). Knowledge about the role of some of these agents is summarized below.

EGF activity during liver growth

In the mouse, EGF functions as an endocrine agent which has profound effects on liver regeneration. In this species, EGF is produced mainly in salivary glands and is abundant in male animals. Removal of salivary glands delays the peak of DNA synthesis after PH by 24 h (Noguchi et al. 1991). EGF administration to sialoadenectomized mice restores EGF blood concentrations and eliminates the delay in DNA synthesis after PH. In mice with intact salivary glands, EGFR mRNA and receptor binding activity increases during the first 8 h after PH and is down regulated thereafter (Noguchi et al. 1992). Although EGF is present in the blood of normal mice, it apparently acts as a hepatocyte mitogen only in regenerating livers. It is conceivable that to make circulating EGF become mitogenic for hepatocytes after PH, a change in the receptor is required to permit ligand binding and activation of signal transduction. Lack of circulating EGF in sialoadenectomized mice alters the timing of DNA synthesis after PH but does not decrease the proportion of hepatocytes which replicate during the process. In contrast, data by Jones et al. (1995) show that removal of salivary glands in rats leads to complete blockage of liver regeneration suggesting that in rats EGF may be essential for liver regeneration. Synthesis of EGF mRNA and peptide have been detected in rat liver very shortly after PH (Mulhaupt et al. 1994), indicating that in these animals EGF may act by both autocrine and endocrine mechanisms. At this time no data are available on EGF activity in humans in vivo but it has been shown that EGF is a potent stimulator of DNA synthesis for cultured human hepatocytes.

TGF-α expression during liver development and regeneration: Relationship with hepatocyte replication

Expression of TGF-α in the liver is associated with hepatocyte proliferation (Mead and Fausto 1989; Fausto and Webber 1994; Evarts et al. 1992; Russell et al. 1993; Sandgren et al. 1990). In contrast to EGF and HGF, TGF-α does not function through endocrine mechanisms. Instead, it exerts its effect on hepatocytes by an autocrine loop, that is, TGF-α is produced by hepatocytes which can respond to the factor because they contain the specific receptor (EGFR). The autocrine loop of TGF-α synthesis is stimulated in liver cell cultures as well as in vivo by TGF-α itself or EGF, providing an amplification mechanism for TGF-α synthesis (Webber et al. 1993; Wu et al. 1994a). It is not known whether this amplification mechanism has physiological importance in vivo. TGF-α is synthesized as a 160 amino acid precursor that is anchored in the cell membrane. The extracellular domain of the precursor contains the 50 amino acid processed (diffusable) form bounded by alanine/valine residues at each end which are sites for cleavage by elastases. The precursor also has a transmembrane domain and a 35 amino acid cytoplasmic domain. The C-terminal valine residue of the intracellular domain serves as a signal site for cleavage of processed TGF-α peptide from the precursor molecule. TGF-α has 35 percent homology with EGF and binds to the same receptor (EGFR). The six cysteines (three disulfide bridges) in TGF-α and EGF share positional homology.

During liver regeneration after PH in rats, TGF-α mRNA increases starting at about 4 h after PH and reaches a maximum before the peak of DNA synthesis. Peptide levels are increased at 24 and 48 h after the operation (Webber et al. 1993).

Interestingly, the 50 amino acid diffusable form of TGF-α is detected only at 48 h, at the time at which the major wave of hepatocyte replication has taken place (Russell et al. 1993). These observations imply that membrane-anchored, nondiffusable forms of TGF-α may be active in hepatocytes, and may account for a significant proportion of the total TGF-α activity. However, hepatocytes stimulated to proliferate in culture release active TGF-α into the culture medium and apparently rely less on the activity of the membrane bound TGF-α precursor.

Constitutive expression of TGF-α is associated with hepatocyte proliferation during the postnatal phase of liver growth and the decline of hepatocyte proliferative activity in weeks three and four of postnatal life is accompanied by an abrupt decline in the levels of the peptide. In culture, hepatocytes from one week old rats produce considerable amounts of TGF-α and have a high rate of replication. After four weeks of age, cultured rat hepatocytes make little TGF-α and have a low rate of replication in the absence of growth factors. Cultured adult hepatocytes respond vigorously to TGF-α and reach levels of DNA synthesis which are equal or higher than those of neonatal rats (Fausto et al. 1995).

A model to study the effects of constitutive overexpression of TGF-α in the liver of adult mice was provided by transgenic mouse lines which overexpress human TGF-α developed by Merlino (Jhappan et al. 1990) and Sandgren (Sandgren et al. 1990). Mice of transgenic line MT42 established by Merlino show major changes in liver growth which may be divided into three phases (Webber, Wu et al. 1994). During the first month of life, hepatocytes of TGF-α transgenic mice have proliferative indices which are two to three times higher than normal and their livers are 25–40 percent larger than in nontransgenic animals. In addition, the shift to higher levels of ploidy, which is completed by 45 days of life in normal mice, is greatly delayed in TGF-α transgenics. In both normal and transgenic mice there is a decrease in DNA replication after the first month of life but the decline is of much smaller magnitude in transgenic mice. At the second phase, which roughly encompasses the period between three and eight months of life, labeling indices of hepatocytes of transgenic mice are six- to eight-fold higher than normal. At three to five months of age the hepatocyte labeling indices are 12 percent and 2 percent for transgenic and normal mice, respectively but, surprisingly, despite the higher levels of hepatocyte replication, livers of transgenic mice are not enlarged in comparison to nontransgenic animals. The absence of enlargement in these highly proliferative livers occurs because the enhanced replication is compensated by high cell turnover. Hepatocytes isolated from these animals have the same sensitivity as normal hepatocytes to the blockage DNA synthesis caused by TGF-β. In the third phase (from 8 to 15 months of life) hepatocyte replication and high turnover continue but hepatocyte dysplasia becomes apparent (Lee et al. 1992). Liver morphology becomes progressively more abnormal and by 15 months of age approximately 85 percent of mice develop hepatic tumors. The observations summarized above demonstrate that overexpression of TGF-α can make adult hepatocytes become replicating cells and that in this process the cells do not lose their differentiated traits. In this situation, the proliferative activity of adult hepatocytes remains a regulated process that responds to physiologic stimuli. The high rate of hepatocyte proliferation exhibited by these animals is eventually compensated by increased cell turnover. It is only when these compensatory mechanisms (which presumably involve a high rate of apoptosis) become deficient that overt malignancy becomes apparent.

Given that the high expression of a liver mitogen converted hepatocytes in vivo into a highly proliferative cell, we explored the possibility of creating continuously proliferating cell lines using hepatocytes from TGF-α transgenics. Hepatocytes from TGF-α transgenic mice maintained in serum containing medium formed small colonies of replicating cells after about 30 days in primary culture. By replating individual colonies which produced albumin, we developed cell lines of replicating differentiated hepatocytes which express albumin, α-1-antitrypsin, transferrin and hepatocyte connexins (Wu et al. 1994; Wu, Merlino and Fausto 1994). When maintained in serum-free medium, hepatocytes from TGF-α transgenic mice undergo DNA replication in the absence of any other growth factor (Wu et al. 1994). Addition of EGF, TGF-α or HGF had no effect on DNA synthesis in these cultures, indicating they are already close to their maximal replicative capacity. Replicating hepatocytes release very large amounts of TGF-α in the medium and the conditioned medium stimulates DNA synthesis of normal hepatocytes, an effect which is inhibited by TGF-α-antibodies. In serum free medium, hepatocytes from transgenic mice die after three rounds of replication, an outcome that can be prevented by addition of nicotinamide of the culture medium (Wu et al. 1994). How nicotinamide may act to maintain cell survival is a matter of speculation, suggestions having been made that its main effects are on ADP-ribosylation, DNA repair, or maintenance of NAD levels. In any event, nicotinamide proved to be essential for the establishment of replicating lines of differentiated hepatocytes, which have now been maintained for more than two years in serum free medium. Continuously proliferating, differentiated hepatocyte lines have also been established from nontransgenic mice using a similar strategy, that is, maintenance of cells in serum free medium containing nicotinamide and growth factor (Wu et al. 1994) and several investigators have now been successful in maintaining normal hepatocytes as replicating cells in long standing cultures (Mitaka et al. 1992; Lee et al. 1989). In summary, studies of replicative capacity of hepatocytes from TGF-α transgenic mice both in vivo and in vitro demonstrated that TGF-α overexpression makes adult, normally quiescent hepatocytes become proliferating cells, while retaining differentiated traits. Other types of experiments using a transgenic mouse model in which the capacity of transplanted hepatocytes to reconstitute a damaged liver can be assessed, demonstrated that hepatocytes in vivo also have a great replicative potential. In these animals it was shown that 10 percent of the hepatocytes of a mouse can replenish a whole liver and replicate more than ten times in this process (Rhim et al. 1995).

HGF expression during liver regeneration, hepatic injury and liver development

HGF is a heterodimeric glycoprotein consisting of a heavy (α) and a light (β) chain of approximate molecular weights of 64,000 and 32,000, respectively. The heterodimeric form is generated from a single chain precursor peptide with a molecular weight of 87,000–92,000. The α chain has four kringle domains (double-loop structure with three disulfide bridges) with 40 percent homology with plasminogen. The β chain has homology with serine proteases but has no proteolytic activity of its own because of amino acid substitutions in the catalytic site residues (Michalopoulos and Zarnegar 1992; Matsumoto and Nakamura 1992).

On a molar basis, HGF is the most potent of the liver mitogens. The factor is not produced by hepatocytes or other epithelial cells but is made by mesenchymal cells throughout the body. In the liver it is made by Ito cells, Kupffer cells and endothelial cells (Schirmacher et al. 1992; Maher 1993). After PH, blood levels of HGF increase sharply during the first 4–6 h (Lindroos et al. 1991). In addition, HGF mRNA produced by nonparenchymal cells, increases and reaches maximum levels 18–24 h after the operation. Thus, HGF may act on hepatocytes during liver regeneration by endocrine and/or paracrine mechanisms. Although the rapid increase in circulating levels of HGF shortly after PH indicates that the factor plays a role in the early events of the process, more precise experiments need to be done to determine whether the rise in circulating HGF triggers liver regeneration (see below). In addition, more data are needed to properly define the relationships between blood levels of HGF and hepatocyte replication. In addition, because HGF is produced both intra- and extrahepatically it is important to determine if synthesis of HGF in these various sites has a common mechanism of induction and whether the endocrine or paracrine activity of HGF is the most important for inducing hepatocyte replication.

Blood levels of HGF also increase rapidly after CCl_4 or galactosamine injection in rats (Michalopoulos and Zarnegar 1992) but maximal hepatic DNA synthesis during these processes occurs later than PH (1 day and 3 days later for CCl_4 and galactosamine respectively compared to PH). These observations suggest that the relationship between blood levels of HGF and DNA synthesis may not be a direct one, a conclusion supported by the finding that in acute liver failure in humans the very high levels of HGF correlate inversely with patient survival (Hughes et al. 1994; Shiota et al. 1995). The difficulty in establishing a direct correlation between HGF blood levels and hepatocyte replication may perhaps be resolved by taking into account that HGF is inactive in its precursor form and requires proteolytic cleavage to be activated (Naldini et al. 1992). Various enzyme systems have now been shown to act on this cleavage. These enzymes may control the local production of active HGF as well as the amount of mitogenically active HGF present in the blood during growth processes (Mars et al. 1993). An interesting feature of HGF activity is that, although the factor circulates and is mitogenic for many different cell types, proliferative responses are confined to a single tissue. Thus, circulating levels of HGF increase after both PH and unilateral nephrectomy but the mitogenic response occurs only in liver or kidney, respectively, after these procedures (Matsumoto and Nakamura 1993). This indicates that HGF activation may take place only in the affected organ and suggests that it is a local event regulated at the receptor level (Comoglio 1993). If local control of HGF activity does indeed exist, it may explain why there may not be a direct relationship between HGF blood levels and hepatocyte proliferation.

HGF overexpression in the liver has major effects on hepatic growth. Earlier observations indicated that transgenic mice which overexpress HGF had a large number of small diploid hepatocytes in the liver (Shiota et al. 1994). After PH, the liver remnant of these animals regained normal weights faster than nontransgenic animals. More recent observations by Merlino (personal communication) show that HGF overexpression at a higher level than those obtained by Shiota et al. , causes profound effects on liver cell composition and growth. Moreover, HGF overexpression causes marked alterations in other organs, particularly the kidney and mammary glands of these animals. Two recent reports show that mice in which the HGF gene has been inactivated ("knockouts") die during embryonic development. Uehara et al. (1995) attributed lethality to a placental defect and did not detect hepatic abnormalities in the embryos while Schmidt et al. (1995) concluded that HGF knockouts have a major defect in liver development. Schmidt et al. (1995) concluded that HGF may be essential for liver morphogenesis and considered the defect found in HGF knockouts to be similar to that described in mice with inactive c-jun

(Hilberg et al. 1993). Knockout mice with c-jun deficiency die during embryonic development and show almost complete failure of liver parenchymal formation. This feature appears to differ from the findings reported in HGF knockout mice. A more detailed analysis of these phenotypes are necessary before definitive conclusions are reached, but the results indicate HGF has an important role as mediator of epithelial mesenchymal interactions in the liver and other organs. Both in vivo and in vitro, hepatocyte gene expression is modulated by cellular matrix components (Rana et al. 1994; Zaret 1994) and it is likely that HGF participates in these interactions as well as in processes requiring branching morphogenesis during liver development. Recent observations indicate that EGF and TGF-α also have morphogenetic properties for some cells in culture but the activities of these two growth factors are weaker than that of HGF (Barros et al. 1995).

Although HGF and TGF-α are potent liver mitogens, lack of activity of the respective genes in knockout animals has very different effects. In contrast to HGF knockouts which, as mentioned above, die during embryonic development, TGF-α knockouts develop normally and grow into healthy adults which display only hair growth abnormalities. Liver regeneration is not impaired in TGF-α knockout mice (Russell et al. 1996). The most likely explanation for these findings is that EGF probably replaces TGF-α in most if not all of its functions. These animal models raise the important question of whether hepatocyte mitogens are redundant in their functions or have specific modes of action in promoting hepatocyte replication. Nevertheless, at least some HGF functions in embryonic development must be nonredundant because their absence results in death. Whether these unique functions pertain to the mitogenic, morphogenic or motogenic ("scatter factor") properties of HGF is not known at this time.

TUMOR NECROSIS FACTOR (TNF) AND ITS ROLE IN LIVER REGENERATION

The rapid activation of NF-κB after PH indicates that a signal for gene activation has been received in the hepatocyte nucleus almost immediately after the operation. Thus, the identification of agents responsible for NF-κB activation at the start of liver regeneration is likely to uncover at least part of the sequence of events that initiate hepatocyte replication after PH. It is known from work in cell cultures that TNF induces NF-κB activation. Recent work showed that intraperitoneal injection of 5 μg of TNF to intact rats caused 30 min after the injection, a strong induction of NF-κB in the liver similar to that found after PH (FitzGerald et al. 1995). A similar inductive effect of TNF on NF-κB· DNA binding was observed in cultured liver cells. Diehl and colleagues have concluded from experiments using TNF antibodies that TNF may cause elevation of c-jun and jun-kinase after PH and that blockage of TNF activity inhibits liver regeneration (Akerman et al. 1992; Diehl et al. 1994). It is thus possible that TNF may contribute to the initiation of liver regeneration by activating two transcription factors that is, by acting on the activation of NF-κB and through its effect on c-jun, also inducing AP1. It should be kept in mind that NF-κB can be activated by many other factors besides TNF and that the activation is ultimately controlled by phosphorylation and proteolytic steps which cause the degradation of the inhibitor IκB. Thus any agent which directly acts on either of these steps would also be capable of activating NF-κB at the start of liver regeneration. Phosphorylation of IκB is modulated by the redox state of the cell while its proteolytic cleavage requires proteasome activity (Meyer et al. 1994; Pahl and Bauerle 1994). In the context of NF-κB activation, TNF as well as intracellular signals involving the generation of reactive oxygen intermediates and proteolytic activity could contribute to the initiation of liver regeneration after PH.

HOW IS REGENERATION INITIATED?

We have outlined above a series of sequential events that takes place almost immediately after PH and indicated that a major goal of the search for initiators of liver regeneration is the identification of molecular events that activate transcription factors. We have singled out NF-κB, AP1 and STAT3 as the transcription factors likely to be involved at the start of liver regeneration and described the mechanism of NF-κB activation. Research on the initiation of liver regeneration has traditionally assumed that there is a single event which triggers the growth process. Given the multiplicity of pathways that are activated shortly after PH, attention should be given to the possibility that multiple events occurring in parallel are required for triggering a complete replicative response. Furthermore, it is possible that the initial triggering events which make hepatocytes leave their quiescent state might not be the most critical ones which determine whether replication will occur. An alternative possibility is that a key step of hepatocyte DNA synthesis is the linkage between initiating events and cell cycle progression.

Both HGF and TGF-α are potent hepatocyte mitogens whose levels increase after PH. HGF blood concentrations increase rapidly after PH and production of HGF mRNA in nonparenchymal cells increases between 6 and 18 h after PH. Production of TGF-α mRNA increases 4–6 h after PH and recent data indicate that the EGF mRNA levels increase in the liver in the first hour after PH. In addition, ligand binding to the EGF receptor is rapidly increased after PH. The buildup of HGF in the blood as well as early events involving EGFR and EGF itself are likely to be important events in the initiation of the growth response. However, although HGF, TGF-α and EGF markedly increase DNA synthesis in cultured hepatocytes, their effect on the replication of hepatocytes in the intact liver in vivo is relatively weak (Webber et al. 1994). Thus, infusion of these factors into the portal vein or their injection into normal rats either fail to produce a significant mitogenic response in hepatocytes or do so only after multiple injections or prolonged exposure (Fujiwara et al. 1993). These findings indicate that intact hepatocytes are not very sensitive to growth factor effects. Several studies have shown, however, that hepatocytes can be "primed" to respond to growth factors and that such priming can be elicited by nutritional factors (Mead et al. 1990), 30 percent hepatectomies (Webber et al. 1994) and by perfusion of the liver with collagenase (Liu et al. 1994). In all of these cases, and in particular the last two, hepatocytes readily respond to HGF and TGF-α and show extensive mitogenic activity. The experimental model involving 30 percent hepatectomy is of particular interest because it shows that a small resection of liver tissue does not cause DNA synthesis but alters liver cells making them capable of responding to mitogenic agents. In this experimental situation many of the immediate early genes which increase their expression after two thirds hepatectomy are also activated but somehow hepatocytes do not progress to DNA synthesis. It is conceivable that the immediate early gene response after 30 percent hepatectomy is incomplete or not of a sufficient magnitude to trigger the activation of secondary response genes required for cell cycle progression. This suggests that a rate limiting step in hepatocyte replication is the linkage between the immediate initiating events and cell cycle progression which occurs approximately 4–6 h later.

In summary, the results indicate that hepatocytes need to be primed to become competent to proliferate and to fully respond to growth factors. This process involves the rapid activation of at least three transcription factors within the first hour after PH (NF-κB, AP1 and STAT3). Their activation is regulated by cytokines, the redox state of the cells and perhaps growth factors. We favor a model in which cytokines (such as tumor necrosis factor and IL-6) and oxygen free radicals cause the activation of transcription factors immediately after PH while growth factors act at a later stage providing the stimulus for cell cycle progression and cyclin activation (Figure 9.6, left panel). Nevertheless, further studies are needed to determine whether HGF, which increases in the blood shortly after PH, or other growth factors can function as the earliest initiating agents of liver regeneration and activate in strictly quiescent cells the multiple pathways which lead to hepatocyte replication (Figure 9.6, right panel).

LIVER REGENERATION IN ACUTE HEPATIC FAILURE

Although regeneration after PH or toxic injury in animals has been studied in great detail, little is known about the regulation of hepatocyte proliferation in patients with acute liver failure. A major unresolved issue regards the type of hepatic cells which proliferate under these conditions and give rise to mature hepatocytes. Gerber et al. (1983), Gerber and Thung (1992), and Phillips and Poucell (1981) described the proliferation of duct-like structures which originate around portal spaces and penetrate into the necrotic parenchyma. Gerber et al. (1983) showed that cells of these duct-like structures have a transitional morphology between ductular cells and hepatocytes and referred to them as ductular hepatocytes. Such cells have markers of both hepatocytes and biliary cells and are similar to cells detected in experimental liver injury in rats (Sirica 1995). The origin of these cells is the subject of long standing debate. It has been proposed that they may originate from precursor ("stem") cells, from biliary cells or from metaplasia of hepatocytes. Although various cell types (including hepatocytes) replicate in acute liver cell failure, the ultimate developmental fate of the cells during this process is largely unknown. However, as in the case of hepatic injury in rodents in which there is extensive proliferation of oval cells (Fausto 1994), it is likely that cellular replenishment in the liver in acute failure may depend both on maturation of precursor cells as well as hepatocyte replication.

The identification of growth factors which make precursor cells and hepatocytes proliferate in acute hepatic failure is a subject of major practical importance. Acute failure patients have very high levels of blood HGF and its concentration was found to be inversely proportional to prognosis. Recent data demonstrate that synthesis of HGF mRNA in the liver in patients with acute hepatic failure is low (P. Harrison, personal communication).

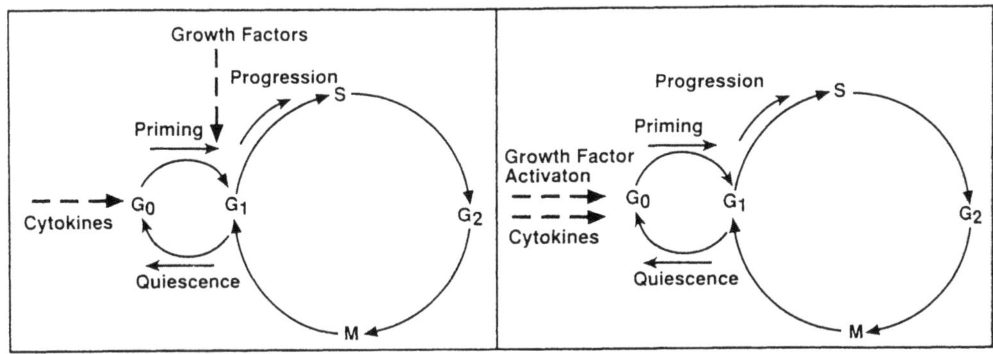

Figure 9.6 Models for the activation of the cell cycle in hepatocytes after partial hepatectomy. The cell cycle is divided into two major phases: priming which represents the G_0 to G_1 transition and progression which represents the G_1 to S transit. Two models are proposed: the left panel shows a model in which priming is induced by cytokines and growth factors act on hepatocytes which have acquired proliferative competence. In the right panel, both cytokine and growth factors are shown as inducers of the priming events on G_0 cells.

These observations suggest that HGF present in the blood of these patients is produced in extrahepatic sites and reaches high levels because of diminished liver uptake. However, it has not been determined whether HGF production in extrahepatic sites is increased above normal levels or if large amounts of HGF are released from the liver during massive hepatic necrosis. It has been suggested that HGF in an inactive form may be bound to extracellular matrix components and stored in normal livers in relatively large amounts. In any event, it is important to establish whether viable cells in livers of patients with acute hepatic failure have the HGF receptor (c-met protooncogene) and whether such cells are capable of responding to circulating HGF. One possibility is that although the surviving cells can respond to HGF they are prevented from doing so by an inhibitor of the growth factor (Yamada et al. 1994). Alternatively, cell proliferation in the liver of these patients may already be high but not sufficient to replenish the liver because of enhanced cell death (Wolf and Michalopoulos 1992). In this case high cell turnover rather than a low proliferative rate would be the major defect which prevents successful regeneration in these patients. Based on these views, prevention of cell death and attempting to increase the mitogenic and differentiation response of the liver in acute failure by growth factors other than HGF (e.g. EGF, TGF-α, HB-EGF, KGF), are therapeutic strategies that should be evaluated. However, it is unlikely that this approach will be successful without the identification of the cells which proliferate in acute liver failure. This can best be accomplished by isolation of various cell types from biopsy and autopsy specimens and the establishment of cell lines for in vitro studies.

In a series of papers, Roskams and her colleagues (Roskams et al. 1990; 1991; 1993; 1994) found that in both chronic cholestatic liver disease and during regeneration after submassive hepatic necrosis in humans, reactive bile ductules express neuroendocrine markers. At the very early stages of regeneration, even before the bile ductular reaction was clearly evident, Roskams et al. (1991) detected bile ductular structures which were cytokeratin (CK)19 positive and expressed the neuroendocrine markers Leu-19, NKH-1 and chromogranin-A. Single cells, with morphologic features similar to that of rat oval cells, stained for chromogranin-A and CK19. As regeneration progressed, single cells expressing a neuroendocrine phenotype were no longer found but proliferating bile ductules as well as hepatocytes located near portal spaces exhibited these features. Further studies (Roskams et al. 1991) revealed that, in regeneration after submassive necrosis, reactive bile ductules but not portal bile ducts expressed parathyroid hormone-related peptide (PTHrP). This protein is not present in normal adult human liver but strong immunoreactivity for PTHrP was detected in maturing bile ducts during embryonic development and during the first two years of life (Roskams and Desmet 1994). These studies suggest that cells expressing neuroendocrine phenotypes may function as progenitor or stem cells in the regeneration of the human liver after submassive failure. Moreover, it is possible that PTHrP could act as a differentiation agent for bile ductular cells.

Acknowledgments

I thank Ms Tamara Carlson for her skillful assistance. The author's research work discussed in this paper was supported by NCI Grants CA 23226 and CA 35249.

Note added in proof

The following recently published reviews are directly pertinent to the subject of this chapter:

Diehl, A.M. and Rai, R.M. 1996. Regulation of signal transduction during liver regeneration. *FASEB J* 10: 215–27.

Fausto, N., Laird, A.D. and Webber, E.M. 1995. Role of growth factors and cytokines in hepatic regeneration. *FASEB J* 9: 1527–36.

Taub, R. 1996. Transcriptional control of liver regeneration. *FASEB J* 10: 413–27.

REFERENCES

Akerman, P., Cote, P., Yang, S.Q., McClain, C., Nelson, S., Bagby, G.J. and Diehl, A.M. 1992. Antibodies to tumor necrosis factor-α inhibit liver regeneration after partial hepatectomy. *Am J Physiol* 263: G579–85.

Albrecht, J.H., Hoffman, J.S., Kren, B.T. and Steer, C.J. 1993. Cyclin and cyclin-dependent kinase 1 mRNA expression in models of regenerating liver and human liver diseases. *Am J Physiol* 265: G857–64.

Anderson, M.T., Staal, F.J., Gitler, C. and Herzenberg, L.A. 1994. Separation of oxidant-mediated and redox-regulated steps in the NF-kappa B signal transduction pathway. *Proc Natl Acad Sci USA* 91: 11527–31.

Barros, E., Santos, O., Matsumoto, K., Nakamura, T. and Nigam, S. 1995. Differential tubulogenic and branching morphogenetic activities of growth factors: Implications for epithelial tissue development. *Proc Natl Acad Sci USA* 92: 4412–16.

Beg, A. and Baldwin, A.J. 1993. The IκB proteins: multifunctional regulators of Rel/NF-κB transcription factors. *Genes Dev* 7: 2064–70.

Beg, A.A., Sha, W.C., Bronson, R.T., Ghosh, S. and Baltimore, D. 1995. Embryonic lethality and liver degeneration in mice lacking the RelA component of NF-κB. *Nature* 376: 167–70.

Braun, L., Mead, J.E., Panzica, M., Mikumo, R., Bell, G.I. and Fausto, N. 1988. Elevation of transforming growth factor beta mRNA during liver regeneration: A possible paracrine mechanism of growth regulation. *Proc Natl Acad Sci USA* 85: 1534–8.

Bucher, N.L.R. 1963. Regeneration of mammalian liver. In *International Review of Cytology*, eds. G.H. Bourne and J.F. Danielli, 245–300. New York: Academic Press.

Bucher, N.L.R. and Malt, R.A. 1971. *Regeneration of liver and kidney*. Boston: Little, Brown and Co.

Comoglio, P.M. 1993. Structure, biosynthesis and biochemical properties of the HGF receptor in normal and malignant cells. In *Hepatocyte growth factor–scatter factor (HGF–SF) and the c-MET receptor*, eds. I.D. Goldberg and E.M. Rosen, 131–65. New York: Springer-Verlag.

Cressman, D.E., Diamond, R.H. and Taub, R. 1995. Rapid activation of the Stat3 transcription complex in liver regeneration. *Hepatology* 21: 1443–49.

Cressman, D., Greenbaum, L. and Haber, B. 1994. Rapid activation of post-hepatectomy factor/nuclear factor κB in hepatocytes, a primary response in the regenerating liver. *J Biol Chem* 269: 30429–35.

Diehl, A., Yin, M., Fleckenstein, J., Yang, S., Lin, H., Brenner, D., Westwick, J., Bagby, G. and Nelson, S. 1994. Tumor necrosis factor-α induces c-jun during the regenerative response to liver injury. *Am J Physiol* 267: G552–61.

Diehl, A., Yin, M., Fleckenstein, J., Yang, S., Lin, H., Brenner, D., Westwick, J., Bagby, G. and Nelson, S. 1994. Tumor necrosis factor-α induces c-jun during the regenerative response to liver injury. *Am J Physiol* 267: G552–61.

Evarts, R.P., Nakatsukasa, H., Marsden, E.R., Hu, Z. and Thorgeirsson, S.S. 1992. Expression of transforming growth factor-alpha in regenerating liver and during hepatic differentiation. *Mol Carcin* 5: 25–31.

Fausto, N. 1994. Liver stem cells. In *The Liver: Biology and Pathobiology*, 3rd edn., eds. L. Arias, J. Boyer, N. Fausto, W. Jakoby, D. Schachter and D. Shafritz, 1501–18. New York: Raven Press, Ltd.

Fausto, N., Laird, A.D. and Webber, E.M. 1995. Role of growth factors and cytokines in hepatic regeneration. *FASEB J* 9: 1527–36.

Fausto, N. and Mead, J.E. 1989. Regulation of liver growth: protooncogenes and transforming growth factors. *Lab Invest* 60: 4–13.

Fausto, N. and Webber, E. 1994. Liver regeneration. In *The Liver: Biology and Pathobiology*, eds. I. Arias, J. Boyer, N. Fausto, W. Jakoby, D. Schachter and D. Shafritz, 1059–84. New York: Raven Press, Ltd.

FitzGerald, M., Webber, E., Donovan, J. and Fausto, N. 1995. Rapid DNA binding by nuclear factor κB in hepatocytes at the start of liver regeneration. *Cell Growth Diff* 6: 417–27.

Francavilla, A., Zeng, Q. and Polimeno, L. 1994. Small-for-size liver transplanted into larger recipient: a model of hepatic regeneration. *Hepatology* 19: 210–16.

Fujiwara, K., Nagoshi, S., Ohno, A., Hirata, K., Ohta, Y., Mochida, S., Tomiya, T., Higashio, K. and Kurokawa, K. 1993. Stimulation of liver growth by exogenous human hepatocyte growth factor in normal and partially hepatectomized rats. *Hepatology* 18: 1443–9.

Gerber, M., Thung, S.N., Shen, S., Stromeyer, F.W. and Ishak, K.G. 1983. Phenotypic characterization of hepatic proliferation. Antigen expression by proliferating epithelial cells in fetal liver, massive hepatic necrosis and nodular transformation of the liver. *Am J Pathol* 110: 70–4.

Gerber, M.A. and Thung, S.N. 1992. Cell lineages in human liver development, regeneration, and transformation. In *The Role of Cell Types in Hepatocarcinogenesis*, ed. A.E. Sirica, 209–26. Boca Raton: CRC Press.

Grilli, M., Chiu, J.-S. and Lenardo, M. 1993. NF-κB and Rel: participants in a multiform transcriptional regulatory system. *Int Rev Cytol* 143: 1–62.

Grisham, J.W. 1962. A morphologic study of deoxyribonucleic acid synthesis and cell proliferation in regenerating rat liver; autoradiography with thymidine-H^3. *Cancer Res* 22: 842–9.

Haber, A.H., Mohn, K.L., Diamond, R.H. and Taub, R. 1993. Induction patterns of 70 genes during nine days after hepatectomy define the temporal course of liver regeneration. *J Clin Invest* 91: 1319–26.

Hilberg, F., Aguzzi, A., Howells N. and Wagner, E. 1993. c-jun is essential for normal mouse development and hepatogenesis. *Nature* 365: 179–81.

Housley, R., Morris, C., Boyle, W., Ring, B., Bitz, R., Tarpley, J., Aukerman, S., Devine, P., Whitehead, R. and Pierce, G. 1994. Keratinocyte growth factor induces proliferation of hepatocytes and epithelial cells throughout the rat gastrointestinal tract. *J Clin Invest* 94: 1764–77.

Hughes, R.D., Zhang, L., Tsubouchi, H., Daikuhara, Y. and Williams, R. 1994. Plasma hepatocyte growth factor and biliprotein levels and outcome in fulminant hepatic failure. *J Hepatol* 20: 106–11.

Ito, N., Kawata, S., Tamura, S., Kiso, S., Tsushima, H., Damm, D., Abraham, J., Higashiyama, S., Taniguchi, N. and Matsuzama, Y. 1994. Heparin-binding EGF-like growth factor is a potent mitogen for rat hepatocytes. *Biochem Biophys Res Comm* 198: 25–31.

Jakowlew, S.B., Mead, J.E., Danielpour, D., Wu, J., Roberts, A.B. and Fausto, N. 1991. Transforming growth factor-β (TGF-β) isoforms in rat liver regeneration: messenger RNA expression and activation of latent TGF-β. *Cell Reg* 2: 535–48.

Jhappan, C., Stahle, C., Harkins, R.N., Fausto, N., Smith, G.H. and Merlino, G.T. 1990. TGFα overexpression in transgenic mice induces liver neoplasia and abnormal development of the mammary gland and pancreas. *Cell* 61: 1137–46.

Jones, D.E.J., Tran-Patterson, R., Cui, D.M., Davin, D., Estell, K.P. and Miller, D.M. 1995. Epidermal growth factor secreted from the salivary gland is necessary for l regeneration. *Am J Physiol* 268: G872–G878.

Kam, I., Lynch, S., Svanas, G., Todd, S., Polimeno, L., Francavilla, A., Penkrot, R.J., Takaya, S., Ericzon, B.G., Starzl, T.E. and Van Thiel, D.H. 1987. Evidence that host size determines liver size: studies in dogs receiving orthotopic liver transplants. *Hepatology* 7: 362–6.

Lee, G.H., Sawada, N., Mochizuki, Y., Nomura, K. and Kitagawa, T. 1989. Immortal epithelial cells of normal C3H mouse liver in culture: possible precursor populations for spontaneous hepatocellular carcinoma. *Cancer Res* 49: 403–9.

Lee, G.H., Merlino, G. and Fausto, N. 1992. Development of liver tumors in transforming growth factor alpha transgenic mice. *Cancer Res* 52: 5162–70.

Lindroos, P.M., Zarnegar, R. and Michalopoulos, G.K. 1991. Hepatocyte growth factor (hepatopoietin A) rapidly increases in plasma before DNA synthesis and liver regeneration stimulated by partial hepatectomy and carbon tetrachloride administration. *Hepatology* 13: 743–9.

Liou, H.-C. and Baltimore, D. 1993. Regulation of the NF-κB/rel transcription factor and IκB inhibitor system. *Curr Opin Cell Biol* 5: 477–87.

Liu, M.-L., Mars, W., Zarnegar, R. and Michalopoulos, G. 1994. Collagenase pretreatment and the mitogenic effects of hepatocyte growth factor and transforming growth factor-α in adult rat liver. *Hepatology* 19: 1521–7.

Loyer, P., Glaise, D., Cariou, S., Baffet, G., Meijer, L. and Guguen-Guillouzo, C. 1994. Expression and activation of cdks (1 and 2) and cyclins in the cell cycle progression during liver regeneration. *J Biol Chem* 269: 2491–500.

Lu, X., Koch, K., Lew, D., Dulic, V., Pines, J., Reed, S., Hunter, T. and Leffert, H. 1992. Induction of cyclin mRNA and cyclin-associated histone H1 kinase during liver regeneration. *J Biol Chem* 267: 2841–4.

Maher, J.J. 1993. Cell-specific expression of hepatocyte growth factor in liver. *J Clin Invest* 91: 2244–52.

Mars, W., Zarnegar, R. and Michalopoulous, G. 1993. Activation of hepatocyte growth factor by the plasminogen activators uPA and tPA. *Am J Pathol* 143: 949–58.

Matsumoto, K. and Nakamura, T. 1992. Hepatocyte growth factor: molecular structure, roles in liver regeneration, and other biological functions. *Crit Rev Oncogen* 3: 27–54.

Matsumoto, K. and Nakamura, T. 1993. Roles of HGF as a pleiotropic factor in organ regeneration. In *Hepatocyte Growth Factor-Scatter Factor (HGF-SF) and the c-Met Receptor*, eds. I. Goldberg and E. Rosen, 226–49. Basel: Birkhäuser Verlag.

Mead, J.E. and Fausto, N. 1989. Transforming growth factor α may be a physiological regulator of liver regeneration by means of an autocrine mechanism. *Proc Natl Acad Sci USA* 86: 1558–62.

Mead, J.E., Braun, L., Martin, D.A. and Fausto, N. 1990. Induction of replicative competence ("priming") in normal liver. *Cancer Res* 50: 7023–30.

Meyer, M., Pahl, H.L. and Baeurle, P.A. 1994. Regulation of the transcription factors NF-κB and AP-1 by redox changes. *Chem-Biol Interact* 91: 91–100.

Michalopoulos, G.K. 1990. Liver regeneration: molecular mechanisms of growth control. *FASEB J* 4: 176–87.

Michalopoulos, G. and Zarnegar, R. 1992. Hepatocyte growth factor. *Hepatology* 15: 149–55.

Mitaka, T., Mikami, M., Sattler, G., Pitot, H. and Mochizuki, Y. 1992. Small cell colonies appear in the primary culture of adult rat hepatocytes in the presence of nicotinamide and epidermal growth factor. *Hepatology* 16: 440–7.

Morello, D., FitzGerald, M.J., Babinet, C. and Fausto, N. 1990. c-myc, c-fos, and c-jun regulation in the regenerating livers of normal and H-2K/c-myc transgenic mice. *Mol Cell Biol* 10: 3185–93.

Morello, D., Lavenu, A. and Babinet, C., 1990. Differential regulation and expression of jun, c-fos and c-myc proto-oncogenes during mouse liver regeneration and after inhibition of protein synthesis. *Oncogene* 5: 1511–19.

Mullhaupt, B., Feren, A., Fodor, E. and Jones, A. 1994. Liver expression of epidermal growth factor RNA. Rapid increases in immediate-early phase of liver regeneration. *J Biol Chem* 269: 19667–70.

Naldini, L., Tamagnone, L., Vigna, E., Sachs, M., Hartmann, G., Birchmeier, W., Daikuhara, Y., Tsubouchi, H., Blasi, F. and Comoglio, P.M. 1992. Extracellular proteolytic cleavage by urokinase is required for activation of hepatocyte growth factor/scatter factor. *EMBO J* 11: 4825–33.

Noguchi, S., Ohba, Y. and Oka, T. 1991. Influence of epidermal growth factor on liver regeneration after partial hepatectomy in mice. *J. Endocrinol* 128: 425–31.

Noguchi, S., Ohba, Y. and Oka, T. 1992. The role of transcription and messenger RNA stability in the regulation of epidermal growth factor receptor gene expression in regenerating mouse liver. *Hepatology* 15: 88–96.

Oberhammer, F.A., Pavelka, M., Sharma, S., Tietenbacher, R., Purchio, A.F., Bursch, W. and Schulte-Hermann, R. 1992. Induction of apoptosis in cultured hepatocytes and in regressing liver by transforming growth factor β1. *Proc Natl Acad Sci USA* 89: 5408–12.

Ogasawara, K., Hata, Y., Une, Y., Sasaki, F., Nakajima, Y., Uchino, J., Ito, Y. and Kawai, T. 1994. Preoperative and postoperative variations of human hepatocyte growth factor (hHGF) in hepatectomized patients. *J Jpn Surg Soc* 95: 521–7.

Pahl, H.L. and Baeuerle, P.A. 1994. Oxygen and the control of gene expression. *BioEssays* 16: 497–502.

Palombella, V.J., Rano, O.J. and Goldberg, A.L. 1994. The ubiquitin-proteasome pathway is required for processing the NF-κB1 precursor protein and the activation of NF-κB. *Cell* 78: 773–85.

Phillips, M.J. and Poucell, S. 1981. Modern aspects of the morphology of viral hepatitis. *Hum Pathol* 12: 1060–84.

Rana, B., Mischoulon, D., Xie, Y., Bucher, N. and Farmer, S. 1994. Cell-extracellular matrix interactions can regulate the switch between growth and differentiation in rat hepatocytes: reciprocal expression of C/EBPα and immediate-early growth response transcription factors. *Mol Cell Biol* 14: 5858–69.

Rhim, J., Sandgren, E., Palmiter, R. and Brinster, R. 1995. Complete reconstitution of mouse liver with xenogeneic hepatocytes. *Proc Natl Acad Sci USA* 92: 4942–6.

Roskams, T., Campos, R. V., Drucker, D.J. and Desmet, V.J. 1993. Reactive human bile ductules express parathyroid hormone-related peptide. *Histopathology* 23: 11–19.

Roskams, T., De Vos R., van den Oord, J.J. and Desmet, V.J. 1991. Cells with neuroendocrine features in regenerating human liver. *APMIS* 23(Suppl): 32–9.

Roskams, T. and Desmet, V.J. 1994. Parathyroid hormone-related peptide and development of intrahepatic bile ducts in man. *Int Hepatol Comm* 2: 121–7.

Roskams, T., van den Oord, J.J., De Vos, R. and Desmet, V.J. 1990. Neuroendocrine features of reactive bile ductules in cholestatic liver disease. *Am J Pathol* 137: 1017–25.

Russell, W., Dempsey, P., Sitaric, S., Peck, A. and Coffey, R., Jr. 1993. Transforming growth factor-alpha (TGF alpha) concentrations increase in regenerating rat liver: evidence for a delayed accumulation of mature TGF alpha. *Endocrinology* 133: 1731–8.

Russell, W.E., Kaufmann, W.K., Sitaric, S., Luetteke, N.C. and Lee, D.C. 1996. Liver regeneration and hepatocarcinogenesis in transforming growth factor-alpha-targeted mice. *Mol Carcinogenesis* 15: 183–9.

Sandgren, E., Luetteke, N., Palmiter, R., Brinster, R. and Lee, D. 1990. Overexpression of TGFα in transgenic mice: induction of epithelial hyperplasia, pancreatic metaplasia, and carcinoma of the breast. *Cell* 61: 1121–35.

Schirmacher, P., Geerts, A., Pietrangelo, A., Dienes, H.P. and Rogler, C.E. 1992. Hepatocyte growth factor/hepatopoietin A is expressed in fat-storing cells from rat liver but not myofibroblast-like cells derived from fat-storing cells. *Hepatology* 15: 5–11.

Schmidt, C., Bladt, F., Goedecke, S., Brinkmann, V., Zschiesche, W., Sharpe, M., Gherardi, E. and Birchmeier, C. 1995. Scatter factor/hepatocyte growth factor is essential for liver development. *Nature* 373: 699–702,

Schulte-Hermann, R., Bursch, W. and Kraupp-Grasl, B. 1993. Cell proliferation and apoptosis in normal liver and preneoplastic foci. *Env Health Perspect* 101: 87–90.

Schwall, R., Robbins, K., Jardieu, P., Chang, L., Lai, C. and Terrell, T. 1993. Activin induces cell death in hepatocytes in vivo and in vitro. *Hepatology* 18: 347–56.

Shiota, G., Wang, T., Nakamura, T. and Schmidt, E. 1994. Hepatocyte growth factor in transgenic mice: Effects on hepatocyte growth, liver regeneration and gene expression. *Hepatology* 19: 962–72.

Shiota, G., Okano, J.-I., Kawasaki, H., Kawamoto, T. and Nakamura, T. 1995. Serum hepatocyte growth factor levels in liver diseases: Clinical implications. *Hepatology* 21: 106–12.

Sirica, A. 1995. Ductular hepatocytes. *Histol Histopathol* 10: 433–56.

Tanahashi, T., Imamura, T. and Suzuki, M. 1994. Re-evaluation of FGF-1 as a potent mitogen for hepatocytes. *In Vitro Cell Dev* 30A: 139–41.

Tewari, M., Dobrzanski, P., Mohn, K.L., Cressman, D.E., Hsu, J.-C., Bravo, R. and Taub, R. 1992. Rapid induction in regenerating liver of RL/IF-1 (an IκB that inhibits NF-κB, RelB-p50, and c-Rel-p50) and PHF, a novel κB site-binding complex. *Mol Cell Biol* 12: 2898–908.

Uehara, Y., Minowa, O., Mori, C., Shiota, K., Kuno, J., Noda, T. and Kitamura, N. 1995. Placental defect and embryonic lethality in mice lacking hepatocyte growth factor/scatter factor. *Nature* 373: 702–5.

Webber, E.M., FitzGerald, M.J., Brown, P.I., Bartlett, M.H. and Fausto, N. 1993. TGFα expression during liver regeneration after partial hepatectomy and toxic injury, and potential interactions between TGFα and HGF. *Hepatology* 18: 1422–31.

Webber, E.M., Godowski, P.J. and Fausto, N. 1994. In vivo response of hepatocytes to growth factors requires an initial priming stimulus. *Hepatology* 19: 489–97.

Webber, E.M., Wu, J.C., Wang, L., Merlino, G. and Fausto, N. 1994. Overexpression of transforming growth factor-alpha causes liver enlargement and increased hepatocyte proliferation in transgenic mice. *Am J Pathol* 145: 398–408.

Willemse, P.J.A., Ausema, L., Terpstra, O.T., Krenning, E.P., ten Kate, F.W.J. and Schalm, S.W. 1992. Graft regeneration and host liver atrophy after auxiliary heterotopic liver transplantation for chronic liver failure. *Hepatology* 15: 54–7.

Wolf, H.K. and Michalopoulos, G.K. 1992. Hepatocyte regeneration in acute fulminant and nonfulminant hepatitis: a study of proliferating cell nuclear antigen expression. *Hepatology* 15: 707–13.

Wu, J.C., Merlino, G., Cveklova, K., Mosinger, B., Jr. and Fausto, N. 1994. Autonomous growth in serum-free medium and production of hepatocellular carcinomas by differentiated hepatocyte lines that overexpress transforming growth factor alpha 1. *Cancer Res* 54: 5964–73.

Wu, J.C., Merlino, G. and Fausto, N. 1994. Establishment and characterization of differentiated, nontransformed hepatocyte cell lines derived from mice transgenic for transforming growth factor alpha. *Proc Natl Acad Sci USA* 91: 674–8.

Yamada, H., Toda, G., Yoshiba, M., Hashimoto, N., Ikeda, Y., Mitsui, H., Kurokawa, K., Sugata, F., Hughes, R.D. and Williams, R. 1994. Humoral inhibitor of rat hepatocyte DNA synthesis from patients with fulminant liver failure. *Hepatology* 19: 1133–40.

Yamanaka, N., Okamoto, E. and Kawamura, E. 1993. Dynamics of normal and injured human liver regeneration after partial hepatectomy as assessed on the basis of computed tomography and liver function. *Hepatology* 18: 79–85.

Yasuda, H., Mine, T., Shibata, H., Eto, Y., Hasegawa, Y., Takeuchi, T., Asano, S. and Kojima, I. 1993. Activin A: An autocrine inhibitor of initiation of DNA synthesis in rat hepatocytes. *J Clin Invest* 92: 1491–6.

Zaret, K. 1994. Genetic control of hepatocyte differentiation. In *The Liver: Biology and Pathobiology*, 3rd edn., eds. I.M. Arias, J.L. Boyer, N. Fausto, W.B. Jakoby, D.A. Schachter and D.A. Shafritz, 53–68. New York: Raven Press.

PART THREE Intensive Care Management

10 Medical management of acute liver failure

William M. Lee

INTRODUCTION

Over the past 25 years, a more thorough understanding of the unique problems of patients with acute liver failure has resulted in improved intensive care and better overall survival. The crucial management decisions for the patient with acute liver failure begin in the emergency room, and the outcome is frequently determined in the first 12 h. Thus, the overall outcome is determined by the initial management strategy adopted, as much as it is by the intensive care administered later on. Acute liver failure is not hard to diagnose, but because it is infrequent, the diagnosis is often missed by the first medical contact. For example, a young person presenting with acute hepatitis symptoms who is ambulatory and has a prothrombin time more than 4 s prolonged should be considered to have developed one important warning sign for acute liver failure. The evolution to encephalopathy in this setting is not a certainty but is likely enough to warrant hospital admission for observation and management. Physicians underestimate the severity of illness in such cases either because they may not have seen a case recently, or because the age of the patient and their apparent excellent general health lulls them into a false sense of security. Moreover, the pace of deterioration in hospital is often extremely rapid and may surprise even the most experienced clinician. This is one situation where there is little time for contemplation or leisurely assessment.

This chapter will cover the initial management decisions that are needed, as well as practical information on intensive care management, therapy for the overall condition of acute liver failure (most of which has been dismally unsuccessful), and special considerations for the smaller hospital as well as the specialist center. This topic has been reviewed previously by several authors (Williams and Gimson 1991; Hawker 1993; Lee 1993; Munoz 1993).

EMERGENCY CARE

Altered mentation and coagulopathy are the hallmarks of the diagnosis of acute liver failure, and usually begin simultaneously or in quick succession (Trey and Davidson 1970). The diagnosis of acute liver failure can be made rapidly in a patient when clinical evidence of hepatitis coincides with the presence of confusion or agitation. A prothrombin time is always available in the emergency room and its rapid turnaround time is valuable to confirm the initial assessment. Patients with severe hepatitis should not be discharged from the emergency area before the prothrombin time is available. If the prothrombin time is more than 4 s prolonged (INR 1.8), (or any alteration in mental status is observed), the diagnosis of acute liver failure is secure and admission to hospital (and usually to the intensive care unit) is mandated. A meticulous search for the etiology and consideration of the possible need for transplantation must begin immediately.

HISTORY TAKING

Since the patient's mental functioning may deteriorate rapidly, all necessary information must be obtained from the patient on the first attempt. The questioner should review all medications ingested in the previous 2–4 weeks, including over-the-counter and herbal preparations, specifically asking about acetaminophen (paracetamol)-containing products, glue or other hydrocarbon exposure (Ruprah, Mank and Flanagan 1985), cocaine (Silva et al. 1991; Van Thiel and Perper 1992), "ecstasy" (Henry, Jeffreys and Dawling 1992), and mushrooms (Klein et al. 1989; Pinson et al. 1990). If a likely hepatotoxin is mentioned, then the exact timing of the ingestion as well as the quantity of drug must be determined. An assessment of other cofactors should also be made, since the toxicity of many agents is heightened by starvation, alcohol, and the use of concomitant drugs (Seeff et al. 1986; Whitcomb and Block 1994; Vale and Proudfoot 1995; Zimmerman and Maddrey 1995). A diligent search for etiology is likely to yield the correct answer in a majority of cases, and this is of crucial importance in considering the use of antidotes and in determining prognosis. If the cause of the illness remains unclear, then little can be said about prognosis except that those with idiopathic fulminant hepatic failure tend to do less well than those with known causes.

Review of possible exposure to viral hepatitis should be undertaken at this point, including needle use, close association with jaundiced individuals, and travel to countries where hepatitis A or E are endemic. A careful review of systems will uncover evidence of heart disease, an occasional cause of ischemic injury (Nouel et al. 1980; Hoffman et al. 1990), or evidence for concomitant acute renal failure (implicating acetaminophen or solvent exposure), or chronic renal failure which might potentiate drug-induced injury. Generally, chronic liver diseases are easily recognized, but an occasional patient with cirrhosis due to Wilson's disease or autoimmune chronic hepatitis may present in acute hepatic failure (McCullough et al. 1983; Berman et al. 1991; Sallie et al. 1992). An infiltrating tumor is implicated if there is massive hepatomegaly in a patient with a previous history of cancer, particularly of the breast, or lymphoma or melanoma.

PHYSICAL EXAMINATION

A thorough examination of the patient may disclose important points which enhance the anamnesis. Fever is uncommon in viral hepatitis and somewhat more common in drug-induced cases. Tachycardia, hypotension, and tachypnea are often impressive and suggest the magnitude of the initial circulatory alterations (and possible acidosis), which is usually in part due to dehydration. Severe hypotension which does not improve promptly should alert the physician to vascular collapse with ischemic injury due to cocaine, ecstacy, nicotinic acid, heart failure or heat stroke. Look for evidence of chronic liver disease such as spider angiomata or caput medusa, or the presence of ascites which often heralds a subacute course. A rash or lymphadenopathy will be seen in cases with phenytoin- or carbamazepine-induced hepatitis. Look for intravenous needle marks, particularly if the history is difficult to obtain or appears unreliable. Occasional patients will not be icteric when the course is truly fulminant; many patients are deeply icteric on admission. Mercaptans in the exhaled breath speak much about future encephalopathy, whether the patient is encephalopathic currently or not. Asterixis is only occasionally present in acute liver failure patients compared to their cirrhotic counterparts, while agitation and bizarre behavior is more common. Check thoroughly for signs of hemorrhage, including epistaxis, or vaginal or upper gastrointestinal bleeding.

LABORATORY INVESTIGATIONS

Initial emergency room tests should include prothrombin time, glucose, arterial blood gasses, complete blood count, toxicology screen, as well as a chemistry profile. Ten percent glucose should be given intravenously after blood is drawn in any patient with altered mental status prior to a clear etiology or blood glucose result being confirmed.

A summary of the lab values usually obtained and their relevance follows.

Test	Relevance
Complete blood count	
WBC	Normal, unless elevated due to infection
Hgb/Hct	Normal, unless gastrointestinal bleeding present
platelet count	Low in nearly 80 percent, frequently less than 100,000/mm^3
Serum chemistries	
Na	Normal (low if there has been excess water intake)
K	Usually low due to renal loss of K^+
Cl	Normal
CO_2	Low due to central hyperventilation (or acidosis)
BUN	Usually low, even in presence of concomitant renal failure; serum creatinine a better measure
Glucose	May be dangerously low, causing mental changes.
AST	Typically >500, may be greater than 10,000 units/l
ALT	Typically >500, may be greater than 10,000 units/l
Albumin	Variably low due to poor synthetic function, may be normal early in ALF
Total protein	Low, for the same reason. High globulins suggest chronicity or autoimmune hepatitis.
Ca^{++}	Low, due to low albumin, markedly low if active pancreatitis
PO_4^{--}	Usually very low, requires vigorous replacement
Mg^{++}	Low depending on recent nutritional state, needs replacement
Bilirubin	Typically high, less so in some hyperacute cases. Very high in Wilson's disease due to hemolysis, or in those with longstanding disease or renal failure. Values >30 mg/dl (510 mmol/l) indicate renal failure or hemolysis
Alkaline phosphatase	Normal to slightly increased: if low suggests Wilson's disease, if elevated, think of lymphoma or other metastatic tumor, or Budd–Chiari syndrome
Amylase, lipase	Should be normal, elevated values signify pancreatitis due to acetaminophen overdose, or, occasionally may be observed in any form of acute liver failure
Alpha-fetoprotein	May be elevated in low 100 range, due to active regeneration of hepatocytes. Values above 1000 suggest hepatocellular carcinoma.
Coagulation studies	
Prothrombin time	Typically several seconds or more prolonged. Depends on laboratory. INR may not be particularly helpful.
PTT	Variably prolonged
Arterial blood gasses	
pH	Often 7.5 or greater due to respiratory alkalosis, but if significant acidosis is present (pH <7.3), a bad prognostic sign
P_{CO_2}	Low due to hyperventilation and/or acidosis
P_{O_2}	Normal, low values are also a bad prognostic sign
Viral serologies	
Hepatitis A IgM	Positive only in acute hepatitis A cases
HBsAg	Positive in many different settings (see Table 10.1)
Anti-HCV antibody	Positive test may be seen, but rarely causes ALF
Anti-HDV antibody	Order mainly in patients positive for HBsAg, may be associated with rapidly progressive or fulminant hepatitis (see Chapter 2).
Toxicology screening tests	
Acetaminophen	When elevated, in early phases, quantitation may provide a rough guide to likely severity, but if the

Table 10.1. *Presentations of acute liver failure associated with hepatitis B*

Several different forms of hepatitis B virus infection lead to liver failure. Each of these differs in serological pattern from the other presentations highlighted here. The most common forms in most areas of the world are the first three listed. The important message to remember is that HBsAg may be negative in certain patients with early clearance. This is presumed due to the very active immune response observed, and is often a good prognostic sign. Such patients can only be diagnosed by obtaining anti-HBc IgM which will be positive in the absence of other markers. If transplant is needed for these "early clearance" patients, their prognosis is good since they seldom reinfect their new liver graft. Many intravenous drug users will be found to have combined HBV and HDV or HBV and HCV infections. These combination infections carry a higher morbidity than either alone, although HBV and HCV rarely causes true acute liver failure. The combination of acute hepatitis B with acute HDV infection is also uncommon, since clearance of hepatitis B infection aborts any continued delta infection, and each virus appears to inhibit replication of the other to some extent, thus facilitating clearance of both (see Chapter 2).

	HBsAg	anti-HBc IgM	anti-delta	HBcAg
Acute viral hepatitis B	+	+	–	+ or –
Acute viral hepatitis B (early clearance)	–	+	–	–
Acute delta hepatitis (HDV) (chronic HBV carrier)	+	–	+	+ or –
Hepatitis B mutant	+	+ or –	–	–
Hepatitis B plus C (anti-HCV +)	+	–	–	+ or –

	value obtained is low, the level should not lead to a false sense of security. Once ALF is established, values are of no help, since typically they are low or undetectable.
Ethanol	When positive, suspect other agents such as acetaminophen, or polysubstance abuse or overdose.
Drug screen	Cocaine may cause acute liver failure, but positive drug screen also may suggest virus exposure (intravenous drug use likely).

Other etiologic tests:

Ceruloplasmin	Should be strikingly low in Wilson's disease, otherwise low normal or normal. Urinary copper may be helpful, particularly after patient has received penicillamine challenge.
Creatine kinase, aldolase	Simultaneous muscle necrosis may falsely elevate transaminase values, but also provides clue to etiology. If muscle enzymes are elevated, consider cocaine, "ecstasy", ischemic necrosis, heat stroke, or shock.

Lumbar puncture is not usually needed unless fever or stiff neck indicate a process other than acute hepatic failure is occurring. Chest radiograph, electrocardiogram and urinalysis will be performed as routine measures, but will typically be normal on admission.

THE INITIAL ASSESSMENT

At this point, with all tests ordered and most of the data not yet received, it is important to make an initial assessment of severity and prognosis so that appropriate consultations, precautions, and plans can be made. This is where experience is the best guide, and few absolutes apply. Decisions to be made include: whether to place in an intensive care unit; whether or not to transfer immediately to a transplant center; and whether to list the patient for transplant, if already in the transplant facility. With only the prothrombin time and an arterial blood gas one usually can make a fairly astute assessment. Based on the King's College Hospital criteria, patients who have consumed acetaminophen and who enter the hospital with an arterial pH <7.3 should be immediately transferred to a transplant center and listed for transplantation (O'Grady et al. 1989). Patients with a normal pH who are relatively alert but have prolonged prothrombin times form a larger group, however, and their management and decision to list for transplantation should be based on evidence of deterioration as indicated in the O'Grady or French criteria (O'Grady et al. 1989; and see Chapter 14). The best single prognostic guide is the prothrombin time, although factor V levels have also been used.

Admission to the intensive care unit (ICU) is mandated for anyone with altered mentation. It is best to consider anyone with grade I or II encephalopathy for transfer to a transplant facility at this time (Ede and Williams 1986; Davenport, Will and Davidson 1990). This does not mean that transplant must be performed simply because transfer has been accomplished, or that the patient will necessarily be listed for transplant. It is necessary simply because transportation of a comatose patient becomes hazardous and is virtually impossible once grade III or IV coma has set in.

A plan for triage of patients with acute liver failure is illustrated in Figure 10.1. It is necessary to make prompt and definite decisions early, based on overall clinical assessment, including social, financial, and other considerations, and to continue to reassess the situation on a daily basis. Distance from the transplant center should not preclude consideration of transfer, nor should the fact that a suicide attempt led to the present dilemma. In general, single suicide attempts represent cries for help and do not preclude transplantation. A repeated pattern of suicidal behavior or a proven long term pattern of substance abuse will color consideration for transplantation. At the time of the initial assessment, it is important to establish rapport with the patient's family and particularly to emphasize the gravity of the situation. This will often be shocking news, since the patient typically will have been totally well only a few days before. The family or next of kin can be extremely helpful in establishing the etiology for the episode and in helping to secure funding for transplantation if this is not immediately at hand, but to do so, they must grasp the seriousness of the condition from the beginning.

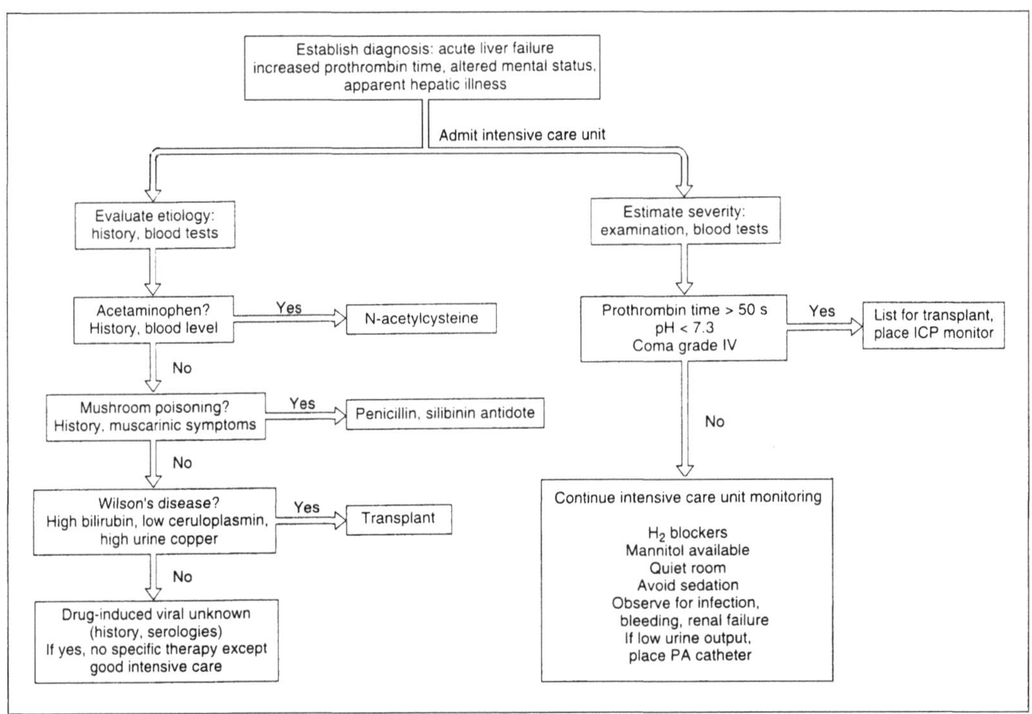

Figure 10.1 Algorithm for triage, diagnosis and treatment of the patient with acute liver failure. It is first necessary to perform the three "E's" – establish the diagnosis, evaluate the etiology, and estimate the severity of the illness.

ANTIDOTES

There are only a few toxins which affect the liver in a dose-related fashion and these same compounds are usually amenable to antidote therapy. In most instances, the antidote is easily obtained and given, with lifesaving results. It is imperative that the correct diagnosis be made on admission if there is any hope of reversing a potentially fatal condition with the antidote prescribed.

Controversy still surrounds the appropriate use of *N*-acetylcysteine (NAC) for acetaminophen poisoning (see Chapter 4), but in general, there is little harm in using this agent and great theoretical risk in withholding a lifesaving measure (Mitchell et al. 1973; Douglas, Hamlyn and James 1976; Prescott et al. 1976, 1979; Smilkstein et al. 1988; Harrison et al. 1990b; Keays et al. 1991; Vale and Proudfoot 1995). NAC is given in all instances where either the dose ingested or the blood level suggest the possibility of toxicity. Oral NAC has few side effects (occasional nausea and vomiting). Opinions vary as to the reliability of nomograms for interpreting acetaminophen blood levels. This is because use of the nomogram depends on an accurate notion of the time of ingestion, and that the ingestion has occurred all at one time. Toxicity may be present despite low blood levels in the alcoholic or fasting patient who takes acetaminophen over several hours or days without suicidal intent, or in the patient with established ALF (Vale and Proudfoot 1995; Zimmerman and Maddrey 1995).

The dose of oral *N*-acetylcysteine which is usually recommended is 140 mg/kg as an initial dose followed by 17 doses of 70 mg/kg at 4 h intervals. The usual intravenous dose is 150 mg/kg intravenously over one hour in 5 percent dextrose, followed at 4 h intervals by 70 mg/kg intravenously over one hour for 12 doses. Reactions resembling anaphylaxis have been reported, which respond readily to antihistamines (Vale and Proudfoot 1995). Although cimetidine has theoretical validity as an antidote since it binds to P4502E1, little clinical experience is available to warrant its recommendation for routine use.

Mushroom poisoning caused by the species *Amanita phalloides* also represents a situation amenable to rapid resuscitation and antidote use. Since there is no blood test to confirm the presence of *Amanita* toxins, the diagnosis rests on an accurate history accompanied, if possible, by identification of the offending mushroom by an expert or by obtaining identification of the toxin in urine samples. One must deal with the immediate antimuscarinic effects: nausea, vomiting, diarrhea, and sweating. After gastric lavage and administration of 50 g of activated charcoal via the nasogastric tube, fluid and electrolyte resuscitation becomes the immediate goal. Antidotes given simultaneously are penicillin 300,000 to 1,000,000 units/kg/day intravenously in divided doses, plus silibinin (a water-soluble form of silymarin), which is administered intravenously at a dose of 20–50 mg/kg/day. Renal function may deteriorate and hypoglycemia is not uncommon in this condition. Transplantation may be the only option, particularly if diagnosis and treatment is initiated later than 8–10 h after ingestion (Klein et al. 1989; Pinson et al. 1990).

Acute hydrocarbon ingestion such as carbon tetrachloride (CCl_4), or trichlorethylene results in a syndrome of concomitant hepatic and renal failure, usually with antecedent gastrointestinal or neurologic symptoms (Baerg and Kimberg 1970; Zimmerman 1978). Fortunately, these seem to be infrequent occurrences in the 1990s. NAC has been recommended as an antidote, although extensive testing has not been performed (Ruprah, Mant and Flanagan 1985).

Activated charcoal or syrup of ipecac as well as gastric lavage may also be considered for patients with a very recent drug ingestion, in whom evidence of toxicity has not yet evolved. These measures are probably without benefit after 12–24 h or if liver injury is already present. Gastric lavage carries the risk of aspiration in the somnolent patient.

THERAPY FOR THE OVERALL CONDITION, ACUTE LIVER FAILURE

Despite evidence that there is a common pathway to multiple organ failure which is followed in most patients with acute hepatic necrosis, there is no universal antidote or therapy which is beneficial for all patients. Numerous attempts to find such an agent have yielded discouraging results (Table 10.2). As early as 1972, Professor Jean-Pierre Benhamou expressed the frustration of all investigators in this field who have seen initial encouraging results in small trials, only to have their hopes dashed when a formal, controlled trial was undertaken:

". . . authors tend to publish isolated cases with a favorable outcome attributed to a given therapy, but not to publish cases in which therapy has failed. In fact it might be argued that the best future one can wish for a sufferer from SAHF (acute liver failure) is to undergo a new treatment and have his case published — 'be published or perish!'" (Benhamou, Rueff and Sicot 1972).

Systemic treatment with corticosteroids demonstrated no efficacy, but it was years before physicians were certain of this conclusion (Ware et al. 1974; EASL Study Group 1979; Rakela et al. 1991). In retrospect, it was intuitively unlikely that steroid therapy would be efficacious, given the variety of causes of acute liver failure. At the time, overexuberant inflammation was thought to underly all types of hepatic necrosis. Another form of therapy which was thought to have possible benefit for hepatic necrosis was heparin, based on the observation that many patients appeared to have disseminated intravascular coagulation, presumably occurring within the liver itself. Most patients with acute liver failure do have a profound coagulopathy, with diminished synthesis of coagulation factors as well as consumption of platelets and the appearance in the blood of fibrin split-products. Heparin was given in a small successful trial (Rake et al. 1971). However, further study over the ensuing years from the same unit failed to disclose any evidence for efficacy.

Table 10.2. *Ineffective treatments for acute liver failure*

Corticosteroid therapy
Exchange transfusions
Pig cross-perfusions
Total body washout with saline (cardiopulmonary bypass)
Spouse cross-perfusions
Heparin infusions
Hemodialysis and hemoperfusions
Charcoal hemoperfusion
Dialysis and activated charcoal
Insulin or glucagon infusions
Prostaglandin infusions

Reprinted with permission from Lee, W.M. 1996. Acute Liver Failure in Gastroenterology and Hepatology: A comprehensive visual text, eds. M. Feldman and W.C. Maddrey, *Current Medicine*, Philadelphia, p.7.11.

More recently, use of prostaglandins followed a similar course, with animal studies (Abecassis et al. 1987) and early small trials (Sinclair et al. 1989) suggesting that there was a general beneficial effect, which was not seen subsequently in a controlled trial from the same unit and elsewhere (Bernuau et al. 1990; Sheiner et al. 1992). Interferon has been used in one study with no obvious improvement in outcome (Levin et al. 1989).

The rationale for these initial trials was the quest for the universal antidote, despite evidence that loss of hepatic parenchymal function with resulting hepatic failure was the problem. A more modest goal, that of supporting the liver by removing toxins and prolonging survival until the liver could regenerate, was the principle behind exchange transfusions and several dramatic variations on this theme. Improvement in mentation could be observed in patients who were subjected to exchange transfusions. In the 1970s, when these procedures were initially performed, no automated equipment was available to carry the blood, the logistics were not easy and the risks to health care personnel were significant (Berger et al. 1966). No overall benefit could be demonstrated in controlled trials, and risks to patients from hypovolemia or to staff from extensive exposure to potentially viremic blood limited further progress. Use of autologous pig perfusion, or even cross-perfusion with another human circulation, proved disastrous as might have been expected (Burnell et al. 1965; Watts et al. 1967).

A unique chapter in treatment of this condition was the "total body washout" technique (Klebanoff 1973). With this method, a near-complete exchange of the patient's blood volume was undertaken by diluting out the blood volume with cold saline while the patient was attached to cardiopulmonary bypass. Hematocrits were said to reach 1 percent before reconstitution of normal blood parameters via transfusion. As with other early methods, a few early successes with this technique led to reports of successful outcomes. No further evidence of efficacy or use of the technique occurred beyond the pioneering institution.

The confusing results and occasional striking successes observed probably sprang from the highly variable prognosis observed for ALF. While the overall outcome statistics have improved for acute liver failure patients over the past 25 years, it is now clear that prognosis varies greatly among different etiologies (Hughes, Wendon and Gimson 1991). Thus, it is likely that the early successes observed with new modalities were more related to favorable patient selection (or to study patients receiving more attentive care), than to the efficacy of the procedure or therapy under study. More recently, high volume plasma exchanges, hemodialysis or plasmapheresis, have been shown to lead to improvement in coma grade, but to no long term benefit if liver cell mass is not reconstituted (Denis et al. 1978; Rakela, Kurtz and McCarthy 1988; Shin et al. 1989; Ramos and Almario 1990; Davenport, Will and Davidson 1993; and Chapter 22).

Efforts aimed at finding a method of restoring hepatic mass arose from the perception that the final failure of the liver was a failure of hepatocyte regeneration. Insulin and glucagon in combination have been shown to have stimulatory effects on hepatic regeneration (Jaspan, Landau and Schneider 1984; Harrison et al. 1990a; and Chapter 9), but in small clinical trials in acute liver failure this mode showed no efficacy, and has been abandoned. Although hepatocyte growth factor has been synthesized by recombinant technology, no clinical trials have been published. The levels of hepatocyte growth factor are already considerably elevated in acute liver failure, so the rationale for increasing the levels further is unclear (Tsubouchi et al. 1989; Gohda et al. 1991; and Chapter 9).

Other experimental therapies are considered in detail in the later chapters of this book (Chapters 18–22), but no treatment (short of transplantation) has yet been found which successfully reverses the overall syndrome of acute liver failure.

INTENSIVE CARE

Lacking specific treatments of proven efficacy (except for toxin antidotes), the best care is superior care of the comatose patient. Exact criteria for placement in the intensive care unit may vary considerably between institutions. As a general rule, any patient with altered mental status or evidence of significant coagulopathy (>4–6 s prolongation of the prothrombin time) warrants intensive care on the basis that his or her condition is likely to deteriorate rapidly. Observation of the liver failure patient for falling urine output, hypotension or the development of cerebral edema is less than ideal in the hospital ward setting.

Management of acute liver failure in the intensive care unit comprises four main areas of concern, which represent the most common systemic effects of the failure of the liver itself: neurological changes, hemodynamic considerations, infectious complications, and gastrointestinal bleeding. The intensive care plan should be aimed at avoidance of complications in each of these four areas, the first three of which are covered in more detail in individual chapters elsewhere in this book. A checklist of areas needing attention and the agents usually used is given in Table 10.3.

Table 10.3. *Therapeutic interventions in acute liver failure*

This list summarizes the current status concerning a variety of therapeutic measures used in intensive care of the patient with acute liver failure. Most are discussed in detail in the text, but this table provides a check list of the variety of treatments which may be considered.

Toxin antidotes
- Acetaminophen (*N*-acetylcysteine, see also Chapter 4)
- *Amanita* poisoning (silymarin, penicillin)
- Hydrocarbons (*N*-acetylcysteine?)

Encephalopathy/cerebral edema (see also Chapters 11 and 12)
- For encephalopathy (lactulose, neomycin, flumazenil all dubious value)
- Mannitol (standard treatment)
- Corticosteroids (no efficacy)
- Thiopental (second line, but controversial)
- Diuretics (second line, probably little efficacy)
- Hyperventilation (rarely used, since patients are already hyperventilating)

Renal failure/hypotension
- Volume replacement (universally needed, colloid most commonly used)
- Diuretics (Furosemide may be useful)
- *N*-acetylcysteine (may improve oxygen delivery, not available i.v. in USA)
- Prostacyclin (may be used to improve hemodynamics, but controversial)
- Dopamine (renal dose, controversial)
- Norepinephrine, other pressors (used for hypotension, if fluid replacement ineffective)
- Dialysis (may be used for acidosis, hyperkalemia, to decrease mannitol load)

Coagulopathy
- Fresh frozen plasma (only for active bleeding)
- Platelets (may be used if platelet count $<$20,000/ml)
- Heparin, DDAVP (no proven value)
- H_2 receptor blockers (given for bleeding prophylaxis)

Metabolic replacement
- Glucose (routine for blood glucose $\leq$60 mg/dl)
- Potassium (typically, large quantities required)
- Phosphate (also depleted in virtually all patients)
- Magnesium (also frequently depleted)

Infection
- Prophylactic antibiotics (controversial, see Chapter 13)

GENERAL CONSIDERATIONS

All patients admitted to the intensive care unit should have a Foley catheter placed, cardiac monitoring, triple lumen intravenous catheters, and (in most instances) an arterial line for pressure monitoring and blood sampling. Swan–Ganz pulmonary artery pressure monitoring and measurement of cardiac output is undertaken in anyone with evidence of hypotension, vasomotor instability (where pressors may be used), or where urine output is inadequate. In the presence of coagulopathy or thrombocytopenia, a jugular vein insertion is safer than use of the subclavian vein. Intracranial monitoring (discussed in detail in Chapters 6 and 13) is reserved for patients in grade III or IV coma, but is usually limited to those who are listed for transplantation, since important changes in intracerebral pressure accompany induction of anesthesia in these patients. Bleeding is the main risk of intracerebral monitor placement. Cerebral blood flow may be measured indirectly by transcranial Doppler studies or by measurement of oxygen extraction via jugular bulb sampling. With this technique, it is necessary to place a retrograde jugular vein catheter, and the use of these devices at present is probably best restricted to research units. Feeding tubes should be placed in all patients in grade III or IV coma.

CNS CONSIDERATIONS

Of utmost importance is the maintenance of adequate cerebral perfusion, since the occurrence of anoxic brain damage precludes any meaningful recovery. An occasional patient will recover fully but be saddled with permanent neurological sequelae (O'Brien et al. 1987). Conversely, evidence of severe injury is not always irreversible. General measures include placement of the patient in a quiet area, since intracerebral pressure is increased by stimulation of any kind. The head is kept at only 10 to 20 degrees elevated above the horizontal, and should not be at 45 degrees as had been advocated in the past (Davenport et al. 1990). In general, sedation of any kind is avoided in the early stages of coma. Benzodiazepines, which are often given mistakenly in the emergency room if the patient is agitated, may linger for days after a single dose and cloud the physician's ability to assess mental status. Agitation is a problem on occasion, but the patient's condition so frequently evolves to a deeper level of coma that simple restraints are usually enough during the agitated phase. Nursing assessments of mental status should be made hourly and guidelines for treatment established with all personnel according to predetermined criteria, specifically when and how to use mannitol if signs of impending uncal herniation appear. Most patients with early grades of encephalopathy will not need respiratory support, since central hyperventilation provides a respiratory alkalosis with low Pco_2 and adequate oxygenation.

Although mechanical hyperventilation is used in brain trauma patients, it has not been shown to improve intracerebral pressure consistently in acute liver failure. Similarly, thiopental which has been used in neurosurgery, may establish a level of coma in which intracerebral pressure and brain metabolism are diminished. However, controversy exists as to the value of such treatment since systemic blood pressure (and cerebral perfusion pressure) may be decreased as well by thiopental (Forbes et al. 1989).

The right way to manage patients with advanced grades of coma is unclear. If the patient has not been transported to a transplant center or if consideration will not be given to transplantation, then observation without assisted ventilation may be adequate even in patients with grade III coma since the gag reflex is usually well-preserved. At some point between grade III and grade IV, the risk of major complications becomes greater, and intubation to protect the airway should be performed. Problems such as vascular instability, gastrointestinal hemorrhage and cerebral edema are likely to require full intensive support for a significant length of time. In addition to endotracheal intubation, placement of a feeding tube, as well as pulmonary artery catheter should be performed, if these have not already been undertaken.

Assisted ventilation should be undertaken in virtually all patients with grade III to IV coma, but may be required in patients with lesser grades if hypoxia is present. With placement of an endotracheal tube to protect the airway and assist ventilation, consideration is given to sedation and paralysis. A traumatic intubation may induce a sudden rise in intracranial pressure and thus provoke uncal herniation. The use of sedation will mask the assessment of mental state, but is mandated for comfort and to avoid periods of agitation. Controlled ventilation has the added value of allowing more precise management of acid–base changes, and affords the ability to counteract the central hyperventilation (which may itself decrease liver blood flow) while decreasing the energy requirements of the actively hyperventilating patient.

Standard ventilator settings should generally provide a respiratory rate of 14–18 breaths per minute, with a tidal volume in liters of 12 times the patient's weight in kg. Some hypercatabolic patients or those with sepsis may require higher than predicted minute volumes. Inspired oxygen requirements vary but the usual starting point is an Fio_2 of 40 to 60 percent. Positive end expiratory pressure (PEEP) levels are usually maintained at 2–4 mmHg, with an inspiration period of 25–33 percent and a pause time of 10 percent of the total cycle. Initial ventilation is usually undertaken with spontaneous intermittent volume (SIMV) controlled ventilation, although this may be ineffective due to the tachypnea and shallow tidal volumes frequently observed in these patients. Tidal volumes should be decreased in the presence of high airway pressures such as are seen in bronchospasm or adult respiratory distress syndrome (ARDS) since barotrauma may result. If the CO_2 level elevates, then the respiratory drive will require paralysis. Similarly, volume-controlled ventilation usually demands that the patient be comatose or paralyzed. SIMV is the normal mode for weaning patients from the ventilator, using a gradual reduction of the respiratory rate, while monitoring arterial blood gasses. If the patient tolerates this, then extubation can usually be performed or the patient switched to pressure support ventilation or continuous positive airway pressure before extubation.

The presence of hypoxia with high airway pressures in this setting should lead to a search for bronchospasm, mucous plugging, cuff leak, pneumothorax, or ARDS. Check for mechanical problems, listen for adequate gas movement and recheck the chest radiograph. ARDS must be identified by chest radiograph, and can be managed by judicious restriction of fluid, use of colloid rather than crystalloid for fluid replacement, as well as increase inspired O_2 concentrations and positive end expiratory pressure. Development of ARDS is uncommon, but usually signals advanced severe multiorgan disease or massive fluid overload (MacNaughton and Evans 1992). For patients with severe lung injury, volume controlled ventilation is better than SIMV, starting with higher FIO_2 (70 percent) and PEEP values (10–14 cmH_2O). It is necessary to monitor cardiac output as PEEP is increased. If ventilatory settings seem appropriate, a search must be made for other causes of inadequate gas exchange. Oxygen extraction at the tissue level is typically increased (Bihari, Gimson, Lindridge and Williams 1985a; Bihari, Gimson and Williams 1986), but this is usually met with ease by increased exchange at the alveolar capillary. Lactulose had been routinely used via nasogastric tube, although no clear evidence of efficacy has been proven for this treatment, and some units do not use lactulose because of this and the concern over fluid losses. If used, 30 to 60 ml lactulose may be given every 8 h, adjusting the dose to provide no more than two loose stools per day. Use of short-acting benzodiazepine antagonists such as flumazenil is not recommended although occasional patients may show transient responses.

Mannitol should be available, preferably in a syringe at the bedside for use at a moment's notice. The initial dose is 0.5 g/kg (at least 30 g) by rapid bolus infusion. This may be repeated twice over the next 4–8 h if needed for intracerebral pressure greater than 30–40 mmHg on intracerebral monitoring, or for signs of neurologic deterioration (unequal pupils, change in breathing pattern, decerebrate posturing). All nursing staff should have received specific instructions in its use, since waiting for a physician's order could cause inordinate delay. The value of diuretics such as furosemide remains controversial in the management of cerebral edema (see Chapter 13).

HEMODYNAMIC CONSIDERATIONS

Liver failure patients arriving in the intensive care unit tend to be tachycardic and hypotensive for several reasons (Wendon et al. 1991). First, any patient who is obtunded has had poor recent oral intake, and will be dehydrated and hemoconcentrated. Second, the presence of a capillary leak, and vasodilatation due to the underlying circulatory changes which accompany liver failure or Gram-negative sepsis, will result in hypotension and an increased cardiac output. In addition, most patients will have increased overall muscle tone and stress- or hypoglycemia-induced epinephrine release. Despite these conflicting features, the overall condition is typically characterized by hypotension and warm dry skin. Volume resuscitation can begin immediately while central line or pulmonary artery catheter placement is under way, since these will ultimately allow for a more careful assessment of cardiac index and volume status. Fresh frozen plasma (FFP) or 4.5 percent albumin may be used as replacement fluid; plasma is not indicated in any standard regimen for coagulopathy per se without evidence of active hemorrhage. In milder cases, it is useful to avoid FFP so that the prothrombin time accurately reflects the state of liver cell synthetic function, since this will be used prognostically in determining the need for transplantation. Although vitamin K is frequently given, there is little evidence of vitamin K depletion in most patients. If vitamin K is used, give intravenously rather than intramuscularly to avoid intramuscular hematomas. Once the pulmonary artery catheter is in place, replacement fluids (which should be primarily colloids) can be given, aiming at a pulmonary capillary wedge pressure of 12–14 mmHg. Crystalloid solutions containing 10 percent glucose may be needed if blood glucose levels are diminished. Hemodynamic measurements should be made at least every 8 h, or after any change in vasopressor medication. For systemic hypotension, norepinephrine is given with the aim of maintaining mean arterial pressure in the range of at least 50–60 mmHg.

In terms of fluid balance, there are many similar features in the acute liver failure patient to chronic liver failure: avid renal retention of salt and water is the rule with loss of fluid into the ascites compartment and the interstitium. As in the cirrhotic patient, therefore, use of salt solutions as volume replacement should be sparing unless a large volume deficit is apparent.

The addition of vasodilators such as prostacyclin, or of *N*-acetylcysteine to increase oxygenation, remains controversial. Epoprostenol (5 ng/kg/min) may be given and this infusion is usually commenced in the seriously ill patient in whom pressors are already in use. *N*-acetylcysteine (in nonacetaminophen cases) has been shown to improve peripheral oxygen extraction, and may be of value in this same setting. Available intravenously in the United Kingdom and Europe, *N*-acetylcysteine appears to improve cardiac output, and oxygen delivery. The dose is 150 mg/kg as a loading dose intravenously over 30 min, followed by a maintenance dose of 150 mg/kg/24 h (Harrison et al. 1991). Oral *N*-acetylcysteine (Mucomyst®, Bristol-Meyers Institutional Products, Evansville, IN) is the only form available in the United States (and is the mainstay antidote in acetaminophen cases). The lack of an intravenous formulation has precluded use of *N*-acetylcysteine for improving cardiovascular support in North American patients.

Hepatectomy has been advocated based on uncontrolled studies as a method of improving the circulatory abnormalities in patients with advanced acute liver failure. Transplant surgeons were the first to introduce such drastic therapy, based on the observation that mean arterial pressure appears to improve following removal of the native liver in the transplant setting (Ringe et al. 1993; Rozga et al. 1993; So et al. 1993), suggesting that liver-derived toxins perpetuate the circulatory abnormalities. The typical situation in which hepatectomy has been performed is the patient who has sustained massive liver trauma or has severe graft dysfunction following transplantation. Nevertheless, removal of the liver without the availability of a suitable donor liver seems futile, since the likelihood of finding a replacement in a short time interval is uncertain. Life support in the absence of a liver has been maintained for up to 60 h with a satisfactory outcome. Wider use of total hepatectomy with extracorporeal liver assist devices and/or with intensive plasmapheresis awaits more careful study in animal models before it can reasonably be applied to man (Lee 1994b).

INFECTION

Severe immuncompromise typifies acute liver failure and the prevention of infection is a major goal in caring for these patients. Fever and leukocytosis may be absent in the presence of systemic infection, or present due to noninfectious causes. Surveillance typically includes obtaining cultures of blood, urine and sputum on admission and roughly every other day. Chest radiographs are usually done on a daily basis to assess evidence for pneumonia, fluid overload, or pulmonary hemorrhage. Gram-positive infections are particularly common, and probably iatrogenic, since the patient invariably has had many invasive procedures (Wyke et al. 1982; Rolando et al. 1990). Ascites, if present, must be tapped periodically to identify the appearance of spontaneous or secondary peritonitis. The efficacy of prophylactic antibiotics has not been established; they appear to decrease morbidity if not mortality (see Chapter 12).

BLEEDING DIATHESIS

Stress ulceration is known to occur in patients with fulminant hepatic failure, and the use of H_2 blockers has been accepted therapy since 1977 (MacDougall et al. 1977; MacDougall and Williams 1978). More recently, the role of acid suppression in fostering growth of gastric nosocomial organisms which can then find their way to the lungs or blood stream has lead to the use of sucralfate in preference to acid-suppressing drugs. The starting dose is 2 g by mouth or via nasogastric tube every 8 h. Treatment of the coagulopathy with fresh frozen plasma or platelets is generally not undertaken in the absence of bleeding (Gazzard, Henderson and Williams 1975). Use of prophylactic platelets is recommended for platelet counts below 30,000/mm^3. Active gastrointestinal hemorrhage should be treated in conventional fashion, with plasma and red blood cell replacement as appropriate. Endoscopic intervention may be necessary, and should be performed early; prophylactic antibiotics may be given to cover bacteremia. Gastrointestinal bleeding was formerly a dreaded complication, but judicious use of resuscitation and endoscopy has made it a relatively infrequent cause of death.

METABOLIC CONSIDERATIONS

A number of further metabolic derangements need mention. Blood glucose levels should be monitored at least every 4–6 h, particularly if hypoglycemia has been detected previously. Phosphate levels are frequently very low in patients, even when nutrition prior to hospitalization appeared adequate. Similarly, magnesium levels are also found to be low. It is generally wise to replace phosphate and magnesium losses early. Values in the low normal range may still require supplementation if there is a history of malnutrition, a long hospital course or the presence of seizures: 16 mmol of magnesium sulfate may be given in 250 ml 5 percent dextrose over an 8 h period. Tube feedings may begin with a suitable balanced liquid diet, and severe protein restriction should be avoided (60 g protein/24 h is a reasonable starting program). No role for specialized high branched-chain amino acid solutions has been determined. Phosphate levels may require ongoing supplementation throughout the hospitalization.

PROBLEM-SOLVING IN THE ICU

Central to the management of patients with acute liver failure is the experience of the staff caring for the patient. Consultants with special expertise should be used as appropriate, but, in general, the hepatologist will have more specific knowledge of the needs of the ALF patients, than say, the anesthesiologist or nephrologist, who are involved in the care of liver failure patients only rarely. It is generally wise to replace phosphate and magnesium losses early. The following are specific troubleshooting hints for evaluation and treatment of specific problems frequently encountered. Contacting a transplant center or other hepatologists with specific expertise in this condition may be of value in addressing specific issues not covered in this text.

Hypotension

Persistent volume depletion is the first consideration in hypotensive patients. If pulmonary artery pressures are diminished, then further volume repletion is necessary. If systemic vascular resistance is low, this suggests the hyperdynamic circulation associated with acute liver failure, possibly complicated by sepsis, whether fungal or bacterial. Treat the underlying cause if it can be identified, or consider broad-spectrum antibiotics. Norepinephrine may be needed to restore arterial pressure, particularly when no etiology for the low mean arterial pressure is elicited.

Acidosis

Lactic acidosis, like hypotension, may be the result of tissue hypoxia due to circulatory failure despite resuscitation. This may be the hardest problem to treat (Bihari et al. 1985a; Bihari and Wendon 1991). Further studies are needed to validate the improvement observed with epoprostenol or *N*-acetylcysteine in initial studies (Harrison et al. 1991; Wendon et al. 1992). A search for other causes of acidosis must also be considered: measure lactate, ketoacids and salicylates. Consider urinary bicarbonate loss as well as concomitant renal failure. Phosphate depletion will also exacerbate acidosis and replacement should help this problem as well as protect against the evolution of ARDS. Bicarbonate will be of limited value unless there is profound renal bicarbonate wasting. Hemodialysis or hemodiafiltration may be of value in reversing the acidosis, particularly in the presence of renal failure.

Low cardiac index

The patient with acute liver failure typically has a high cardiac index (Cardiac index = cardiac output/body surface area), associated with low peripheral vascular resistance. The presence of a *low* cardiac index (<4.5 l/min) suggests the presence of a separate confounding problem. Consider blood loss, pneumothorax, excess PEEP, acidosis, or cardiac tamponade. Based on these possible problems, a chest radiograph, cardiogram and analysis of airway pressures should highlight the problem. Intravenous dobutamine should be started if no other problem can be elicited. Low cardiac index is a bad prognostic sign (Shoemaker, Kram and Appel 1990).

Arrhythmias are reportedly rare in acute liver failure, but may occur due to electrolyte imbalance, passage of pulmonary artery catheter through the right ventricle, or may be due to underlying unrelated heart disease (Rosenbloom 1991).

CARE IN THE COMMUNITY HOSPITAL

In many instances, the community hospital is the site of care for these very sick and complex patients. Reasons for not transferring patients to a major transplant center may include lack of funding, presence of a pattern of recurrent substance abuse or simply the distance from a transplant center. Whatever the reason, it may be necessary to support the patient in the best possible way short of transfer. In this instance, most of the general considerations above apply, except that the most invasive measures may not be practical or indicated. For example, mannitol should still be at the bedside, but use of intracerebral monitoring will not be feasible. Nor will a pulmonary artery catheter necessarily be indicated or obtainable. Nevertheless, support should continue with vigorous attention to fluid balance, pulmonary status, and surveillance for infection. Evidence for irreversible brain damage will be present if fixed dilated pupils appear, or loss of spontaneous breathing patterns develop in patients who are not sedated or paralyzed. Confirmation of loss of brain function can be sought via electroencephalogram. With the finding of two consecutive flat electroencephalograms, it is appropriate to consider discontinuation of respiratory support. A cautionary word concerning irreversible brain damage was offered by a recent paper in which a patient who appeared to have no active brain function was seen to make a full recovery (Davies, Mutimer, Lowes, Elias and Neuberger 1994). Nevertheless, this is an unusual occurrence and must be put in perspective with the overall outcome of such patients.

TIMING OF LIVER TRANSPLANTATION

One of the most vexing problems for all physicians dealing with acute liver failure is determining the precise timing of liver transplantation given the limited organ availability. While liver transplantation is listed as "the only definitive treatment," only one in ten patients who might benefit from a transplant ultimately receives a graft. In some instances, even those patients who are grafted receive their organ too late and have sustained permanent brain damage. The overall survival for acute liver failure patients approaches that for those with chronic liver disease, probably reflecting the good general health of the recipients on one side and the occasional failure to obtain a graft in a suitable time interval on the other. The acute liver failure patient, who is generally young with a well-preserved nutritional state, lacking portal hypertension and all its complications, is a near-optimal transplant candidate. Unfortunately, the urgency of the situation, once transplantation is considered, as well as the logistics involved in obtaining funding, transportation to the transplant center and an organ all in a timely fashion, presents a series of hurdles to a successful outcome. This not only limits the number of such patients transplanted, but impairs their recovery when the liver arrives too late to be of optimal benefit. The decision to transplant is considered in Chapters 14–16 (Lee 1994a). Optimal timing is only possible if the correct diagnosis is made early and if the severity of the condition is appreciated at the time of the initial assessment, so that arrangements for transfer and securing funding can be made in a timely fashion.

REFERENCES

Abecassis, M., Falk, J.A., Makowka, L., Dindzans, V.J., Falk, R.E. and Levy, G.A. 1987. 16,16-dimethyl prostaglandin E_1 prevents the development of fulminant hepatitis and blocks the induction of monocyte/macrophage procoagulant activity after murine hepatitis virus strain 3 infection. *J Clin Invest* 80: 881–9.

Baerg, R.D. and Kimberg, D.V. 1970. Centrilobular hepatic necrosis and acute renal failure in glue sniffers. *Ann Intern Med* 73: 713–20.

Benhamou, J.P., Rueff, B. and Sicot, C. 1972. Severe hepatic failure: a critical study of current therapy. In *Liver and Drugs*, eds. F. Orlandi and A.M. Jezequel, 213. New York: Academic Press.

Berger, R.L., Liversage, R.M., Chalmers, T.C., Graham, J.H., McGoldrick, D.M. and Stohlman, F. 1966. Exchange transfusion in the treatment of fulminating hepatitis. *N Engl J Med* 274: 497–500.

Berman, D.H., Leventhal, R.I., Gavaler, J.S., Cadoff, E.M. and Van Thiel, D.H. 1991. Clinical differentiation of fulminant Wilsonian hepatitis from other causes of hepatic failure. *Gastroenterology* 100: 1129–31.

Bernuau, J., Babany, G., Bourliere, M. et al. 1990. Prostaglandin E1 (PGE1) has no beneficial effect in patients with either severe or fulminant hepatitis B (abst.) *Hepatology* 12: 875.

Bihari, D., Gimson, A.E., Lindridge, J. and Williams, R. 1985a. Lactic acidosis in fulminant hepatic failure. Some aspects of pathogenesis and prognosis. *J Hepatol* 1: 405–16.

Bihari, D., Gimson, A.E.S., Waterson, M. and Williams, R. 1985b. Tissue hypoxia in fulminant hepatic failure. *Crit Care Med* 13: 1034–9.

Bihari, D. and Wendon, J. 1991. Tissue hypoxia in fulminant hepatic failure. In *Acute Liver Failure: Improved Understanding and Better Therapy*, eds. R. Williams and R.D. Hughes, 42–4. London: Miter Press.

Bihari, D.J., Gimson, A.E.S. and Williams, R. 1986. Cardiovascular, pulmonary and renal complications of fulminant hepatic failure. *Sem Liver Dis* 6: 119–28.

Burnell, J.M., Thomas, E.D., Ansell, J.S. et al. 1965. Observations on cross circulation in man. *Am J Med* 38: 832–6.

Davenport, A., Will, E.J. and Davidson, A.M. 1993. Improved cardiovascular stability during continuous modes of renal replacement therapy in critically ill patients with acute hepatic and renal failure. *Crit Care Med* 21: 323–8.

Davenport, A., Will, E.J. and Davidson, A.M. 1990. Effect of posture on intracranial pressure and cerebral perfusion pressure in patients with fulminant hepatic and renal failure after acetaminophen self-poisoning. *Crit Care Med* 18: 286–9.

Davies, M.H., Mutimer, J.D., Lowes, J., Elias, E. and Neuberger, J. 1994. Recovery despite impaired cerebral perfusion in fulminant hepatic failure. *Lancet* 343: 1329–30.

Denis, J., Opolon, P., Nusinovici, V., Granger, A. and Darnis, F. 1978. Treatment of encephalopathy during fulminant hepatic failure by haemodialysis with high permeability membrane. *Gut* 19: 787–93.

Douglas, A.P., Hamlyn, A.N. and James, O. 1976. Controlled trial of cysteamine in treatment of acute paracetamol (acetaminophen) poisoning. *Lancet* i: 111–15.

EASL Study Group. 1979. Randomised trial of steroid therapy in acute liver failure. *Gut* 20: 620–3.

Ede, R.J. and Williams, R. 1986. Hepatic encephalopathy and cerebral edema. *Sem Liver Dis* 6: 107–18.

Forbes, A., Alexander, G.J.M., O'Grady, J.G. et al. 1989. Thiopental infusion in the treatment of intracranial hypertension complicating fulminant hepatic failure. *Hepatology* 10: 306–10.

Gazzard, B., Henderson, J. and Williams, R. 1975. Early changes in coagulation following paracetamol overdose and a controlled trial of fresh frozen plasma therapy. *Gut* 16: 617–20.

Gohda, E., Tsubouchi, H., Nakayama, H., et al. 1991. Purification and partial characterization of hepatocyte growth factor in blood of patients with fulminant hepatic failure. *Dig Dis Sci* 36: 785–90.

Harrison, P.M., Hughes, R.D., Forbes, A., Portmann, B., Alexander, G.J.M. and Williams, R. 1990a. Failure of insulin and glucagon to stimulate liver regeneration in fulminant hepatic failure. *J Hepatol* 110: 332–6.

Harrison, P.M., Keays, R., Bray, G.P., Alexander, G.J.M. and Williams, R. 1990b. Improved outcome of paracetamol-induced fulminant hepatic failure by late administration of acetylcysteine. *Lancet* 335: 1572–3.

Harrison, P.M., Wendon, J.A., Gimson, A.E.S., Alexander, G.J.M. and Williams, R. 1991. Improvement by acetyl cysteine of hemodynamics and oxygen transport in fulminant hepatic failure. *N Engl J Med* 324: 1852–7.

Hawker, F. 1993. Fulminant hepatic failure. In *The Liver*, ed. F. Hawker, 71–135. London: Saunders.

Henry, J.A., Jeffreys, K.J. and Dawling, S. 1992. Toxicity and deaths from 3,4-methylene-dioxymethamphetamine ("ecstacy"). *Lancet* 340: 384–7.

Hoffman, B.J., Pate, M.B., Marsh, W.H. and Lee, W.M. 1990. Cardiomyopathy unrecognized as a cause of hepatic failure. *J Clin Gastroenterol* 12: 306–9.

Hughes, R.D., Wendon, J. and Gimson, A.E.S. 1991. Acute liver failure. *Gut* (Suppl.), S86–9.

Jaspan, J.B., Landau, R.L. and Schneider, J. 1984. Insulin and glucagon infusion in the treatment of liver failure. *Arch Intern Med* 144: 2075–8.

Keays, R., Harrison, P.M., Wendon, J.A. et al. 1991. A prospective controlled trial of intravenous *N*-acetylcysteine in paracetamol-induced fulminant hepatic failure. *BMJ* 303: 1024–9.

Klebanoff, G. 1973. Early experience with total body washout for hepatic coma. *Gastroenterology* 64: 156–8.

Klein, A.S., Hart, J., Brems, J.J., Goldstein, L., Lewin, K. and Busuttil, R.W. 1989. Amanita poisoning: treatment and the role of liver transplantation. *Am J Med* 86: 187–93.

Lee, W.M. (1994a). Acute liver failure: Is anything really effective short of transplantation? In *Difficult Decisions in Gastroenterology*, eds. J.S. Barkin and A.I. Rodgers, 141–6.

Lee, W.M. (1994b). Selected summaries: Total hepatectomy for acute liver failure: don't take out my liver! *Gastroenterology* 107: 894–7.

Lee, W.M. 1993. Medical progress: Acute liver failure. *N Engl J Med* 329: 1862–74.

Levin, S., Leibowitz, E., Torten, J. and Hahn, T. 1989. Interferon treatment in acute progressive and fulminant hepatitis. *Israel J Med Sci* 25: 364–72.

MacDougall, B. and Williams, R. 1978. H_2 receptor antagonists in the prevention of upper gastro-intestinal hemorrhage in fulminant hepatic failure. *Gastroenterology* 74: 464–5.

MacDougall, B.R.D., Bailey, R.J. and Williams, R. 1977. H_2-receptor antagonists and antacids in the prevention of acute gastrointestinal haemorrhage in fulminant hepatic failure. *Lancet* i: 617–19.

MacNaughton, P.D. and Evans, T.W. 1992. Management of adult respiratory distress syndrome. *Lancet* 339: 469–71.

McCullough, A.J., Fleming, R., Thistle, J.L., et al. 1983. Diagnosis of Wilson's disease presenting as fulminant hepatic failure. *Gastroenterology* 84: 161–7.

Mitchell, J.R., Jollow, D.J., Potter, W.Z., Gillette, J.H. and Brodie, B.B. 1973. Acetaminophen-induced hepatic necrosis. IV. protective role of glutathione. *J Pharmacol Exp Ther* 187: 211–17.

Munoz, S.J. 1993. Difficult management problems in fulminant hepatic failure. *Sem Liver Dis* 13: 395–413.

Nouel, O., Henrion, J., Bernuau, J. et al. 1980. Fulminant failure due to transient circulatory failure in patients with chronic heart disease. *Dig Dis Sci* 25: 49–52.

O'Brien, C.J., Wise, R.J.S., O'Grady, J.G. and Williams, R. 1987. Neurological sequelae in patients recovered from fulminant hepatic failure. *Gut* 28: 93–5.

O'Grady, J.G., Alexander, G.J.M., Hayllar, K.M. and Williams, R. 1989. Early indicators of prognosis in fulminant hepatic failure. *Gastroenterology* 97: 439–45.

Pinson, C.W., Daya, M.R., Benner, K.G., et al. 1990. Liver transplantation for severe *Amanita phalloides* mushroom poisoning. *Am J Surg* 159: 493–9.

Prescott, L.F., Illingworth, R.N., Critchley, J.A.J.H., Stewart, M.J., Adam, R.D. and Proudfoot, A.T. 1979. Intravenous *N*-acetyl cysteine: the treatment of choice for paracetamol poisoning. *BMJ* ii: 1097–100.

Prescott, L.F., Sutherland, G.R., Park, J., Smith, I.J. and Proudfoot, A.T. 1976. Cysteamine, methionine and penicillamine in the treatment of paracetamol poisoning. *Lancet* 2: 109–13.

Rake, M.O., Shilkin, K.B., Winch, J., Flute, P.T., Lewis, M.L. and Williams, R. 1971. Early and intensive therapy of intravascular coagulation in acute liver failure. *Lancet* 1: 1215–18.

Rakela, J., Kurtz, S.B. and McCarthy, J.T. 1988. Postdilution hemofiltration in the management of acute hepatic failure: a pilot study. *Mayo Clin Proc* 63: 113–18.

Rakela, J., Mosley, J.W., Edwards, V.M., Govindarajan, S. and Alpert, E. 1991. A double-blinded randomized trial of hydrocortisone in acute hepatic failure. *Dig Dis Sci* 36: 1223–8.

Ramos, C.P. and Almario, J.S. 1990. Hemodialysis-hemoperfusion in fulminant viral hepatitis. *Biomater Artif Cells Artif Org* 18: 689–92.

Ringe, B., Lubbe, N., Kuse, E., Frei, U. and Pichlmayr, R. 1993. Management of emergencies before and after liver transplantation by early total hepatectomy. *Transpl Proc* 235: 1090.

Rolando, N., Harvey, F., Brahm, J., Philpott-Howard, J., Alexander, G., Gimson, A., Casewell, M., Fagan, E. and Williams, R. 1990. Prospective study of bacterial infection in acute liver failure: an analysis of fifty patients. *Hepatology* 11: 49–53.

Rosenbloom, A.J. 1991. Massive ST-segment elevation without myocardial injury in a patient with fulminant hepatic failure and cerebral edema. *Chest* 100: 870-2.

Rozga, J., Podesta, L., LePage, E. et al. 1993. Control of cerebral oedema by total hepatectomy and extracorporeal liver support in fulminant hepatic failure. *Lancet* 342: 898–9.

Ruprah, M., Mant, T.G.K. and Flanagan, R.J. 1985. Acute carbon tetrachloride poisoning in 19 patients: implications for diagnosis and treatment. *Lancet* 1: 1027–9.

Sallie, R., Katsiyannakis, L., Baldwin, D., et al. 1992. Failure of simple biochemical indexes to reliably differentiate fulminant Wilson's disease from other causes of fulminant hepatic failure. *Hepatology* 16: 1206–11.

Seeff, L.B., Cuccerina, B.A., Zimmerman, H.J., Adler, E. and Benjamin, S.B. 1986. Acetaminophen toxicity in alcoholics. *Ann Intern Med* 104: 399–404.

Sheiner, P., Sinclair, S., Greig, P., Logan, A., Blendis, L.M. and Levy, G. 1992. A randomized controlled trial of prostaglandin E_2 (PGE_2) in the treatment of fulminant hepatic failure (FHF). *Hepatology* 16: 88A.

Shin, K., Nagai, Y., Hirano, C., Kataoka, N. and Ono, I.

1989. Survival rate in children with fulminant hepatitis improved by a combination of twice daily plasmapheresis and conservative therapy. *J Pediatr Gastroenterol* 9: 163–9.

Shoemaker, W., Kram, H.B. and Appel, P.L. 1990. Therapy of shock based on pathophysiology, monitoring, and outcome prediction. *Crit Care Med* 18S: 19–25.

Silva, M.O., Roth, D., Reddy, K.R., Fernandez, J.A., Albores-Saavedra, J. and Schiff, E.R. 1991. Hepatic dysfunction accompanying acute cocaine intoxication. *J Hepatol* 12: 312–15.

Sinclair, S.B., Greig, P.D., Blendis, L.M. et al. 1989. Biochemical and clinical response of fulminant viral hepatitis to administration of prostaglandin E. *J Clin Invest* 84: 1063–9.

Smilkstein, M.J., Knapp, G.L., Kulig, K.W. and Rumack, B.H. 1988. Efficacy of oral *N*-acetylcysteine in the treatment of acetaminophen overdose. *N Engl J Med* 319: 1557–62.

So, S.K.S., Barteau, G.A., Perdrizet, G.A. and Marsh, J.W. 1993. Successful retransplantation after a 48-hour anhepatic state. *Transpl Proc* 25: 1962–3.

Trey, C. and Davidson, C.S. 1970. The management of fulminant hepatic failure. In *Progress in Liver Diseases*, eds. H. Popper and F. Schaffner, 282. New York: Grune and Stratton.

Tsubouchi, H., Hirono, S., Gohda, E. et al. 1989. Clinical significance of human hepatocyte growth factor in blood from patients with fulminant hepatic failure. *Hepatology* 9: 875–81.

Vale, J.A. and Proudfoot, A.T. 1995. Paracetamol (acetaminophen) poisoning. *Lancet* 346: 547–52.

Van Thiel, D.H. and Perper, J.A. 1992. Hepatotoxicity associated with cocaine abuse. *Rec Dev Alcoholism* 10: 335–41.

Ware, A.J., Jones, R.E., Shorey, J.W. and Combes, B. 1974. A controlled trial of steroid therapy in massive hepatic necrosis. *Am J Gastroenterol* 62: 130–3.

Watts, J.McK., Douglas, M.C., Dudley, HAF, Curr, F.W. and Owen, J.A. 1967. Heterologous liver perfusion in acute hepatic failure. *BMJ* 2: 341–7.

Wendon, J., Alexander, G.J.M. and Williams, R. 1991. Cardiovascular monitoring and local blood flow. In *Acute Liver Failure: Improved Understanding and Better Therapy*, eds. R. Williams and R.D. Hughes, 39–41. London: Miter Press.

Wendon, J.A., Harrison, P.M., Keays, R., Gimson, A.E., Alexander, G.J.M. and Williams, R. 1992. Effects of vasopressor agents and epoprostenol on systemic hemodynamics and oxygen transport in fulminant hepatic failure. *Hepatology* 15: 1067–71.

Whitcomb, D.C. and Block, G.D. 1994. Association of acetaminophen hepatotoxicity with fasting and alcohol use. *JAMA* 272: 1845–50.

Williams, R. and Gimson, A.E.S. 1991. Intensive liver care and management of acute hepatic failure. *Dig Dis Sci* 36: 820–6.

Wyke, R.J., Canalese, J.C., Gimson, A.E.S. and Williams, R. 1982. Bacteraemia in patients with fulminant hepatic failure. *Liver* 2: 45–52.

Zimmerman, H.J. and Maddrey, W.C. 1995. Acetaminophen (paracetamol) hepatotoxicity with regular intake of alcohol: analysis of instances of therapeutic misadventure. *Hepatology* 22: 767–73.

Zimmerman, H.J. 1978. Syndromes of enviornmental hepatotoxicity. In *Hepatotoxicity. The Adverse Effects of Drugs on the Liver*, 279–302. New York: Appleton Century Crofts.

11 Circulatory derangements, monitoring, and management: heart, kidney, and brain

Julia A. Wendon and Antony J. Ellis

INTRODUCTION

Significant hemodynamic changes are seen in acute liver failure (ALF) which resemble those seen in sepsis, including an elevated cardiac output and lowered systemic vascular resistance (Bihari et al. 1986). Patients with critical illness frequently demonstrate a covert tissue oxygen debt despite apparently adequate blood pressure and arterial oxygen saturation (Haupt et al. 1985). In a healthy individual, adjustments are made in pulmonary gas exchange, cardiac output, hemoglobin, oxygen binding, capillary resistance, and oxygen extraction ratio to maintain an adequate supply of oxygen to the cell in the face of changing energy demands. Failure to maintain an adequate oxygen uptake to cells appears to be related to a combination of factors resulting in an inability to regulate delivery and extraction of oxygen at a cellular level.

MICROCIRCULATORY DYSFUNCTION

The basis for the microcirculatory dysfunction in critical illness is poorly understood, but evidence is accumulating to suggest the importance of interactions between the endothelium, exogenous factors, such as bacterial toxins and cytokines, specifically tumor necrosis factor (TNF) and interleukins (IL-1, IL-6). Endotoxin and other bacterial toxins lead to the production of cytokines by activated macrophages and may be maintained in the circulation because of impaired Kupffer cell function. Activation and consumption of platelets with formation of microthrombi within various organs, may lead to endothelial damage and release of further vasoactive compounds. This series of events, together with increased adhesion of activated leukocytes to endothelial cells, causes microcirculatory plugging with blood being shunted through non-nutritive arteriovenous channels. Endothelial derived relaxant factor (EDRF) and prostacyclin are important endothelial derived factors whose role in control of microcirculatory flow is being recognized increasingly. Patients with ALF have been demonstrated to have elevated levels of the end products of EDRF, nitrite and nitrate (Wendon, Harrison, Heaton and Williams 1994) and have also been shown to have elevated levels of cyclic GMP (cGMP) and citrulline (Chase et al. 1978) suggesting activation of the EDRF pathway.

It is proposed that circulating cytokines are released as a consequence of liver damage and/or sepsis and initiate microcirculatory abnormalities which result in tissue hypoxia. The ability of the endothelium to release PGI2 or EDRF has an important bearing on the evolution of tissue hypoxia as endothelial interactions may limit release of prostacyclin (PGI2) and EDRF, thus further potentiating tissue hypoxia and end-organ damage.

In healthy individuals, physiologic supply-dependency of oxygen only occurs when oxygen delivery (Do_2) falls below a level of 330 ml/min/m^2 (Haupt et al. 1985). Any additional fall in delivery below this critical level will result in a fall in tissue oxygen uptake (Vo_2), with the subsequent development of tissue hypoxia, anaerobic metabolism and build up of lactate (Figure 11.1). Observations in patients with impaired cardiac function, pulmonary hypertension, and while under general anesthesia are also consistent with a supply-dependent pattern of oxygen utilization when delivery falls below a critical lower limit. A normal oxygen delivery (Do_2) is around 525–675 ml/min/m^2, and with a tissue oxygen extraction of 20–25 percent this results in a consumption of 110–150 ml/min/m^2. At deliveries between 300 and 525 ml/min/m^2, the oxygen consumption is maintained at normal levels by increasing the extraction ratio in the periphery. In patients who are critically ill, such as those with severe sepsis, multiple trauma, adult respiratory distress syndrome, and those with ALF "pathological supply-dependency" for oxygen is observed (Figure 11.1). In these patients, oxygen consumption is dependent upon delivery over a far greater range than is seen in normals, such that an increase in Do_2 will frequently result in an increase in Vo_2. An appropriate level for Vo_2 is difficult to estimate in patients with critical illness but is likely to be higher than that seen in the resting healthy state due to the presence of fever, sepsis, inflammatory foci or increased levels of circulating catecholamines. Measured baseline levels of Vo_2 in the critically ill are often lower that those seen in normal individuals but increases in delivery will frequently result in increases in Vo_2 above and beyond that seen in normals.

Work by Bihari and Gimson has demonstrated the presence of pathologic supply-dependency for oxygen in patients with ALF. After infusion of prostacyclin, a microcirculatory vasodilator, a fall in systemic vascular resistance was demonstrated. Mean arterial pressure was maintained by virtue of a significant increase in cardiac output. This resulted in an increase in oxygen delivery or

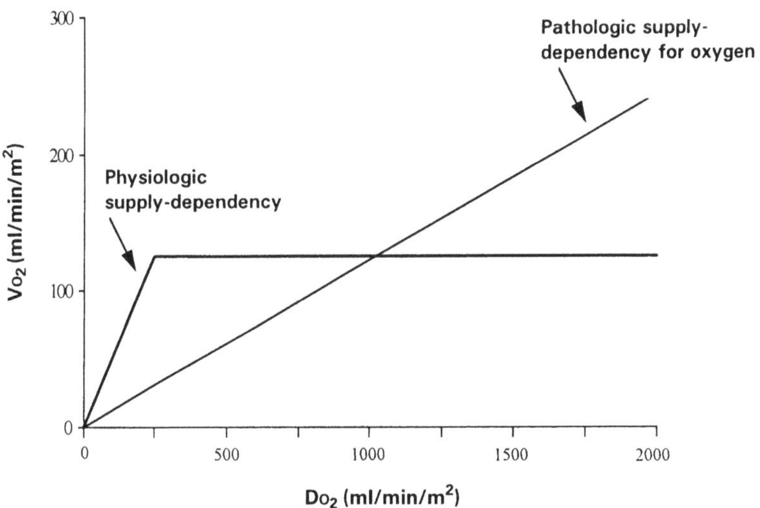

Figure 11.1 Relationship between oxygen delivery (Do_2) and oxygen consumption (Vo_2) in healthy individuals and patients with critical illness.

dispatch from the left ventricle and a significant increase in oxygen consumption (Bihari et al. 1986), suggesting a pre-existing tissue oxygen debt. The patients with ALF who failed to survive had both a lower baseline Vo_2 than survivors and greater increases in Vo_2 following infusion of prostacyclin, suggesting that these sicker patients had a greater tissue oxygen debt. It was also noted by these workers that mixed venous lactate correlated inversely with systemic vascular resistance index, mean arterial pressure and oxygen extraction ratio (Bihari et al. 1986).

The degree of intervention that is required to monitor the circulation in ALF will be dictated by the patient's clinical condition. All but the most stable subfulminant patient will require insertion of a central venous line to facilitate appropriate fluid therapy. The hemodynamic disturbances seen in patients with acute liver failure are similar to those of patients with sepsis, with an elevated cardiac output and lowered systemic vascular resistance index (Bihari et al. 1986). Relative hypovolemia secondary to vasodilatation is frequent in ALF, and a pulmonary artery flotation catheter is often required to optimize fluid replacement. Colloid loading is best achieved with either 4.5 percent human albumin solution or blood. Crystalloid, to cover maintenance requirements, should be given in the form of dextrose only. The role of other synthetic colloid solutions in ALF is unclear, since there is some evidence that their use may result in impaired Kupffer cell function, which may be detrimental with respect to infection. Intravascular depletion will rapidly result in the development of hypotension, renal failure and potentially worsening tissue perfusion with metabolic acidosis and ongoing organ failure.

USE OF INOTROPIC AND VASOPRESSOR AGENTS

Agents such as dobutamine, a predominantly beta agonist, are not normally effective in increasing mean arterial pressure in patients with ALF owing to the presence of an already elevated cardiac output and such agents should only be used in the hypotensive patient who has associated cardiac dysfunction with a low output state. The most efficacious agents to improve mean arterial pressure are either epinephrine or norepinephrine, commencing at a dose of 0.1 μg/kg/min. The findings of a recent study demonstrated that administration of either of these agents led to a significant improvement in mean arterial pressure. Cardiac index and oxygen delivery, however, were not improved and there was a significant fall in oxygen consumption owing to a fall in oxygen extraction (Wendon et al. 1992). These findings were seen in all of the patients studied regardless of etiology. The detrimental effects of epinephrine and norepinephrine on tissue oxygen transport seen in this study probably relate to constriction of nutrient, as well as resistance, arterioles, thus reducing local blood flow to tissues despite an increase in perfusion pressure. Therapeutic maneuvers which aim to increase mean arterial pressure in isolation may result in a decrease in tissue oxygen uptake with the potential to worsen tissue hypoxia.

Prostacyclin is unlike other commonly used vasodilators because it increases vasomotor tone in the microcirculation, aids dispersal of platelet aggregates, inhibits platelet aggregation (Slotman et al. 1983), aids fibrinolysis (Utsunomiya et al. 1980) and decreases post-capillary tone. Thus, it has the potential to both increase nutrient flow and decrease interstitial edema. Co-infusion of prostacyclin in addition to either epinephrine or norepinephrine in the above-mentioned study was associated with a marked increase in oxygen consumption, owing to a rise in oxygen delivery and oxygen extraction ratio. The tendency for improvement in arterial pH following the addition of the prostacyclin adds further evidence to the hypothesis that nutritive blood flow is improved (Table 11.1). Infusion of prostacyclin caused a deterioration in alveolar–arterial (A–a) gradient, as might be expected due to the pulmonary vasodilatation

Table 11.1. *Effects of epinephrine and norepinephrine plus prostacyclin on heart rate, mean arterial pressure, cardiac index, systemic and pulmonary vascular resistance indices, A–a gradient, pH, left and right stroke work indices (mean ± SD)*

	Baseline (n=10)	Norepinephrine (n=10)	Norepinephrine + PGI2 (n=10)
Heart rate, bpm	100 ± 7	104 ± 7	108 ± 7
Mean arterial pressure, mmHg	47 ± 3	62 ± 3[b]	62 ± 3
Cardiac index, $l/min/m^2$	6.8 ± 0.3	6.2 ± 0.4	7.1 ± 0.6[b]
Systemic vascular resistance index, dyne sec cm^5 m^2	491 ± 52	683 ± 37[b]	610 ± 39[a]
Oxygen delivery	811 ± 124	785 ± 48	862 ± 58[a]
A–a gradient, mmHg	298 ± 38	317 ± 36	334 ± 34
pH	7.246 ± 0.05	7.27 ± 0.04	7.29 ± 0.04
Oxygen consumption	139 ± 23	112 ± 27[b]	145 ± 36[b]
Oxygen extraction	17 ± 2.8	14 ± 2.5	17 ± 4

[a] $P < 0.05$, [b] $P < 0.01$.

and an increased ventilation–perfusion mismatch. This, however, was not detrimental, since cardiac output and overall oxygen delivery to tissues was significantly enhanced. Other vasodilators, such as nitroglycerin and sodium nitroprusside do not have their predominant effects on the microcirculation.

We have also recently examined the effects of blockade of NO using L-N-nonomethylarginine (L-NMMA). This agent was effective in increasing mean arterial pressure and systemic vascular resistance, although larger doses were required than those previously administered in studies of patients with sepsis. Cardiac output fell in association with the increase in afterload and oxygen consumption was observed to fall as well. It may be that agents which selectively inhibit the inducible enzyme nitric oxide synthase alone may be more attractive as therapeutic agents in patients with hypotension and multiple organ failure.

In patients who require vasopressor support, *N*-acetylcysteine (NAC) is given in addition to prostacyclin. The rationale for this treatment arose from the observation that patients receiving late NAC treatment following acetaminophen (paracetamol) overdose after the period during which it should act as an antidote have a better prognosis than those who do not receive it. A lower incidence of renal failure and less progression to deeper levels of coma were observed despite similar prolongation of prothrombin times (Harrison et al. 1990). These findings have been confirmed in a prospective study. Treated patients displayed less hypotension and less cerebral edema (Keays et al. 1991). The beneficial mechanism of action of *N*-acetylcysteine is unclear. Recent work has demonstrated that infusion of *N*-acetylcysteine results in an increase in cardiac output, oxygen delivery, oxygen extraction ratio and hence oxygen consumption in patients (Harrison, Wendon, Gimson et al. 1991).

Several potential actions of *N*-acetylcysteine may account for these observations; NAC is a potent antioxidant and as such may stabilize the effects of endothelial derived relaxant factor (EDRF) and prevent endothelial damage by free radicals. *N*-acetylcysteine, by repleting tissue sulfhydryl groups either directly or by its action of increasing cysteine levels (Burgunder et al. 1989), could restore full EDRF activity by a similar mechanism to its reversal of tolerance to nitrates (Horowitz et al. 1988). However, the relative roles of constitutive and inducible EDRF require further definition. The role of other antioxidants such as superoxide dismutase and desferrioxamine require further clarification in their role in increasing oxygen extraction in ALF and other forms of multiple organ failure.

Other potential beneficial therapies have been investigated by the Copenhagen group who have demonstrated marked improvements in patients' hemodynamic status following the institution of high volume plasmapheresis in patients' with ALF (Kondrup et al. 1992; and Chapter 21). They have observed increases in mean arterial pressure and systemic vascular resistance, in addition to improved neurological status following plasmapheresis (Larsen et al. 1994). The mode of action of plasmapheresis in this setting may be related to removal of putative vasorelaxant compounds which accumulate in patients with ALF.

The application of monoclonal antibodies to a variety of cytokines in the clinical setting is intuitively attractive as a novel mode of prevention of the cycle of multiple organ failure in patients with ALF. Unfortunately, however, many trials of such agents in patients with other forms of critical illness have been disappointing. One of the problems may be early identification of suitable patients for such treatments.

TEN IMPORTANT POINTS IN MANAGEMENT AND MONITORING

1. Maintain hemoglobin level at least at 8–10 g/dl with appropriate transfusions.
2. Maintain central venous pressure (CVP) or pulmonary capillary wedge pressure (PCWP) of 10–14 mmHg.

   CVP may not be an accurate measure of intravascular filling in patients with tense ascites and is difficult to interpret with the marked swings in intrathoracic pressure seen as a result of respiratory distress.

   Optimal fluid loading on the basis of the PCWP needs to be individualized to any given patient on the basis of Starling response and oncotic pressure. Some patients may require a PCWP of 18 mmHg or more.
3. Crystalloid is required to account for the patients' insensible losses and for any other source of crystalloid loss.
4. *N*-acetylcysteine (150 mg/kg over 30 min as a loading dose followed by 150 mg/kg per 24 h maintenance) should be considered in all patients regardless of the etiology of their ALF.
5. Maintain serum K and Mg in the normal range.
6. With the development of hypotension, insert a pulmonary artery flotation catheter, volume load and consider reloading with acetylcysteine (150 mg/kg). Measure hemodynamic variables.
7. If hypotension persists, a vasopressor agent should be commenced, either epinephrine or norepinephrine. In patients with relatively lower cardiac output (<5.5 l/min/m^2) epinephrine may be the preferred agent providing arrhythmias have not been troublesome. Hemodynamic and oxygen transport variables should be measured again following institution of vasopressor therapy and if oxygen extraction and oxygen consumption have fallen the patient is started on prostacyclin (5 ng/kg/min) in addition to NAC. The PCWP needs to be maintained with colloid while the drug is commenced to mitigate against further falls in blood pressure.
8. A specific cause of the hypotension should always be sought: sepsis (the commonest), bleeding, pneumothorax etc. Blood cultures should be taken and the patient's antibiotics either changed or commenced. In patients with associated multiple organ failure, systemic antifungal therapy may also be started. Doses of inotropic agents above 0.5 μg/kg/min may be given but are associated with a very poor prognosis unless there is an eminently treatable cause for the ALF or the patient is proceeding to transplantation.
9. Oxygen transport values should not be used to direct increasing delivery alone, as dispatch of oxygen from the left ventricle is usually adequate; agents should ideally be instituted to improve the availability and utilization of oxygen to tissues.
10. Plasmapheresis may be considered in some patients.

CEREBRAL MANAGEMENT OF ACUTE LIVER FAILURE

Increases in intracranial pressure (ICP) may be caused by increases in volume of any of the three main components within the skull, namely brain tissue, cerebrospinal fluid (CSF) and the cerebral vessels. The increased volume of CSF is not thought to be important; indeed the ventricular system is usually collapsed at CT scanning (Adrogue et al. 1989). An increase in the volume of the brain tissue is reported to occur in up to 80 percent of patients progressing to grade IV (Ede et al. 1986).

The clinical signs of cerebral edema, systemic hypertension, decerebrate posturing, and abnormal pupillary reflexes, are generally attributed to brain stem compression. In our experience, however, cerebellar or uncal herniation is comparatively rare with present day therapies. In fact, these findings were present at autopsy in only 25 percent of patients with cerebral edema (Ware et al. 1971), suggesting that other factors are involved. The development of cerebral edema in any given setting is probably dependent on a variety of causative events. Increased permeability of the blood brain barrier will result in leakage of protein rich fluid into the extracellular space of the brain. The efficacy of mannitol in the management of patients with a raised ICP suggests that intracellular cytotoxic cerebral edema is also important in addition to vasogenic mechanisms. The role of hyponatremia in ALF remains to be clarified, though it is no doubt important in the evolution of cerebral edema in some clinical settings (see Chapter 12).

Until recently it was thought that cerebral blood flow (CBF) was significantly increased in patients with ALF and contributed to the raised ICP. Indeed, treatment measures were devised to decrease CBF. This concept has been examined in several animal studies. Trewby et al. noted in a pig model that increases in ICP were associated with falls in CBF, a finding in contrast to the perceived view that raised ICP was always associated with an elevated CBF (Trewby et al. 1978). A more recent series of experiments in a rat model of ALF demonstrated a linear fall in CBF before a rise in ICP (Blei 1991).

Although early studies in man suggested that CBF was elevated in ALF, more recent studies have demonstrated marked variation in CBF between patients with ALF (Almdal et al. 1989; Ede et al. 1986; Kramer et al. 1991; Sari et al. 1990).

Almdal et al. were the first group to describe a fall in CBF as the level of coma deepened (Almdal et al. 1989). These findings were confirmed by others (Sari et al. 1990). Subsequent studies have demonstrated more variable levels of CBF, but the observed values have always been within the normal range (40–70 ml/min/100 g brain tissue). Investigators have questioned whether this level of CBF, in patients who are deeply comatose is actually in excess of the demand. In examining the relationship between CBF and cerebral metabolic rate for oxygen ($CMRO_2$), investigators found the latter to be low at 1.6 ml/min/100 g. In this group, 25 percent studied had CBF values of greater than 50 ml/min/100 g, suggestive of a level of CBF greater than that required, while 52 percent had a reduced CBF (Aggarwal et al. 1994). By contrast, Kramer et al. have reported that cerebral hyperemia precedes or coincides with the presence of cerebral edema on CT scanning (Kramer et al. 1991). The Copenhagen group has suggested that an increase in CBF, as assessed by middle cerebral artery Doppler studies, was associated with an improvement in neurological status, inferring that CBF had previously been inadequate for metabolic demands (Larsen et al. 1994). The increase in CBF, however, was achieved by the use of plasmapheresis and it may be that this increase was due to removal of postulated "neurotoxins" resulting in an increase in cerebral metabolic activity and the subsequent rise in CBF.

In our own studies, CBF was measured in patients in grade IV coma using a radioactive xenon technique. A catheter was also inserted into the jugular venous bulb and blood sampled for oxygen content, lactate and glucose. CBF varied widely between 12 and 50 ml/min/100 g (Figure 11.2). In those patients who had developed clinical signs of cerebral edema, CBF was higher and correlated significantly with $CMRO_2$, a feature not observed in patients who did not develop cerebral edema (Figure 11.3). These findings appear at variance with those observed in normal individuals where changes in CBF are

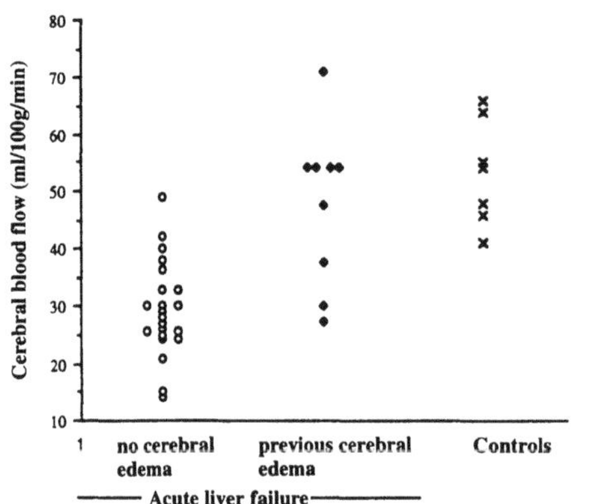

Figure 11.2 Cerebral blood flow in controls and patients with and without cerebral edema.

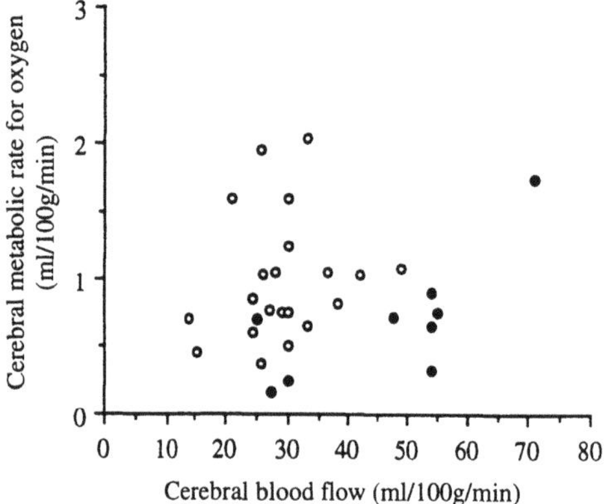

Figure 11.3 Relationship between cerebral blood flow and cerebral metabolic rate for oxygen in patients with cerebral edema (closed circles) and those without (open circles).

counterbalanced by reciprocal changes in the proportion of oxygen extracted so that $CMRO_2$ remains unchanged (Wendon, Harrison, Keays and Williams 1994). Although the levels of CBF measured have been thought to be adequate for the metabolic demands of patients in deep coma, the observation that many of these patients had cerebral lactate production is more suggestive of an inadequate delivery of substrate for metabolic demand.

Substantial increases in CBF can be demonstrated following the infusion of mannitol and acetylcysteine (Figures 11.4 and 11.5) and are associated with a rise in $CMRO_2$ and a fall in anaerobic metabolism. Infusion of prostacyclin was also shown to increase CBF, suggesting that, providing mean arterial pressure is maintained, this agent may also be beneficial. A fall in CBF was seen following hyperventilation confirming the findings of previous studies (Ede et al. 1988; Sari et al. 1990). These studies confirmed that cerebrovascular reactivity to changes in carbon dioxide tension is maintained in patients with grade IV encephalopathy. The fall in CBF, however, was accompanied by a fall in $CMRO_2$ and an increase in cerebral lactate production demonstrating that, in ALF, $CMRO_2$ appears to be dependent on CBF and that CBF is frequently inadequate. We were unable to assess whether the increase in CBF following mannitol, epoprostenol and acetylcysteine was due to cerebral arteriolar vasodilatation or a fall in intracranial pressure. It is of interest, however, that infusion of mannitol to patients with traumatic head injury has been shown to increase CBF without changing mean arterial or intracranial pressures (Jafar et al. 1986). Acetylcysteine, by enhancing oxygen delivery, has also been shown to have a beneficial effect in oxygen uptake in the peripheral circulation (Harrison et al. 1991).

This implicates cerebral hypoxia as one of the potential precipitating events in the development of cellular swelling. Cerebral hypoxia may lead to cell membrane damage which, in association with impaired Na/K ATPase activity (Ede et al. 1987; Seda et al. 1984) could result in increased brain water thus exacerbating the cerebral edema. Cerebral hypoxia has not previously been implicated in the pathogenesis of cerebral edema in ALF (Berk and Popper 1978), but results from the above studies demonstrate that inadequate cerebral oxygenation is frequently seen in patients in grade IV encephalopathy. The effects of NAC on CBF and $CMRO_2$ are most likely responsible for the lower incidence of cerebral edema seen (Harrison, Keays, Bray, Alexander and Williams 1990; Keays et al. 1991).

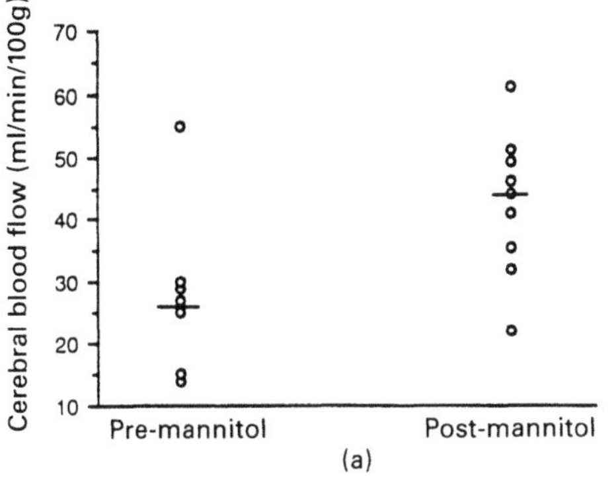

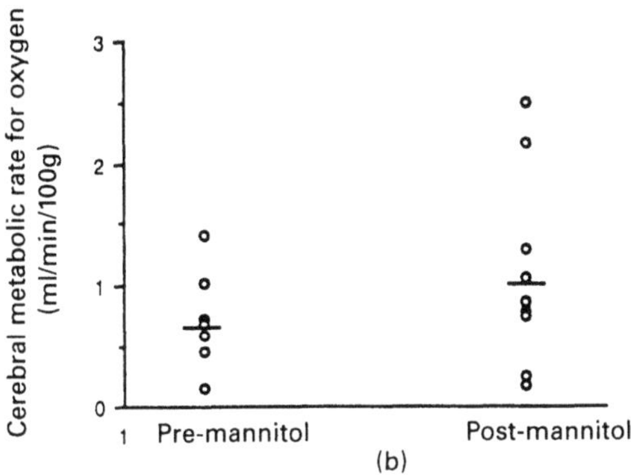

Figure 11.4 Effect of a mannitol infusion on cerebral blood flow (a) and metabolic rate for oxygen (b) in patients with acute liver failure.

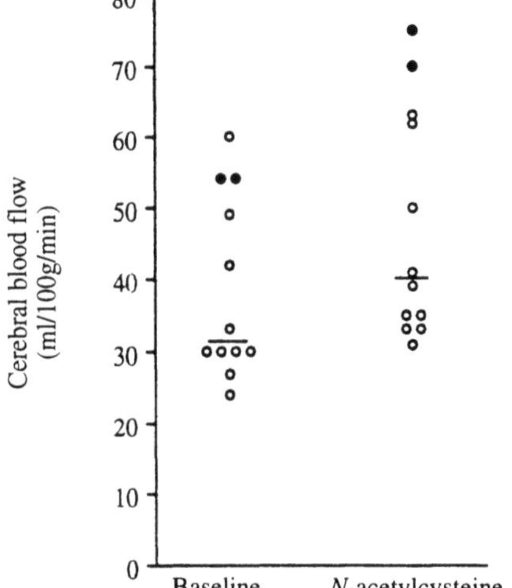

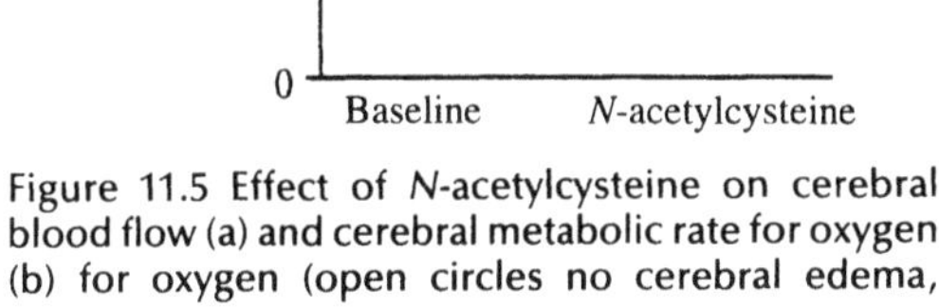

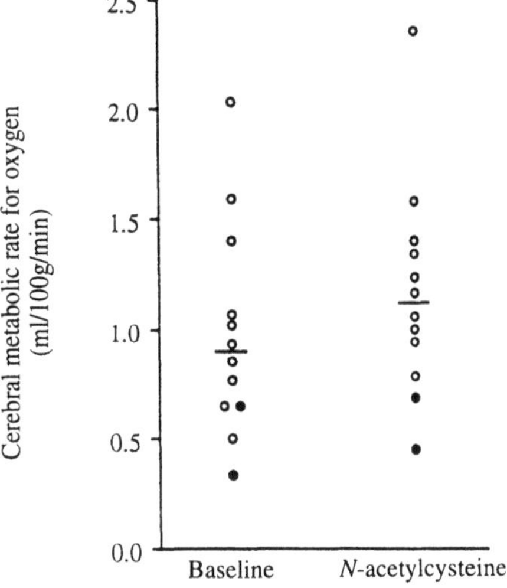

Figure 11.5 Effect of *N*-acetylcysteine on cerebral blood flow (a) and cerebral metabolic rate for oxygen (b) for oxygen (open circles no cerebral edema, closed circles cerebral edema) in patients with acute liver failure.

THE MANAGEMENT OF PATIENTS WITH GRADE III/IV ENCEPHALOPATHY

Elective ventilation following development of grade III encephalopathy is required in order to control the airway and frequently also in the aggressive and agitated patient to allow appropriate treatment. Patients should be nursed at 10 to 20 degrees head-up in order to maximize the cerebral perfusion pressure (Davenport et al. 1990). Our practice is to institute ICP monitoring in all patients who have demonstrated either pupillary abnormalities or unexplained systolic hypertension or who have developed grade III/IV coma and are proceeding to liver transplantation. In the latter group, monitoring is continued for 24–48 h after transplantation when cerebral edema may still be a problem. Prior to insertion of an ICP bolt, we administer sufficient fresh frozen plasma to achieve a prothrombin ratio (INR) of two and infuse one adult dose of platelets if the count is less than 50×10^9/l. Subsequent supplementation is not given. In those cases where cerebral edema is difficult to control and a donor liver has become available, hepatectomy with formation of a temporary end-to-side portocaval shunt may be carried out with good effect on both ICP and inotrope requirement, thus prolonging the time interval during which transplantation may be considered (Muñoz et al. 1991; Ringe et al. 1988; Rozga et al. 1993; see also Chapters 10 and 11).

In the management of patients at risk of cerebral edema, the preservation of an adequate cerebral perfusion pressure is critical if survival is to be maximized. For patients without ICP monitoring, a mean arterial pressure of 60 mmHg should be maintained using epinephrine or norepinephrine in the presence of NAC (150 mg/kg over 24 h) and prostacyclin (5 ng/kg/min) infusions. The additional information given by intracranial pressure monitoring allows the cerebral perfusion pressure (CPP) to be quantified. The decision as to what is the minimum CPP tolerable which will allow a full neurological recovery to take place is controversial. Shaw et al. have stated that a CPP of less than 40 mmHg for more than 2 h is a contraindication to transplantation due to severe neurological damage (see Chapters 12 and 16). Cases have been reported, however, demonstrating full recovery despite continued low CPP values of below 40 mmHg for more than 24 h (Davies et al. 1994). Complications of ICP monitoring may be significant (Blei et al. 1993).

The placement of a catheter within the jugular bulb allows for jugular venous bulb blood sampling for oxygen saturation and arteriojugular lactate difference as an indirect marker of cerebral oxygen consumption and extraction. Such information, in addition to hemodynamic data, can aid the manipulation of further therapy. In patients in whom the jugular venous saturation is between 55 and 75 percent and the lactate difference is not greater than 0.35 mmol/l, CBF and CPP may be considered to be adequate. If the CPP falls due to a fall in mean arterial pressure and the jugular venous saturation also falls below 55 percent, vasopressor therapy should be instituted. In those where the fall in CPP is predominantly due to an increase in ICP, mannitol (0.5 g/kg) is the treatment of choice. Provided that cerebral perfusion pressure is maintained, jugular venous oxygen saturation is greater than 55 percent, and pupillary signs are not present, we would not treat modest elevations in ICP, saving the use of mannitol to treat sudden surges in ICP.

Cerebral function monitoring (CFM) is also of considerable value in detecting subclinical epileptiform activity, a very detrimental occurrence resulting in increased metabolic demand, in the face of potentially limited substrate delivery. The use of routine CFM has, in our hands, demonstrated a high incidence of epileptiform activity. This explains the observed clinical situation in which marked pupillary abnormalities occur in the presence of a relatively low jugular venous saturation, with only a marginal increase in ICP. It has also been suggested by the Vienna group (Madl et al. 1994) that sensory evoked potentials may be useful, especially in assessment of outcome.

The successful use of thiopental given as 50 mg boluses followed by an infusion of 50 mg/h for up to 6 h in the treatment of intractable cerebral hypertension has been reported (Forbes et al. 1989). Certainly this agent may be useful though its tendency to decrease mean arterial pressure has to be monitored. Thiopental is an anticonvulsant and much of its activity may be attributable to this action, by decreasing cerebral metabolic requirements if seizures are prevented.

Hyperventilation should not be routinely advocated. There may be a role for short periods of hyperventilation in patients with raised jugular venous saturation and ICP suggestive of hyperemia.

RENAL HEMODYNAMICS AND MANAGEMENT

Renal failure (urine output of less than 300 ml/24 h and serum creatinine of greater than 300 mmol/l) in the presence of adequate intravascular filling pressures is seen to occur in up to 70 percent of patients with ALF (O'Grady et al. 1988). The development of hypovolemia and reduced intravascular filling pressures are important factors in the development of renal failure, as is the occurrence of sepsis. In addition, factors such as altered levels of vasodilators and constrictors within the renal vasculature play an important role. Patients in whom acetaminophen (paracetamol) is the cause of the ALF may have renal failure due to direct renal toxicity of the ingested drug. In some patients, renal blood flow autoregulation may be lost and a low mean arterial pressure may also contribute to a declining urine output. Thus, the etiology of renal failure in ALF is usually multifactorial comprising prerenal factors, hepatorenal failure, acute tubular necrosis, and direct nephrotoxicity.

Initial management should consist of aggressive volume loading as guided by intravascular filling pressures utilizing colloid and crystalloid as already described. If oliguria persists, "renal dose" dopamine (2.5 μg/kg/min) or a furosemide infusion (10 mg/h) may be tried. The role of renal dose dopamine has recently come under scrutiny in the general intensive care literature. Current opinion is that its role is very limited and that the effects which may ensue, with regard to suppression of all aspects of pituitary function, render furosemide a more attractive alternative (Thompson and Cockrill 1994). Whether this is the case in ALF has not been examined. If the patient increases urine output with volume loading and infusion of either agent, treatment should continue with this regime; neither dopamine nor furosemide will be effective in an anuric patient. Renal replacement therapy of some form will need to be instituted in patients if acidosis, hyperkalemia, fluid overload, or a rising creatinine develop. This should also be instituted in any patient who is oliguric and shows signs of cerebral edema, or in patients with hyponatremia. Access for renal replacement therapy is normally achieved through a double lumen catheter placed in either the femoral or internal jugular vein.

Continuous arteriovenous hemodiafiltration (CAVHD) or pumped veno–venous hemodiafiltration (CVVHD) is the best form of renal replacement therapy in ALF (Davenport et al. 1989). High volume hemofiltration may also be utilized but care must be taken in the choice of replacement fluid, since patients will not be able to metabolize many of the standard solutions in which lactate or acetate are the predominant buffers, while a bicarbonate buffered solution will be well tolerated. Intermittent machine driven hemodialysis should be avoided in ALF, since hypotension is a frequent complication and this may result in significant falls in CPP. This technique is useful in patients who have undergone transplantation or those following ALF who are hemodynamically stable and no longer at risk of cerebral edema.

Anticoagulation in patients with ALF can be difficult since these patients have large sticky platelets and are antithrombin III deficient, and, despite their coagulopathy, may clot off circuits rapidly. Anticoagulation is accomplished with heparin unless patients are actively bleeding or have an intracranial pressure monitor in situ. An initial heparin bolus of 1000–2000 units is usually administered followed by an infusion of heparin to achieve an activated clotting time (ACT) of 150–180 s. In patients in whom heparin is contraindicated, prostacyclin may be infused at 5 ng/kg/min.

APPENDIX

Formulae and calculations

Cardiac index
Cardiac output divided by surface area, l/m^2

Stroke volume index (SVI)
Cardiac index divided by heart rate × 10^4, ml/beat

Systemic vascular resistance index (SVRI)
({mean arterial pressure − right atrial pressure} divided by cardiac index) × 79.9, dyne.s.cm^5.m^2

Pulmonary vascular resistance index (PVRI)
({mean pulmonary artery pressure − pulmonary capillary wedge pressure} divided by cardiac index) × 79.9, dyne.s.cm^5.m^2

Left ventricular stroke work index
(mean arterial pressure − pulmonary capillary wedge pressure) × SVI × 0.0136, g.beat.m^2

Right ventricular stroke work index
(mean pulmonary artery pressure − right atrial pressure) × SVI × 0.0136, g.beat.m^2

Oxygen content (arterial)
{hemoglobin × 1.34 × percentage saturation arterial} + {arterial oxygen tension (mmHg) × 0.0031}, ml/dl

Oxygen content (mixed venous)
{hemoglobin × 1.34 × percentage saturation pulmonary artery} + {pulmonary artery oxygen tension (mmHg) × 0.0031}, ml/dl

Oxygen delivery (Do_2)
cardiac index × arterial oxygen content × 10, ml.min.m^2

Oxygen uptake index/consumption (Vo_2)
obtained from the reverse Fick relationship: cardiac index × {arterial − mixed venous oxygen content difference} × 10, ml.min.m^2

Oxygen extraction index (OER)
calculated by dividing the arteriovenous oxygen content difference by the arterial oxygen content × 100 percent.

REFERENCES

Adrogue, H., Rashad, M., Gorin, A., Yacoub, J. and Madias, N. 1989. Assessing acid–base status in circulatory failure. Differences between arterial and central venous blood. *N Engl J Med* 320: 1312–16.

Aggarwal, S.K.D., Yonas, H., Obrist, W., Kang, Y., Martin, M. and Policare, R. 1994. Cerebral hemodynamic and metabolic changes in fulminant hepatic failure: A retrospective study. *Hepatology* 19: 80–7.

Almdal, T., Schroeder, T. and Ranek, L. 1989. Cerebral blood flow and liver function in patients with encephalopathy due to acute and chronic liver diseases. *Scand J Gastroenterol* 24: 299–303.

Berk, P. and Popper, H. 1978. Fulminant hepatic failure. *Am J Gastroenterol* 69: 349–400.

Bihari, D.J., Gimson, A.E. and Williams, R. 1986. Cardiovascular, pulmonary and renal complications of fulminant hepatic failure. *Sem Liver Dis* 6: 119–28.

Blei, A. 1991. Cerebral edema and intracranial hypertension in acute liver failure: distinct aspects of the same problem. *Hepatology* 13: 376–9.

Blei, A., Olafsson, S., Webster, S. and Levy, R. 1993. Complications of intracerebral pressure monitoring in fulminant hepatic failure. *Lancet* 341: 157–8.

Burgunder, J.M., Varriale, A. and Lauterburg, B.H. 1989. Effect of *N*-acetylcysteine on plasma cysteine and glutathione following paracetamol administration. *Eur J Clin Pharmacol* 36: 127–31.

Chase, R., Davies, M., Trewby, P., Silk, D. and Williams, R. 1978. Plasma amino acid profiles in patients with fulminant hepatic failure treated by repeated polyacrylonitrile membrane hemodialysis. *Gastroenterology* 75: 1033–40.

Davenport, A., Will, E., Davidson, A.M., Swindells, S., Cohen, A.T. et al. 1989. Changes in intracranial pressure during machine and continuous haemofiltration. *Int J Artif Org* 12: 439–44.

Davenport, A., Will, E.J. and Davison, A.M. 1990. Effect of posture on intracranial pressure and cerebral perfusion pressure in patients with fulminant hepatic and renal failure after acetaminophen self-poisoning. *Crit Care Med* 18: 286–9.

Davies, M.H., Mutimer, D., Lowes, J., Elias, E. and Neuberger, J. 1994. Recovery despite impaired cerebral perfusion in fulminant hepatic failure. *Lancet* 343: 1329–30.

Ede, R.J., Gimson, A.E., Bihari, D. and Williams, R. 1986. Controlled hyperventilation in the prevention of cerebral oedema in fulminant hepatic failure. *J Hepatol* 2: 43–51.

Ede, R.J., Gove, C.D., Hughes, R.D., Marshall, W. and Williams, R. 1987. Reduced brain Na+, K+-ATPase activity in rats with galactosamine-induced hepatic failure: relationship to encephalopathy and cerebral oedema. *Clin Sci* 72: 365–71.

Ede, R.J. Moore, K.P., Marshall, W.J. and Williams, R. 1988. Frequency of pancreatitis in fulminant hepatic failure using isoenzyme markers. *Gut* 29: 778–81.

Forbes, A., Alexander, G.J., O'Grady, J.G., Keays, R., Gullan, R., Dawling, S. and Williams, R. 1989. Thiopental infusion in the treatment of intracranial hypertension complicating fulminant hepatic failure. *Hepatology* 10: 306–10.

Harrison, P., O'Grady, J., Alexander, G. and Williams, R. 1990. Serial prothrombin times: a prognostic indicator in paracetamol-induced fulminant hepatic failure. *BMJ* 301: 964–6.

Harrison, P.M., Keays, R., Bray, G.P., Alexander, G.J.M. and Williams, R. 1990. Improved outcome of paracetamol-induced fulminant hepatic failure by late administration of acetylcysteine. *Lancet* i: 1572–3.

Harrison, P.M., Wendon, J.A., Gimson, A.E.S., Alexander, G.J.M. and Williams, R. 1991. Improvement by acetylcysteine of hemodynamics and oxygen transport in fulminant hepatic failure. *N Engl J Med* 324: 1852–8.

Haupt, M.T., Gilbert, E.M. and Carlson, R.W. 1985. Fluid loading increases oxygen consumption in septic patients with lactic acidosis. *Am Rev Respir Dis* 131: 912–16.

Horowitz, J.D., Henry, C.A., Syrjanen, M.L., Louis, W.J., Fish, R.D., Antman, E.M. and Smith, T.W. 1988. Nitroglycerine/*N*-acetylcysteine in the management of unstable angina pectoris. *Eur Heart J* 9 (Suppl.) A: 95–100.

Jafar, J.J., Johns, L.M. and Mullan, S.F. 1986. The effect of mannitol on cerebral blood flow. *J Neurosurg* 64: 754–9.

Keays, R., Harrison, P.M., Wendon, J.A., Gimson, A.E.S., Alexander, G.J.M. and Williams, R. 1991. Intravenous acetylcysteine in paracetamol induced fulminant hepatic failure: a prospective controlled trial. *BMJ* 303: 1026–9.

Kondrup, J.A.T., Vilstrup, H. and Tygstrup, N. 1992. High volume plasma exchange in fulminant hepatic failure. *Int J Artif Org* 11: 669–76.

Kramer, D., Aggarwal, M., Darby, J., Obrist, W., Rosenblum, A., Murray, G., Linden, P. and Miro, A. 1991. Management options in fulminant hepatic failure. *Transpl Proc* 23: 1895–8.

Larsen, F.S., Jorgensen, L.G., Secher, N.H., Bondesen, S., Linkis, P., Hjortrup, A., Kirkegaard, P., Agerlin, N., Kondrup, J. and Tygstrup, N. 1994. Cerebral blood flow velocity during high volume plasmapheresis in fulminant hepatic failure. *Int J Artif Org* 17: 353–61.

Madl, C., Grimm, G., Ferenci, P., Kramer, L., Yeganehfar, W., Oder, W., Steininger, R., Zauner, C., Ratheiser, K.,

Stockenhuber, F. and Lenz, K. 1994. Serial recording of sensory evoked potentials: A noninvasive prognostic indicator in fulminant liver failure. *Hepatology* 20: 1487–94.

Muñoz, S., Robinson, M., Northup, B., Bell, R., Moritz, M., Jarrell, B., Martin, P. and Maddrey, W. 1991. Elevated intracranial pressure and computed tomography of the brain in fulminant hepatocellular failure. *Hepatology* 209–12.

O'Grady, J.G., Gimson, A.E., O'Brien, C.J., Pucknell, A., Hughes, R.D. and Williams, R. 1988. Controlled trials of charcoal hemoperfusion and prognostic factors in fulminant hepatic failure. *Gastroenterology* 94: 1186–92.

Ringe, B., Pichlmayr, R., Lubbe, N., Bornscheuer, A. and Kuse, E. 1988. Total hepatectomy as a temporary approach to acute hepatic or primary graft failure. *Transpl Proc* 552–7.

Rozga, J., Podesta, L., LePage, E., Hoffman, A., Morsiani, E., Sher, L., Woolf, G.M., Makowka, L. and Demetriou, A.A. 1993. Control of cerebral edema by total hepatectomy and extracorporeal liver support in fulminant hepatic failure. *Lancet* 342: 898–9.

Sari, A., Yamashita, S., Ohosita, S., Ogasahara, H., Yamada, K., Yonei, A. and Yokota, K. 1990. Cerebrovascular reactivity to CO_2 in patients with hepatic or septic encephalopathy. *Resuscitation* 19: 125–34.

Seda, H.W., Hughes, R.D., Gove, C.D. and Williams, R. 1984. Inhibition of rat brain Na^+,K^+-ATPase activity by serum from patients with fulminant hepatic failure. *Hepatology* 4: 74–9.

Slotman, G., Machiedo, G., Novak, R. and Bush, B. 1983. The hemodynamic effect of profound hypercapnia on acute hypoxic respiratory failure. *Circ Shock* 11: 187–94.

Thompson, B.T. and Cockrill, B.A. 1994. Renal-dose dopamine: a siren song? *Lancet* 344: 7–8.

Trewby, P.N., Hanid, M.A., Mackenzie, R.L., Mellon, P.J. and Williams, R. 1978. Effects of cerebral oedema and arterial hypotension on cerebral blood flow in an animal model of hepatic failure. *Gut* 19: 999–1005.

Utsunomiya, T., Krauz, M., Valeria, C., Shepro, D. and Hechtman, H. 1980. The treatment of pulmonary embolus with epoprostenol. *Surgery* 88: 25–8.

Ware, A.J., D'Agostino, A.N. and Combes, B. 1971. Cerebral edema: A major complication of massive hepatic necrosis. *Gastroenterology* 61: 877–84.

Wendon, J., Harrison, P., Keays, R., Gimson, A., Alexander, G. and Williams, R. 1992. Effects of vasopressor agents and epoprostenol on systemic hemodynamics on oxygen transport variables in patients with fulminant hepatic failure. *Hepatology* 15: 1067–71.

Wendon, J., Harrison, P., Keays, R. and Williams, R. 1994. Cerebral blood flow and metabolism in fulminant hepatic failure. *Hepatology* 19: 1407–13.

Wendon, J.A., Harrison, P., Heaton, N. and Williams, R. 1994. Serum nitrates as markers of postoperative morbidity. *Lancet* 344: 410–11 (letter).

12 Brain edema and intracranial hypertension in acute liver failure

Andres T. Blei

INTRODUCTION

The development of neurological complications is a critical turning point in the course of acute liver failure (ALF). Hepatic encephalopathy can quickly progress from mild alterations of consciousness to deep coma, and intracranial hypertension as a result of brain swelling can be a major cause of death in this syndrome (O'Grady et al. 1989). At a time when liver transplantation appears as an effective therapy for patients with a low likelihood of spontaneous recovery, management of the neurological picture acquires a new urgency. The goal of this chapter is to discuss current views on the pathogenesis of brain edema, its clinicial manifestations and current therapeutic options.

HISTORY

The importance of alterations in mental state in the course of acute jaundice have been recognized since antiquity. The description of the neurological symptomatology of "acute yellow atrophy" by Frerichs in the 19th century is rich with details that are still valid today (quoted in Adams and Foley 1953). Neuropathologic descriptions of hepatic coma have lumped together the few cases of acute failure with those of cirrhosis. However, it was only in the 1940s that separation between the clinical manifestations of encephalopathy in acute liver failure from those of cirrhosis became more clearly demarcated, with delirium and convulsions a feature of acute liver disease that was seldom observed in the "quiet" evolution of coma in chronic liver failure (Greene 1940).

Although the first report on brain swelling dates to 1944 (Lucké 1944), autopsy cases of acute liver failure were reported where the patients had findings consistent with brain edema and intracranial hypertension; namely, increased brain weight and evidence of temporal lobe or uncal herniation (Ware et al. 1971). These observations were subsequently confirmed in other liver centers. In 1977, a combined conference of neurologists and hepatologists interested in acute liver failure discussed the specificity of purported brain swelling (Berk and Popper 1978). Prominent neurologists expressed concern that the reports of brain edema may simply represent an agonal phenomenon. Twenty years later, knowledge acquired through intracranial pressure measurements in vivo, experimental models of acute liver failure, and the experience with liver transplantation have established brain edema as a major complication of acute liver failure. The challenge now resides in deciphering its pathogenesis so that rational therapy and prophylaxis can be instituted.

NEUROPATHOLOGY

There are few reports that have systematically examined the neuropathology of patients dying with brain edema and intracranial hypertension in ALF. In an autopsy series of 132 patients, 92 subjects underwent a neuropathological examination (Gazzard et al. 1975). In 38 brains, the dura was tense and the brain swollen with flattening of the gyri, suggesting the presence of edema. More dramatically, twelve of these subjects had evidence of herniation of the cerebellar tonsils and eight of the temporal lobes, a factor that can be deemed the cause of death. In another autopsy series, brain swelling was recorded at autopsy in approximately half of the 35 cases (Ware et al. 1971). In both series, many patients also exhibited renal failure, had been on artificial ventilatory support and had variable lengths of duration of coma, factors that could contribute to neuropathologic findings.

It is in experimental models of ALF where additional information has been provided on the neuropathology of brain edema. Using perfusion methods to rapidly fix the brain in situ, some of the variables that cloud neuropathologic studies in humans can be overcome. The results have been similar across species and across types of liver injury: In galactosamine-induced ALF in the rat (Dixit and Chang 1990) and rabbit (Traber et al. 1986), in hepatectomized rats (Livingstone et al. 1977) and in rats after hepatic devascularization (Traber et al. 1989), brain edema can be detected using sensitive methods, such as the density gradient technique, that measure water content in small brain samples. In our study, swelling was detected in the cerebral cortex (rich in cells) while it was not observed in the white matter (Traber et al. 1986). Detailed studies, including electron microscopy, indicate that cortical astrocytes appear swollen (Potvin et al. 1984), with hydropic foot processes and vacuolation of organelles (Traber et al. 1987). White matter astrocytes did not appear affected.

Astrocytes are the most numerous cellular element in the brain and occupy one-third of the volume of the cerebral cortex (Fedoroff and Vernadakis 1986; Norenberg et al. 1988). Their anatomical features, with a small cellular body and extensions that surround blood vessels, axons and neuronal elements, led to prior views that defined this cell simply as a structural support element in the brain. More recent views have emphasized a multifunctional role for what is in reality a syncitium of cells, joined via gap junctions, in a structure that allows easy amplification of signals. Astrocytes have important functions in regulating the extracellular concentrations of ions and transmitters, important for neuronal signaling. They participate in water regulation in the brain, they confer impermeable properties to the blood–brain barrier and modulate inflammatory responses. Specific enzyme systems are present in this cell, such as glutamine synthetase, that allow the detoxification of ammonia and other potential neurotoxins.

Astrocytes have been recognized as affected in other forms of encephalopathy associated with liver diseases, including the classic Alzheimer type II astrocytosis seen in cirrhotic patients dying in hepatic coma (reviewed in Norenberg 1994). Using immersion-fixation techniques, the Alzheimer type II change is seen as an enlarged, clear nucleus with a marginated chromatin. Its presence has been observed in young primates challenged with an ammonia load (Voorheis et al. 1983). It is not seen when the brain is processed with techniques of perfusion-fixation (Cavanagh and Kyu 1971). Astrocyte swelling, on the other hand, is also seen in the first weeks after portacaval anastomosis in the rat (Zamora et al. 1973; Swain et al. 1991), to be replaced by degenerative changes as time elapses. This suggests that glial swelling may be a manifestation of the initial reaction of the brain to exposure to toxin(s) present in liver disease. In brain biopsies of patients dying with ALF obtained immediately after death, astrocyte swelling could also be detected (Kato et al. 1992).

It should be noted that astrocyte swelling is not a specific finding in ALF. It can occur as an early response to injury from multiple etiologies, including other metabolic etiologies, ischemia, and trauma. Furthermore, a leaky capillary endothelial cell is associated with glial swelling, as astrocytes take up excess water and protein (Klatzo et al. 1980). Thus, are the astrocyte changes seen in ALF a primary phenomenon or a secondary change to a disrupted blood–brain barrier? This question will be discussed in the next section.

PATHOGENESIS

Background

Brain edema leading to intracranial hypertension appears as a complication of the encephalopathy of acute liver failure and not of cirrhosis. Within the spectrum of acute liver failure, brain edema is more prominent in those cases where there is a short interval between the onset of jaundice and the development of encephalopathy (O'Grady et al. 1993). In cirrhosis, there have been reports of decerebrate posturing in patients in hepatic coma (Conomy and Swash 1986), as well as scattered reports of raised intracranial pressure (ICP) in this setting (Crippin et al. 1992). However, death from intracranial hypertension is rare. Although in a recent preliminary report evidence of brain herniation was seen at autopsy in a few cirrhotic subjects in deep coma (Donovan et al. 1990), earlier but much larger anatomopathologic series do not record such observations (Adams and Foley 1953).

Why then are brain edema and intracranial hypertension unique to acute liver failure? An immediate answer could be that they originate from products of the acutely necrotic liver. This possibility can be now re-examined with a limited clinical experience using total hepatectomy in the treatment of ALF. Several groups have reported an improvement in the cardiovascular instability that characterizes advanced stages of ALF (Ringe et al. 1993; Williams 1995). In one series, the hyperdynamic circulatory syndrome was improved after removal of the injured liver (Noun et al. 1995). The impact on intracranial events has been less well documented. Cerebral hyperperfusion was corrected after hepatectomy (Ejlersen et al. 1994) but its effects on intracranial hypertension remain unknown. Furthermore, as in some reports hypothermia has been instituted in combination with the hepatectomy (Rozga et al. 1994), lowering of body temperature can have beneficial effects on intracranial hypertension per se (Traber et al. 1989).

In the experimental animal, the effects of removal of the liver have been studied in the rat and the pig. Several groups have reported the development of brain swelling in rats 10–18 h after hepatectomy (Livingstone et al. 1977; Olafsson et al. 1995). In one series, water in brain samples was measured using the dry-weight method and values as high as 3.5 percent swelling were seen (Livingstone et al. 1977), coupled with changes in the permeability of the blood–brain barrier (Potvin et al. 1984). In a more recent work, using the more sensitive density gradient method, swelling of up to 1 percent was noted (Olafsson et al. 1995), with a rise in intracranial pressure as measured in the cisterna magna. A preliminary experience in the pig, however, notes no elevation of intracranial pressure after hepatectomy (Chen et al. 1995); brain water values were not reported. In no experimental study has a failing liver been removed once the full neurological syndrome has developed. At this time, the role of products originating from liver cell necrosis in the genesis of part or the entire neurological picture of ALF remains unanswered.

On the other hand, brain edema and intracranial hypertension are detected only in the last stages of hepatic encephalopathy in ALF. This suggests a relationship between the mechanisms that account for the alteration in mental state and the increase in brain water and intracranial pressure. If not, if truly both phenomena were independent from each other, the rise in intracranial pressure would occur on a more random basis. To answer this question and with the impossibility of serially measuring brain water in humans, the temporal sequence of changes needs to be studied in the experimental animal. The rat after hepatic devascularization has been well characterized as a model of brain edema and intracranial hypertension (Traber et al. 1989). At a time when the righting reflex is lost (rodents turn immediately when placed on their backs), an increase in water of the cortical gray matter could be detected using the density gradient method (Swain et al. 1992). Water continued to increase until loss of the corneal reflex. This process lasts approximately two hours (Table 12.1). When intracranial pressure was continuously measured from the onset of ALF (Webster et al. 1991), the rise in pressure also occurred in the last two hours and became severe only in the last 30 min, culminating with the development of intracranial pressure waves, that displace brain tissue and result in brain herniation (Figure 12.1). It would appear, then, that the process that results in an increase in brain water occurs in parallel to the one that results in worsening encephalopathy and culminates in the appearance of intracranial hypertension.

Astrocyte swelling, a primary or secondary phenomenon?

We have discussed how in different experimental models of ALF astrocytes appear swollen. Two possible scenarios explain this finding.

An increase in intracellular osmolarity

In several other clinical conditions associated with brain edema, the driving force for water accumulation in the brain is a change in intracellular osmolarity. For example, the accumulation of sorbitol in diabetic brain may explain the development of brain edema during rapid correction of hyperglycemia (Burg and Kador 1988). In ALF, an increase in two intracellular osmoles has been proposed as an explanation of brain swelling.

Sodium

This would increase as a consequence of circulating inhibitors of Na^+-K^+ ATPase that interfere with the function of this key membrane pump for extrusion of sodium from the cellular interior. Using rat brain plasma membranes, sera from patients in stage III–IV encephalopathy inhibited the activity of Na^+-K^+ ATPase in this preparation (Seda et al. 1984). These inhibitors could also interfere with the Na^+-K^+ ATPase activity in other tissues, such as leucocytes (Sewell et al. 1982). Plasma levels of digoxin-like immunoreactive substances are elevated in ALF of different etiologies (Yang et al. 1988), and have been proposed as a possible explanation for the inhibition of Na^+-K^+ ATPase activity.

Proposed in the 1980s, the nature of this inhibitory activity remains elusive. In an experimental model of ALF, there was no relation between the activity of Na^+-K^+ ATPase and the degree of swelling (Ede et al. 1987). Cross-reactivity with bile acids may explain findings in the radioimmunoassay for digoxin (Day and James 1989). Furthermore, why circulating inhibitors would selectively involve the astrocytes of the cerebral cortex remains unexplained. More recently, brain ischemia (see later) has been proposed as a mechanism responsible for brain swelling (Wendon et al. 1994); in this scenario, inhibition of Na^+-K^+ ATPase could occur as a result of decreased oxygen supply.

Glutamine

This amino acid is generated within astrocytes as result of the combination of ammonia with glutamate, a reaction catalyzed by glutamine synthetase, an enzymatic activity localized to astrocytes (Martinez-Hernandez et al. 1977). The brain lacks other systems for ammonia detoxification (such as the urea cycle) and the concentration of glutamine markedly increases in the brain in experimental models of ALF (Maus et al. 1989; Swain et al. 1992)

Table 12.1. *Temporal sequence of changes in mental state, brain water and intracranial pressure (rat after hepatic devascularization)*

Time (min)	Mental state	Brain water (%)	ICP (mmHg)
	Normal	*80.26 ± 0.22*	*1–6*
−120	Loss of righting reflex	80.88 ± 0.15[a]	10 ± 2
−60	Coma		18 ± 2
−30	Loss of corneal reflex	81.74 ± 0.25[b]	24 ± 2
0	Respiratory arrest	82.46 ± 0.06[b]	Pressure waves[c]

All values are mean ± SD. ICP = intracranial pressure. [a] $P < 0.05$, [b] $P < 0.01$ versus sham-operated animal.
[c] Pressure waves refer to a sudden rise in ICP to values greater than 50 mmHg. Adapted from Webster et al. 1991; Swain et al. 1992.

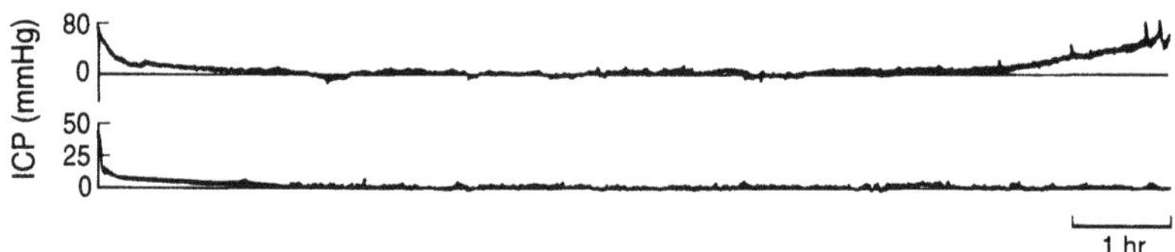

Figure 12.1 A progressive rise in intracranial pressure occurs in a rat with acute liver failure (top panel) due to hepatic devascularization in the last hour of evolution. The initial decrease reflects stabilization of pressure after placement of the transducer. The bottom panel reflects values in a sham-operated rat.

as well as in human autopsy material (Record et al. 1976). Glutamine exerts osmolar effects in other tissues, such as the liver (Haussinger and Schliess 1995), and changes in its cerebral concentration adapt to chronic changes in serum osmolarity, such as hyponatremia (Lien et al. 1990).

If this is correct, ammonia, a key factor in the pathogenesis of hepatic encephalopathy (Mousseau and Butterworth 1994) would also be linked to the pathogenesis of brain swelling. There is a body of experimental and clinical evidence that supports this connection.

- "Pure" hyperammonemic conditions in humans are associated with brain edema. These include children with urea cycle enzyme deficiencies who exhibit an acute rise of plasma ammonia (Brusilow 1985) and in adults, a postchemotherapy associated hyperammonemia (Watson et al. 1985); in both, brain swelling and intracranial hypertension have been documented.
- A continuous infusion of ammonia over several hours is associated with brain edema or intracranial hypertension in the rat (Takahashi et al. 1991) and primates (Voorhies 1983).
- An increase in cellular volume is observed after addition of ammonia to brain slices (Ganz et al. 1989) or cultured astrocytes (Norenberg et al. 1991).
- Inhibition of glutamine synthesis with methionine-sulfoximine results in a decrease in ammonia-induced cellular swelling in vitro (Norenberg and Bendor 1994) and of brain swelling in vivo (Takahashi et al. 1991; Blei et al. 1994).

In nature, cells adapt to chronic changes in their osmolar environment by activating short-term and long-term regulatory mechanisms (reviewed in McManus et al. 1995). In the case of cellular swelling, regulatory volume decrease brings about the restoration of cellular volume. Immediate reactions include the loss of ions, such as KCl via separate channels or via a cotransporter at the level of the plasma membrane, and of organic osmolytes. This term refers to a group of compounds, for the most part noncritical intermediates in cellular metabolic pathways, such as amino acids (taurine, alanine), polyalcohols (myoinositol, sorbitol) and methylamines (betaine, glycerylphosphocholine). The acute egress of these compounds from the cell occurs via passive efflux through a volume-activated channel. For chronic adaptation to swelling, a membrane transporter involved in the entry of organic osmolytes to the brain is down-regulated over several days.

Teleologically, chronic changes in cellular ionic concentration carry the potential for alterations in intracellular pH and multiple enzymatic processes. Altering the levels of organic osmolytes is a more efficient way to cope with volume stress throughout nature. Organic osmolytes are "nonperturbing" solutes and changes in their intracellular concentration do not primarily affect cell function.

Preliminary reports of measurements of organic osmolytes in ALF using NMR spectroscopy reveal the expected increase in glutamine without changes in myo-inositol concentration (McConnell et al. 1995). This is in contrast to observations in patients with cirrhosis, where the increase in glutamine is accompanied by a decrease in myo-inositol (Haussinger et al. 1994). In isolated astrocytes, an acute addition of ammonia results in the loss of intracellular taurine (Albrecht et al. 1994), while exposure over several days reduces the uptake of myo-inositol (Norenberg and Bendor 1994). These observations have led to a further refinement of the "glutamine" hypothesis in the pathogenesis of brain edema. It is not only the fact that astrocytes would gain glutamine, but that there is insufficient time to compensate for this increase by losing other organic osmolytes, that results in the development of brain swelling. This time-dependency could explain the more frequent development of brain edema in the hyperacute forms of acute liver failure as well as account for the lack of brain swelling in cirrhosis, where glutamine also markedly increases.

An increased permeability of the blood–brain barrier

An increased permeability of the barrier explains brain swelling in diverse clinical conditions, where the integrity of the endothelial cell is altered, the "vasogenic" mechanism of brain edema. Even in conditions of altered cellular osmoregulation, the "cytotoxic" etiology of brain edema, a net increase of water must occur into brain in order for edema to occur. In brain trauma, primary or secondary tumors or after brain ischemia, passage of solutes and water can occur via a breakdown of the tight intercellular junctions or through activation of transcellular pathways (Klatzo 1994). In response to changes in the extracellular milieu, compensatory mechanisms are activated, that include the uptake of protein and water by astrocytes. Astrocyte swelling can be prominent in this setting. In ischemic injury, neuronal release of the neuroexcitatory neurotransmitter, glutamate, is observed and reuptake into astrocytes, a Na^+ coupled process, may result in the development of glial swelling (Kimelberg et al. 1989). Of note, increased concentrations of extracellular glutamate have been noted in experimental ALF using microdialysis techniques (de Knejt, Gramsbergen et al. 1994); higher extracellular glutamate could lead to an entry of calcium into cells via receptor-mediated and voltage-operated calcium channels. However, calcium content in the brain of rabbits with ALF was not increased (de Knejt, Schalm et al. 1994). A role for glutamate in the pathogenesis of brain edema in ALF has not been fully explored.

In experimental models of ALF, an increased entry into the brain of compounds to which the barrier is normally impermeable has been documented. In two different rat models, passage of inulin and sucrose (Zaki et al. 1984) or of Evans Blue (Dixit and Chang 1990) has been reported. In rabbits with galactosamine-induced ALF, passage of gamma-isoaminobutyric acid, as measured with autoradiography, occurred in the later stages of the course (Basett et al. 1990). Curiously, the highest counts were present in the basal ganglia and not in the cortex, where brain edema is most prominent (Traber et al. 1986). In this same model, no increased uptake of horseradish peroxidase, an electron-dense protein, could be demonstrated using electron microscopy (Traber et al. 1987). An increase of GABA uptake was not seen in the rat (Lo et al. 1987; Knudsen et al. 1988).

If this information in the experimental animal appears conflicting, clinical evidence does not support the existence of a gross breakdown of the blood–brain barrier in humans. Brain biopsies at the time of death do not show alterations in the integrity of tight junctions (Kato et al. 1992). CT scanning is for the most part unremarkable (Muñoz et al. 1991) and even the reports of swollen brain do not show the patchy change characteristic of a broken barrier (Wijdicks et al. 1995). Therapeutic observations in ALF patients are also important. It could be argued that the beneficial effects of mannitol indicate the ability of this molecule to exert an osmotic gradient across the barrier; however, mannitol is also effective in conditions of vasogenic edema by allowing further room for brain expansion via removal of water from normal brain tissue. More compelling is the observation that corticosteroids, effective in cases of endothelial cell disruption, are unhelpful in relieving brain swelling in ALF (Canalese et al. 1982).

To summarize this aspect, the evidence does not suggest a primary event at the level of the endothelial cell to account for brain swelling. It is possible that at the later stages of evolution, secondary changes in the permeability of the barrier may amplify abnormalities that primarily develop within the brain. Whether abnormalities in astrocyte function in ALF result in secondary changes in endothelial cell function has not been determined. In this regard, it is of interest that in cocultured preparations, the astrocyte allows the expression of activities of the capillary endothelial cell that are not seen when the latter is cultured alone (Abbott et al. 1992).

Intracranial hypertension

Pressure can rise within the rigid skull from the expansion of any of its volume compartments. Traditional views point to three major compartments: brain tissue, cerebrospinal fluid and blood volume. More recently, a four compartment model has been proposed, where brain tissue is divided between interstitial and cellular sections. This approach is based on observations that point to the maintenance of intracellular volume in the face of alterations of the extracellular space (McManus et al. 1995). In any case, the increase in pressure in ALF is associated with an expansion of brain tissue volume. This is well documented in animal models (reviewed in Blei 1995) and corresponds to neuropathological observations of "heavy" brains in human ALF (Ware et al. 1971; Gazzard et al. 1975). The progressive rise in pressure culminates in the development of intracranial pressure waves that result in brain displacement and can culminate in herniation (see Figure 12.1).

The volume of cerebrospinal fluid has not been measured, but is highly unlikely to be expanded in ALF. Repeatedly, CT exams at the time of elevated intracranial pressure have shown unchanged or compressed ventricular spaces (Muñoz et al. 1991; Wijdicks et al. 1995). The exact role of cerebral blood volume remains to be defined, as repeated measurements of this space are difficult to obtain both in humans and the experimental animal. A rise in cerebral blood volume can increase intracranial pressure without a change in tissue water, as seen with arterial vasodilators (Hirayama et al. 1994). In ALF, the role of cerebral blood volume may be important towards the end of the course, where the compliance characteristics of the brain change and small increases in volume can result in large increases in pressure. Cerebral blood flow has been used as an indirect marker, with the assumption that hyperemia could be equated with increased cerebral blood volume. Errors in this assumption exist when increased cerebral blood volume is associated with decreased flow, as in the case of venous outflow obstruction.

A reduced cerebral blood flow, seen in the experimental animal (Shah et al. 1993), appears to be present in the majority of patients with ALF (Almdal et al. 1989). It has been postulated that this decrease induces brain ischemia. The reduction in oxygen consumption (the product of blood flow and arteriovenous oxygen difference) and the apparent production of lactate by the brain support this view (Wendon et al. 1994). Furthermore, the apparent beneficial effects of *N*-acetylcysteine (NAC) on the development of brain edema in acetaminophen (paracetamol)-induced ALF (Keays et al. 1991) have been postulated to arise from an improvement in the cerebral microcirculation. These include the antioxidant properties of NAC (counteracting the effects of free radicals produced during ischemia) as well as the generation of nitrosothiols, compounds that stimulate the release of nitric oxide.

Some patients, especially those who develop intracranial hypertension, appear to exhibit cerebral hyperemia (Aggarwal et al. 1994). A low arteriovenous oxygen difference was interpreted as an indicator of increased cerebral blood flow, although this interpretation may be incorrect in the face of changes in cerebral oxygen consumption (Schmidt 1992). More detailed studies suggest the presence of a "luxury perfusion" syndrome, where the volume of flow exceeds the metabolic needs of the brain (Larsen et al. 1995). It is possible that a failure of blood flow autoregulation may underlie this phenomenon (Paulson et al. 1990). The ability of blood flow to remain constant in the face of variation in blood pressure has been studied in an experimental model as well as in humans and failure of autoregulation was observed (Larsen et al. 1994; 1995). In humans, the response of blood flow to variations in CO_2 has shed further light on mechanisms that may underlie the abnormal cerebral circulation (Durham et al. 1995). A decrease in Pco_2 was associated with the expected vasoconstriction and reduction in blood flow. On the other hand, an increase in Pco_2 did not result in vasodilatation, suggesting the presence of an already dilated cerebral vascular territory. Whether this vasodilatation is part of the generalized hyperdynamic circulatory syndrome seen in ALF (Bihari et al. 1985) remains to be determined. In any case, it is in such a vasodilated setting that hyperemia, failure of cerebrovascular autoregulation and/or an increase in cerebral blood volume may contribute to the increase in intracranial pressure.

DIAGNOSIS

Clinical aspects

Brain edema and intracranial hypertension develop in patients with acute liver failure at stages III-IV of hepatic encephalopathy. Cerebral swelling without a rise in intracranial pressure is for the most part clinically silent. It is the displacement of brain structures during an elevation of intracranial pressure that results in clinical manifestations. Signs of increased pressure within the skull include pupillary alterations in response to light, lack of response to heat stimuli during caloric ear testing and decerebrate posturing (Langfitt 1982). However, these signs are not a sensitive tool; in patients with head trauma, elevations of intracranial pressure of up to 60 mmHg can go clinically undetected. Frequent monitoring of clinical signs is not a practical alternative for a rapidly changing clinical picture. Other signs of chronic elevation of pressure, such as papilledema, are usually absent. The rise of intracranial pressure can result in agitation, elevation of arterial pressure (the Cushing response) and bradycardia. Agitation can be on occasion accompanied by seizures. An elevation of brain quinolinic acid has been found in patients who died in acute liver failure, and it has been proposed that such changes could predispose patients to seizures (Basile et al. 1995). Of note, both in the experimental animal (Webster et al. 1991) and in humans (Keays et al. 1993) the response of the arterial pressure to the rise of intracranial pressure has an influence on the clinical course. With a larger increase in arterial pressure, death is delayed in rats with ischemic hepatic failure and patients appear to have a better prognosis.

Monitoring of intracranial pressure

Monitoring has become increasingly widespread, especially in patients awaiting liver transplantation. Placement of a pressure device simplifies the management of patients though its ultimate goal, to improve patient survival, appears only marginally achieved (Jenkins et al. 1987; Lidofsky et al. 1992; Keays et al. 1993). Knowledge of intracranial pressure values allows better use of therapy, permits detection of pressure waves (harbingers of brain herniation) and may signal the need for therapeutic measures of last resort, such as barbiturate coma. Its role in the decisions that surround emergency liver transplantation is discussed in the next section.

The type of intracranial pressure monitor has received intense scrutiny. In a retrospective survey of academic medical centers in the United States, the use of epidural monitors resulted in 5 percent of hemorrhagic complications as compared to 18–22 percent when the dura was pierced, either for placement of a subdural bolt or an intraparenchymal monitor (Blei et al. 1993). On the other hand, epidural devices are by their nature less precise and have potential for zero shift; subdural bolts allow calibration to atmospheric pressure. In any case, deaths from intracranial hemorrhage have been reported with all devices. Measures to reduce the risk of hemorrhage include the correction of coagulopathy, plasmapheresis (Muñoz 1993), use of very small diameter transducers placed against the brain surface (Armstrong et al. 1993) and avoiding placement at a late stage in the clinical course, when intracranial pressure may be already high (Aldersley et al. 1995). Experience with this procedure is also a critical element and in many centers, hepatologists and intensivists have found it difficult to convince their neurosurgical colleagues that the risk of hemorrhage can be overcome. Due to the relatively short duration of the clinical course, infectious complications are seldom seen.

Computed tomography

The need for alternative, less invasive methods of monitoring intracranial events is obvious. Two reports note the lack of diagnostic changes with computed tomography at the time of elevated intracranial pressure (Muñoz et al. 1991; Lidofsky et al. 1992). In a recent report, however, some evidence of brain swelling could be detected at encephalopathy stages II and III (Wijdicks et al. 1995). All subjects had marked changes during stage IV encephalopathy, as evidenced by effacement of sulci, compression of the white matter and changes in cisternal appearance. The inability to serially image the brain in critically ill patients in whom mobilization to radiology departments is a major undertaking, limits the usefulness of CT scanning. The procedure may be helpful in ruling out other intracranial pathology prior to placement of intracranial pressure monitors.

Cerebral blood flow and oxygen consumption

We have discussed a recent view where cerebral ischemia has been postulated as a cause of brain swelling (Wendon et al. 1994). However, any increase in intracranial pressure has the risk of resulting in secondary brain ischemia as a result of the reduction of cerebral perfusion. A diagnosis of brain ischemia can be obtained by measurements of cerebral perfusion coupled to the ability of the organ to extract oxygen, the arteriovenous oxygen difference. Both parameters can be clinically determined.

Cerebral blood flow can be measured using radioactive xenon as a marker of a freely diffusible substance whose appearance in the brain thus depends on cerebral perfusion. However, repeated injections of radioactive material is not well suited for multiple measurements. Employing Doppler flowmetry, insonation of the middle cerebral artery has been used as a bedside technique to measure blood flow (Ringelstein 1986). The Doppler signal allows calculation of velocity, which is converted to flow by multiplying the cross-sectional area of the artery. Validation of

Doppler flowmetry in ALF is needed and its impact on patient management awaits further studies. For measurements of arteriovenous oxygen difference, the internal jugular vein is cannulated in a retrograde fashion and the sampling catheter placed in the jugular bulb; for calculations, the oxygen content from a peripheral artery as well as from the jugular sample are needed. In any case, experience with this approach has been limited (Wendon et al. 1994; Aggarwal et al. 1994; Larsen et al. 1995) and proof of its usefulness is needed before it could replace current measures that include intracranial pressure monitoring.

Somatosenory evoked potentials

Evoked potentials have been postulated recently as a tool to predict the neurological course in ALF (Madl et al. 1994). In this neurophysiological method, the integrated electroencephalographic response to a peripheral stimulus is recorded in a series of characteristic wave patterns. Loss of the P20 potential was associated with death or lack of neurological recovery post-transplantation. Of note, changes in these potentials could be correlated to the development of brain edema. The exact role for this methodology awaits additional studies.

THERAPY

At this time, we cannot offer our patients a prophylactic approach to the problem of brain swelling. Nor is available treatment based on interrupting the abnormal pathophysiology. The therapeutic strategy (Cordoba and Blei, 1995) is based on: appropriate treatment of the multiorgan complications of ALF; avoidance of factors that increase intracranial hypertension; administration of drugs that decrease ICP; and decisions that surround the performance of emergency liver transplantation.

The development of brain edema occurs in the setting of very ill patients, in whom infections, renal failure and metabolic acidosis are also a major cause of morbidity/mortality. The vasodilatory circulatory state present in ALF can result in a decrease in arterial pressure that worsens the cerebral perfusion pressure. Fever will increase intracranial pressure as a result of cerebral hyperemia (Muñoz et al. 1993). The presence of renal failure will complicate volume replacement; if dialysis is instituted, shifts may occur that can affect water and osmolar regulation in the brain.

The importance of nursing care in the management of patients with neurological complications cannot be emphasized enough. Local factors that increase intracranial pressure include the Valsalva maneuver, head turning and moving and neck vein compression. A recent study indicates that a head position at 30 degrees is of benefit to patients with ALF (Herrine et al. 1995). Patients in stage III–IV encephalopathy are intubated with the concern that a sudden respiratory arrest may develop; respiratory suctioning should be done with care. Treatment of psychomotor agitation, a feature in the earlier stages of ALF, requires the administration of drugs that will inevitably decrease the sensorium; on the other hand, this agitation can be harmful to the patient and requires therapy. Myoclonic or generalized seizures, a feature seen in some patients with ALF, will aggravate the rise in intracranial pressure and should be promptly recognized and treated.

It is common to start treatment of intracranial hypertension when values of ICP are above 25 mmHg. The development of pressure waves requires prompt attention, as it signals imminent herniation. Osmotherapy with mannitol is the mainstay of therapy. The drug is given as a bolus, 0.5–1 gm/kg, but not at fixed dosage intervals. After repeated treatments, plasma osmolarity should be checked as values should not rise above 320 mOsm/l. If renal failure is present, dialysis may be required to eliminate mannitol in order to administer more drug. Hyperventilation is of limited use (Ede et al. 1986) as patients already exhibit respiratory alkalosis with hypocapnia.

For intractable intracranial hypertension, barbiturate infusion is administered. Published experience with thiopental (Forbes et al. 1989), infused at a dose of 10 μg/kg/min, indicates beneficial effects that are thought to arise from the reduction in brain metabolism induced by the drug. As clinical assessment is not possible, monitoring of plasma levels and electrophysiologic recordings should guide therapy. Arterial hypotension may develop from the drug's vasodilatory effects and vasoconstrictive agents may be required to maintain cerebral perfusion pressure (CPP). Induction of hypothermia can also be considered. In the experimental animal, hypothermic animals with ALF do not develop brain swelling (Traber et al. 1989) or a rise in intracranial pressure (McGrath et al. 1995). Lowering of body temperature with its resultant reduction in cerebral blood flow and metabolism has been used therapeutically in other neurosurgical conditions associated with increased intracranial pressure (Maher and Hachinski 1993).

Additional modalities of therapy, such as connection to a liver assist device (Hughes and Williams 1995), to an extracorporeal pig or human liver (Fox et al. 1995), or performance of a hepatectomy (Rozga et al. 1993; Ringe et al. 1993) are still in the experimental arena and should be conducted only within the framework of a controlled evaluation (Lee 1994). They are discussed elsewhere in this volume. Of note, the major beneficial effect of a liver assist device that employs pig hepatocytes was a reduction in intracranial pressure (Rozga et al. 1994). The beneficial effects of i.v. *N*-acetylcysteine to improve cerebral microcirculatory parameters, as discussed in an earlier section, awaits further confirmation.

Liver transplantation is the definitive solution for refractory intracranial hypertension in ALF. This aspect is discussed elsewhere in this volume. One of the most difficult decisions in hepatology is to cancel the life-saving operation due to concerns about irreversible brain damage being present after surgery. Indeed, neurological deficits can occur after transplantation for ALF (O'Brien et al. 1987). Some centers use a prolonged reduction of CPP (<40 mmHg for 2 h) as an indicator of prolonged cerebral ischemia. With such values, children with Reye's syndrome (Jenkins et al. 1987) and adults with ALF (Schafer and Shaw Jr 1989) have impaired neurological recovery or do not survive the acute injury. It has been recommended that such a reduction of cerebral perfusion pressure is a contraindication to emergency liver transplantation (Donovan et al. 1992). More recently, this view has been questioned. In a small group of patients transplanted with a CPP <40 mmHg for more than 2 h, full neurological recovery occurred (Davies et al. 1994); similar findings were reported in a preliminary observation (Aldersley et al. 1995). At the bedside, facing such critical decisions, the first step is to exclude malfunctioning of the pressure monitor. If values are correct, decisions about transplantability should use CPP as one of the clinical criteria. Ischemia is the concern; thus, it is likely that changes in cerebral oxygenation, with repeated measurements of flow and arteriovenous oxygen difference to determine cerebral oxygen consumption, may provide additional useful information.

CONCLUDING REMARKS

There are two areas where future efforts in cerebral edema should be concentrated. Unraveling the mechanisms that lead to the development of brain edema and intracranial hypertension should lead to effective therapy as well as opening the possibility of prophylactic measures. Furthermore, links between the alteration of mental state seen in acute liver failure with that of cirrhosis suggest that insight into the pathogenesis of hepatic encephalopathy may also be forthcoming (Cordoba and Blei 1996).

On the other hand, validation of noninvasive or minimally invasive procedures to supplement and even replace intracranial pressure measurements is critical. The goal of such information should be to improve management and to facilitate decisions regarding the timing of liver transplantation. The results of ongoing investigations are eagerly awaited.

REFERENCES

Abbott, N.J., Revest, P.A. and Romero, I.A. 1992. Astrocyte–endothelial interaction: physiology and pathology. *Neuropathol Appl Neurobiol* 18: 424–33.

Adams, R.D. and Foley, J.M. 1953. The neurological disorders associated with liver disease. *Proc Assoc Res Nerv Ment Dis* 32: 198–235.

Aggarwal, S., Kramer, D., Yonas, H., Obrist, W., Kang, Y., Martin, M. and Policare, R. 1994. Cerebral hemodynamic and metabolic changes in fulminant hepatic failure: a retrospective study. *Hepatology* 19: 80–7.

Albrecht, J., Bender, A.S. and Norenberg, M.D. 1994. Ammonia stimulates the release of taurine from cultured astrocytes. *Brain Res* 660: 282–92.

Aldersley, M.A., Juniper, M., Richardson, P., Howdle, P.D. and O'Grady, J.A. 1995. Inability of intracranial pressure monitoring to select patients with acute liver failure for transplantation. *Hepatology* 22: 208A.

Almdal, T., Shroeder, T. and Ranek, L. 1989. Cerebral blood flow and liver function in patients with encephalopathy due to acute and chronic liver diseases. *Scand J Gastroenterol* 24: 299–303.

Armstrong, I.R., Pollok, A. and Lee, A. 1993. Complications of intracranial pressure monitoring in fulminant hepatic failure. *Lancet* 341: 690.

Basile, A.S., Saito, K., Al-Mardini, H., Record, C.O., Hughes, R.D., Harrison, P., Williams, R., Li, Y. and Heyes, M.P. 1995. The relationship between plasma and brain quinolinic acid levels and the severity of hepatic encephalopathy. *Gastroenterology* 108: 818–23.

Bassett, M.L., Mullen, K.D., Scholz, B., Fenstermacher, J.D. and Jones, E.A. 1990. Increased brain uptake of gamma-aminobutyric acid in a rabbit model of hepatic encephalopathy. *Gastroenterology* 98: 747–57.

Burg, M.B. and Kador, P.F. 1988. Sorbitol, osmoregulation and the complications of diabetes. *J Clin Invest* 81: 635–40.

Berk, P.D. and Popper, H. 1978. Fulminant hepatic failure. *Am J Gastroenterol* 69: 349–400.

Bihari, D., Gimson, A.E., Waterson, M. and Williams, R. 1985. Tissue hypoxia during fulminant hepatic failure. *Crit Care Med* 13: 1034–9.

Blei, A.T., Olafsson, S., Therrien, G. and Butterworth, R.F. 1994. Ammonia-induced brain edema and intracranial hypertension in rats after portacaval anastomosis. *Hepatology* 19: 1431–44.

Blei, A., Olafsson, S., Webster, S. and Levy, R. 1993. Complications of intracranial pressure monitoring in fulminant hepatic failure. *Lancet* 341: 157–8.

Blei, A.T. 1995. Pathogenesis of brain edema in fulminant hepatic failure. *Prog Liver Dis* 13: 311–29.

Brusilow, S.W. 1985. Inborn errors of urea synthesis. In *Genetic and Metabolic Disease in Pediatrics*, eds. J. Lloyd and C. Scriver, 140–65. London: Butterworths.

Canalese, J., Gimson, A.E.S., Davies, C., Melton, P.J., Davis, M. and Williams, R. 1982. Controlled trial of dexamethasone and mannitol for the cerebral edema of fulminant hepatic failure. *Gut* 23: 625–9.

Cavanagh, J.B. and Kyu, M.H. 1971. Type II Alzheimer changes experimentally produced in astrocytes in the rat. *J Neurol Sci* 12: 63–75.

Chen, S., Watanobe, F.D., Wang, C.C., Eguchi, S., Demetriou, A.A. and Rozga, J. 1995. Presence of liver necrosis is needed for development of intracranial hypertension in acute liver failure. *Hepatology* 22: 381A.

Conomy, J. and Swash, M. 1986. Reversible decerebrate and decorticate postures in hepatic coma. *N Engl J Med* 278: 876–9.

Cordoba, J. and Blei, A.T. 1995. Cerebral edema and intracranial pressure monitoring. *Liver Transpl Surg* 1: 187–94.

Cordoba, J. and Blei, A.T. 1996. Brain edema and hepatic encephalopathy. *Semin Liv Dis* (in press).

Crippin, J.S., Gross, J.B. Jr. and Lindor, K.D. 1992. Increased intracranial pressure and hepatic encephalopathy in chronic liver disease. *Am J Gastroenterol* 87: 879–82.

Davies, M.H., Mutimer, D., Lowes, J., Elias, E. and Neuberger, J. 1994. Recovery despite impaired cerebral perfusion in fulminant hepatic failure. *Lancet* 343: 1329–30.

Day, C.P. and James, O.F. 1989. Digoxin-like factors in liver disease. *J Hepatol* 9: 281–4.

de Knejt, R.J., Gramsbergen, J.B. and Schalm, S.W. 1994. $_{45}Ca\ CL_2$ autoradiography in brain from rabbits with encephalopathy from acute liver failure or acute hyperammonemia. *Metabol Brain Dis* 9: 153–60.

de Knejt, R.J., Schalm, S.W., Van der Ryt, C.C., Fekkes, D., Dalm, E. and Hekking-Weyma, I. 1994. Extracellular brain glutamate during acute liver failure and during acute hyperammonemia simulating acute liver failure: an experimental study based on in vivo brain dialysis. *J Hepatol* 20: 19–26.

Dixit, V. and Chang, T.M. 1990. Brain edema and the blood–brain barrier in galactosamine-induced fulminant hepatic failure rats: an animal model for evaluation of liver support systems. *ASAIO Trans.* 36: 21–7.

Donovan, J.P., Quigley, EMM, Sorell, M.F., Zetterman, R.E., Castaldo, P., Markin, R.S. and Shaw, B.W. 1990. Cerebral edema as a complication of chronic liver disease. (Abstract). *Hepatology* 12: 60.

Donovan, J.P., Shaw, B.W., Langnas, A.V. and Sorrell, M. 1992. Brain water and acute liver failure: The emerging role of intracranial pressure monitoring. *Hepatology* 16: 267–8.

Durham, S., Yonas, H., Aggarwal, S., Darby, J. and Kramer, D. 1995. Regional cerebral blood flow and CO_2 reactivity in fulminant hepatic failure. *J Cerebr Blood Flow Meth* 15: 329–35.

Ede, R.J., Gove, C.D., Hughes, R.D., Marshall, W. and Williams, R. 1987. Reduced brain Na+-K+ ATPase activity in rats with galactosamine-induced hepatic failure; relationship to encephalopathy and cerebral oedema. *Clin Sci* 72: 365–71.

Ede, R.J., Gimson, A.E.S., Bihari, D. and Williams, R. 1986. Controlled hyperventilation in the prevention of cerebral edema in fulminant hepatic failure. *J Hepatol* 2: 43–51.

Ejlersen, E., Larsen, F.S., Pott, F., Gyrtrup, H.J., Kirkegaard, P. and Secher, N.H. 1994. Hepatectomy corrects cerebral hyperperfusion in fulminant hepatic failure. *Transpl Proc* 26: 1794–5.

Fedoroff, S. and Vernadakis, A. eds. 1986. *Astrocytes, Vol 1–3*. Orlando: Academic Press.

Forbes, A., Alexander, G.J., O'Grady, J.G., Keays, R., Gullan, R., Dawling, S. and Williams, R. 1989. Thiopental infusion in the treatment of intracranial hypertension complicating fulminant hepatic failure. *Hepatology* 10: 306–10.

Fox, I.J., Collin, D., Merrill, J., Langhas, A., Dixon, R.S., Fristoe, L., Heffron, T.G. and Shaw, B.W. Jr. 1995. Extracorporeal liver perfusion with human and porcine livers for the treatment of fulminant hepatic failure. *Hepatology* 22: 148A.

Ganz, R., Swain, M., Traber, P., Dal Canto, M., Butterworth, R. and Blei, A.T. 1989. Ammonia-induced swelling of rat cerebral cortical slices: implications for the pathogenesis of brain edema in acute hepatic failure. *Metabol Brain Dis* 4: 213–23.

Gazzard, B.G., Portman, B., Murray-Lyon, I.M. and Williams, R. 1975. Causes of death in fulminant hepatic failure and relationship to quantitative histological assessment of parenchymal damage. *Quart J Med* 44: 615–26.

Greene, C.H. 1940. Liver and biliary tract, review for 1940. *Arch Intern Med* 67: 867–88.

Haussinger, D., Laubenberger, J., Von Dahl, S., Ernst, T., Bayer, S., Langer, M., Gerok, W. and Hennig, J. 1994. Proton magnetic resonance spectroscopy studies on human brain myoinositol on hyposmolarity and hepatic encephalopathy. *Gastroenterology* 107: 1475–80.

Haussinger, D. and Schliess, F. 1995. Cell volume and hepatocellular function. *J Hepatol* 22: 94–100.

Herrine, S.K., Northrup, B., Bell, R. and Muñoz, S.J. 1995. The effect of head elevation of cerebral perfusion pressure in fulminant hepatic failure. *Hepatology* 22: 289A.

Hirayama, T., Katayama, Y., Kemo, T. and Tsubokawa, T. 1994. Control of systemic hypertension with diltiazem, a calcium antagonist, in patients with a mildly elevated intracranial pressure; a comparative study. *Neurol Res* 16: 97–100.

Hughes, R.D. and Williams, R. 1995. Evaluation of extracorporeal bioartificial liver devices. *Liver Transpl Surg* 1: 200–6.

Jenkins, J.G., Glasgow, J.F., Black, G.W., Fannin, T.F., Hicks, E.M., Keilty, S.R. and Crean, P.M. 1987. Reye's syndrome: assessment of intracranial pressure monitoring. *BMJ* 294: 337–8.

Kato, M.D., Hughes, R.D., Keays, R.T. and Williams, R. 1992. Electron microscopic study of brain capillaries in cerebral edema from fulminant hepatic failure. *Hepatology* 15: 1060–6.

Keays, R.T., Alexander, G.J.M. and Williams, R. 1993. The safety and value of extradural intracranial pressure monitors in fulminant hepatic failure. *J Hepatol* 18: 205–9.

Keays, R.T., Harrison, P.M., Wendon, J.A., Forbes, A., Gove, C., Alexander, G.J. and Williams, R. 1991. Intravenous acetylcysteine in paracetamol induced fulminant hepatic failure: a prospective controlled trial. *BMJ* 303: 1026–9.

Kimelberg, H.K., Pang, S. and Treble, D.H. 1989. Excitatory amino acid-stimulated uptake of $^{22}Na+$ in primary astrocyte cultures. *J Neurosci* 9: 1141–9.

Klatzo, I., Chui, E., Fujiware, K. and Spatz, M. 1980. Resolution of vasogenic brain edema. *Adv Neurol* 28: 359–73.

Klatzo, I. 1994. Evolution of brain edema concepts. *Acta Neurochir* (Suppl) 60: 3–6.

Knudsen, G.M., Poulson, H.E. and Paulson, O.B. 1988. Blood–brain barrier permeability in galactosamine-induced hepatic encephalopathy: no evidence for increased GABA transport. *J Hepatol* 6: 187–92.

Langfitt, T.W. 1992. Increased intracranial pressure and the cerebral circulation. In *Neurological Surgery*, ed. J.R. Youngmans, 846–76. Philadelphia: W.B. Saunders.

Larsen, F.S., Eljissen, E., Hausen, B.E., Knudsen, G.M., Tygstrup, N. and Secher, N.H. 1995. Functional loss of cerebral blood flow autoregulation in patients with fulminant hepatic failure. *J Hepatol* 23: 212–17.

Larsen, F.S., Knudsen, G.T., Paulson, O.B. and Vilstrup, H. 1994. Cerebral blood flow autoregulation is absent in rats with thioacetamide-induced hepatic failure. *J Hepatol* 21: 491–5.

Lee, W.M. 1994. Total hepatectomy for acute liver failure: don't take out my liver! *Gastroenterology* 107: 894–7.

Lidofsky, S.D., Bass, N.M., Prager, M.C., Washington, D.E., Read, A.E., Wright, T.L., Ascher, N.L., Roberts, J.P., Scharschmidt, B.F. and Lake, J.R. 1992. Intracranial pressure monitoring and liver transplantation for fulminant hepatic failure. *Hepatology* 16: 1–7.

Lien, Y.H., Shapiro, J. and Chan, L. 1990. Effects of hypernatremia on organic brain osmoles. *J Clin Invest* 85: 1427–35.

Livingstone, A.S., Potvin, M., Goresky, C.A., Finlayson, M.H., Hinchey, E.J. 1977. Changes in the blood–brain barrier in hepatic coma after hepatectomy in the rat. *Gastroenterology* 73: 697–704.

Lo, W.D., Ennis, S.R., Goldstein, G., McNeely, D. and Betz, L.A. 1987. The effects of galactosamine-induced hepatic failure upon blood–brain barrier permeability. *Hepatology* 7: 452–6.

Lucké, B. 1944. Pathology of fatal epidemic hepatitis. *Am J Pathol* 20: 471–593.

Madl, C., Grimm, G., Ferenci, P., Kramer, L., Yeganehfar, W., Oder, W., Steininger, R., et al. 1994. Serial recording of sensory evoked potentials; a noninvasive prognostic indicator in fulminant liver failure. *Hepatology* 20: 1487–94.

Maher, J. and Hachinski, V. 1993. Hypothermia as a potential treatment for cerebral ischemia. *Cerebrovasc Brain Met Rev* 5: 277–300.

Martinez-Hernandez, A., Bell, K.P. and Norenberg, M.D. 1977. Glutamine synthetase: glial localization in brain. *Science* 195: 1356–85.

Maus, A.M., Saunders, S.J., Kirsh, R.E. and Biebryck, J.F. 1989. Correlation of plasma and brain amino acid and putative neuro-transmitter alterations during acute hepatic coma in the rat. *J Neurochem* 32: 285–92.

McConnell, J.R., Antonson, D.L., Ong, C.S., Chu, W.K., Fox, I.J., Heffron, T.G., Langnas, A.N. and Shaw, B.W. 1995. Proton spectroscopy of brain glutamine in acute liver failure. *Hepatology* 22: 69–74.

McGrath, M.F., Rozga, J., Kong, L.B. and Demetriou, A.A. 1995. Metabolic, hemodynamic and intracranial pressure and cerebral perfusion pressure changes in hepatic and ischemic liver failure animals. *Surg Forum* 46: 419–20.

McManus, M.L., Churchwell, K.B. and Strange, K. 1995. Regulation of cell volume in health and disease. *N Engl J Med* 333: 1260–6.

Mousseau, D.D. and Butterworth, R.F. 1994. Current theories on the pathogenesis of hepatic encephalopathy. *Proc Soc Exp Biol Med* 206: 329–44.

Muñoz, S.J. 1993. Difficult management problems in fulminant hepatic failure. *Sem Liver Dis* 13: 395–413.

Muñoz, S.J., Moritz, M., Bell, R., Northup, B. et al. 1993. Factors associated with severe intracranial hypertension in candidates for emergency liver transplantation. *Transplantation* 55: 1071–4.

Muñoz, S.J., Robinson, M., Northrup, B., Bell, R., Moritz, M., Jarrel, B., Martin, P. and Maddrey, W.C. 1991. Elevated intracranial pressure and computed tomography of the brain in fulminant hepatocellular failure. *Hepatology* 13: 209–12.

Norenberg, M.D. 1994. Astrocyte responses to CNS injury. *J Neuropath Esp Neurol* 53: 213–20.

Norenberg, M.D. and Bendor, A.S. 1994. Astrocyte swelling in liver failure: Role of glutamine and benzodiazepines. *Acta Neurochir* (Suppl) 60: 24–7.

Norenberg, M.D., Baker, L., Norenberg, L.-O.B., Blicharska, J., Bruce-Gregorios, J.H. and Neary, J.T. 1991. Ammonia-induced astrocyte swelling in primary culture. *Neurochem Res* 16: 833–6.

Norenberg, M.D., Hertz, L. and Schousboe, A., eds. 1988. *The Biochemical Pathology of Astrocytes.* New York: Alan Liss.

Noun, R., Zante, E., Sauvanet, A., Durand, F., Bernau, J. and Belghiti, J. 1995. Liver devascularization improves the hyperkinetic syndrome in patients with fulminant and subfulminant hepatic failure. *Transpl Proc* 27: 1256–7.

O'Brien, C.J., Wise, R.J., O'Grady, J.G. and Williams, R. 1987. Neurological sequelae in patients recovered from fulminant hepatic failure. *Gut* 28: 93–5.

O'Grady, J., Alexander, G.J., Hayllar, K.M. and Williams, R. 1989. Early indicators of prognosis in fulminant hepatic failure. *Gastroenterology* 97: 439–45.

O'Grady, J., Schalm, S.W. and Williams, R. 1993. Acute liver failure: redefining the syndromes. *Lancet* 342: 273–5.

Olafsson, S., Gottstein, J. and Blei, A.T. 1995. Brain edema and intracranial hypertension in rats after total hepatectomy. *Gastroenterology* 108: 1097–103.

Paulson, O.B., Strandgaard, S. and Edvinsson, L. 1990. Cerebral autoregulation. *Cerebrovasc Brain Met Rev* 2: 161–92.

Potvin, M., Finlayson, M.H., Hinchey, E.J., Lough, J.O. and Goresky, C.A. 1984. Cerebral abnormalities in hepatectomized rats with acute hepatic coma. *Lab Invest* 50: 560–4.

Record, C.O., Buxton, B., Chase, R.A., Curzon, G., Murray-Lyon, I.M. and Williams, R. 1976. Plasma and brain amino acids in fulminant hepatic failure and their relationships to hepatic encephalopathy. *Eur J Clin Invest* 6: 387–94.

Ringe, B., Lubbe, N., Kuse, E., Frei, U. and Pichlmayr, R. 1993. Total hepatectomy and liver transplantation as two-stage procedure. *Ann Surg* 218: 3–9.

Ringelstein, E.B. 1986. Transcranial Doppler monitoring. In *Transcranial Doppler Sonography,* ed. R. Aaslid. 149–63. Vienna: Springer Verlag.

Rozga, J., Podesta, L., LePage, L., Hoffman, A., Morriani, E., Sher, L., Woolf, G.M., Makowka, L. and Demetriou, A.A. 1993. Control of cerebral edema by total hepatectomy and extracorporeal liver support in fulminant hepatic failure. *Lancet* 342: 898–99.

Rozga, J., Podesta, L., LePage, E., Morsiani, E., Moscioni, A.D., Hoffman, A., Sher, L., Villamil, F., Woolf, G., McGath, M., Vierling, J. and Demetriou, A. 1994. A bioartificial liver to treat severe acute liver failure. *Ann Surg* 219: 538–46.

Schafer, D.F. and Shaw, J.R., B.W. 1989. Fulminant hepatic failure and orthotopic liver transplantation. *Sem Liver Dis* 9: 189–95.

Schmidt, J.F. 1992. Changes in human cerebral blood flow estimated by the (A-V) O_2 difference method. *Dan Med Bull* 39: 335–42.

Seda, H.M.V., Hughes, R.D., Gove, C.D. and Williams, R. 1984. Inhibition of rat brain Na+ –K+ ATPase activity by serum from patients with fulminant hepatic failure. *Hepatology* 4: 74–9.

Sewell, R.B., Hughes, R.D., Poston, L. and Williams, R. 1982. Effects of serum from patients with fulminant hepatic failure on leucocyte sodium transport. *Clin Sci* 63: 237–42.

Shah, V., Webster, S., Gottstein, J. and Blei, A. 1993. Reduction of cerebral perfusion precedes the rise of intracranial pressure in rats with ischemic fulminant liver failure. *Hepatology* 17: 1117–21.

Swain, M.S., Blei, A.T., Butterworth, R.F. and Kraig, R.P. 1991. Intracellular pH rises and astrocytes swell after portacaval anastomosis in rats. *Am J Physiol* 261: R1491–6.

Swain, M., Butterworth, R.F. and Blei, A.T. 1992. Ammonia and related amino acids in the pathogenesis of brain edema in acute ischemic liver failure in rats. *Hepatology* 15: 449–53.

Takahashi, H., Koehler, R.C., Brusilow, S.W. and Traystman, R.J. 1991. Inhibition of brain glutamine accumulation prevents cerebral edema in hyperammonemic rats. *Am J Physiol* 261: G825–9.

Traber, P.G., DalCanto, M., Ganger, D.R. and Blei, A.T. 1989. Effect of body temperature on brain edema and encephalopathy in the rat after hepatic devascularization. *Gastroenterology* 96: 885–91.

Traber, P.G., DalCanto, M., Ganger, D.R. and Blei, A.T. 1987. Electron microscopic evaluation of brain edema in rabbits with galactosamine-induced fulminant hepatic failure: Ultrastructure and integrity of the blood–brain barrier. *Hepatology* 7: 1272–7.

Traber, P.G., Ganger, D.R. and Blei, A.T. 1986. Brain edema in rabbits with galactosamine-induced fulminant hepatitis. *Gastroenterology* 91: 1347–56.

Voorheis, T.M., Ehrlich, M.E., Duffy, T.E., Petito, C.K. and Plum, F. 1983. Acute hyperammonemia in the young primate: physiologic and neuropathologic correlates. *Pediatr Res* 17: 970–5.

Ware, A.J., D'Agostino, A.N. and Combes, B. 1971. Cerebral edema: A major complication of massive hepatic necrosis. *Gastroenterology* 61: 877–84.

Watson, A.J., Chambers, T., Karp, J.E., Risch, V.R., Walker, W.G. and Brusilow, S.W. 1985. Transient idiopathic hyperammonemia in adults. *Lancet* 328: 1271–4.

Webster, S., Gottstein, J., Levy, R. and Blei, A.T. 1991. Intracranial pressure-waves and intracranial hypertension in rats with ischemic acute hepatic failure. *Hepatology* 14: 715–20.

Wendon, J.A., Harrison, P.M., Keays, R. and Williams, R. 1994. Cerebral blood flow and metabolism in fulminant hepatic failure. *Hepatology* 19: 1407–13.

Wijdicks, E.F.M., Plevak, D.J., Rakela, J. and Wiesner, R.H. 1995. Clinical and radiological features of cerebral edema in fulminant hepatic failure. *Mayo Clin Proc* 70: 119–24.

Williams, R. 1995. Treatment of acute liver failure. In *Therapeutics in Hepatology,* eds. J. Rodes, J. Bosch and V. Arroyo, 365–73. Barcelona: Masson.

Yang, S.S., Hughes, R.D. and Williams, R. 1988. Digoxin-like immunoreactive substances in severe acute liver disease due to viral hepatitis and paracetamol overdose. *Hepatology* 8: 93–7.

Zaki, A.E.O., Ede, R.J., Davis, M. and Williams, R. 1984. Experimental studies of blood–brain barrier permeability in acute hepatic failure. *Hepatology* 4: 359–63.

Zamora, A.J., Cavanagh, J.B. and Kyu, M.H. 1973. Ultrastructural responses of the astrocytes to portocaval anastomosis in the rat. *J Neurosci* 18: 25–45.

13 Management of infection in acute liver failure

Nancy Rolando, John Philpott-Howard and Roger Williams

INTRODUCTION

Patients with acute liver failure (ALF) require multiple invasive procedures and are at risk of the wide range of nosocomial and opportunistic infections commonly associated with intensive care. Furthermore, these patients are known to have several immunological defects that increase their suspectibility to infection, and are probably more immunocompromised than other groups of susceptible patients such as those with neutropenia. Study of the efficacy of a variety of antimicrobial strategies to reduce the very high infection-related mortality in ALF patients has resulted in the selection of antimicrobial prophylaxis and therapy for these patients. This has been based upon three important factors: knowledge of the immunological abnormalities present in this condition; the risk factors associated with the clinical management of organ failure; and the incidence, timing and microbiological nature of these infections.

NATURE OF DEFECTS IN HOST DEFENSE MECHANISMS

Several defects of host immune function arise as a direct consequence of ALF. The liver is the major site of complement synthesis, and reduced levels of serum complement (mainly C3 and C5 components) are found in ALF (Wyke et al. 1980). Low levels of complement correlate with a low opsonization index against bacteria and yeasts, and opsonization is significantly impaired in both children and adults (Wyke et al. 1980; Larcher et al. 1981; Wyke, Yousif-Kadaru et al. 1982). In addition, serum from these patients is a poor chemoattractant for normal polymorphs. This correlates with C5 levels and is independent of the etiology of the liver failure and the presence of bacterial infection (Wyke, Canalese et al. 1982). A significant reduction in neutrophil adherence to nylon fiber has been reported (Altin et al. 1993) and abnormalities in neutrophil adherence in ALF may increase susceptibility to infection. Although impaired phagocytosis and intracellular killing by polymorphs have been reported in patients with ALF (Bailey et al. 1976; Alam et al. 1978), these functions improve when a heat-labile fraction of normal serum is added (Wyke et al. 1980). This again suggests that the major immunological defect in ALF is related to complement deficiency. Optimal phagocytosis by neutrophils of *Candida albicans* and bacteria requires the presence of both antibody and complement (Gelfand et al. 1978; Wyke et al. 1980).

In a recent study, isolated neutrophils were stimulated in vitro by zymosan opsonized with either control serum or autologous patient's serum. Neutrophils from ALF patients were defective in the production of superoxide and hydrogen peroxide when compared with controls (Rolando, unpublished observations). Encephalopathy, renal failure and infection did not appear to be related to the production of superoxide and hydrogen peroxide by neutrophils, and this defect appears to be cellular and opsonic in origin.

The low concentrations of plasma fibronectin found in ALF may explain why phagocytosis of micro-organisms by Kupffer cells is impaired, since adhesion and ingestion is enhanced if the organisms are coated with fibronectin (Gonzales-Calvin et al. 1982; Proctor 1984). Imawari et al. (1985) reported a correlation between low plasma fibronectin and impaired Kupffer cell function, as assessed by the systemic clearance of microaggregated albumin. The degree of dysfunction of Kupffer cells and hepatocytes has been shown to reflect the severity of liver damage; Canalese et al. (1982) reported an impairment in ^{125}I-labeled microaggregated albumin and galactose clearance. Furthermore, in patients with similar hepatocyte dysfunction but not encephalopathy, Kupffer cell function was not significantly different from controls. In patients who recovered from ALF, Kupffer cell and hepatocyte function returned to normal within 10 days of ingestion of acetaminophen (paracetamol) at about the same time as the prothrombin time returned to near-normal values.

The impairment of the Kupffer cells may contribute indirectly to patient sepsis since these cells clear endotoxin and other gut-derived bacterial toxins from the portal circulation. It has been known for over 50 years that intestinal bacteria have an adverse effect on hepatic necrosis. In animal models, eradication of gut organisms with nonabsorbed sulfonamides reduces the severity of hepatic damage induced by carbon tetrachloride (Leach and Forbes 1941; Leduc 1973). The protective effect of sulfonamides was found to be related to a reduction in endotoxin derived from intestinal Gram-negative bacteria (Broitman et al. 1964). Normally, endotoxin which enters the portal circulation is cleared by Kupffer cells. In acute and chronic liver disease, levels of endotoxin in the circulation are raised and endotoxemia may have a role in the development of hepatorenal syndrome in ALF (Nolan 1975; Passavanti et al. 1987). In a recent study, endotoxin levels were found to be elevated in 37 out of 38 ALF patients, although the levels were considerably lower than those usually seen in patients with Gram-negative sepsis (Alexander et al. 1991). Furthermore, there was no correlation between the levels of endotoxin and the presence of Gram-negative sepsis, as all infected patients had similar levels regardless of whether the infection was caused by Gram-negative or Gram-positive bacteria, or fungi.

If endotoxins are not cleared by the liver, they may cause induction of cytokines and associated hemodynamic disturbances characteristic of septic shock. Cytokines are significantly elevated in ALF, and those patients with very high levels are more likely to develop multiorgan failure and death (Sheron et al. 1990).

Finally, translocation of bacteria from the intestinal lumen into the bloodstream may be another mechanism by which ALF patients develop sepsis and shock. However, there are no studies of this phenomenon in ALF, although uncontrolled hemorrhage, a complication seen in some ALF patients, has been shown to be associated with bacterial translocation in an animal model (Katouli et al. 1994).

RISK FACTORS FOR INFECTION DURING MANAGEMENT

Arterial, central venous pressure and Swan–Ganz lines have been implicated as important sources of bacteremia in ALF patients (Rolando et al. 1990). In addition, approximately 50 percent of patients require treatment by hemodialysis, and the risk of bacteremia during hemodialysis has been reported in other intensive care patients

(Nsouli et al. 1979). Endotracheal intubation and ventilation is necessary in up to 80 percent of cases, and there is a well-recognized association between endotracheal intubation and chest infection in these patients (Rolando et al. 1990). The endotracheal tube by-passes the upper respiratory tract defense mechanisms and the tube itself readily becomes colonized with an abnormal microbial flora, such as coliform bacteria and *Pseudomonas* (Sottile et al. 1986). The increase in pH of gastric acid is also thought to be a predisposing factor for endotracheal colonization and subsequent pneumonia (Stoutenbeek et al. 1984).

Cerebral edema in ALF patients precludes chest physiotherapy and the subsequent accumulation of secretions may increase the risk of chest infection. Insertion of an intracranial pressure (ICP) monitor provides a further portal of entry for infection. Some workers have proposed that intravenous vancomycin should be given prophylactically in order to prevent Gram-positive infection in patients who have an ICP monitor inserted (Muñoz 1993). However, we have not seen significant local infection associated with such monitors. Urethral catheters are another risk factor for infection and should be removed in anuric patients.

In a study by MacDougall et al. (1977) H_2 antagonists were used to prevent gastric ulceration and gastrointestinal bleeding in ALF, but there was no evidence of increased sepsis in patients receiving these drugs. However, other studies in general intensive care unit patients have shown an association between H_2 antagonists and the development of infection with aerobic Gram-negative bacilli and yeasts (Penn et al. 1981; Triger et al. 1981; Goularte et al. 1986). Ventilated patients receiving H_2 antagonists may develop gastric and oropharyngeal colonization with aerobic Gram-negative bacilli and this commonly precedes the development of nosocomial pneumonia (Johanson et al. 1969; Johanson, Pierce, Sanford and Thomas 1972; Craven et al. 1986).

Another important factor is the suppression of the normal bacterial gut flora by broad-spectrum antibiotics. This may allow the proliferation of yeasts that can then translocate from the gut lumen to the bloodstream (Krause 1969; Stone et al. 1974). Finally, when corticosteroids were used for the treatment of cerebral edema, an association with development of disseminated aspergillosis was described (Walsh and Hamilton 1983).

THE COURSE OF INFECTION: INCIDENCE, TIMING AND MICROBIOLOGICAL CHARACTERISTICS

Bacterial infections

In a retrospective autopsy study, major sepsis (including endocarditis, meningitis, peritonitis and empyema), were considered to have contributed to death in 11 percent of 105 cases of ALF (Gazzard et al. 1975). In other studies, bacteremia has been reported in up to 36 percent of adults with ALF (Mummery et al. 1971; Nusinovici et al. 1977; Wyke, Yousif-Kadaru et al. 1982) and 47 percent of children (Larcher et al. 1982). More recent prospective studies of infection have shown a high incidence and wide spectrum of infections. In one such study, extensive microbiological surveillance was carried out and this highlighted the magnitude of the problem. Bacteriologically proven infection was recorded in 80 percent of patients and, in a further 10 percent infection was suspected on clinical grounds (Rolando et al. 1990). An elevation in the core body temperature or the peripheral white blood cell count were shown to be poor indicators of infection, and were absent in 30 percent of infected patients (Figure 13.1). In addition, 14 percent of infected patients had more than one episode of infection, and 8 percent had concomitant infections at different sites. The most common infections were pneumonia, accounting for nearly 50 percent of episodes, followed by bacteremia (26 percent) and urinary tract infection (22 percent) (Figure 13.2). Characteristically, infection occurs early in the course of ALF, with a median onset of

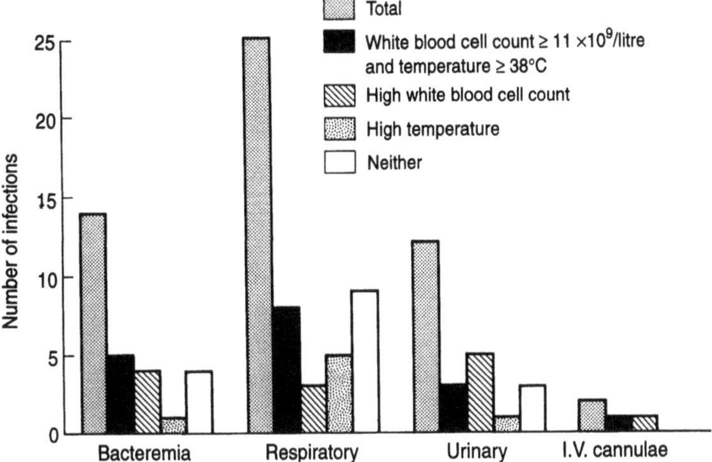

Figure 13.1 Analysis of clinical indicators of infection in acute liver failure patients.

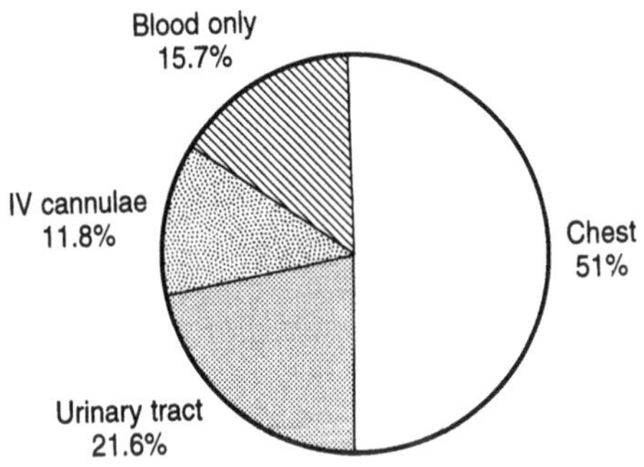

Figure 13.2 Sites of infection in acute liver failure.

five days for pneumonia, three days for bacteremia and two days for urinary tract infection. Infection was present in the majority of deaths occurring during the first four days. Late death was directly attributable to overwhelming infection in a quarter of the cases (Rolando et al. 1990).

In an analysis of 50 patients who were not given antibiotics until they had evidence of infection, the predominant bacterial pathogens isolated were *Staphylococcus aureus*, coagulase-negative staphylococci and *Escherichia coli*. Gram-positive bacteria were responsible for 70 percent of bacterial infections and *S. aureus* was the cause of three-quarters of the pneumonias (Rolando et al. 1990). *Escherichia coli* was the most common cause of Gram-negative infection, predominantly of the urinary tract. Pneumonia was on four occasions caused by *Pseudomonas aeruginosa*, as might be expected in intensive care patients.

Fungal infections

An assessment of the incidence of fungal infection in autopsy studies almost certainly underestimates the true incidence in this condition. In a retrospective study in pediatric patients, fungal infections were implicated as the cause of death in 13 percent (Larcher et al. 1982). In a prospective study fungal infection was present in 32 percent of patients (Rolando et al. 1991), the majority of fungal infections in ALF being caused by yeasts. Virtually all fungal infections were caused by *Candida albicans* and concomitant bacterial infection was always present. Disseminated aspergillosis is rare in ALF and has been reported in a few cases, including patients with subacute hepatic necrosis who received corticosteroids as part of their management (Park et al. 1982; Sesma et al. 1984).

The diagnosis of fungal infection when there is tissue invasion is difficult in these patients since biopsy of tissue for microscopy and culture is often prohibited by clotting abnormalities. Fungal infection is diagnosed when fungi are isolated from significant clinical sites, together with a clinical syndrome characterized by: deterioration in coma grade after an initial improvement; pyrexia (>38°C) unresponsiveness to broad-spectrum antibiotics; white cell count exceeding 20 × 10^9/l; and acute renal failure. In some cases the diagnosis of fungal infection is made only at autopsy. The most common sites of infection were the chest and bloodstream. Although candida pneumonia is rare in other intensive care unit patients, it is particularly common in ALF. Fungal infection develops mainly in the second week after admission and is not related to duration of antibiotic therapy. Mortality from fungal infection is high, 69 percent of the patients died in one study (Rolando et al. 1991).

APPROACHES TO THE TREATMENT AND PREVENTION OF INFECTION

Antibiotic treatment when infection is suspected or established

The wide range of pathogens and the high mortality attributable to infection are clear indications for the use of broad-spectrum antimicrobial agents. To evaluate the efficacy of two broad-spectrum approaches, 50 patients with ALF were randomized to receive either aztreonam with vancomycin, or piperacillin with gentamicin (Rolando et al. 1992). Antimicrobials were only commenced when cultures yielded significant isolates or when bacterial infection was suspected. In the 36 evaluable patients, there were 42 episodes of microbiologically documented infection. The overall rate of bacterial infection during this study was 80 percent and the rate of fungal infection 17 percent. In either arm of the study, antibacterial therapy had to be modified: in 63 percent of the patients in the aztreonam/vancomycin arm; and in 70 percent in the piperacillin/gentamicin arm. The main indication for treatment modification was persisting pyrexia, despite in vitro sensitivity of significant isolates to the trial drugs. Overall, the numbers of deaths attributable to infection were similar in both groups. It was notable that in each group there was a high incidence of *S. aureus* infection, principally pneumonia, with a poor clinical response to gentamicin and vancomycin despite the antistaphylococcal activities of these antibiotics.

Use of selective parenteral and enteral antimicrobial regimen (SPEAR)

The failure of appropriate broad-spectrum antibiotics when infection was suspected or established, suggests the use of antimicrobial prophylaxis. The use of SPEAR (Selective Parenteral and Enteral Antimicrobial Regimen) in the general intensive care setting has shown a reduction of infection rates in some series although the use of these regimens is controversial (Stoutenbeek et al. 1984; 1987; Unertl et al. 1987). In a recent study patients considered on admission to be infected were allocated to receive either intravenous cefuroxime (group 1) or SPEAR (group 2). If there was no evidence of infection, either SPEAR was given on admission (group 3), or antibiotics were withheld until clinically indicated (group 4) (Figure 13.3). The SPEAR regimen comprised local oral and enteric nonabsorbed antimicrobials designed to reduce the aerobic Gram-negative and fungal gut flora (colistin, tobramycin and amphotericin B); in addition, an intravenous cephalosporin was given to provide systemic antimicrobial cover during the first five days of the regimen, whilst selective gut decontamination was established. Intravenous cefuroxime was used in place of cefotaxime, the most commonly used cephalosporin in SPEAR. In addition, nasal mupirocin ointment was applied in order to eradicate nasal carriage of *S. aureus* (Casewell and Hill 1986) together with vaginal clotrimazole for anticandidal prophylaxis in women.

The results of this prospective randomized controlled study (Figure 13.3, Rolando et al. 1993) showed that in patients allocated to the "noninfected" arm of the study there was a statistically significant reduction in episodes of infection in the patients that received SPEAR

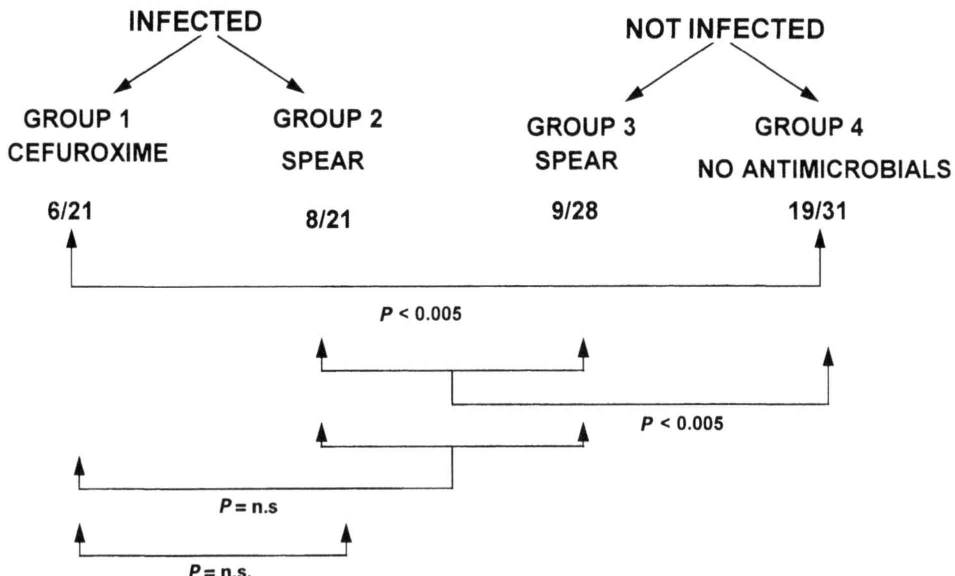

Figure 13.3 Selective parenteral and enteral antisepsis regimen (SPEAR) in acute liver failure.

(group 3), compared with those that received antimicrobials only when clinically indicated (group 4). This difference was not observed in patients already infected on admission. All patients receiving SPEAR (groups 2 and 3) had a significant reduction in rates of infection compared with those not given antibiotics initially (group 4). All groups receiving any early antimicrobial treatment had a lower incidence of infection than controls.

Interestingly, there was no statistically significant difference in the rates of infection between patients given antibiotics from admission (group 1) and those receiving the full SPEAR regimen (groups 2 and 3). The incidence of fungal infection was higher in the patients that did not receive SPEAR, although this was not statistically significant. Overall survival was 56 percent and the proportion of survivors was higher in the groups receiving SPEAR (62 percent compared with the control group, 45 percent), although this was not statistically significant. Death related to sepsis was less frequent in those receiving SPEAR compared with the controls. The suitability of patients for liver transplantation was higher in patients receiving SPEAR or early antimicrobials. Thirty-six patients fulfilled the criteria for transplantation. Of these, 18 proceeded to liver transplantation: 15 out of 24 patients (62.5 percent) receiving SPEAR or early antimicrobials, compared with 3/12 (25 percent) of the remaining patients ($P=<0.05$). SPEAR did not alter the length of stay in the Liver Failure Unit or result in a significant cost benefit: the mean of length of stay was 8.9 days in SPEAR patients compared with 7.5 days in other patients, and the mean cost of antimicrobials was $427.50 and $355.00 respectively. Overall, the reduction of infection episodes in groups receiving SPEAR or antibiotics alone compared with the control group (group 4, Figure 13.3) seemed more closely related to the time of initiation of antimicrobials rather than to the gut decontamination per se.

In a separate study of enteric decontamination in ALF, reported from Spain, neomycin and colistin (or norfloxacin) were administered with nystatin (Salmeron et al. 1992). A 35 percent infection rate was found, compared with 58 percent in the controls, although these were historical controls. A large proportion of infections were caused by Gram-negative bacilli whereas Gram-positive bacteria predominated in our study.

Prophylactic use of antimicrobials with and without gut decontamination

In the study described above, the overall rate of infection was 45 percent, about half the rate found previously. However, the number of patients in all groups was relatively low. In order to determine whether early antimicrobials alone would be sufficient, a further study was performed comparing use of early antimicrobial treatment with the full SPEAR regimen (Rolando et al. 1996). One hundred and eight patients with ALF or severe acetaminophen hepatotoxicity were studied (Table 13.1); these patients were randomized on admission to receive i.v. ceftazidime and flucloxacillin plus either oral and gut decontamination with colistin, tobramycin and amphotericin B (group 1), or oral amphotericin B only (group 2).

There were 15 episodes of infection in 10 patients in group 1, and 17 episodes in 12 patients in group 2. There were no differences between the groups in the number of clinical episodes of chest infection. Three episodes of infection were caused by multiply resistant bacteria: two were gentamicin-resistant *Klebsiella* spp., and one was a vancomycin-resistant *Enterococcus fecium*. Two infections were caused by *Candida albicans*.

The overall rate of infection in this study was 20 percent and the mortality was 33 percent. There was no significant difference in mortality between the two groups. All the deaths were in patients who had developed grade III or IV encephalopathy. Infection was present or contributed to death in 21 percent of patients in group 1 and in 27 percent in group 2. This study showed that the administration of oral nonabsorbable antibacterials did not confer any additional benefit over prophylactic systemic antibacterials. This may be explained by the length of time required for the selective gut decontamination regimen to become effective in a disease that usually has a short and fulminating course.

The emergence of multiresistant bacteria, particularly *Klebsiella* and *Enterobacter* species, has become a problem. The inclusion of a third generation cephalosporin in this recent study regimen may in part account for this, together with cross-infection. Although there was no demonstrable additional benefit with the use of gut decontamination, it is clear that antimicrobial prophylaxis does dramatically reduce the risk of infectious complications in ALF (Figure 13.4). Such an improvement in overall survival results has to be considered in relation to improvements in the care of ALF patients. For example, late infusion of *N*-acetylcysteine in patients with ALF due to acetaminophen overdose reduces progression

Table 13.1. *Infections, deaths and transplantation among patients with acute liver failure who received intravenous antibiotics alone (Group 1) or in combination with SPEAR (Group 2)*

	Group 1 Ceftazidime & flucloxacillin plus oral & enteral amphotericin B, colistin & tobramycin (SPEAR) $n = 47$	Group 2 Ceftazidime & flucloxacillin plus enteral amphotericin alone $n = 61$
Microbiologically proven infection	15/17	47/47
Clinical episodes of chest infection	8/47	16/61
Total infections	23	33
Transplanted patients	5	10
Deaths	18	18

SPEAR = selective parenteral and enteral antimicrobial regimen.

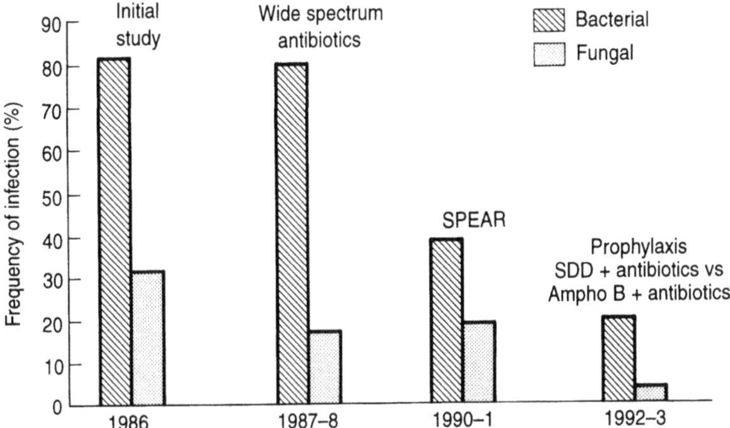

Figure 13.4 Effect of different anti-infective strategies in the frequency of infection in acute liver failure at King's College Hospital, UK.

to grade 3 or 4 coma (Harrison et al. 1990; Keays et al. 1991). In addition, infusion of *N*-acetylcysteine regardless of etiology, results in a reduction in cerebral edema and hypotension, and an increase in cardiac output, oxygen delivery and oxygen consumption (Harrison et al. 1991). These developments, combined with a reduction in infections, have had a significant impact on overall mortality (Makin et al. 1995).

We have also observed important effects of these different regimens on the microbiological pattern of infections (Table 13.2; Rolando, unpublished observations). As noted earlier staphylococci and aerobic Gram-negative rods predominate when antibiotics are not given until the patient is clinically infected. Patients receiving SPEAR or prophylactic antibiotics alone have a reduced incidence of infection. The incidence of infection caused by *S. aureus* is reduced by two thirds, as are infections caused by antibiotic-sensitive aerobic Gram-negatives such as *E. coli*. However, more resistant pathogens such as methicillin-resistant *S. aureus* (MRSA), vancomycin-resistant *Enterococcus fecium* and multiply-resistant *Klebsiella* spp. have appeared in a small number of patients and caused bacteremia and chest infection, and have required additional measures for infection control. It is notable that in all of these studies that anaerobic bacteria were a rare cause of infection.

GUIDELINES FOR THE PREVENTION AND MANAGEMENT OF BACTERIAL AND FUNGAL INFECTION

General guidelines for the prevention and management of infection are similar to those applicable to patients with multiple organ failure in intensive care units. Close liaison between clinicians, nursing staff and the medical microbiologist is essential in the prevention of infection. Infection control policies relating to handwashing, environmental cleaning, disinfection and sterilization, should be reviewed regularly. Handwashing is undoubtedly one of the most cost-effective procedures. Permanent staff on the unit should wash their hands in a topical skin disinfectant (such as aqueous chlorhexidine) on starting their work shift, and use a disinfectant hand rub such as alcoholic chlorhexidine after close patient contact throughout the day. Other staff must use an alcoholic hand rub on entry to the unit and on leaving. Aseptic techniques are the first line of defense against infection and should be strictly enforced particularly when inserting or manipulating intravascular catheters or other invasive monitoring devices. Intravascular catheters should be changed every five days and the catheter tips routinely sent for culture.

Table 13.2. *Analysis of microbiological causes of bacteremias and chest infections in patients with acute liver failure who received: no antibiotics until clinically infected; SPEAR on admission; or prophylactic intravenous antibiotics without SPEAR*

	Antibiotics given when patient clinically infected		SPEAR		Patients receiving prophylactic antibiotics without SPEAR	
	Bacteremia	Chest infection	Bacteremia	Chest infection	Bacteremia	Chest infection
Staphylococcus aureus	6	17		6	2	1
Coagulase-negative staphylococci	8	1	4		3	
Enterococcus fecium			1		3	
Enterococcus fecalis	1	1			2	
Streptococcus pneumoniae	1	1				
Streptococcus sanguis	1	1				
Streptococcus agalactiae	1					
Escherichia coli	2	1			1	
Klebsiella spp	1	1		3		1
Hemophilus spp		2		1		
Pseudomonas aeruginosa		4		2		2
Proteus spp				1		
Acinetobacter spp	2					
Stenotrophomonas maltophilia				1		
Candida spp	3	10		2	1	2
Aspergillus spp		1				1
Total	23	42	6	16	12	7

SPEAR = selective parenteral and enteral antimicrobial regimen.

Microbiological monitoring

Monitoring should be carried out daily, at least during the first week of admission or until recovery from coma. Daily cultures of blood, urine and other samples as indicated are justified since positive results can be obtained for one or two days after initiating antibiotic treatment (Rolando et al. 1990). In addition, later colonization or infection with multiply-resistant bacteria or fungi may be detected (Rolando et al. 1991). In units caring for considerable numbers of patients with ALF, and where antimicrobial usage is extensive, surveillance for the emergence of bacteria resistant to clinically important antimicrobials is essential. The identification of patients colonized or infected with resistant organisms will allow early implementation of policies to prevent cross-infection. Weekly surveillance includes swabs of nose, throat, axillae and wounds for methicillin-resistant *S. aureus;* surveillance for resistant enterobacteria includes superficial swabs and urine samples when available. Rectal swabs are not performed since this requires unnecessary movement of patients with cerebral edema. This kind of surveillance has allowed us to document and to attempt to control the emergence of both vancomycin-resistant *Enterococcus fecium and Enterococcus fecalis* (Wade et al. 1992). Other important multiply-resistant bacteria in patients with ALF may include *Stenotrophomonas (Xanthomonas) maltophilia, Acinetobacter* and *Enterobacter* species.

Measures to control colonization and infection with resistant bacteria may require changes in antimicrobial policies to reduce the selective antibiotic pressure that encourages microorganisms to develop resistance. When choosing a prophylactic regimen, it is important to balance the benefit of the regimen in high risk ALF patients with the risk of selecting resistant organisms through over-use of certain antibiotics. Cephalosporins may be particularly responsible for the emergence of broad-spectrum bacterial beta-lactamases. In general, the prophylactic regimen should be adjusted to match the microbiological problems being encountered in each center.

A suggested algorithm to follow in the infection-related management of ALF patients is shown in Figure 13.5. On admission to the unit, clinical cultures are performed as described above, together with a screen for MRSA, resistant Gram-negative rods, enterococci and yeasts. Prophylaxis is commenced with intravenous antibiotics, oral amphotericin B and vaginal clotrimazole in females. The antibiotics selected for systemic prophylaxis may be varied according to current resistance patterns in the unit, and culture results from the referring hospital. In the Liver Failure Intensive Care Unit at King's, an antibiotic with some anti-staphylococcal activity is used. After 24–48 h, antibiotic therapy may be modified in the light of significant clinical cultures or a positive microbiological screen. If a patient is listed for transplantation, intravenous amphotericin B is added. If the patient has just been started on antibiotics these are continued as prophylaxis for the transplant procedure, otherwise the antibiotics are changed to a different regimen at the time of the anesthetic premedication or induction. In general, antibiotic prophylaxis or treatment is discontinued five days after transplantation although intravenous amphotericin is continued for 21 days.

INFECTION AFTER TRANSPLANTATION FOR ALF

Between 15 and 20 percent of patients with ALF require treatment by liver transplantation. In a recent prospective study of 284 transplants (Wade et al. 1995), the findings in 51 patients transplanted for ALF were compared with results from 233 patients having a transplant for chronic liver disease (CLD) (Table 13.3). Patients transplanted for ALF had more episodes of infection, 1.6 per patient, compared with 0.92 in those transplanted for CLD. In addition, 33 percent of the ALF patients had three or more episodes of infection, compared with 3 percent of those in the CLD group. The incidence of chest infection was higher in patients transplanted for ALF, 0.29 episodes per patient compared with 0.10 in the CLD patients (relative risk 2.9), and bacteremia was also more frequent (0.41 versus 0.20 respectively, relative risk 2.0). Univariate analysis of post-transplantation sequelae showed that return to operating room, reintubation and tracheostomy were more common in ALF patients (Table 13.3) and they were more likely than their CLD counterparts to have had antibiotics and cryoprecipitates preoperatively. Treatment for suspected or proven fungal infection was five times commoner amongst the ALF transplants than the CLD transplant group, an incidence of 60 percent versus 12 percent respectively. For this reason, we now give intravenous amphotericin B 1 mg/kg routinely for 21 days after transplantation, whatever the clinical state.

FUTURE DEVELOPMENTS

The combination of antimicrobial prophylaxis and measures to prevent infection has been shown to improve the outcome in multiorgan failure with sepsis. This is difficult to establish in ALF because of the number of inter-related factors and improvements in the management of other complications (e.g. encephalopathy, renal failure, etc.) that have affected the morbidity and mortality. Overall meticulous prophylaxis does appear to have contributed to a significant improvement in outcome for those patients.

In these severely immunocompromised patients, other approaches aimed at improving the underlying immunological defects seem rational. Currently, we are evaluating the effects of granulocyte-colony stimulating factor (G-CSF) on neutrophils from ALF patients. By improving the microbicidal

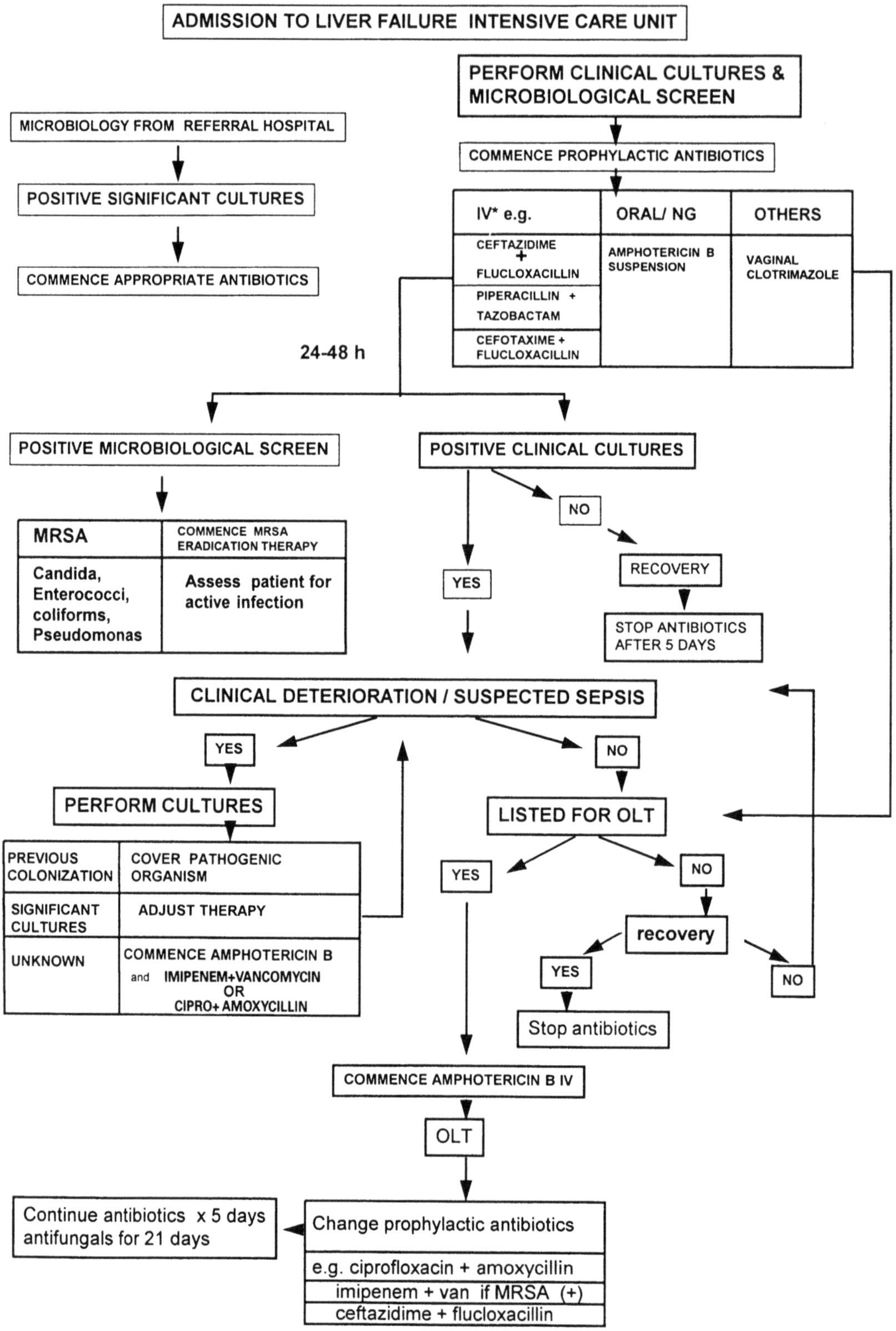

ADMISSION TO LIVER FAILURE INTENSIVE CARE UNIT

MICROBIOLOGY FROM REFERRAL HOSPITAL

POSITIVE SIGNIFICANT CULTURES

COMMENCE APPROPRIATE ANTIBIOTICS

PERFORM CLINICAL CULTURES & MICROBIOLOGICAL SCREEN

COMMENCE PROPHYLACTIC ANTIBIOTICS

IV* e.g.	ORAL/ NG	OTHERS
CEFTAZIDIME + FLUCLOXACILLIN	AMPHOTERICIN B SUSPENSION	VAGINAL CLOTRIMAZOLE
PIPERACILLIN + TAZOBACTAM		
CEFOTAXIME + FLUCLOXACILLIN		

24-48 h

POSITIVE MICROBIOLOGICAL SCREEN

MRSA	COMMENCE MRSA ERADICATION THERAPY
Candida, Enterococci, coliforms, Pseudomonas	Assess patient for active infection

POSITIVE CLINICAL CULTURES

NO

RECOVERY

STOP ANTIBIOTICS AFTER 5 DAYS

YES

CLINICAL DETERIORATION / SUSPECTED SEPSIS

YES

PERFORM CULTURES

PREVIOUS COLONIZATION	COVER PATHOGENIC ORGANISM
SIGNIFICANT CULTURES	ADJUST THERAPY
UNKNOWN	COMMENCE AMPHOTERICIN B and IMIPENEM+VANCOMYCIN OR CIPRO+ AMOXYCILLIN

NO

LISTED FOR OLT

YES

NO

recovery

YES

Stop antibiotics

NO

COMMENCE AMPHOTERICIN B IV

OLT

Change prophylactic antibiotics
e.g. ciprofloxacin + amoxycillin
imipenem + van if MRSA (+)
ceftazidime + flucloxacillin

Continue antibiotics x 5 days antifungals for 21 days

Figure 13.5 Algorithm for the prevention and treatment of infection in acute liver failure patients.

Table 13.3. *Univariate analysis of variables after orthotopic liver transplantation (OLT) in patients with acute liver failure and chronic liver disease*

	OLT for acute liver failure (n = 51)	OLT for chronic liver disease (n = 233)	P
Return to theatre	19 (37.3)	42 (18.0)	< 0.0020
Reintubation	23 (45.1)	44 (18.9)	< 0.0001
Tracheostomy	8 (15.7)	6 (2.6)	< 0.0001
Cryoprecipitates	6.52 ± 7.3	3.22 ± 5.2	< 0.0013
Antibiotics (pre-OLT)	1.47 ± 1.65	0.8 ± 2.01	< 0.0001
Bacteremia	23 (45)	44 (19)	0.030
Chest infection	15 (29)	25 (11)	0.047
Cholangitis	10 (20)	37 (16)	0.006
Fungal infection	30 (60)	28 (12)	< 0.000001

Values in parentheses are percentages.

activity, the incidence of infection may be reduced. The use of G-CSF in other clinical conditions has been shown to enhance neutrophil adhesion (Young and Linch 1992), and Kitagawa et al. (1987) showed that G-CSF increased superoxide release within granulocytes. The chemotactic activity of G-CSF, that induces migration of neutrophils, was demonstrated by Wang et al. in 1988. The administration of G-CSF rapidly increases expression of C3bi receptors on circulating granulocytes, thereby improving opsonization (Yuo et al. 1989). Other workers have reported that the phago-cytic and bactericidal activity of normal and defective neutrophils is enhanced by G-CSF (Roilides et al. 1990; Roilides et al. 1991).

In addition to research on colony stimulating factors, other studies are needed to clarify the potential for treatment with cytokines and other newly available drugs such as antitumor necrosis factor, anti-interleukin-6, interleukin-1 receptor antagonists and nitric oxide synthase inhibitors. However, with the relatively small number of ALF patients in any one center, it is likely that these novel therapies will first become established in commoner conditions with multiorgan failure admitted to intensive care units.

REFERENCES

Alam, A.N., Poston, L.P., Wilkinson, S.P., Golindano, C.G. and Williams, R. 1978. A study in vitro of the sodium pump in fulminant hepatic failure. *Clin Sci Mol Med* 55: 355–63.

Alexander, G.J.M., Goka, A.J. and Sheron, N. 1991. The relationship between sepsis, endotoxaemia and cytokines in patients with acute liver failure. In *Acute Liver Failure: Improved Understanding and Better Therapy. 1990.* eds. R. Williams and R.D. Hughes, 22–5. London: Miter Press.

Altin, M., Rajkovic, I., Hughes, R. and Williams, R. 1983. Neutrophil adherence in chronic liver disease and fulminant hepatic failure. *Gut* 24: 746–50.

Bailey, R.J., Woolf, I.L., Cullens, H. and Williams, R. 1976. Metabolic inhibition of polymorphonuclear leucocytes in fulminant hepatic failure. *Lancet* i: 1162–3.

Broitman, S.A., Gottlieb, L.S. and Zamcheck, N. 1964. Influence of neomycin and ingested endotoxin in the pathogenesis of choline deficiency cirrhosis in the adult rat. *J Exp Med* 119: 633–41.

Canalese, J., Gove, C.D., Gimson, A.E.S., Wilkinson, S.P., Wardle, E.N. and Williams, R. 1982. Reticuloendothelial system and hepatocyte function in fulminant hepatic failure. *Gut* 23: 265–9.

Casewell, M.W. and Hill, R.L.R. 1986. Elimination of nasal carriage of *S. aureus* with mupirocin ('Pseudomonic acid') – a controlled trial. *J Antimicrob Chemother* 17: 365–72.

Craven, D.E., Kunches, L.M., Kilinsky, V., Lichtenberg, D.A., Make, B.J. and McCabe, W.R. 1986. Risk factors for pneumonia and fatality in patients receiving continuous mechanical ventilation. *Am Rev Respir Dis* 133: 792–6.

Gazzard, B., Portmann, B., Murray-Lyon, I.M. and Williams, R. 1975. Causes of death in fulminant hepatic failure and relationship to quantitative histological assessment of parenchymal damage. *Quart J Med* 176: 615–26.

Gelfand, J.A., Hurley, D.L., Fauci, A.S. and Frank, M.M. 1978. Role of complement in host defences against experimental candidiasis. *J Infect Dis* 138: 9–16.

Gonzales-Calvin, J., Scully, M.F., Sanger, Y., Fok, J., Kakkar, V.V., Hughes, R.D., Gimson, A.E.S. and Williams, R. 1982. Fibronectin in fulminant hepatic failure. *BMJ* 285: 1231–2.

Goularte, T.A., Lichtenberg, D.A. and Craven, D.E. 1986. Gastric colonization in patients receiving antacids and mechanical ventilation: a mechanism for pharyngeal colonization. *Am J Infect Contr* 14: 88.

Harrison, P.M., Keays, R., Bray, G.P., Alexander, G.J.M. and Williams, R. 1990. Improved outcome of paracetamol-induced fulminant hepatic failure by late administration of acetylcysteine. *Lancet* 335: 1572–3.

Harrison, P.M., Wendon, J.A., Gimson, A.E.S., Alexander, G.J.M. and Williams, R. 1991. Improvement by acetylcysteine of hemodynamics and oxygen transport in fulminant hepatic failure. *N Engl J Med* 324: 1852–8.

Imawari, M., Hughes, R., Gove, C. and Williams, R. 1985. Fibronectin and Kupffer cell function in fulminant hepatic failure. *Dig Dis Sci* 30: 1028–33.

Johanson, W.G., Pierce, A.K. and Sanford, J.P. 1969. Changing pharyngeal bacterial flora of hospitalized patients. Emergence of Gram-negative bacilli. *N Engl J Med* 281: 1137–40.

Johanson, W.G., Pierce, A.K., Sanford, J.P. and Thomas, G.D. 1972. Nosocomial respiratory infections with Gram-negative bacilli: The significance of colonization of the respiratory tract. *Ann Intern Med* 77: 701–6.

Katouli, M., Bark, T., Ljungqvist, O., Svenberg, T. and Mollby, R. 1994. Composition and diversity of intestinal coliform flora influence bacterial translocation in rats after hemorrhagic stress. *Infect Immun* 62: 4768–74.

Keays, R., Harrison, P.M., Wendon, J.A., Forbes, A., Gove, C., Alexander, G.J.M. and Williams, R. 1991. Intravenous acetylcysteine in paracetamol induced fulminant hepatic failure: a prospective controlled trial. *BMJ* 303: 1026–9.

Kitagawa, S., You, A., Souza, L.M., Saito, M., Miura, Y. and Takaku, F. 1987. Recombinant human granulocyte colony-stimulating factor enhances superoxide release in human granulocytes stimulated by chemotactic peptide. *Biochem Biophys Res Comm* 144: 1143–6.

Krause, W., Matheis, H. and Wulf, K. 1969. Fungemia and funguria after oral administration of *Candida albicans*. *Lancet* i: 598–9.

Larcher, V.F., Wyke, R.J., Mowat, A.P. and Williams, R. 1981. Mechanisms of serum defect in yeast opsonisation in children with fulminant hepatic failure. *Clin Exp Immunol* 46: 406–11.

Larcher, V.F., Wyke, R.J., Mowat, A.P. and Williams, R. 1982. Bacterial and fungal infection in children with fulminant hepatic failure: possible role of opsonisation and complement deficiency. *Gut* 23: 1037–43.

Leach, B.E. and Forbes, J.C. 1941. Sulfonamide drugs as protective agents against carbon tetrachloride poisoning. *Proc Soc Exp Biol Med* 48: 361–3.

Leduc, E.H. 1973. Sulfoguanidine protection of mouse liver from carbon tetrachloride induced necrosis. *Lab Invest* 29: 186–96.

MacDougall, B.R.D., Bailey, R.J. and Williams, R. 1977. H_2-receptor antagonists and antacids in the prevention of acute gastrointestinal haemorrhage in fulminant hepatic failure. *Lancet* i: 617–19.

Makin, A.J., Wendon, J. and Williams, R. 1995. A 7-year experience of severe acetaminophen-induced hepatotoxicity (1987–1993). *Gastroenterology* 109: 1907–16.

Mummery, R.V., Bradley, J.M. and Jeffries, D.J. 1971. Microbiological monitoring of patients in hepatic failure with particular reference to extracorporeal porcine liver perfusion. *Lancet* ii: 60–1.

Muñoz, S.J. 1993. Difficult management problems in fulminant hepatic failure. *Semin Liver Dis* 13: 395–413.

Nolan, J.P. 1975. The role of endotoxin in liver injury. *Gastroenterology* 69: 1346–56.

Nsouli, K.A., Lazarus, J.M., Schoenbaum, S.C., Gottlieb, M.N., Lowrie, E.G. and Shocair, M. 1979. Bacteremic infection in haemodialysis. *Arch Intern Med* 139: 1255–8.

Nusinovici, V., Crucibille, C., Opolon, P., Touboul, J.P., Darnis, F. and Caroli, J. 1977. Hepatittes fulminantes avec coma. Revue de 137 cas. I Complications. *Gastroenterologie Clinique et Biologique (Paris)*. 1: 861–73.

Park, G.R., Drummond, G.B., Lamb, D., Durie, T.B., Milne, L.J., Lambie, A.T. and Cameron, E.W.J. 1982. Disseminated aspergillosis occurring in patients with respiratory, renal and hepatic failure. *Lancet* ii: 179–83.

Passavanti, G., Coratelli, P., Munno, I., Fumarola, D. and Amerio, A. 1987. Role of endotoxin in hepatorenal syndrome. *Adv Exp Med Biol* 212: 162–77.

Penn, R.G., Sanders, W.E., and Sanders, C.C. 1981. Colonization of the oropharynx with Gram negative bacilli: a major antecedent to nosocomial pneumonia. *Am J Infect Contr* 9: 25–34.

Proctor, R.A. 1984. Fibronectin: A brief overview of its structure, function and physiology. *Rev Infect Dis* 9: S317–21.

Roilides, E., Mertins, S., Eddy, J., Walsh, T.J., Pizzo, P.A. and Rubin, M. 1990. Impairment of neutrophil chemotactic and bactericidal function in HIV-infected children and partial reversal after *in vitro* exposure to granulocyte-macrophage colony-stimulating factor. *J. Pediatr* 117: 531–40.

Roilides, E., Walsh, T., Pizzo, P.A. and Rubin, M. 1991. Granulocyte colony-stimulating factor enhances the phagocytic and bactericidal activity of normal and defective human neutrophils. *J Infect Dis* 163: 579–83.

Rolando, N., Harvey, F., Brahm, J., Philpott-Howard, J., Alexander, G., Gimson, A.E.S., Casewell, M. and Williams, R. 1990. Prospective study of bacterial infection in acute liver failure: an analysis of fifty patients. *Hepatology* 11: 49–53.

Rolando, N., Harvey, F., Brahm, J., Philpott-Howard, J., Alexander, G., Casewell, M. and Williams, R. 1991. Fungal infection: a common, unrecognised complication of acute liver failure. *J Hepatol* 12: 1–9.

Rolando, N., Wade, J.J., Fagan, E., Philpott-Howard, J., Casewell, M.W. and Williams, R. 1992. An open, comparative trial of aztreonam with vancomycin and gentamicin with piperacillin in patients with fulminant hepatic failure. *J Antimicrob Chemother* 30: 215–20.

Rolando, N., Gimson, A.E.S., Wade, J.J., Philpott-Howard, J., Casewell, M. and Williams, R. 1993. Prospective controlled trial of selective parenteral and enteral antimicrobial regimen in fulminant liver failure. *Hepatology* 17: 196–201.

Rolando, N., Wade, J., Stangou, A., Gimson, A., Wendon, J., Philpott-Howard, J. Casewell, M. and Williams, R. 1996. Prospective study comparing the efficacy of prophylactic parenteral antimicrobials, with or without enteral decontamination, in patients with acute liver failure. *Liver Transpl Surg* 2: 8–13.

Salmeron, J.M., Tito, L., Rimola, A., Mas, A., Navasa, M.A., Lach, J., Gines, A., Gines, P., Arroyo, V., Rodes, J. 1992. Selective intestinal decontamination in the prevention of bacterial infection in patients with acute liver failure. *J Hepatol* 14: 280–5.

Sesma, P., Alvarez, J., Linares, P. and Suarez, M.D. 1984. Disseminated aspergillosis complicating hepatic failure. *Arch Intern Med* 858: 141–4.

Sheron, N., Goka, J., Wendon, J., Keays, R., Keane, H., Alexander, G. and Williams, R. 1990. Highly elevated plasma cytokines in fulminant hepatic failure: correlation with multi-organ failure and death. (Abstract). *Hepatology* 12: 939.

Sottile, F. D., Marrie, T.J., Prough, D.S., Hobgood, C.D., Gower, D.J., Webb, L.X., Costerton, J.W. and Gristina, A.G. 1986. Nosocomial pulmonary infection: possible etiologic significance of bacterial adhesion to endotracheal tubes. *Crit Care Med* 14: 265–70.

Stone, H.H., Kolb, L.D., Currie, C.A., Geheber, C.E. and Cuzzell, J.Z. 1974. Candida sepsis: Pathogenesis and principles of treatment. *Ann Surg* 179: 697–710.

Stoutenbeek, C.P., van Saene, H.K.F., Miranda, D.R. and Zandstra, D.F. 1984. The effect of selective decontamination of the digestive tract on colonisation and infection rate in multiple trauma patients. *Intens Care Med* 10: 185–92.

Stoutenbeek, C.P., van Saene, H.K.F., Miranda, D.R., Zandstra, D.F. and Langrehr, D. 1987. The effect of oropharyngeal decontamination using topical non absorbable antibiotics on the incidence of nosocomial respiratory tract infections in multiple trauma patients. *Trauma* 27: 357–64.

Triger, D.R., Slater, D.N., Goepel, J.R. and Underwood, J.C.E. 1981. Systemic candidiasis complicating acute hepatic failure in patients treated with cimetidine. *Lancet* ii: 837–8.

Unertl, K., Ruckdeschel, G., Selbmann, H.K., Jensen, U., Forst, H., Lenhart, F.P. and Peter, K. 1987. Prevention of colonization and respiratory tract infections in long-term ventilated patients by administration of local antimicrobial prophylaxis. *Intens Care Med* 13: 106–13.

Wade, J., Baillie, L., Rolando, N. and Casewell, M. 1992. Pristinamycin for *Enterococcus faecium* resistant to vancomycin and gentamicin. *Lancet* 339: 312–13.

Wade, J., Rolando, N., Hayllar, K., Philpott-Howard, J., Casewell, M.W. and Williams, R. 1995. Bacterial and fungal infections after liver transplantation: An analysis of 284 patients. *Hepatology* 21: 1328–36.

Walsh, T.J. and Hamilton, S.R. 1983. Disseminated aspergillosis complicating hepatic failure. *Arch Intern Med* 143: 1189–91.

Wang, J.M., Chen, Z.G., Collela, S., Bonilla, M.A., Welte, K., Bordigon, C. and Montovani, A. 1988. Chemotactic activity of recombinant human granulocyte colony-stimulating factor. *Blood* 72: 1456–60.

Wyke, R.J., Canalese, J.C., Gimson, A.E.S. and Williams, R. 1982. Bacteraemia in patients with fulminant hepatic failure. *Liver* 2: 45–52.

Wyke, R.J., Yousif-Kadaru, A.G.M., Rajkovic, I.A., Eddleston, A.L.W.F. and Williams, R. 1982. Serum stimulatory activity and polymorphonuclear leucocyte movement in patients with fulminant hepatic failure. *Clin Exp Immunol* 50: 442–9.

Wyke, R.J., Rajkovic, I.A., Eddleston, A.L.W.F. and Williams, R. 1980. Defective opsonisation and complement deficiency in serum from patients with fulminant hepatic failure. *Gut* 21: 643–9.

Young, K.L. and Linch, D.C., 1992. Differential effects of granulocyte- and granulocyte-macrophage colony-stimulating factors (G-and GM-CSF) on neutrophil adhesion in vitro and in vivo. *Eur J Haematol* 49: 251–9.

Yuo, A., Kitagawa, S., Ohsaka, A., Ohta, M., Miyasono, K., Okabe, T., Urabe, A., Saito, M. and Takaku, F. 1989. Recombinant human granulocyte colony-stimulating factor as an activator of human granulocytes: Potentiation of responses triggered by receptor-mediated agonist and stimulation of 3Cbi receptor expression and adherence. *Blood* 74: 2144–9.

PART FOUR Transplantation

14 Prognosis and consideration of transplantation

John Devlin and Roger Williams

INTRODUCTION

Liver transplantation is an important treatment option in the management of severe cases of acute liver failure (ALF). The process of selecting appropriate patients for transplantation rather than relying on intensive conservative medical therapy remains problematic (Van Thiel 1993). Before reaching a decision in favor of surgical intervention, clinicians have to be able to identify those patients in whom the prognosis is otherwise poor and in whom the likely outcome will be considerably improved by transplantation. The practical importance of accurate determination of prognosis has stimulated several centers to examine systematically their outcomes experience in patients with ALF (Iwatsuki et al. 1985; Emond et al. 1989). Several different prognostic variables have been derived from these studies (Christensen et al. 1984; Bernuau et al. 1986; O'Grady et al. 1989). However, paradoxically, the sickest patients who carry the worst prognosis, are also those in whom the complications of the liver failure render them least likely to survive a transplant.

In this chapter, we will review the clinical and laboratory characteristics which are associated with a poor prognosis in ALF and which accordingly serve as a useful basis for selecting candidates for transplantation. Thereafter, we will consider the equally difficult issue of identifying those clinical features present before transplantation, which are associated with unfavorable post-transplant outcomes. These features, if validated, could serve as relative contraindications to proceeding with a liver graft.

PROGNOSIS OF LIVER FAILURE

A thorough understanding of the natural history and prognosis of the different clinical and etiological variants of acute liver failure is mandatory if an informed decision on the likelihood of spontaneous recovery and survival, with conservative management, is to be made. The published data on the prognosis of liver failure discussed below has predominantly emerged from those centers with large experience such as Boston and Los Angeles in the USA and the Paris group and our own experience at King's College, in Europe. Particular attention will be given to the study from this unit by O'Grady which employed logistic analysis and prognostic modeling in a population of 588 patients (O'Grady et al. 1989).

Course of illness

The significance of the rate of onset of illness is a cardinal feature of acute liver failure and is the basis for the recently proposed classification from this group (see Chapter 1) (Gimson et al. 1986; Takahashi and Shimizi 1991; O'Grady et al. 1993). The interval between the onset of jaundice and development of encephalopathy was the second most important variable found in our study. This paradoxical influence of the rapidity of the onset of encephalopathy is reflected in the favorable outcome of patients in whom this complication develops within 7 days of the onset of jaundice (so-called *hyperacute liver failure*). The survival of a cohort of 81 cases in this group managed conservatively was 36 percent; a figure which compares favorably with the survival rate of patients experiencing *acute liver failure* (encephalopathy developing 8–28 days after jaundice) at 7 percent, or *subacute liver failure* (jaundice to encephalopathy time 4–12 weeks) at 14 percent. Deeper grades of hepatic encephalopathy have long been regarded as being associated with a worse prognosis. However, the above data alert clinicians that at least early in the illness this does not necessarily hold, with those who are initially not encephalopathic and who subsequently deteriorate to grade 3 or 4 coma having the worst prognosis. Once this level of encephalopathy is established, an increased mortality is seen secondary to the direct hazards of cerebral edema and infarction and to the other attendant risks of severe liver failure (Trey 1972). Fluctuation in coma grade, the influence of concomitant medication and difficulty in assessment once a patient is sedated and/or paralyzed can limit the value of this clinical sign.

Etiology and age

The etiology of liver failure was the single most important and independent static variable predicting outcome in the King's study. Cases categorized as of indeterminate (NANB) origin account for the largest proportion of the two unfavorable acute and subacute liver failure groups in the new classification. A fulminant presentation of Wilson's disease is invariably fatal, as are many cases of drug-induced liver failure although antituberculous drug cases may have a somewhat better prognosis (Sternleib 1984). The rare fulminant presentation of an autoimmune hepatitis carries a similarly poor prognosis with medical therapy alone. An acute presentation of Budd–Chiari syndrome is a rare cause of ALF and although comparison of outcome with emergency decompressive surgery is not available, liver replacement will be the only option for survival if liver structure as well as function is severely deranged. The best prognosis is seen in acetaminophen (paracetamol) hepatotoxicity and acute fatty liver of pregnancy. Amongst the viral hepatitides, hepatitis A virus has the best outcome, hepatitis B intermediate and, indeterminate (NANB), which comprises the largest group in many series, the worst (Figure 14.1) (Trey 1972; Rakela 1979). In the King's series, the survival in these groups was 44.7 percent, 34.4 percent and 9 percent, respectively. These figures in relation to reported cases of acute hepatitis correspond to case mortality rates of approximately 0.3 percent, 1 percent and 2 percent as reported by the large Viral Hepatitis Surveillance Program (VHSP) (n=169,666 cases) and the smaller but more accurate Sentinel Counties Study (n=11,226 cases) (Alter et al. 1990; Centers for Disease Control 1991). *Amanita phalloides* hepatotoxicity causes a hyperacute liver failure. Prognostic indicators of this condition have been difficult to determine (Klein et al. 1989).

Mortality is increased in patients at the extremes of age (Trey 1972). The large VHSP study found that mortality in acute hepatitis was higher in patients older than 50 years or younger than 5 years. This corresponds to our experience in non-acetaminophen induced liver failure (the majority were cases of acute hepatitis), where mortality rates were raised in those patients less than 10 or more than 40 years old.

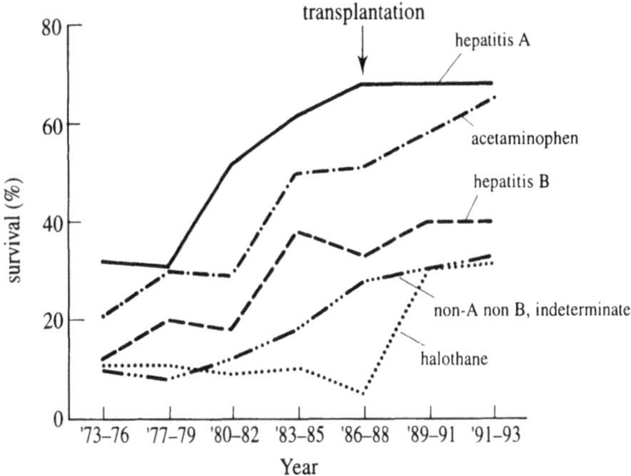

Figure 14.1 Improving survival of all etiological categories of acute liver failure (whether managed conservatively or with transplantation).

Laboratory parameters

Several readily available laboratory variables have also been identified as having prognostic value (Table 14.1). The height of total serum bilirubin is recognized as the most important indicator in viral and drug cases. This relationship which was first recognized in the study from Christensen (1984) was subsequently confirmed by this unit. In our study, the height of the bilirubin level in non-acetaminophen patients was related to the duration of illness (in itself an unfavorable parameter), although with a correlation coefficient of only 0.48. An exception to this relationship exists in acetaminophen cases which is probably explained by the close association of increased bilirubin levels and duration of illness in this particular group; those patients with the highest levels have survived the crisis phase of severe hepatotoxicity. Perhaps unexpectedly, liver enzymes (both hepatocellular and biliary) have not been found in any study to have a major influence on outcome. Low arterial pH (reflecting a metabolic acidosis) was found in the King's study to be of foremost importance in acetaminophen cases and of value in other causes of liver failure. The exact causes underlying this metabolic derangement are unclear but are considered to reflect the combined influences of severe hepatic necrosis, systemic tissue hypoxia and renal impairment. In some series, derangement of quantitative liver function tests, arterial ketone body ratios and serum α-fetoprotein, used as an index of liver regeneration, have been correlated with outcome (Karvountzis and Redeker 1974; Tygstrup and Ranek 1986; Scaiola et al. 1990; Saibara et al. 1991).

Liver biopsy and volume assessment

Histologic assessment of a liver biopsy has also been proposed to be of value in determining prognosis in ALF and in assisting selection for transplantation (Van Thiel 1993). In particular, Van Thiel has proposed that the presence of submassive necrosis in 50 percent or more of the hepatic lobules should be interpreted as indicating a need for transplantation. This presently unvalidated assertion has several potential limitations. Performing a liver biopsy in this clinical context is potentially hazardous because of the associated coagulopathy and thrombocytopenia (Scotto et al. 1973). Sample size, which would be restricted if the biopsy was taken by the transjugular route, is important given the potentially misleading histologic heterogeneity of necrosis and regenerative nodules which especially characterizes subacute liver failure.

Van Thiel also bases the decision to transplant on the extent of reduction in size of the liver as determined by CT scanning at the time

Table 14.1. *Significant laboratory parameters of prognosis (univariate analysis)*

	Acetaminophen (paracetamol)		Viral / drugs	
Parameter	Survivors	Nonsurvivors	Survivors	Nonsurvivors
Prothrombin time				
Admission (s)	72 (35)	93 (51)[b]	51 (31)	81 (57)[b]
Peak (s)	73 (36)	104 (58)[c]	52 (32)	96 (67)[c]
Bilirubin				
Admission (μmol/l)	162 (85)	133 (84)[a]	299 (205)	404 (188)[c]
Peak (μmol/l)	317 (194)	185 (140)[b]	373 (230)	460 (222)[b]
AST: Admission (units/l)			948 (1181)	1409 (2291)[a]
pH: Admission (units/l)	7.41 (0.1)	7.31 (0.15)[c]	7.43 (0.09)	7.39 (0.1)[a]
Creatinine				
Admission (μmol/l)	241 (180)	351 (234)[b]		
Peak (μmol/l)	374 (286)	439 (262)[b]	322 (442)	279 (268)[a]
WCC: Admission (×10⁹/l)	12.5 (9.2)	14.6 (8.5)[a]	11.4 (5.6)	13.6 (6.3)[a]
Platelets: *n* (×10⁹/l)	93 (75)	112 (89)[a]	138 (87)	159 (112)[a]

AST, aspartate aminotransferase; WCC, white cell count. Values are mean (SD).
[a] $P < 0.05$. [b] $P < 0.01$. [c] $P < 0.001$.

when an organ becomes available (Van Thiel 1993). Patients with a liver volume of less than 700 cm^3 are listed for transplantation immediately whilst those with volumes of 700–900 cm^3 can be observed but are likely to require transplantation. This parameter again has not been subjected to extensive study. A Japanese group which used computed tomography to assess both liver size and functional volume found that although a correlation with survival existed, it was insufficiently precise to discriminate survivors from nonsurvivors (Kumahara et al. 1989). Moving a patient with ALF can be hazardous, particularly if they are developing cerebral edema.

Coagulation abnormalities

Changes in coagulation factor levels are widely used, particularly in Europe, for assessment of the severity of liver injury in ALF. The prolongation of prothrombin time and the more-recently introduced international normalized ratio (INR) was shown in our multivariate analysis to be an independent predictor of outcome regardless of etiology. Although in the acetaminophen overdose group, no particular prognostic cut off level of INR could be determined, a rise in INR from day 3 to 4 following ingestion was associated with a 7 percent compared to a 79 percent survival in those whose INR fell at that time (Harrison et al. 1990). Measurement of specific coagulation factors has been advocated by the French group. In a study of 115 patients with fulminant hepatitis B, factor V levels were lower in those who died. Multivariate analysis confirmed this to be the most predictive indicator of outcome (Bernuau et al. 1986). However, in a detailed study of 22 patients with acetaminophen-induced ALF carried out in this unit, although factor V levels were lower in the patients who died there was considerable overlap with the survivors. The prognostic value was considerably improved if the ratio factor VIII/V was employed. The value was less than 30 in all patients who survived with values greater than 30 in ten of eleven patients who died (Pereira et al. 1992).

IDENTIFYING POTENTIAL TRANSPLANT CANDIDATES

Any proposed scheme for assessing prognosis in ALF needs to be judged against several principles if it is to be useful in the process of consideration and selection for transplantation (Table 14.2). The criteria should be simple and easily reproduced, achieve a high index of sensitivity and specificity in discriminating

Table 14.2. *Ideal characteristics for selection criteria*

Derived from large mixed population
Prospectively validated
Simple and reproducible
Applicable early in course of illness
High positive and negative predictive values
On-going validation and refinement

survivors and nonsurvivors and, most importantly, be valid early in the hospital admission given the rapid deterioration often observed in this condition. Furthermore, all criteria have to be judged within the clinical context of the study population from whch they were derived since the likely variations in clinical expertise, quite apart from etiological case mix, will also affect outcome. Finally, there needs to be on-going prospective validation and refinement of criteria reflecting the continued advances in management. For example, advances in the control of infection and manipulation of hemodynamic derangements may well improve outcome. It is our experience that the overall survival of patients with ALF is improving annually (Figure 14.1).

Selection criteria

On the basis of their findings, the Clichy group uses the presence of encephalopathy and measurement of factor V levels in identifying candidates for transplantation (see Chapter 10). At this center, we have developed guidelines which are based predominantly on two principles: the guidelines must be applicable early in the hospital admission, and they must employ readily available clinical or laboratory parameters. In acetaminophen patients, arterial pH can be employed irrespective of encephalopathy. In those who have developed encephalopathy, a combination of significant elevation in prothrombin time and serum creatinine are used (Table 14.3). In non-acetaminophen patients, other criteria are required reflecting an often quite different clinical course. In these patients, we note the etiology, the speed of onset of encephalopathy

Table 14.3. *Criteria adopted for identifying patients who are considered for transplantation at King's College Hospital, London*

Acetaminophen (paracetamol)
pH <7.30 (irrespective of grade of encephalopathy)
or
prothrombin time >100 s and serum creatinine >300 μmol/l if in grade III or IV coma
Non-acetaminophen
prothrombin time >100 s (irrespective of grade of encephalopathy)
or
any three of the following (irrespective of grade of encephalopathy):
etiology – NANB (indeterminate) hepatitis, halothane hepatitis, idiosyncratic drug reactions
age <10 or >40 years
jaundice to encephalopathy interval > 7 days
prothrombin time >50 s
serum bilirubin > 300 μmol/l

and the degree of liver impairment (Table 14.3). All the criteria in the latter patients are independent of the grade of encephalopathy and have been shown to be applicable early in the course of the illness (Pauwels et al. 1993).

Limitations to current criteria

The above "first-generation criteria" fail to reach the ideal characteristics for selection criteria to varying degrees. For example, the issue of low sensitivity compared to their high specificity for death is acknowledged as a short-coming. In our criteria for acetaminophen ALF (the group in which this problem is most evident), an arterial pH below 7.30 on admission has a sensitivity for death of less than 0.50. If less stringent criteria with good positive predictive values could be developed, the overall survival figure (whether transplanted or managed conservatively) could improve. However, striving in particular for a higher post-transplant survival figure by that approach may be flawed, unless the criteria are matched by improved negative predictive values (i.e. identifying patients likely to live), since it could also result in a higher proportion of unneccessary transplants being performed.

Although with the King's criteria the aim is

to identify patients as early as possible, if not at the time of hospital admission, satisfying the criteria may lead to delays in listing for transplant in a significant proportion of patients. For example, in 79 non-acetaminophen transplant cases recently reviewed, the interval from admission to transplant was 132 (9–264) hours and from listing to transplant 65 (7–216) hours. This interval for the most part reflects the delay in patients attaining the defined criteria. Similarly, in acetaminophen cases, delays from admission to listing for transplantation are often inevitable with present criteria. We have recently noted an increasing reliance on the second set of criteria, which require attainment of grade 3–4 encephalopathy, since there appear to be fewer patients with an arterial pH less than 7.30 than we had observed previously. The latter criterion (arterial pH) has the advantage of being determinable on admission, independent of encephalopathy and has a higher specificity and sensitivity for death. Likely reasons for the reduced frequency of the latter variable include improved referral hospital care at presentation and greater use of *N*-acetylcysteine.

Present selection criteria do not address the manner in which different clinical etiologies and degrees of severity of ALF will benefit from transplantation. It can be speculated that survival figures will relate to both the level of liver impairment which is judged of sufficient severity to proceed with transplantation and the criteria used for removing patients from emergency lists due to systemic complications and general pre-transplant clinical status (i.e. centers' definition of absolute and relative contraindications).

CONTRAINDICATIONS TO LIVER TRANSPLANTATION

Although attempts are made to proceed to transplantation as soon as possible once a patient is listed, delays in organ allocation are likely to result in the development of further complications in this critically ill group. As a consequence, a significant proportion of patients initially considered appropriate are removed from lists. Despite this, those who are transplanted have a survival rate inferior to elective liver recipients. In the recent King's adult series (1992–1994), just over half the patients who fulfilled our transplant criteria (39 of 77 cases) were ultimately transplanted (Table 14.4). Indeed, due to predominantly medical contraindications, only 53 of the 77 patients with a poor prognosis were actually listed for super-urgent priority in the first instance. As already indicated, the assessment of contraindications is based often on clinical judgment and experience in the absence of defined unfavorable parameters. In this section, we will discuss those complications of ALF traditionally regarded as contraindications to transplantation and then describe parameters which, on a recent analysis, we found correlated with the post-transplant outcome. During these considerations, the determination of trends rather than single time-point assessments tends to be more useful.

Sepsis

Active on-going infection is normally considered an absolute contraindication to proceeding with a transplant. However, if the patient has received 24 h of antibiotics and his or her clinical course is stable, then it may be reasonable to proceed. The presence of a rising white blood cell count or temperature extremes are poor prognostic indicators. The advent of continuous renal replacement therapy systems has made interpretation of temperature trends more difficult, since treatment on an extracorporeal circuit will frequently render the patients normo- or hypothermic. Severe sepsis during the course of ALF is often manifest by development of hemodynamic instability, and which normally precludes transplantation.

Table 14.4. *Development of contraindications significantly reduces the population of patients who meet criteria to those listed and eventually transplanted*

	Admission	Fulfilled criteria	Listed	Transplanted
Acetaminophen toxicity	252	44 (17.5)	29 (11.5)	21 (8.3)
Viral hepatitis	46	27 (58.7)	18 (39.1)	13 (28.3)
Idiosyncratic reactions / others	46	6 (13.0)	6 (13.0)	5 (10.9)

Values in parentheses are percentages.

Cardiovascular disturbances and respiratory failure

In ALF, systemic vascular resistance falls secondary to both deteriorating liver function and worsening sepsis. The requirement for vasopressor agents per se is not an absolute contraindication, since hemodynamic indices nearly always improve following removal of the necrotic liver. Nevertheless, rapidly increasing requirements for vasopressor support should be considered a relative contraindication. Progressive deterioration in respiratory function with increasing oxygen requirements and arterial–alveolar gradients are more important than absolute values. Chest radiograph changes and sputum bacteriological results must be considered in addition to oxygenation requirements. Adult respiratory distress syndrome requiring an inspired oxygen fraction of greater than 0.6 to achieve adequate saturation is generally regarded as an absolute contraindication to proceeding with transplantation.

Cerebral edema

Isolated episodes of raised intracranial pressure/dilated pupils that respond to treatment should not be considered a contraindication but the development of fixed pupils for prolonged periods of time (two hours or more) or prolonged elevations of intracranial pressure to levels greater than 35 mmHg certainly are contraindications. The cerebral perfusion pressure may be a more reliable indicator than the intracranial pressure is in isolation (Schafer and Shaw 1989). A reduction in this pressure below 40 mmHg for two hours is accompanied by a high rate of irretrievable neurological deficit whereas aggressive maintenance of perfusion pressure above 50 mmHg has reduced peritransplant cerebral deaths (Inagaki et al. 1992; Ascher et al. 1993).

Age and psychiatric state

Age alone should not preclude transplantation but in patients older than 65 years there is a higher risk of impaired cardiorespiratory reserve. Psychiatric stability (which is relevant in acetaminophen cases) is, however, often difficult to assess fully at the time transplantation is being considered. In our experience, major psychiatric sequelae, although rare, do sometimes occur in acetaminophen cases and often culminate in noncompliance with immunosuppression.

THE KING'S EXPERIENCE IN DETERMINING UNFAVORABLE PRETRANSPLANT PARAMETERS

In an analysis of the first 100 patients transplanted for ALF, we specifically examined the influence of pretransplant clinical status on postoperative outcome (Devlin et al. 1995). We considered the pretransplant condition to be especially relevant in this critically ill population since not only was it likely to be an important determinant of outcome, but unlike other unfavorable variables, such as impaired organ viability or severe rejection, it was determinable (and therefore to an extent avoidable) prior to transplantation.

The 100 patients reported represented 13 percent of consecutive cases with acute liver failure (n=759) admitted over an 8 year period. The etiological categories were hepatitis A virus 6/36 (11 percent), non-A non-B/ indeterminate 51/125 (41 percent), acetaminophen overdose 21/446 (5 percent), fulminant Wilson's disease 9/14 (64 percent), idosyncratic drug hepatotoxicity 7/26 (26 percent) and miscellaneous causes (hepatitis B virus 1, halothane toxicity 2, fulminant presentation of autoimmune hepatitis 2 and Budd–Chiari syndrome 1, 6/83 (7 percent). Over the 8 year study period, the increase in the median Apache 111 scores at the time of transplantation appeared to be a reflection of the increasingly ill patients being put forward for this option (Figure 14.2).

Reflecting the progressive nature of the condition in these patients selected for transplantation and the delays in listing (see above), a significant deterioration in the majority of clinical and laboratory parameters was observed during the interval from admission to the time of transplantation (Table 14.5). By the time of transplantation, approximately two thirds of patients were in either grade III or IV hepatic coma and there was ongoing evidence of severe liver impairment as reflected by elevated prothrombin times and serum bilirubin levels. In addition to specific liver indices, the mean Apache 111 score (an index of critical illness) had increased from 38 to 50 in non-acetaminophen cases (group 1) and from 49 to 74 in the acetaminophen cases (group 2) with 32 of the 100 patients requiring renal replacement therapy.

Patient and graft outcome

Two month patient survival for the whole series was 68 percent (66 percent in group 1 and 76 percent in group 2). Among those patients experiencing fulminant hepatic failure who were selected for transplantation on the basis of our criteria for a poor prognosis since 1988, 38 of 58 (66 percent) were alive at two months. In patients with non-acetaminophen liver failure, a significant variation in patient survival in relation to etiology was noted (Figure 14.3). An excellent prognosis was seen in patients transplanted for fulminant Wilson's disease in contrast to those with idiosyncratic drug reactions in whom only one of seven survived. For the other etiological categories, no significant variations in outcome were seen. In patients with non A non B/indeterminate hepatitis, the two-month patient survival rate was 69 percent with no significant difference in outcome between fulminant or late-onset presentations (67 percent and 71 percent respectively). Retransplantation was required in nine patients within the first 2 months, and was only successful in two.

Of the 32 deaths during the first two months post-transplant, the largest proportion were due to systemic sepsis developing as a primary complication (13 [41 percent]). Fungal infection was detected in eight patients and was associated with death in seven. Possible disease recurrence from viral graft reinfection in six cases of non A non B hepatitis was noted and usually led to death within the first two weeks post-transplant. Technical or rejection events caused death in four cases. Miscellaneous events leading to early two-month mortality were neurological complications in three patients (cerebral edema/infarction [2], intracerebral hematoma [1], graft versus host disease [1], primary graft non-function [1], aortic dissection [1], myocardial infarction [1] and a gastrointestinal bleed [1]).

Preoperative risk factors for early (two month) post-transplant mortality

A trend toward a reduction in patient survival was seen with increasing coma grade pretransplant. Two-month survival rates were 80 percent for patients transplanted in grade I, 81 percent in grade II, 63 percent in grade III and 59 percent in grade IV. Given the distinct clinical picture of acetaminophen-induced ALF, the outcome for these patients with respect to pretransplant illness was analyzed separately from the other etiologies (Table 14.6).

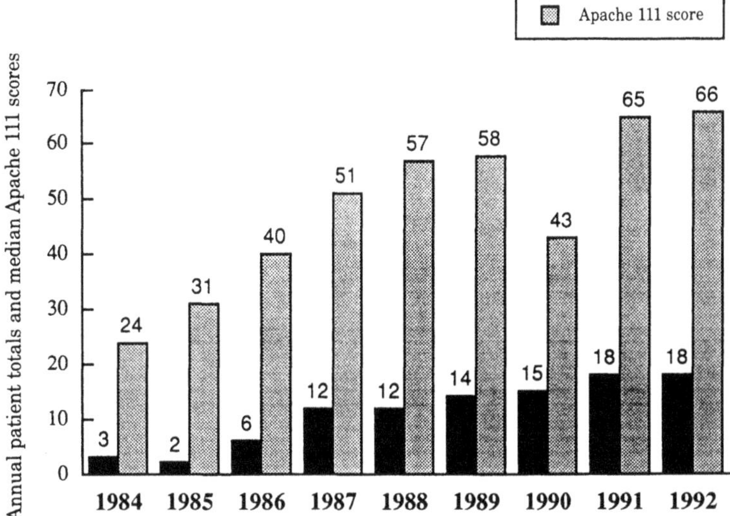

Figure 14.2 Distribution of the 100 recipients with regard to year of transplantation (March 1984 to September 1992). The median Apache III score, at the time of transplantation, is also shown. It is clear these are tending to rise annually, probably reflecting the increased use of emergency transplantation in severe acetaminophen hepatotoxicity and lengthening delays in organ allocation.

Table 14.5. *Clinical parameters on admission and at transplantation in both groups: (nonacetaminophen liver failure [group 1] and severe acetaminophen hepatotoxicity [group 2]). Deterioration in a range of important indices (particularly encephalopathy and multisystem illness) was apparent during this variable interval*

	Group 1 (*n*=79)		Group 2 (*n*=21)	
Variable	Admission mean (SD)	Transplantation mean (SD)	Admission mean (SD)	Transplantation mean (SD)
Bilirubin (μmol/l)	443 (190)	485 (193)[b]	104 (13.9)	146 (19)[a]
(mg/dl)	26.1 (11.2)	28.5 (11.4)	6.1 (0.8)	8.6 (1.1)
AST (units/l)	518 (582)	470 (809)	3214 (1892)	2034 (2057)
Prothrombin time (INR)	4.6 (3.4)	6.0 (4.1)[c]	8.1 (3.3)	8.2 (4.0)
Albumin (mg/dl)	3.0 (0.6)	3.3 (0.7)[b]	3.8 (0.8)	4.0 (0.7)
Encephalopathy grade[d]	1	3[c]	1	4[c]
Cerebral edema (%)	4.2	22[b]	9.5	43[c]
Creatinine (μmol/l)	131 (88)	153 (122)	272 (148)	349 (176)
(mg/dl)	1.75 (1.17)	2.04 (1.63)	3.62 (1.97)	4.65 (2.35)
White cells (× 10^9)	12.4 (7.0)	12.4 (6.2)	17.2 (6.6)	10.1 (5.5)[c]
Platelets (× 10^9)	201 (132)	160 (162)[c]	154 (98)	68 (52)[c]
Organ system failures[d]	0	1[c]	0	2[b]
Apache 111	38 (18)	50 (22)[c]	49 (23)	74 (21)[c]
Arterial pH	—	—	7.28 (0.14)	7.35 (0.10)

[a] $P<0.05$, [b] $P<0.01$, [c] $P<0.001$. [d] Encephalopathy grade and organ system failures expressed as median.

In non-acetaminophen-induced liver failure, no static variable other than etiology (fulminant Wilson's disease and idiosyncratic drug reactions as described above) were significantly related to two-month survival. Of the dynamic variables examined *on admission* to the Unit, the serum creatinine (2.1 [1.6] mg/dl nonsurvivors versus 1.4 [0.6] mg/dl survivors, P=0.02) was the only parameter significantly different in a univariate analysis.

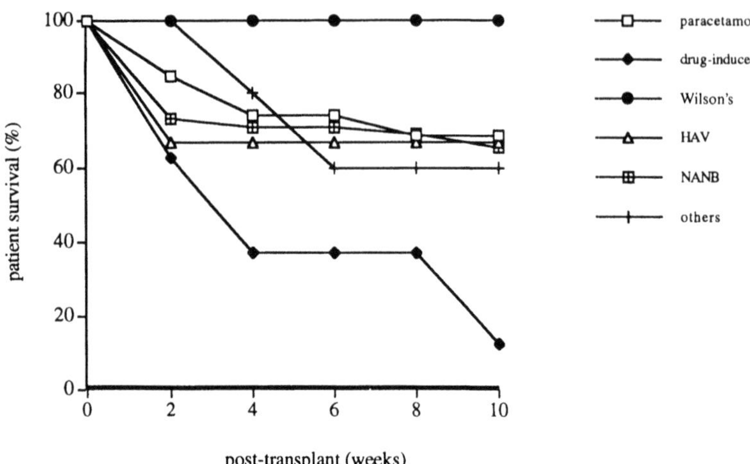

Figure 14.3 Early actuarial patient survival following transplantation in the different etiological categories (1984–1992 inclusive). With the exception of idiosyncratic drug reactions and fulminant Wilson's disease (filled symbols), the outcome was independent of etiology.

Table 14.6. *Summary of clinical and laboratory data in groups 1 and 2 for survivors and nonsurvivors at two months post-transplant, calculated at the time of transplantation*

Variable	Group 1		Group 2	
	Survivors (n=52) mean (SD)	Nonsurvivors (n=27) mean (SD)	Survivors (n=16) mean (SD)	Nonsurvivors (n=5) mean (SD)
Bilirubin (μmol/l)	504 (192)	443 (181)	121 (47)	233 (126)[b]
(mg/dl)	29.6 (11.3)	26.1 (10.6)	7.1 (2.8)	13.7 (7.4)
AST (units/l)	418 (354)	654 (1315)	1782 (1593)	2791 (3292)
Prothrombin time (INR)	5.8 (3.8)	6.7 (4.8)	8.9 (4.6)	7.9 (2.5)
Albumin (mg/dl)	3.2 (0.7)	3.4 (0.7)	4.5 (0.9)	3.8 (0.6)
Encephalopathy grade[d]	2	3[a]	4	3
Cerebral edema (%)	23	26	44	40
Creatinine (μmol/l)	117 (81)	190 (147)[a]	333 (167)	402 (214)
(mg/dl)	1.56 (1.08)	2.53 (1.96)	4.44 (2.22)	5.36 (2.85)
White cells (× 10^9)	11.6 (5.5)	12.0 (5.8)	9.1 (5.3)	13.1 (5.7)
Platelets (× 10^9)	155 (116)	153 (117)	67 (36)	74 (94)
Organ system failures[d]	0.5	1[a]	2	2
Apache 111	48 (20)	58 (23)[a]	68 (19)	92 (16)[a]
Arterial pH	—	—	7.36 (0.09)	7.26 (0.13)

[a] P <0.05, [b] P <0.01. [d] Encephalopathy grade and organ system failures expressed as median.

In contrast, by the time of *transplantation,* in addition to serum creatinine which remained significantly elevated in nonsurvivors, the two intensive care indices of systemic critical illness (organ system failure and Apache 111 score) also discriminated survivors from nonsurvivors (Table 14.6). When these significant parameters were entered into a stepwise logistic regression model to predict two-month mortality, serum creatinine at the time of transplantation was the only independent variable (r=0.33). A serum creatinine >2.7 mg/dl (200 μmol/l) at transplantation had a 42 percent sensitivity and a 92 percent specificity for a fatal outcome at two months.

In acetaminophen-induced liver failure, the "time from ingestion to transplantation/hepatectomy" was significantly different between survivors: four [±1] days versus nonsurvivors, six [±1] days ($P<0.01$). No patient transplanted at day seven or greater from the time of drug ingestion survived to two months. The "time from admission to transplantation/hepatectomy" also approached statistical significance with survivors waiting for a graft on average less than nonsurvivors, 41 [±14] h versus 67 [±52] h ($P=0.09$). With respect to other dynamic variables on admission, no parameter examined could significantly distinguish survivors from nonsurvivors. However, by the time of transplantation, total serum bilirubin and Apache 111 score were significantly different in survivors versus nonsurvivors (Table 14.6). Significant correlations between serum bilirubin and "time from overdose to transplantation/hepatectomy" existed ($r=0.56$) with a lesser association between the bilirubin level and Apache 111 score ($r=0.29$). In a stepwise logistic regression with the significant variables above entered, the Apache 111 score at the time of transplantation was the only independent determinant ($r=0.51$). If one patient who died from a technical complication (severe postoperative bleeding on day 3) was excluded from the analysis, arterial pH would have been the strongest parameter by a significant margin. In a univariate analysis, the mean (median) pH at transplantation in nonsurvivors was 7.21 (7.23) versus 7.38 (7.37) in survivors ($P<0.001$). A pH below 7.30 at transplantation had a sensitivity of 80 percent and a specificity of 94 percent for the two-month mortality figure.

What lessons have been learned?

The development of systemic sepsis is the greatest threat to a successful outcome. This susceptibility to infection, present in patients with ALF from an early stage, is continued and possibly initially aggravated in the early post-transplant period by the introduction of immunosuppression regimens which include high dose corticosteroids. Use of inferior donor livers or those which are ABO incompatible (as conventional strict criteria are set aside through necessity) will further predispose to this complication (see Chapter 15). Improved control of infection (especially fungal) is required (Brems et al. 1988). Whether benefit will derive from antimicrobial prophylaxis regimens and/or immunosuppression regimens with lower corticosteroid cumulative exposure, such as are possible when tacrolimus rather than cyclosporin is used as the primary immunosuppressive agent, remain to be determined (Devlin et al. 1994). Retransplantation, given the poor results, should be reserved for highly selected patients.

The results of our analysis and data from other series serve to highlight both the hazards which particularly relate to pretransplant status and those areas of management which need to be improved. Surprisingly, clinical characteristics of the primary liver disease were poor discriminators of survival. Liver failure from idiosyncratic drug reactions managed conservatively is similarly associated with a high mortality. Excellent results are achievable in fulminant Wilson's disease recipients possibly reflecting the benefits of patients being fit and young and listed for transplant as soon as the diagnosis is made. In relation to the two largest etiological groups, no significant difference in patient survival between non-A non-B/indeterminate liver failure and acetaminophen hepatotoxicity was detected despite this latter group having the worst indices of both liver damage and systemic critical illness (Apache 111 scores). The similar outcomes may reflect the use of a prognostic scoring system which identifies patients in these groups with a similarly poor prognosis (approximately 10 percent survival) if managed conservatively. It might be expected that their prognosis would improve similary post-transplant. The two-month survival of approximately 68 percent in these groups represents a considerable improvement on medical management. The documented recurrence of viral hepatitis in the graft should not influence selection for transplantation.

No relationship between outcome and the

year in which the transplant was carried out was noted in our analysis. This initially surprising result is in line with the recent "plateauing" of outcome, a phenomenon as yet not adequately explained, reported for liver transplantation by the registries. The explanation may be the significant increases in Apache III scores in patients being transplanted. The increasing necessity to use suboptimal organs, as indicated above, is also likely to prevent further improvements in outcome, particularly in ALF where the rapid restoration of adequate hepatic function is so crucial to a successful outcome.

Systemic illness at the time of transplantation is as important an indicator of post-transplant outcome as more conventional indices of liver function. Determination of the Apache III score, as part of the clinical review at the time of proposed transplantation, would appear to allow a subjective appraisal of post-transplant outcome. Athough critical illness scoring systems are not widely applied in liver failure/transplant programs, adoption of these scores in general intensive care units has considerably improved the accuracy of clinical judgments on likely patient hospital mortality. Our data show that considerable deterioration in patients selected for transplantation occurs between the time of listing and the eventual transplant. The clear detrimental effect of this delay has prompted some programs to develop novel experimental maneuvers to either by-pass this interval (employing living-related organ donation) or offset the sequelae of having a necrotic liver in-situ by undertaking hepatectomy prior to organ availability (Ringe et al. 1988; Matsunami et al. 1992). Although the early results appear encouraging, the potential clinical role of these procedures have yet to be medically or ethically defined.

The length of the period from admission to transplantation is of critical importance. Prolongation of this interval leads to a greater opportunity to develop serious complications (such as the unfavorable parameters of deeper encephalopathy and worsening renal impairment in the nonacetaminophen cases) and inevitably an inferior outcome. Our results reinforce the continued need for a super-urgent category in graft allocation.

The final decision to proceed to transplantation when a donor liver becomes available needs to be separated from the initial selection of potential candidates. With the likelihood of greater delays in organ availability, the definition of prospectively validated risk factors at the time of transplantation may permit a more informed basis for deciding which patients are too ill to have a successful outcome. In our initial report on liver transplantation for acetaminophen overdose, we described the "window period" of opportunity for a successful outcome (O'Grady et al. 1991). Such an approach can also be applied to other etiologies of ALF.

REFERENCES

Ascher, N.L., Lake, J.R., Emond, J.C. and Roberts, J.P. 1993. Liver transplantation for fulminant hepatic failure. *Arch Surg* 128: 677–82.

Alter, M.J., Margolis, H.S., Krawczynski, K. et al. 1990. The changing epidemiology of hepatitis B in the United States: need for alternative vaccination strategies. *JAMA* 263: 1218–22.

Bernuau, J., Goudeau, A., Poynard, T., Dubois, F., Lesage, G., Yvonnet, B., Degott, C. et al. 1986. Multivariate analysis of prognostic factors in fulminant hepatitis B. *Hepatology* 6: 648–51.

Brems, J.J., Hiatt, J.R., Klein, A.S., Hart, J. et al. 1988. Disseminated aspergillosis complicating orthotopic liver transplantation for fulminant hepatic failure refractory to corticosteroid therapy. *Transplantation* 46: 479–81.

Centers for Disease Control. 1991. Summary of notifiable diseases. *MMWR* 40: 53.

Christensen, E., Bremmelgaard, A., Bahnsen, M., Andreasen, P.B. and Tygstrup, N. 1984. Prediction of fatality in fulminant hepatic failure. *Scand J Gastroenterol* 19: 90–6.

Devlin, J., Wong, P., Williams, R. et al. 1994. FK506 primary immunosuppression following emergency liver transplantation for fulminant hepatic failure. *Transpl Int* 7: 64–9.

Devlin, J., Wendon, J., Heaton, N., Tan, K.C. and Williams, R. 1995. Pretransplantation clinical status and outcome of emergency transplantation for acute liver failure. *Hepatology* 21: 1018–24.

Emond, J.C., Aran, P.P., Whitington, P.F., Broelsch, C.E. and Baker, A.L. 1989. Liver transplantation in the management of fulminant hepatic failure. *Gastroenterology* 96: 1583–8.

Gimson, A.E., O'Grady, J., Ede., R.J., Portmann, B. and Williams, R. 1986. Late onset hepatic failure: clinical, serological and histological features. *Hepatology* 6: 288–94.

Harrison, P., O'Grady, J., Alexander, G. and Williams, R. 1990. Serial prothrombin times: a prognostic indicator in acetaminophen-induced fulminant hepatic failure. *BMJ* 301: 964–6.

Inagaki, M., Shaw, B., Schafer, D. et al. 1992. Advantages of intracranial pressure monitoring in patients with fulminant hepatic failure. *Gastroenterology* 102: A826 (abstract).

Iwatsuki, S., Esquivel, C.O., Gordon, R.D., Shaw, B.J., Starzl, T.E., Shade, R.R. and Van, T.D. 1985. Liver transplantation for fulminant hepatic failure. *Sem Liver Dis* 5: 325–8.

Karvountzis, G.G. and Redeker, A.G. 1974. Relation of alpha-fetoprotein in acute hepatitis to severity and prognosis. *Ann Intern Med* 80: 156–60.

Klein, A.S., Hart, J., Brems, J.J., Goldstein, L., Lewin, K. and Busuttil, R.W. 1989. Amanita poisoning: treatment and the role of liver transplantation. *Am J Med* 86: 187–93.

Kumahara, T., Muto, Y., Moriwaki, H., Yoshida, T. and Tomita, E. 1989. Determination of an integrated CT number of the whole liver in patients with severe hepatitis: an indicator of the functional reserve of the liver. *Gastroenterol Jpn* 24: 290–7.

Matsunami, H., Makuuchi, M., Kawasaki, S., Ishizone, S., Mizusawa, Y., Kawarasaki, H. and Takayama, T. 1992. Living-related liver transplantation in fulminant hepatic failure. *Lancet* 340: 1411–12.

O'Grady, J.G., Alexander, G.J., Hayllar, K.M. and Williams, R. 1989. Early indicators of prognosis in fulminant hepatic failure. *Gastroenterology* 97: 439–45.

O'Grady, J.G., Wendon, J., Tan, K.C., et al. 1991. Liver transplantation after acetaminophen overdose. *BMJ* 303: 221–3.

O'Grady, J.G., Schalm, S. and Williams, R. 1993. Acute liver failure: redefining the syndromes. *Lancet* 342: 273–5.

Pauwels, A., Mostefa, K.N., Florent, C. and Levy, V.G. 1993. Emergency liver transplantation for acute liver failure. Evaluation of London and Clichy criteria. *J Hepatol* 17: 124–7.

Pereira, L., Langley, P., Hayllar, K., Tredger, J.M. and Williams, R. 1992. Coagulation factors V and VIII/V ratio as predictors of outcome in acetaminophen-induced fulminant hepatic failure: relationship to other prognostic indicators. *Gut* 33: 98–102.

Rakela, J. 1979. Etiology and prognosis in fulminant hepatitis: acute hepatic failure study group. *Gastroenterology* 77: A33 (abstract).

Ringe, B., Pichlmayr, R., Lubbe, N., Bornscheuer, A. and Kuse, E. 1988. Total hepatectomy as a temporary approach to acute hepatic or primary graft failure. *Transpl Proc* 20: 552–7.

Saibara, T., Onishi, S., Sone, J., Yamamoto, N., Shimahara, Y., Mori, K., Ozawa, K. and Yamamoto, Y. 1991. Arterial ketone body ratio as a possible indicator for liver transplantation in fulminant hepatic failure. *Transplantation* 51: 782–6.

Schafer, D. and Shaw, B. 1989. Fulminant hepatic failure and orthotopic liver transplantation. *Sem Liver Dis* 9: 189–94.

Scaiola, A., MacMathuna, P., Langley, P.G., Gove, C.D., Hughes, R.D. and Williams, R. 1990. Determination of the ketone-body ratio in fulminant hepatic failure. *Hepatogastroenterology* 37: 413–16.

Scotto, J., Opolon, P., Eteve, J. et al. 1973. Liver biopsy and prognosis in acute liver failure. *Gut* 14: 927–33.

Sternleib, I. 1984. Wilson's disease: indications for liver transplants. *Hepatology* 4 (Suppl): 15S-17S.

Takahashi, Y. and Shimizi, M. 1991. Aetiology and prognosis of fulminant hepatic viral hepatitis in Japan: a multicentre study. *J Gastroenterol Hepatol* 6: 159–64.

Trey, C. 1972. The fulminant hepatic failure surveillance study: brief review of the effects of presumed aetiology and age on survival. *CMAJ* 106: 525–6.

Tygstrup, N. and Ranek, L. 1986. Assessment of prognosis in fulminant hepatic failure. *Sem Liver Dis* 6: 129–37.

Van Thiel, D.H. 1993. When should a decision to proceed with transplantation actually be made in cases of fulminant or subfulminant hepatic failure: at admission to hospital or when a donor organ is made available? *J Hepatol* 17: 1–2.

15 Liver transplantation in patients with acute liver failure: the European experience

Didier Samuel and Henri Bismuth

INTRODUCTION

Before 1986, only a few cases of liver transplantation for acute liver failure (ALF) had been reported (Le Bihan et al. 1982; Williams and Gimson 1984; Iwatzuki et al. 1985; Ringe et al. 1986). By 1988, 85 cases of transplantation for ALF had been listed (European Liver Transplant Registry 1995). The reasons for the low number of successful cases reported were multiple: the indications of liver transplantation as well as the timing of transplantation were not clearly defined; national organizations for organ sharing were not well organized for emergency liver procurement; and there were many technical limitations, such as the inability to correct coagulation defects or to perform transplantation in patients with multiple organ failure (associated anuria, sepsis, etc.). Our center was one of the first in the world to start a program of emergency liver transplantation for ALF, beginning in January 1986. The initial experience with 17 patients transplanted for ALF was reported one year later (Bismuth et al. 1987).

Since then, there has been a dramatic increase in the number of transplants performed in the world for ALF. Between 1988 and 1993, 1390 patients with acute liver failure were transplanted in Europe, representing 12 percent of the primary indications for liver transplantation (European Liver Transplant Registry 1995). Among these 1390 patients, 982 were reported to have fulminant hepatitis, 70 subfulminant hepatitis and 338 acute liver failure of other causes.

DEFINITIONS

One of the difficulties encountered in analyzing the results in the literature is the heterogeneity of definitions for the syndrome of acute liver failure. Three main definitions have been given. Trey and others have defined fulminant hepatitis as acute hepatitis complicated by acute liver failure with hepatic encephalopathy occurring less than 8 weeks after the onset of symptoms (Trey and Davidson 1970). Bernuau and Benhamou have defined fulminant hepatitis as acute hepatitis complicated by acute liver failure with hepatic encephalopathy occurring less than two weeks after the onset of jaundice and subfulminant hepatitis as acute hepatitis complicated by acute liver failure with hepatic encephalopathy occurring two weeks to three months after the onset of jaundice (Bernuau, Rueff and Benhamou 1986). The common points of these two definitions are the occurrence of clinical encephalopathy during the course of an acute hepatitis in a patient without known previous hepatopathy. The definitions varied widely, with some authors including fulminant Wilson's disease in the group although a chronic underlying disease of the liver is present, while other authors do not. Some authors have included in their series patients with severe liver dysfunction without occurrence of encephalopathy. In an attempt to standardize the definition of fulminant hepatitis, a new classification has been proposed (O'Grady et al. 1993). The starting point of the disease is the occurrence of jaundice and patients have been classified in relation to the delay between onset of jaundice and occurrence of encephalopathy. Patients have been classified into three groups: hyperacute liver failure with a jaundice to encephalopathy interval of less than seven days, acute liver failure with a jaundice to encephalopathy interval of seven to 28 days, and subacute liver failure with an interval of 28 to 100 days. A fourth group has been isolated: patients with late onset hepatic failure as defined by the King's College group with a delay of eight weeks to six months between jaundice and encephalopathy. Clearly, there is an overlap between late onset hepatic failure and subacute liver failure (Gimson et al. 1986; Ellis et al. 1995).

One of the other confusing features are the definitions of encephalopathy, coma, and of intracranial hypertension. Some authors are mixing the definitions of coma. We classified hepatic encephalopathy into four grades as suggested previously (Trey and Davidson 1970): grade I: slowed consciousness; grade II: accentuation of grade I and presence of asterixis; grade III: presence of deep confusion or only reactive to vocal stimuli; grade IV: presence of deep coma assessed by at least the absence of reactions to vocal stimuli. Using the above definition, coma is present only in grade III and IV encephalopathy, and is sub-classified by us into four grades (Bismuth et al. 1995): grade 1: reactivity to vocal stimuli; grade 2: absence of reactivity to vocal stimuli with coordinate response to nociceptive stimuli; grade 3: absence of reactivity to vocal stimuli with incoordinate response to nociceptive stimuli; grade 4: brain death. Intracranial hypertension is independent of the stage of encephalopathy or of coma but is rarely seen in patients with grade I or II encephalopathy and is more frequent in the more severe stages of encephalopathy. The clinical signs of intracranial hypertension are: marked hyperventilation, opisthotonus, hyperpronation-adduction of the arms, cardiac arrhythmia, myoclonus, seizures, poorly reactive pupils, asymmetric pupils.

CAUSES OF ACUTE LIVER FAILURE

One of the other differences between reported series from different countries are the causes of the hepatitis. In France, acute viral hepatitis is the major cause of ALF. In a French series (Benhamou 1991), 52 percent of the patients were affected with acute viral hepatitis: hepatitis B virus (HBV), either alone (32 percent), or together with hepatitis D virus (HDV) (13 percent), hepatitis A virus (HAV) 4 percent, non-A non-B non-C hepatitis virus(es) 2 percent, Herpes viruses (1 percent). The other causes were drug-induced in 16 percent, toxic ingestion (*Amanita phalloides* ingestion, massive acetàminophen (paracetamol) ingestion, others) in 4.5 percent, various in 9.5 percent and indeterminate in 18 percent. In our own series of 152 patients referred for liver transplantation from 1986 to 1994, 46 percent of patients were suffering from viral B or B-delta related hepatitis, 18 percent from drug-induced liver failure, and 26 percent from hepatitis of indeterminate etiologies. Precise etiologies are listed in Table 15.1. It should be noted that acetaminophen overdose represented only three patients of this series. In our experience, hepatitis C virus (HCV) infection alone was not responsible for any cases of ALF, however HCV superinfection of a chronic B carrier or coinfection with HBV and HCV have been found in some patients of our series (Feray et al. 1993). In contrast with France, acetaminophen overdose is the main cause of ALF in Great Britain and represented

Table 15.1. *Etiologies of fulminant and subfulminant hepatitis in 152 patients referred to at the Hepatobiliary Center at Paul Brousse Hospital from 1986 to 1994*

Viral	
Viral B	56
Viral B-Delta	14
Viral A	3
Viral Non-A Non-B	2
Herpes virus	1
Nonviral	
Drug-induced	28
Toxic (acetaminophen 3)	5
Acute fatty liver of pregnancy	1
Heatstroke	1
Indeterminate	41

52 percent of the cases amongst 588 patients admitted for fulminant hepatitis at King's College with HBV infection representing only 13 percent (O'Grady et al. 1988). In other European countries, acetaminophen overdoses are much less frequent than in the United Kingdom, and viral hepatitis is the leading cause. Viral hepatitis is clearly the main cause of ALF in countries of the south of Europe such as Italy, Spain, Portugal and Greece. In a recent series from Spain on 67 patients with ALF referred for transplantation, the etiologies were viral in 28 (45 percent) (HBV 18, HDV 7, HAV 3) of the patients, drug-induced in five, due to Wilson's disease in four, various in three and from indeterminate origin in 27 (44 percent) (Castells et al. 1993).

CRITERIA FOR LIVER TRANSPLANTATION FOR PATIENTS WITH ACUTE LIVER FAILURE

The spontaneous overall mortality rate in patients with ALF is around 80 percent (Bernuau et al. 1986). The main cause of death is cerebral edema complicated by brain herniation or by irreversible ischemic brain damage (Ware et al. 1971). The mortality rate is 75 percent to 80 percent in patients with HBV, or HBV-HDV ALF; 80 to 95 percent in those with drug-induced ALF, ALF due to halothane ingestion, ALF of indeterminate cause and so-called non-A non-B ALF. The survival rate is higher in patients with HAV ALF reaching 55 percent and is between 50 and 60 percent in those with acetaminophen overdose (O'Grady et al. 1988). In addition, older patients, or patients with renal failure have a worse prognosis.

Since 20 percent of the patients with ALF will survive with conservative management, it is necessary to determine who will die without transplantation and those who will survive spontaneously. Thus, it is necessary to have reliable criteria for the indications of liver transplantation. In addition, if transplantation is required, these criteria must be applicable early in the course of the hepatitis in order to have time to find a donor. It should be emphasized that when transplantation is decided for a patient, the delay in finding a donor is between 0.5 and 4 days; in addition, the procedure itself can take as long as 12 h.

The indications for liver transplantation used at Paul Brousse Hospital (Bismuth et al. 1987), are the criteria of poor prognosis developed in the hepatology unit of Beaujon Hospital in Clichy (Bernuau, Rueff and Benhamou 1986; Bernuau et al. 1991): that is, confusion or coma combined with a factor V level below 20 percent of normal (in patients less than 30 years old) or below 30 percent of normal (in patients more than 30 years old) independent of the etiology. These criteria indicating the need for liver transplantation are now the criteria used in all transplant centers in France for all adult patients. In children, Devictor et al. considered liver transplantation where there was encephalopathy and a factor V level below 25 percent (Devictor et al. 1992). The group at King's College Hospital in London have shown a higher survival rate in patients with hepatitis due to acetaminophen overdose than in those due to other causes. Their criteria for transplantation of patients with ALF not due to acetaminophen were either a prothrombin time over 100 s, or the presence of any three of the following variables: aged <10 or >40 years; etiology: non-A non-B hepatitis, halothane, drug-induced liver failure; duration of jaundice before onset of encephalopathy >7 days, prothrombin time>50 s, and serum bilirubin> 300 μmol/l (O'Grady et al. 1989). The King's criteria will be discussed in another chapter. Some authors have applied retrospectively the criteria for transplantation of Villejuif and London to their own series of patients. They have found a good positive predictive accuracy of 0.96 and 0.90 using the London and Villejuif criteria. In contrast, the negative predictive accuracy was less good (Pauwels et al. 1993). Thus, for these authors the criteria used in Villejuif and London were not good enough to predict which patients will survive without liver transplantation. However, this last study was retrospective and studied heterogeneous groups of patients included in different protocols. Others consider transplantation according to the daily quantity of fresh frozen plasma required to improve the coagulation defect, and the evolution to stage 4 encephalopathy (Emond et al. 1989). In most centers, patients are considered for transplantation if their general condition deteriorates, especially with regard to neurological status and prothrombin time. In a group from Barcelona, Spain, patients with ALF were considered for transplantation in case of presence of grade 3–4 encephalopathy or when encephalopathy appears to progress after a transient period of improvement. Patients with subfulminant acute liver failure were transplanted when no improvement was observed after three days of supportive management (Castells et al. 1993). Some centers have based their decision on intracranial pressure or cerebral perfusion pressure, patients with raised intracranial pressure are considered for liver transplantation; in contrast, patients with cerebral perfusion pressure below 40 mmHg for one hour are considered too ill, to have probable irreversible brain damage and are excluded for liver transplantation (Schafer and Shaw 1989; Lidofsky et al. 1992). For Van Thiel, all patients referred with ALF should be listed for liver transplantation and the decision should be made when the liver graft is available (Van Thiel 1993). In the intermediate cases, this author proposed to perform transplantation if the liver volume at CT scan is less than 700 cm^3; in patients with liver volume more than 700 cm^3, a liver biopsy may be indicated and transplantation be performed if liver cell necrosis is more than 50 percent (Van Thiel 1993). This attitude is difficult to achieve, since the decision to transplant should be taken rapidly, and moving a patient to a CT scan, or performing a liver biopsy may be dangerous and waste valuable time for the patient. Finally, in our experience liver cell necrosis does not correlate well with the degree of encephalopathy or with prognosis.

Thus, it is difficult from the different published series to have standardized criteria for transplantation. The decision to undertake transplantation is easily made in the majority of cases, but it is difficult in patients with lower grades of encephalopathy or levels of factor V approximating the criteria values. Furthermore, it is difficult to know *a posteriori* if the transplantation was not indicated; in contrast, if the transplantation decision is not made and the patient dies before transplantation, the wrong decision is clearly understood. On the basis of our criteria defined above, among 152 patients referred to our center meeting these criteria, all but one of the patients who were not transplanted died; among the transplanted patients, the neurological status of all but one of our patients either deteriorated or remained stable without improvement until transplantation (Table 15.2). These points argue in favor of the accuracy of our selection. One final point to take into account is the additional problems encountered in obtaining a graft urgently as well and the delay in procuring the graft once the decision is taken. In conclusion, the definition of ALF and the criteria used for decision to transplantation should be strict.

Table 15.2. *Evolution of 152 patients referred to the Hepatobiliary Center at Paul Brousse Hospital from 1986 to 1994 with fulminant and subfulminant hepatitis who met the criteria for transplantation, until transplantation or death related to the neurological status on admission*

	Encephalopathy stage III		Encephalopathy stage IV	
Neurological status on admission	Confusion	Coma Grade 1	Coma Grade 2	Coma Grade 3
Patients admitted (*n*)	24	35	50	43
Patients dying before transplant (*n*)	1	4	5	13
Patients transplanted (%)	23/24 (96)	29/35 (83)	45/50 (90)	30/43 (69)[a]
Grade of coma at transplant				
Patients with Grade 0[b] 1/2/3	7/10/4/2	0/7/13/11	0/0/18/27	0/0/0/29[c]

[a] One recovered and survived without transplant.
[b] Coma grade 0: patients were in encephalopathy stage 3 with marked confusion.
[c] $P < 0.001$.

CONTRAINDICATIONS TO LIVER TRANSPLANTATION IN PATIENTS WITH ACUTE LIVER FAILURE

One of the key questions is: when is transplantation contraindicated in patients with acute liver failure? Indeed, any analysis of the results should take into account the severity of the patients' condition at the time of transplantation. For example, in our experience the one year survival rate after transplantation was 90 percent in patients in encephalopathy stage III and confusion without coma, 77 percent in those who had encephalopathy stage III and grade 1 coma, 79 percent in those who had encephalopathy stage IV and coma grade 2, and 54 percent in those with encephalopathy stage IV and coma grade 3 ($P<0.005$, Table 15.3). Thus, it is clear that results are much improved when more severely ill patients are excluded. In our series, the contraindications for emergency liver transplantation in patients with ALF were: the inability to support the procedure: age more than 65 years, severe cardiac, lung or multiorgan failure; the presence of uncontrolled sepsis, i.e. septic shock, extensive pneumonia (positive blood cultures are not a contraindication); the presence of brain death assessed by the presence of fixed bilateral dilated pupils and flat electroencephalogram. Some centers are reluctant to perform liver transplantation in high risk patients: those with deep coma or hemodynamic instability, since they consider these patients to have a poorer chance of survival after liver transplantation and therefore the graft should be given to a less risky recipient. Some authors have argued against transplantation for patients with cerebral perfusion pressure less than 40 mmHg. This attitude is debatable. It is evident that complete neurologic recovery can occur even in the most severely ill patients: in our center, among patients who survived after transplantation, there were patients who at time of transplantation were in grade 3 coma, with seizures, low cerebral perfusion pressure, asymmetric dilated pupils, hemodynamic instability requiring the use of high doses of epinephrine or norepinephrine. Thus, in our opinion, the neurologic limit to transplantation before death is never known.

THE SEARCH FOR A DONOR

As soon as the decision to proceed with liver transplantation is made, the search for a liver donor should be initiated urgently. In France, there is a national superemergency procedure held by the French Transplant organization which gives an absolute priority to patients with acute liver failure for receiving any donor liver available in the country. This procedure often reduces the waiting time to less than a day. There are some differences between countries, however. Thus, in most European

Table 15.3. *Outcome of 128 patients transplanted at Paul Brousse Hospital from 1986 to 1995 in relation to the grade of coma at time of transplantation*

Encephalopathy stage[a]	Grade of coma	Patients (*n*)	Survival (%)	Peri- or post-transplant brain deaths (*n*)
III	0[b]	7	90	0
III	1	17	77	1
IV	2	35	79	2
IV	3	69	54[c]	10

[a] Trey's classification.
[b] Marked confusion.
[c] $P < 0.00$.

countries, acute liver failure patients are listed on a superemergency list which gives these patients an absolute priority. In countries in the Eurotransplant region, a graft can be obtained within two days in most cases. In Spain, the feasibility of emergency liver transplantation is more difficult (Castells 1993). Likewise, in countries with low rates of donation such as Italy, Greece, Portugal, Israel, the probability of obtaining a graft before the death of the patient is low. In the United States, patients with acute liver failure are classified as UNOS 4 similar to all other patients waiting for a graft in the ICU (including patients with chronic liver disease) and the mean delay to obtain a graft is four days, which may be too long for many acutely ill patients.

In theory, acute liver failure patients require a good quality graft with enough functional liver mass in order to recover very quickly after transplantation. However, these patients are frequently transplanted in an emergency setting. As a result, two policies are emerging: either to accept the first offer of liver donor in order to transplant the patient as quickly as possible whatever the quality, the blood group and the size of the graft, or, by contrast, to wait until a good quality ABO compatible graft is available with the increased risk of clinical deterioration and death due to the additional waiting time. Tables 15.3 and 15.4 show the influence of the degree of severity of coma at transplantation, and the effect of graft quality on the survival after transplantation. Our policy is to accept the first graft offered with the exception of fibrotic grafts, or grafts with cirrhosis. This policy permits transplantation of more patients with ALF listed emergently; however, it proves costly in terms of graft survival with some authors stating that ABO incompatible grafts should not be used and should only be given to blood group compatible elective patients. The feasibility of transplantation should be included in the analysis of the results. Castells et al. have a low feasibility rate of liver transplantation, thus the overall survival of patients who required transplantation remained low because so many patients died awaiting transplantation (Castells 1993). In our own series, patients who met the criteria for liver transplantation, who were in coma grade 3 at admission had a 35 percent overall survival rate in comparison to a 90 percent survival rate in patients who were only confused at admission. This is due to the much higher rate of death before transplantation and after transplantation in the former group (Table 15.5) (Bismuth et al. 1995).

MANAGEMENT OF PATIENTS WITH ACUTE LIVER FAILURE BEFORE TRANSPLANTATION

Despite the fact that nonspecific medical treatment will not cure acute liver failure, it has been suggested that the recent advances in the management of these patients may improve the outcome (O'Grady et al. 1989; Williams and Gimson 1991).

Table 15.4. *Outcome in relation with the quality of the graft. Experience at the Hepatobiliary Center at Paul Brousse Hospital*

	Graft without risk factors	Graft with 1–3 risk factors[a]
Patients (n)	74	54
1-year patient survival (%)	82	50[b]
Retransplantation before 1 year (%)	5.4	24
1-year graft survival (%)	79	35[b]

[a] Risk factors for the graft: blood group ABO incompatibility, size-reduction, poor quality graft.
[b] $P < 0.001$.

Table 15.5. *Overall survival of 152 patients referred to the Hepatobiliary Center at Paul Brousse Hospital from 1986 to 1994 with fulminant and subfulminant hepatitis who met the criteria for transplantation, related to the neurological status on admission*

	Encephalopathy stage III		Encephalopathy stage IV	
Neurological status on admission	Confusion	Coma Grade 1	Coma Grade 2	Coma Grade 3
Patients admitted (n)	24	35	50	43
Patients transplanted (%)	96	83	90	69[a]
Transplant patients alive at 1 year (%)	86	67	71	51
Referred patients alive at 1 year (%)	83	60	64	35[b]

[a] One recovered and survived without transplant.
[b] $P < 0.001$.

Patients should be monitored for glucose level, since they are exposed to hypoglycemia which can worsen cerebral function. It is necessary to maintain the glucose level by the administration of a minimal daily dose of 200 g carbohydrates.

Infection is frequent and should be searched for routinely by performing blood, urine and sputum cultures. Patients with acute liver failure are susceptible to bacteremias, septic shock, and fungal complications especially when liver failure is prolonged for several days (Rolando et al. 1990; Rolando et al. 1991). In our series and in the series from King's College in London, 26 percent of the patients developed bacteremia. In the series from King's College in London, 32 percent of the patients with acute liver failure developed fungal infections (Rolando et al. 1991). The prophylactic use of antimicrobial treatments in patients with ALF has been suggested by some authors. We routinely administer antimicrobial treatments against Gram-negative bacteria as soon as the patient is placed on mechanical ventilation. When liver failure persists for several days we add anti-fungal prophylactic therapy with amphotericin B intravenously or triflu-conazole.

A clinical neurologic examination has to be performed several times a day in order to classify the stage of encephalopathy and to assess for the appearance of clinical signs of intracranial hypertension. When signs of cerebral edema are present, intravenous mannitol, 0.5 g to 1 g/kg body weight/4 h can be used as first line therapy. When renal failure is present, mannitol can be deleterious. We use continuous venovenous hemofiltration or hemodialysis with polyacrylonitrile membranes (Hospal; Lyon, France) when mannitol is inefficient or deleterious. In addition, continuous venovenous hemofiltration can be used during the surgical procedure. Use of thiopental has been suggested for patients refractory to mannitol but has never been used in our center. Profound hypotension, which can be deleterious, has been described with the use of thiopental (Forbes et al. 1989). The monitoring of the intracranial pressure by using an intracranial sensor remains controversial (Schafer and Shaw 1989; Blei 1991; Donovan et al. 1992). For several teams, its use seems helpful in controlling intracranial pressure and maintaining cerebral perfusion pressure (the difference between the mean arterial pressure and the intracranial pressure) during the pre-, peri- and post-transplant phases (Blei 1991; Lidofsky 1992; Bismuth 1995). Some authors consider the cerebral perfusion pressure as a guide in the decision to transplant (Schafer and Shaw 1989; Lidofsky et al. 1992). Liver transplantation may be contraindicated if the cerebral perfusion pressure is below 40 mmHg for several hours (Schafer and Shaw 1989; Lidofsky et al. 1992; Ascher et al. 1993). In our experience, the monitoring of the intracranial pressure has not been used in making the decision to transplant, although it is used for the management of patients for the following reasons: there may be some discrepancies between the clinical symptoms and the degree of intracranial pressure (Hanid et al. 1980); during the surgical procedure under anesthesia, there are no reliable clinical symptoms and the intracranial pressure can vary during the various phases of the procedure (Keays et al. 1991) and after transplantation, brain death can still occur due to persistence of high intracranial pressures, and careful monitoring until the patient is fully awake seems warranted (Bismuth et al. 1987; Keays et al. 1991; Lidofsky et al. 1992; Bismuth et al. 1995). There are also difficulties in the use of intracerebral monitoring: it is an invasive method, and there is a risk of bleeding complications in these patients with major coagulation disorders; these sensors are not completely reliable; and the more reliable sensors (i.e. placed in a subdural or intraventricular position) are probably more dangerous in terms of hemorrhage (Blei et al. 1993). Thus, intracranial pressure monitoring remains controversial mainly because of the risk of severe complications. The Hepatology unit of Beaujon Hospital in Clichy does not use ICP monitoring, insisting that it is an invasive method which is possibly deleterious and without proven advantages (Bernuau et al. 1995). We consider intracranial pressure monitoring to be useful, and we currently use monitors in stage IV encephalopathy patients as soon as the patient is placed on mechanical ventilation. The insertion of the sensor is done in the ICU and should be done with extreme care because of the risk of bleeding. We recommend correction of the coagulation defects before insertion of the sensor and careful control of hemostasis at the insertion point. Like other centers, we currently are using fiberoptic catheters (Camino Laboratories, San Diego CA, USA) which are reliable and easier to use. We, like others (Blei et al. 1993), do not recommend placing the sensor in the intracerebral position and prefer an extradural one.

We avoid the use of sedative drugs prior to transplant so as not to modify the neurologic status or the criteria for indicating the need for liver transplantation. Sedatives are only used when the patient is on mechanical ventilation and cannot be adequately ventilated. The place of sedatives in the management of patients with acute liver failure is debatable. On the one hand, the administration of sedatives may decrease the intracranial pressure and protect the brain, while on the other hand it renders difficult the assessment of prognosis of the patient. We also do not administer fresh frozen plasma (FFP) or other plasma substitutes prior to transplant in order not to alter the level of coagulation factors since they remain one of the main criteria for decision making in liver transplantation. In addition, the risk of spontaneous bleeding is low. Thus, we administer FFP only before insertion of an intracerebral sensor or at the beginning of surgery.

Hemodynamic instability requiring the use of vasopressor drugs such as epinephrine or norepinephrine is generally the consequence of a profound vasodilatation or reflects recognized or unrecognized sepsis. In the presence of hemodynamic instability, the transplantation procedure can be performed with the use of vasopressor infusions, however, the risk of peri- or postoperative death is higher. Some teams have proposed, in these cases, performing a total hepatectomy with temporary portacaval anastomosis in order to improve the hemodynamic condition, hypothesizing that the necrotic liver is the source of toxins causing the shock. After performing the total hepatectomy (Ringe et al. 1988), the patient is placed again in the intensive care unit waiting for a liver graft. Some cases of hemodynamic improvement have been described, however, the postoperative mortality was high (Ringe et al. 1993) and the risk of postoperative death was related to the length of waiting time for the liver graft. The risk of such a procedure is that the patient will still die before a graft can be found. For this reason, the indication for this procedure remains controversial.

COURSE OF PATIENTS PRIOR TO TRANSPLANTATION

Some patients with acute liver failure referred for transplantation die before a transplant can be performed. Brain death occurred in our experience in 70 percent of those who died before transplantation, the other causes of death being sepsis, hemodynamic instability, multiple organ failure, and gastrointestinal bleeding. A few patients may improve before transplantation and can be removed from the waiting list. In our personal experience, improvement occurred in only one out of 152 patients who met criteria for liver transplantation. Thus, it is necessary to re-evaluate the clinical condition of the patient and the last laboratory test results once a donor is found, in order to determine whether a transplant is still indicated. However, as shown in Table 15.2, the clinical condition of all patients who met the criteria for transplantation except one either deteriorated or stabilized between the admission and transplantation.

PERIOPERATIVE MANAGEMENT

In order to correct the coagulation defects, fresh frozen plasma is administered at the beginning of the surgical procedure. It is necessary to maintain a balance between fluid restriction to avoid the increase of brain edema and maintenance of a satisfactory cerebral perfusion pressure. Due to fluid restriction, the clamping of the inferior vena cava and of the portal vein is often poorly tolerated and we advocate the routine use of venovenous bypass during the transplantation in acute liver failure patients in order to maintain a stable hemodynamic status. The venous outflow of the venovenous bypass should not be directed into the jugular vein because of the risk of increasing intracranial pressure but is inserted into the axillary vein. Typically, intracranial pressure increases at the initiation of the bypass and at the discontinuation of the bypass. Another technical solution is to perform a lateral clamping of the inferior vena cava and a temporary portacaval anastomosis during the surgical procedure without using venovenous bypass in order to maintain a stable hemodynamic condition (Belghiti et al. 1995). Patients with anuric renal failure can be transplanted; however, the risk of fluid overload is high and we use perioperative venovenous hemofiltration in these cases. Any rise in intracranial pressure should be treated during surgery.

The surgical procedure itself is generally easy: the coagulation defects can be corrected with infusion of fresh frozen plasma and platelets. The hepatectomy is facilitated because of the presence of a normal or atrophic liver and the absence of severe portal hypertension. However, some difficulties may appear with diffuse bleeding particularly in the absence of immediate graft function at revascularization or when a size-reduction is necessary (Bismuth and Houssin 1984). The combination of several factors such as graft reduction and massive steatosis may increase the risk of abdominal bleeding.

Until January 1994, most transplantations performed for acute liver failure worldwide and all of those in our center, were performed orthotopically. Our first case of liver transplantation for ALF was a heterotopic auxiliary graft which failed (Le Bihan et al. 1982), but successful cases of heterotopic (Metselaar et al. 1990) and auxiliary orthotopic transplantation (Gubernatis et al. 1991; Boudjema et al. 1993; Boudjema et al. 1995) (a procedure that requires partial hepatectomy of the original liver) have been reported. The authors postulated that the native liver would regenerate, with the graft acting as a temporary support. These approaches are interesting, but may have a number of drawbacks: the native liver does not always regenerate correctly, especially in patients with ALF; when hepatitis is due to hepatitis viruses, there is a risk of chronic viral persistence due to the immunosuppressive drugs; and there is only moderate portal hypertension in these patients, and as part of the portal flow must be derived to the graft, the loss of flow could negatively affect the regeneration of the native liver. The main disadvantage of these procedures is that heterotopic and auxiliary orthotopic liver transplantation are technically more difficult and may delay satisfactory graft function, whereas most of these patients do require a functional liver as soon as possible. Recent results have shown that auxiliary liver transplantation may be successful permitting removal of the graft and discontinuation of immunosuppressive therapy (Boudjema et al. 1995 and Chapter 17). However, this procedure may be deleterious in some patients, thus the exact place of auxiliary liver transplantation in the armamentarium of liver transplantation and the indications for this surgical technique should be defined in the future.

RESULTS OF LIVER TRANSPLANTATION FOR ACUTE LIVER FAILURE

Survival

Survival after transplantation for acute liver failure ranges between 50 and 75 percent in different series (Brems et al. 1987; Peleman et al. 1987; Vickers et al. 1988; O'Grady et al. 1989; Rakela et al. 1989; Muñoz et al. 1990; Devictor et al. 1992; Ascher et al. 1993). The actuarial one- and five-year survival rate for 128 patients transplanted between January 1986 and December 1994 at our center was 68 percent and 61 percent respectively (Bismuth et al. 1995) which should be compared to the one- and five-year survival of patients transplanted electively: 85 percent and 75 percent. In the European Liver Transplant Registry the one- and five-year survival was 59 percent and 53 percent respectively. This is much lower than the one- and five-year survival for patients transplanted for liver cirrhosis: 78 percent and 69 percent respectively (European Liver Transplant Registry). As observed in other series the postoperative mortality was high. The survival in our center was related to the condition of the patient at transplantation and to the quality of the graft. According to the grade of coma at admission, the one-year survival was higher in patients who were in encephalopathy stage III with confusion than in those who had encephalopathy stage IV with grade 3 coma (90 percent versus 48 percent, $P<0.05$) (Bismuth et al. 1995). According to the grade of coma at time of transplantation, the actuarial one year survival was 90 percent in the patients who were in encephalopathy stage III but not comatose, 76.9 percent in the patients who had grade 1 coma, 79 percent in the patients with grade 2 coma, and 54 percent in the patients with grade 3 coma ($P<0.05$ between all patients and $P<0.001$ between patients in coma grade 3 and others). Patient survival was not different with regard to etiology of the hepatitis, and was the same in patients transplanted for viral B or B–D hepatitis, drug-induced hepatitis, or hepatitis of indeterminate cause.

The one-year patient and graft survivals according to the quality of the graft are shown in Table 15.4. One-year survival of patients transplanted with an ABO-incompatible, compatible and identical graft was 52.9 percent, 64.7 percent and 76.9 percent, respectively ($P<0.05$ between incompatible and others). The one-year graft survival was 32.4 percent, 64.7 percent and 70.8 percent in ABO-incompatible, -compatible and -identical grafts, respectively ($P<0.001$). In a multivariate analysis, the use of reduced-size or partial liver graft (RR=3.76; $P<0.01$), or of a steatotic graft (RR=2.41; $P<0.05$) were independently predictive of a lower patient survival; grade 3 coma at admission was almost independently predictive of a lower patient survival (RR= 3.45; $P=0.10$), while all other parameters tested were not independently predictive of a lower survival. The use of reduced-size or partial liver graft (Bismuth et al. 1989) (RR= 2.79; $P<0.05$), of a steatotic graft (RR=2.01; $P<0.05$), or ABO blood group incompatibility (RR=2.22; $P<0.01$) were independently predictive of a lower graft survival. The presence of grade 3 coma at admission was almost independently predictive of lower graft survival (RR=2.9; $P=0.10$), while all the other parameters tested were not (Bismuth et al. 1995). It is debatable whether patients with severe coma should be transplanted, given their high post-transplant mortality, and some authors have argued against transplanting patients with cerebral perfusion pressure below 40 mmHg (Schafer and Shaw 1989; Lidofsky et al. 1992; Ascher et al. 1993). In our series, the one-year survival among patients transplanted when in grade 3 coma was 54 percent which is still reasonable considering the severity of their condition. In addition, it appears that complete neurologic recovery can occur even in the most severely ill patients. Our policy to use the first liver donor available even when of an ABO-incompatible group or of poor quality has permitted reduction of the waiting period so that the percentage of patients not transplanted was only 7 percent in recent years. It should, however, be balanced with the risk of nonfunction of a poor quality graft or of irreversible rejection of an ABO-incompatible graft. It is clear from Table 15.4 and from our multivariate analysis, that post-transplant morbidity and mortality was in part related to the quality of the graft and to the blood group compatibility between donor and recipient. In the European Liver Transplant Registry, ABO-incompatible liver transplantations were performed only for emergency cases. The one- and five-year graft survival was 53 percent and 44 percent in ABO-identical emergency transplantation, 51 percent and 44 percent in ABO-compatible emergency transplantations and was 33 percent and 24 percent in ABO-incompatible emergency liver transplantation ($P<0.001$) (European Liver Transplant Registry). Thus, all centers in Europe do not agree with the policy of giving an ABO-incompatible graft to a patient with ALF. In most European countries, use of ABO-incompatible grafts are authorized only for such emergency cases but some centers are still reluctant to do so for the above mentioned reasons.

In our experience, most of the deaths occurred in the first three postoperative months. The main causes of death during and after transplantation were brain death and sepsis. It should be noted that brain death can occur during the surgical procedure or occasionally in the immediate postoperative period. Once again, peri- and postoperative brain deaths are more frequent in patients transplanted in grade 3 coma than in patients with less severe grade of coma.

Sepsis is a main cause of death. This may be due to several causes: as described above, sepsis is common in patients with acute liver failure; patients in coma before transplantation often remain on mechanical ventilation after transplantation for several days, thus increasing the risk of sepsis; the length of ICU stay in fulminant and subfulminant hepatitis patients was longer than in the elective patients; and patients receiving ABO incompatible grafts generally receive higher dose of antirejection therapy which obviously increases the risk of sepsis.

Morbidity

Neurologic sequelae

Neurologic sequelae are sometimes observed after transplantation. This was only rarely described in patients with ALF who survived spontaneously before the era of liver transplantation (O'Brien et al. 1987). Neurologic sequelae can be minor such as memory defects or major including hemiplegia or severe mental deterioration. The neurologic complications may be the direct consequences of the severity of pretransplant coma, since they are more frequently seen in patients with grade 3 coma at transplantation (Ichai et al. 1995). The role of the surgical procedure by itself in the occurrence of these neurologic sequelae remains to be elucidated. Neurologic complications may be the result of the use of intracranial pressure monitoring devices (Blei 1993) since they can induce cerebral bleeding with extradural, subdural or intracerebral hematomas or provoke cerebral abscess formation. The rate of complications due to the sensor was 10 percent in our overall series but was drastically reduced: by the use of fiberoptic catheters permitting a 1–2 mm burr hole in place of a several centimeter burr hole required with other sensors; by correcting the coagulation defects before the insertion of the sensor; and by a procedure performed cautiously by a well trained surgeon involved in the care of these patients.

Sepsis

Sepsis is a frequent complication after liver transplantation for ALF for the reasons described above.

Retransplantation

In our series, the rate of retransplantation for acute liver failure was 13 percent versus 7 percent in the elective series. The main causes of retransplantation were acute rejection, primary graft nonfunction, and intrahepatic biliary strictures. This high rate of retransplantation was mostly due to the emergency conditions surrounding the transplant: the use of ABO incompatible grafts was responsible for a high rate of severe acute rejection episodes and for occurrence of biliary strictures in the graft (Gugenheim et al. 1990; Farges et al. 1995). In the selected group of patients transplanted with an ABO incompatible graft, the rate of retransplantation was 35 percent and the one year graft survival 30 percent. The use of steatotic grafts may also be a factor in the high rate of primary graft nonfunction (Adam et al. 1991). Many complications are related to the quality of the graft or to the graft compatibility. These severely ill patients need a very good graft so that they reverse their liver failure as quickly as possible; however, due to the emergency situation usually involved, they often receive the first liver available which increases the likelihood that it is of poor quality or ABO blood group incompatible.

Viral B recurrence after liver transplantation for fulminant hepatitis B

HBV recurrence can occur after transplantation for HBV ALF but the recurrence rate is much lower than that observed for patients transplanted for chronic liver disease due to HBV. In the multicenter European study, the rate of HBV recurrence was 50 percent in patients who did not receive anti-HBs immunoprophylaxis. The rate of HBV recurrence was 0 percent in the group of patients receiving long-term post-transplant passive immunoprophylaxis (Samuel et al. 1991; Samuel et al. 1993). In our experience, HBV recurrence was generally less severe than that seen in patients with HBV recurrence after transplantation for chronic HBV liver disease. However, most patients transplanted for fulminant hepatitis B who developed recurrence still have chronic liver disease in the graft, and this chronic course was probably facilitated by immunosuppressive therapy.

Viral B recurrence after liver transplantation for ALF due to co-infection B and delta or due to superinfection with delta virus

In the European multicenter study, the rate of HBV recurrence was 40 percent in patients transplanted for fulminant hepatitis due to HBV and delta virus, and this rate was higher than that observed in patients transplanted for chronic liver disease due to hepatitis delta infection (32 percent) (Samuel et al. 1993). In this study, it was impossible to differentiate patients with co-infection B-delta and superinfection with the delta virus. In our own series, patients with fulminant B-delta hepatitis receiving anti-HBs immunoprophylaxis had a 25 percent rate of HBV recurrence.

Quality of life and long term survival

The quality of life of the ALF survivors who are transplanted is generally good and seems similar to that of patients transplanted for chronic liver disease. The majority of the younger patients will return to a normal social life and to work. However, psychological troubles can be observed in the early postoperative period and are thought to be related to pretransplant encephalopathy and to the fact that these patients have not been prepared psychologically for transplantation in contrast to patients transplanted for chronic liver disease. In addition, some patients with ALF have severe social problems before transplantation. Many ALF patients with hepatitis B or B- combined with delta infection were drug-addicts and there is a risk of recidivism of drug addiction. Patients transplanted for ALF due to acetaminophen overdose also may be at risk of attempting suicide again after transplantation. Still other patients have been transplanted for ALF due to antidepressants. All these patients should receive intensive psychological support in the post-transplant period.

Long term survival after transplantation for acute liver failure has been generally good. There are few deaths observed after one year; in our own series, there was only a 7 percent decline of survival between one and five years post-transplantation. This is due in part to the young age of the patients, and the low rate of recurrence of the initial liver disease.

FUTURE

Dramatic improvement in the feasibility and in the results of transplantation have occurred since the first emergency liver transplants were performed for ALF: the most experienced centers are able to transplant successfully patients who were in the past not considered for transplantation: patients in hemodynamic shock, anuric patients, patients with uncontrolled sepsis, and patients with a more severe grade of coma; national organizations for organ sharing have developed in most countries and in Europe, a specific program for these patients has led to the creation of a high priority waiting list. However, stabilization of the survival curve after transplantation of the more critically ill patients is observed. Indeed, the improvement of the results published in some series are more the consequence of selecting the more favorable cases and excluding high risk patients than the consequence of a real improvement of the medical care of these patients. In addition, with the increasing shortage of organs, the tendency of many centers is to avoid liver transplantation in the most severely ill patients. One of the key reasons for the absence of improvement in results is our inability to protect the brain from cerebral edema over a long period of time. In fact, all the available therapeutic measures we have used provide only a transient decrease in intracranial pressure. For all these reasons, the place of bioartificial livers (Rozga et al. 1993; Sussman et al. 1992), of hepatocyte transplantation, or of xenotransplantation should be evaluated in the future for the management of patients with acute liver failure.

REFERENCES

Adam, R., Reynes, M., Johann, M., Astarcioglu, I., Kafetzis, I., Castaing, D. and Bismuth, H. 1991. The outcome of steatotic grafts in liver transplantation. *Transpl Proc* 23: 1538–40.

Ascher, N., Lake, J.R., Emond, J.C. and Roberts, J.P. 1993. Liver transplantation for fulminant hepatic failure. *Arch Surg* 128: 677–82.

Belghiti, J., Noun, R. and Sauvanet, A. 1995. Temporary portocaval anastomosis with preservation of caval flow during orthotopic liver transplantation. *Am J Surg* 169: 277–9.

Benhamou, J.P. 1991. Fulminant and subfulminant liver failure: definition and causes. In *Acute Liver Failure: Improved Understanding and Better Therapy*, eds. R. Williams and R.D. Hughes, 6–10. London UK: Miter Press.

Bernuau, J., Goudeau, A., Poynard, T., Dubois, F., Lesage, G., Yvonnet, B., Degott, C., Bezeaud, A., Rueff, B. and Benhamou, J.P. 1986. Multivariate analysis of prognostic factors in fulminant hepatitis B. *Hepatology* 6: 648–51.

Bernuau, J., Rueff, B. and Benhamou, J.P. 1986. Fulminant and subfulminant liver failure: definition and causes. *Sem Liver Dis* 6: 97–106.

Bernuau, J., Samuel, D., Durand, F. et al. 1991. Criteria for emergency liver transplantation in patients with acute viral hepatitis and factor V below 50 percent of normal: a prospective study. *Hepatology* 14: 49A (Abstract).

Bernuau, J., Durand, F., Werner, P., Sauanet, A., Erlinger, S., Benhamou, J.P. and Belghiti, J. 1995. Management of patients with fulminant or subfulminant hepatic failure (FSLF) without intracranial pressure monitoring (ICPM): A 4-year prospective study. *Liver Transpl Surg* 1: 436 (Abstract).

Bismuth, H. and Houssin, D. 1984. Reduced-sized orthotopic liver graft in hepatic transplantation in children. *Surgery* 95: 367–70.

Bismuth, H., Samuel, D., Gugenheim, J., Castaing, D., Bernuau, J., Rueff, B. and Benhamou, J.P. 1987. Emergency liver transplantation for fulminant hepatitis. *Ann Intern Med* 107: 337–41.

Bismuth, H., Morino, M., Castaing, D., Gillon, M.C., Descorps Descleres, A., Saliba, F. and Samuel, D. 1989. Emergency liver transplantation in 2 patients with one donor liver. *Br J Surg* 76: 722–4.

Bismuth, H., Samuel, D., Castaing, D., Adam, R., Saliba, F., Johan, M., Azoulay, D., Ducot, B. and Chiche, L. 1995. Orthotopic liver transplantation in fulminant and subfulminant hepatitis. The Paul Brousse experience. *Ann Surg* 222: 109–19.

Blei, A.T. 1991. Cerebral edema and intracranial hypertension in acute liver failure: distinct aspects of the same problem. *Hepatology* 13: 376–9.

Blei, A.T., Olafson, S., Webster, S. and Levy, R. 1993. Complications of intracranial pressure monitoring in fulminant hepatic failure. *Lancet* 341: 157–8.

Boudjema, K., Jaeck, D., Simeoni, U., Bientz, J., Chenard, M.P. and Brunot, P. 1993. Temporary auxiliary liver transplantation for subacute liver failure in a child. *Lancet* 342: 778–9.

Boudjema, K., Cherqui, D., Jaeck, D., Chenard-Neu, M.P., Steib, A., Freis, G., Becmeur, F., Brunot, B., Simeoni, U., Bellocq, J.P., Tempe, J.D., Wolf, P. and Cinqualbre, J. 1995. Auxiliary liver transplantation for fulminant and subfulminant hepatic failure. *Transplantation* 59: 218–23.

Brems, J.J., Hiatt, J.R., Ramming, K.P., Quinones-Baldrich, W.J. and Bussutil, R.W. 1987. Fulminant hepatic failure: The role of liver transplantation as primary therapy. *Am J Surg* 154: 137–41.

Castells, A., Salmeron, J.M., Navasa, M., Rimola, A., Salo, J., Andreu, H., Mas, A. and Rodes, J. 1993. Liver transplantation for acute liver failure: analysis of applicability. *Gastroenterology* 105: 532–8.

Devictor, D., Desplanques, L., Debray, D., Ozier, Y., Dubousset, A.M., Valayer, J., Houssin, D., Bernard, O. and Huault, G. 1992. Emergency liver transplantation for fulminant liver failure in infants and children. *Hepatology* 16: 1156–62.

Donovan, J.P., Shaw, B.W., Langnas, A.N. and Sorrell, M.F. 1992. Brain water and acute liver failure: the emerging role of intracranial pressure monitoring. *Hepatology* 16: 267–8.

Ellis, A.J., Saleh, M., Smith, H., Portmann, B., Gimson, A. and Williams, R. 1995. Late onset hepatic failure: clinical features, serology and outcome following transplantation. *J. Hepatol* 23: 363–72.

Emond, J.C., Aran, P.P., Whitington, P.F., Broelsch, C.E. and Baker, A.L. 1989. Liver transplantation in the management of fulminant hepatic failure. *Gastroenterology*. 96: 1583–8.

European Liver Transplant Registry Report: 5/1968–12/1994. Hopital Paul Brousse, Villejuif, France. 1995.

Farges, O., Kalil, A., Samuel, D., Saliba, F., Arulnaden, J.L., Debat, P., Bismuth, A., Castaing, D. and Bismuth, H. 1995. The use of ABO incompatible grafts in liver transplantation: a life saving procedure in highly selected patients. *Transplantation* 59: 1124–33.

Feray, C., Gigou, M., Samuel, D., Reyes, G., Bernuau, J., Reynes, M., Bismuth, H. and Brechot, C. 1993. Hepatitis C virus RNA and hepatitis B virus DNA in serum and liver of patients with fulminant hepatitis. *Gastroenterology* 104: 549–55.

Forbes, A., Alexander, G.J.M., O'Grady, J.G., Keays, R., Gullan, R., Dawling, S. and Williams, R. 1989. Thiopental infusion in the treatment of intracranial hypertension complicating fulminant hepatic failure. *Hepatology* 10: 306–10.

Gimson, A.E.S., O'Grady, J.G., Ede, R.J., Portmann, B. and Williams, R. 1986. Late onset hepatic failure: clinical, serological and histological features. *Hepatology* 6: 288–94.

Gubernatis, G., Pichlmayr, R., Kemnitz, J. and Gratz, K. 1991. Auxiliary partial orthotopic liver transplantation (APOLT) for fulminant hepatic failure: first successful case report. *World J Surg* 15: 660–6.

Gugenheim, J., Samuel, D., Reynes, M. and Bismuth, H. 1990. Liver transplantation across ABO blood group barriers. *Lancet* 336: 519–23.

Hanid, M.A., Davies, M., Mellon, P.J., Silk, D.B.A., Strunin, L., McCabe, J.J. and Williams, R. 1980. Clinical monitoring of intracranial pressure in fulminant hepatic failure. *Gut* 21: 866–9.

Ichai, P., Samuel, D., Chemouilly, P., Saliba, F., Azoulay, D. and Bismuth, H. 1995. Severe neurological sequelae after liver transplantation for fulminant hepatitis. *Liver Transpl Surg* 1: 435 (Abstract).

Iwatzuki, S., Esquivel, C.O., Gordon, R.D., Shaw, B.W., Jr. and Starzl, T.E. 1985. Liver transplantation for fulminant hepatic failure. *Sem Liver Dis* 5: 325–8.

Keays, R., Potter, D., O'Grady, J., Peachey, T., Alexander, G. and Williams, R. 1991. Intracranial and cerebral perfusion pressure changes before, during and immediately after orthotopic liver transplantation

for fulminant hepatic failure. *Quart J Med* 289: 425–33.
Le Bihan, G., Coquerel, A., Houssin, D., Bourreille, J., Szekely, A.M., Bismuth, H., Hemet, J. and Samson, M. 1982. Insuffisance hépatique aigüe mortelle au cours d'un traitement par le valproate de sodium. *Gastroenterol Clin Biol* 6: 477–81.
Lidofsky, S.D., Bass, N.M., Prager, M.C., Washington, D.E., Read, A.E., Wright, T.L., Ascher, N.L., Roberts, J.P., Scharschmidt, B.F. and Lake, J.R. 1992. Intracranial pressure monitoring and liver transplantation for fulminant hepatic failure. *Hepatology* 16: 1–7.
Metselaar, H.J., Hesselink, E.J., De Rave S., Ten Kate, F.J.W., Lameris, J.S., Groenland, T.H.N., Reuvers, C.B., Weimar, W., Terpstra, O.T. and Schalm, S. 1990. Recovery of failing liver after auxiliary heterotopic transplantation. *Lancet* 335: 1156–7.
Muñoz, S.J., Moritz, M., Martin, P. et al. 1990. Liver transplantation for fulminant hepatic failure. *Hepatology* 12: 1019.
O'Brien, C.J., Wise, R.J., O'Grady, J.G. and Williams, R. 1987. Neurological sequelae in patients recovered from fulminant hepatic failure. *Gut* 28: 93–5.
O'Grady, J., Gimson, A.E.S., O'Brien, C.J., Pucknell, A., Hughes, R.D. and Williams, R. 1988. Controlled trials of charcoal hemoperfusion and prognostic factors in fulminant hepatic failure. *Gastroenterology* 94: 1186–92.
O'Grady, J.G., Alexander, G.J.M., Thick, M., Potter, D., Calne, R.Y. and Williams, R. 1988. Outcome of orthotopic liver transplantation in the etiological and clinical variants of acute liver failure. *Quart J Med* New Series 69: 817–24.
O'Grady, J.G., Alexander, G.J.M., Hayllar, K.M. and Williams, R. 1989. Early indicators of prognosis in fulminant hepatic failure. *Gastroenterology* 97: 439–45.
O'Grady, J.G., Hambley, H. and Williams, R. 1991. Prothrombin time in fulminant hepatic failure. *Gastroenterology* 100: 1480–1.
O'Grady, J.G., Schalm, S.W. and Williams, R. 1993. Acute liver failure: redefining the syndromes. *Lancet* 342: 273–5.
Pauwels, A., Mostefa-Kara, N., Florent, C. and Levy, V.G. 1993. Emergency liver transplantation for acute liver failure. Evaluation of London and Clichy criteria. *J Hepatol* 17: 124–7.
Peleman, R.R., Gavaler, J.S., Van Thiel, D.H., Esquivel, C., Gordon, R., Iwatzuki, S. and Starzl, T.E. 1987. Orthotopic liver transplantation for acute or subacute hepatic failure in adults. *Hepatology* 7: 484–9.
Rakela, J., Perkins, J.D., Gross, J.B. et al. 1989. Acute hepatic failure: the emerging role of orthotopic liver transplantation. *Mayo Clin Proc* 64: 424–8.
Ringe, B., Pichlmayr, R., Lauchart, W. and Muller, R. 1986. Indications and results of liver transplantation in acute hepatic failure. *Transpl Proc* 18: 86–8.
Ringe, B., Pichlmayr, R., Lubbe, N., Bornscheuer, A. and Kuse, E. 1988. Total hepatectomy as temporary approach to acute hepatic or primary graft failure. *Transpl Proc* 1(Suppl 1): 552–7.
Ringe, B., Lubbe, N., Kuse, E., Frei, U. and Pichlmayr, R. 1993. Total hepatectomy and liver transplantation as a two-stage procedure. *Ann Surg* 218: 3.
Rolando, N., Harvey, F., Brahm, J., Philpott-Howard, J., Alexander, G., Gimson, A., Casewell, M., Fagan, E. and Williams, R. 1990. Prospective study of bacterial infection in acute liver failure: an analysis of fifty patients. *Hepatology* 11: 49–53.
Rolando, N., Harvey, F., Brahm, J., Philpott-Howard, J., Alexander, G., Gimson, A., Casewell, M., Fagan, E. and Williams, R. 1991. Fungal infections: a common, unrecognised complication of acute liver failure. *J. Hepatol* 12: 1–9.
Rozga, J., Williams, F., Ro, M.S., Neuzil, D.F., Giorgio, T.D., Backfisch, G., Moscioni, A.D., Hakim, R. and Demetriou, A.A. 1993. Development of a bioartificial liver: properties and function of a hollow-fiber module inoculated with liver cells. *Hepatology* 17: 258–65.
Samuel, D., Bismuth, A., Mathieu, D., Arulnaden, J.L., Reynes, M., Benhamou, J.P., Brechot, C. and Bismuth, H. 1991. Passive immunoprophylaxis after liver transplantation in HBsAg positive patients. *Lancet* 337: 813–15.
Samuel, D., Muller, R., Alexander, G., Fassati, L., Ducot, B., Benhamou, J.P., Bismuth, H. and the European Concerted Action on Viral Hepatitis (EUROHEP). 1993. Liver transplantation in European patients with the Hepatitis B surface antigen. *N Engl J Med* 329: 1842–7.
Schafer, D.F. and Shaw, B.W. 1989. Fulminant hepatic failure and orthotopic liver transplantation. *Sem Liver Dis* 9: 189–94.
Sussman, N.L., Chong, M.G., Koussayer, T., He, D.E., Shang, T.A., Whsenhand, H.H. and Kelly, J.H. 1992. Reversal of fulminant hepatic failure using an extracorporeal liver assist device. *Hepatology* 16: 60–5.
Trey, C. and Davidson, C.S. 1970. The management of fulminant hepatic failure. In *Progress in Liver Diseases*, Vol. 3, eds. H. Popper and F. Schaffner, 282–98. New York: Grune and Stratton, and London: Heinemann.
Van Thiel, D.H. 1993. When should a decision to proceed with transplantation actually be made in cases of fulminant or subfulminant hepatic failure: at admission to hospital or when a donor organ is made available? *J Hepatol* 17: 1–2.
Vickers, C., Neuberger, J., Buckels, J., McMaster, P. and Elias, E. 1988. Transplantation of the liver in adults and children with fulminant hepatic failure. *J Hepatol* 7: 143–50.
Ware, A.J., D'Agostino, A. and Combes, B. 1971. Cerebral edema: a major complication of massive hepatic necrosis. *Gastroenterology* 61: 877–84.
Williams, R. and Gimson, A.E. 1984. An assessment of orthotopic liver transplantation in acute liver failure. *Hepatology* 4: 22S–24S.
Williams, R. and Gimson, A.E.S. 1991. Intensive liver care and management of acute hepatic failure. *Dig Dis Sci* 36: 820–6.

16 Transplantation for acute liver failure: the American experience

Byers W. Shaw Jr

INTRODUCTION

For the patient in deep coma secondary to acute liver failure (ALF), liver transplantation offers the best chance for survival. As discussed elsewhere in this book, the prognosis of acute liver failure is highly dependent on many variables, including patient age and the etiology of liver failure. Nevertheless, when a patient progresses to deep stage III coma, the prognosis without transplantation in the absence of effective artificial support is grave.

The first American reports of liver transplantation for the treatment of acute hepatic failure were not very encouraging (Friend et al. 1989; Iwatsuki et al. 1989; Iwatsuki et al. 1985). Patients in these early series with acute liver failure had a one year probability of survival of about 50 percent, substantially lower than the 65–75 percent reported for those with chronic liver disease. For the most part, this high mortality was related to several factors, including late referral and an inability to identify those patients who, at the time of transplantation, had already suffered irreversible brain injury from the cerebral edema associated with acute liver failure.

INTRACRANIAL PRESSURE MONITORS

In 1986, based on previous experience with acute liver failure (Ede and Williams 1986) and with management of Reye's syndrome (Venes et al. 1978), we began using intracranial pressure (ICP) monitoring in the care of patients with acute liver failure (Schafer and Shaw 1989). In the first 31 of these patients, cerebral intracranial pressure monitor data was collected, but not used for selection of patients. Retrospective review of these data revealed that those patients who had a sustained cerebral perfusion pressure lower than 40 mmHg for two hours or more either did not awaken following liver transplantation, or had devastating permanent neurologic injuries. This led us to define this parameter (viz., cerebral perfusion pressure (CPP) <40 mmHg for two hours or more) as a contraindication to liver transplantation. In our subsequent experience with 30 additional patients, all patients awoke following transplantation with only one suffering permanent neurologic injury. However, 10 patients were excluded from transplantation on the basis of low CPP and all of these patients died. There is no evidence that the monitoring of ICP improved the survival of patients with ALF. Rather, it appeared to prevent futile transplantation of patients with irreversible cerebral injury. Furthermore, these data represent a relatively limited experience and may be specific for the use of the LADD extradural monitor for measuring ICP. Extreme caution must be exercised when extending these lessons to the use of other types of ICP monitoring devices. Even more vital to the proper use of any such device is a thorough understanding of the pitfalls associated with the technique, the potential source of erroneous readings and, most relevant, the need to carefully correlate CPP data with other clinical measures of the patient's status. In all cases, we have never abandoned the care of a patient with acute liver failure based on concerns over cerebral status until we had documented unequivocal evidence of brain death.

RAPID DONOR AVAILABILITY: THE KEY TO SUCCESS

Increasingly, others have used intracranial pressure monitoring both to aid perioperative management of patients with cerebral edema and for selection of transplant candidates (Lidofsky et al. 1992; Potter et al. 1989). However, all of these studies reveal the same problem: that early treatment is the key to improving survival with liver transplantation for acute liver failure. The report from the University of California, San Francisco, underscores this dramatically (Ascher et al. 1993). In this series, 35 patients underwent 42 liver transplants for treatment of acute liver failure, and 8 additional patients underwent transplantation for subacute liver failure. With follow-ups ranging from one to 60 months, this group was able to obtain a remarkable 92 percent actuarial one year survival in patients with acute liver failure and 100 percent actuarial survival in those with subacute failure, better survival probabilities than those obtained in their more stable group of chronic patients. The median waiting time for a donor organ in this series was an enviable 42 h, and 28 of the group received donor livers within one to three days of listing for transplantation. The incidence of permanent neurologic injury in the patients was low with only two adults experiencing mild problems long-term. The causes of death included sepsis in two patients and primary nonfunction of the allograft in a third. Two of seven patients with acute type B hepatitis developed recurrence, one patient with non-A non-B non-C hepatitis developed post-transplant type B hepatitis and one patient with an original diagnosis of type A hepatitis developed hepatitis C following transplantation.

This paper emphasizes several important principles: rapid treatment improves the results of liver transplantation for acute liver failure, leading to survival probabilities that potentially could exceed those achieved for patients with chronic liver disease; even with comparatively rapid availability of donor organs, some patients will be excluded from treatment and die, largely the result of delays in treatment; recurrence of type B hepatitis after transplantation for acute hepatitis is relatively infrequent and likely does not represent the same threat as after transplantation for chronic hepatitis.

What remains unanswered is the overall effectiveness of liver transplantation for the treatment of acute liver failure. We do not know, for instance, the number or fate of patients with acute liver failure who were excluded from transplantation by these authors. The authors themselves acknowledge the potential criticism that they may have been too selective, but offer the severe shortage of donor organs as justification.

ACUTE VS. CHRONIC LIVER FAILURE: TREATMENT DECISIONS

A comparison between the manifestations of acute liver failure with those of advanced, end stage chronic liver disease defines an important difference between urgent need and high risk. These are important differences worth examining when considering the allocation of precious donor organs.

By definition, patients with acute liver failure have generally been well within a few weeks of presentation. As such, they are usually well nourished, have intact immune mechanisms, and do not suffer from any of the stigmata, physiological or psychological, of chronic illness. In contrast, patients with advanced chronic liver disease are severely malnourished with profoundly abnormal immune responses, and with virtually all of the stigmata of chronic disease including weakness, depression and longstanding disability. Once coma has progressed to the point that the patient is minimally responsive to noxious stimuli, the course for either patient is likely to be rapidly downhill. In this setting, the patient with acute liver failure is likely to die, if untreated, from cerebral edema. The chronic liver patient, on the other hand, often has sepsis as an underlying cause of the clinical deterioration and will probably die with associated multiorgan failure even if transplantation is performed.

As amply demonstrated by past experience, rapid and early treatment of the patient with acute liver failure, even in the face of deep coma, carries a high probability of success. This is not the case for the patient with chronic liver failure that progresses to deep coma. In development of the RISK scoring system in Pittsburg in 1985, Stage III or IV encephalopathy in association with chronic liver disease was shown to be associated with a very high risk of mortality following transplantation (Shaw et al. 1985). In fact, among the patients in such condition studied in that report, only a few patients whose age was <20 years survived transplantation, suggesting that coma in association with advanced chronic liver disease might be considered a contraindication to transplantation.

The essential point is that coma, if the result of acute liver failure, represents a much different clinical situation than coma attending chronic liver disease. In the former case, coma implies an urgent need for transplantation. When attending advanced chronic liver disease, deep encephalopathy implies great risk of mortality following transplantation, perhaps in part owing to the likelihood that sepsis is an underlying etiologic factor of the observed deterioration. In the latter instance, rather than urgent transplantation, the patient would more properly benefit from aggressive support measures designed to correct the underlying cause of the deterioration.

ROUTINE MANAGEMENT (AND SEVEN HOMILIES)

In evaluating the comatose patient with acute liver failure, very few clinical variables are useful for predicting neurologic recovery following successful transplantation (Schafer and Shaw 1989). Specifically, we have not found computerized tomographic scanning (CT scan), electroencephalogram (EEG), or clinical examination to be of prognostic value (with the exception of an isoelectric EEG or a CT scan documenting uncal herniation). In fact, even in the presence of a profoundly abnormal EEG, complete unresponsiveness on clinical examination and severe loss of gray-white matter distinction on CT scan, patients have recovered full neurologic function following liver transplantation. Thus, we have not found EEG or CT scanning to be a useful monitoring tool, and only repeat them if indicated by clinical condition (e.g., to look for seizure activity or to investigate the etiology of new focal neurologic findings, sudden increases in ICP or to look for evidence of cerebral death).

More recently, we have tested the usefulness of transcranial Doppler ultrasound (TCD) for real-time monitoring of cerebral blood flow in patients with acute liver failure and coma (Sidi and Mahla 1995). Our experience to date remains unpublished and largely anecdotal, however. We have been impressed that: TCD does not add appreciably to the information already provided by ICP monitoring data; the TCD does not appear to show significant diminution of cerebral flow until markedly abnormal CPPs (<40 mmHg) have been observed; and TCD provides confirmatory evidence to that provided by CPP data when the patient develops significant cerebral ischemia. Thus, despite our hopes, we have not found that TCD can replace ICP as a sensitive yet noninvasive indication of changing cerebral blood flow.

The routine measures for management of the patient with acute liver failure deserve re-emphasizing in light of common clinical experience at most busy transplant centers (Table 16.1). These measures are directed toward prevention of the most common causes of morbidity and death in these patients, viz. sepsis, respiratory embarrassment from aspiration, bleeding in association with coagulopathy, acid–base and electrolyte disturbances, hyperosmolality and cerebral edema. Careful and frequently repetitive attention to these matters will buy valuable time necessary to obtain a donor organ needed for definitive liver transplantation.

Experience with these patients has led to the development of other caveats that may be useful to the clinician.

1. Whenever in doubt about the patient's ability to protect his/her own airway, secure endotracheal intubation immediately. This advice should be passed on in the clearest terms possible to the referring center when the patient is to be transferred since many cases of airway misadventure occur during transportation and are related to inadequate airway control.
2. In the case of acetaminophen (paracetamol) overdose, if the patient is still salvageable at the time of presentation, never assume it is too late to administer *N*-acetylcysteine. In the US, most of these cases will recover if treated early and aggressively, even in spite of blood levels that popular nomograms suggest are associated with a poor prognosis.
3. Be very wary of the ICP that changes rapidly or that does not appear to change at all. The epidural models (LADD) of ICP monitors, found to be most popular for use in patients with liver failure because of their lower risk of bleeding and infection, are notorious in the neurosurgery community for their propensity to give false readings related to fluid (blood or serum) accumulation around the sensor. Any sudden change may be related to just such a problem, as may an unwavering ICP value. Periodic inspection, even replacement may be necessary if the patient is maintained with ICP monitoring for days.
4. In most cases, it is advisable to journey to the operating room to place the ICP monitor. Better light, better coagulators and better sterility are benefits that we believe make the operating room a better place than the intensive care unit (ICU) for this procedure. We have not had any clinically significant bleeding complications or infections in over seven years, and nearly 75 cases of the use of ICP monitors for the management of patients with acute liver failure and cerebral edema.
5. In reality, many patients who progress from sleepiness to severe agitation require sedation in order to protect them from themselves. Unfortunately, this often results in changing a patient from late Stage II to Stage III or IV encephalopathy and effectively eliminates mental status examination as a useful tool for assessing the progress of liver failure. In such instances, early placement of an ICP monitor may need to be considered if one wants to observe the earliest signs of cerebral edema in order to initiate early treatment.
6. Despite fairly common understanding of the differences between encephalopathy associated with acute versus chronic liver disease, there appears to exist a great temptation to administer large doses of lactulose, neomycin or other purgatives to the patient with acute liver failure whose stage of encephalopathy is progressing. In addition to not offering any lasting improvements in the patient's state of awareness in acute liver failure, these measures may further complicate the management if abdominal distention results. This is particularly worrisome in the sleepy patient who is not yet intubated but who may not have normal gag reflexes.
7. In the crush to provide the most advanced measures for managing liver failure and cerebral edema, do not overlook the more mundane but nonetheless important routine care matters designed to prevent bed sores, catheter infections, upper airway damage (particularly in small children), Cushing's (stress) ulcers, malnutrition and skin breakdown at puncture sites.

THE DECISIONS TO TRANSFER AND TO TRANSPLANT

Aside from the issues of routine management, the clinician faced with caring for a patient with acute liver failure may face another decision: when to transfer the patient to a transplant center. The easy answer, and one offered by someone working at a transplant center, is: "immediately." But this answer begs the real question being asked, viz. what are the indications and contraindications to transplantation in acute liver failure? I have

Table 16.1. *Initial protocol for acute liver failure patients admitted to a transplant unit*

1. Admit to the intensive care unit.
2. Oral–tracheal intubation for stage II or worse coma or if need for sedation arises.
3. Notify blood bank, laboratory, and consultants (e.g. pulmonology, nephrology, neurology, hematology, neurosurgery) of patient's condition and projected needs.
4. Draw blood for diagnostic serologic and drug testing.
5. Order routine diagnostic blood tests: liver profile and blood cultures every 12 h, blood count and electrolytes every 6 h.
6. Institute bedside profile of neurologic status.
7. Electroencephalogram (EEG) and computed tomography (CT) head scan.
8. Avoid corticosteroid and sedative-hypnotic drug administration.
9. Give vitamin K, prophylactic antibiotics and sufficient H_2-blocker to maintain gastric pH above 5.0.
11. Patients in stage III or IV coma are taken to surgery for placement of a Ladd epidural pressure monitor.
12. If pressure measurements indicate the presence of cerebral edema, the following therapeutic measures are taken in sequence: raise the head of the bed 30–45 degrees; hyperventilate to P_{CO_2} 30 torr; give mannitol if serum osmolality <320 mOsm/l; administer pentobarbital for resistant intracranial hypertension. [Cerebral perfusion pressure (CPP) = mean arterial pressure, (MAP) minus intracranial pressure (ICP).] Maintain CPP >50–60 mmHg.

already stressed the importance of encephalopathy, stating that any patient who develops late stage III or worse coma should be considered a potential candidate. This is primarily based on the observation that the mortality without transplantation exceeds that following transplantation in most cases that progress to deep coma. Nonetheless, equally important considerations include the etiology of liver failure and the age of the patient. In younger patients with acetaminophen poisoning, recovery is the norm even when deep coma develops. However, the progression of acidosis and continued decreases in CPP should prompt one to move forward with transplantation. In contrast, most patients with acute viral hepatitis and a rapid progression to Stage IV coma will not recover without transplantation. The more difficult decision point would involve, for example, a 55-year-old with acetaminophen overdose and a history of some alcohol abuse who laspes into unresponsiveness. Spontaneous recovery seems less likely than in the 20-year-old college student who took too much acetaminophen over a 48 hour period to treat symptoms of a cold, even if total exposure to the toxin is equivalent. A similar dilemma is presented by the 40-year-old woman who presents with two weeks of progressive jaundice in stage II coma, mild coagulopathy, and mild mixed-etiology renal dysfunction with mild acidosis.

Elsewhere in this text, much more scientific information is presented to suggest the value of corroborating laboratory and clinical tests in guiding the difficult decisions regarding when to transfer or transplant the patient. To provide better insight into what we often face at the receiving end in a transplant center, I offer the following step-by-step outline of a normal progression from initial referral to completion of treatment.

1. Community physician calls transplant center describing a 35-year-old high school football coach with 10 days history of progressive jaundice following a flu-like illness. The patient is oriented but somewhat sleepy. He has been vomiting for three days and the physician is considering parenteral nutrition. The prothrombin time is slightly elevated and the patient has a mild metabolic acidosis as indicated by a serum bicarbonate level of 19 mmol/l. The physician has admitted the patient to the hospital, drawn the appropriate serological tests screening for hepatitis A, B and C. He is seeking advice regarding management and whether a transfer is appropriate. The former questions are more easily answered than the latter, yet the latter depends on what the response is to advice about the former! In short, one can usually get an immediate sense regarding how early in the course the patient should be transferred based upon the response on the other end to the litany of suggestions one might have for management.

The following criteria would lead us to recommend early transfer to the transplant center for a patient in this stage of evolution: the referring center is located at a distance from the transplant center that dictates more than one hour travel time by whatever means are available; the preference of the referring physician, indicated either by hesitancy to handle the variety of problems likely to develop or, less likely, by a direct request; the course of deterioration has been noticeable over a period of hours rather than days.

2. If a decision is made not to transfer the patient, then a plan must be made to establish frequent return communications with the referring center on a twice or three-times daily basis until either the patient's condition improves or shows clear signs of progression.
3. The patient is always transferred to the transplant center once the patient enters the later phase of stage II encephalopathy. If the patient becomes increasingly agitated, he will need to be sedated. As stated before, once the need for protective sedation arises, mental status examination becomes unavailable as a useful tool to monitor the course of liver failure. In the initial discussions with the referring physician, the decision regarding the timing of transfer must take into account the capacity of the referring center to manage a patient who becomes increasingly agitated, including the ability to recognize the need for early endotracheal intubation. The arrival at the transplant center of a heavily sedated patient who has been aspirating gastric contents during a one-hour transfer ride represents a particularly disheartening specter to the receiving transplant team.
4. Once the patient arrives, he is admitted to the intensive care unit. Based upon an initial examination of both the patient and his records, we try to make a decision regarding whether to place the patient on the transplant waiting list within the first hour. In reality, with the exception of patients with acetaminophen poisoning, we have rarely seen patients present to our center in whom the question regarding the need for transplantation is difficult. This may be related to the fact that we are geographically distant from many of the centers from which these patients have come, and to the fact that the care of liver failure patients in many areas of the country has improved dramatically in the last several years, leading to both more timely referral (i.e. not too late) and fewer unnecessary referrals. More often, the real issue facing us is whether the patient has a contraindication to transplantation. When the etiology of liver failure is not yet known at the time of transfer, most of the initial few hours after arrival is spent determining what the most likely etiologies are. Provided the differential diagnosis does not include an infectious disease or malignancy (masquerading as acute liver failure alone) that will likely affect other organ systems in a lethal manner, we will almost always place the patient on the waiting list soon after arrival. Note that there is an important difference between the decision to "list" the patient and the decision to perform the transplant.
5. The patient is reassessed frequently and managed as outlined elsewhere. The decision about transplantation is not relevant until a donor organ is referred specifically for the patient. A brief explanation of current organ distribution policies seems in order.

Allocation of donor organs in the United States is controlled by the United Network for Organ Sharing (UNOS) and is based on a "points" system. Patients on the list accumulate points based on blood group compatibility with potential donors, total waiting time on the list, and medical urgency. When a donor organ becomes available, the organ procurement officer at the donor center enters (via remote link) the blood type, height and weight of the donor into the UNOS central computer database in Richmond, Virginia. The UNOS computer then matches these characteristics with all of the potential recipients based on the acceptable weight range and blood type which the transplant centers have listed for their candidates. This large list of candidates is then ranked in order of points. The patient who gets the most points is the one who is the same blood type as the donor, is in the highest of the four medical urgency categories, and has been waiting the longest time. The priorities for distribution are further determined by geographic location. Thus, the donor center will receive a list of ranked candidates for the local area served by that donor center's organ procurement organization (OPO), a second list ranking the candidates in the broader UNOS region, and a third list comprising all of the remaining candidates in the nation. The organ procurement officer then begins a series of phone calls to transplant centers, starting with the one listed as the transplant center for the patient at the top of this ranked list and working down. Local candidates have priority over regional patients, and regional candidates take precedence over the remainder of the candidates in the nation.

Several key points are worth remembering in relation to the discussion of acute liver failure. First, the highest medical urgency status will admit the patient with acute liver failure who requires care in the ICU *and* has any one of the following: stage III or worse encephalopathy; a markedly elevated (>25 s) prothrombin time; renal failure requiring dialysis; hemodynamic instability requiring pressor support; uncontrollable variceal bleeding; ventilator dependency; or primary nonfunction of an allograft. Second, UNOS does not distinguish between acute and chronic liver disease when assigning priority.

6. If the patient's condition continues to deteriorate and cerebral edema begins to develop (as indicated by rising ICP and falling CPP), and if a donor organ is not within a few hours' availability, consideration must be given to one of the methods of artificial support undergoing investigation under the auspices of standard institutional review processes for such matters. One must struggle with the realization that from the time of initial referral of a donor organ and the actual revascularization of the organ in the recipient, more than eight and often more than twelve hours are likely to elapse.
7. If an organ becomes available, the patient is immediately assessed to determine whether transplantation is the best option. If the clinical condition has deteriorated further or is progressing rapidly, the current unavailability of donor livers might force one to make a decision to go ahead and perform transplantation even if there remains some hope for spontaneous recovery. Ironically, however, one is more often faced with the opposite concerns, viz. that the patient's condition has deteriorated to the extent that survival even with transplantation seems untenable. If the effectiveness of auxiliary transplantation were better established, it would likely remove one of the more significant penalties (viz. life-long immunosuppression and a life-long risk of rejection) to more liberal use of liver transplantation for acute liver failure in the earliest stages. This introduces an even greater irony, of course, namely that the greater use of human livers for this purpose makes their availability even more tenuous.
8. The patient who begins to show steady and definite decreases in ICP values with concomitant increases in CPP is probably on the road to recovery, at least from the cerebral edema associated with liver failure. We have found a falling ICP and simultaneous rise in CPP to be the earliest and most reliable sign of the start of recovery and have avoided transplantation in several patients in whom this was the only clinical sign of improvement.
9. The intraoperative management of patients undergoing liver transplantation for acute liver failure must concern itself with a variety of unique problems, most notably cerebral edema, acidosis, hemodynamic instability, pulmonary failure (often manifested as adult respiratory distress syndrome), and severe coagulopathy. As previously noted, the severity of these problems increases in proportion to the delay in providing definitive transplantation.

SOME SPECIAL CONSIDERATIONS IN CHILDREN

The majority of patients in the American reports of transplantation for acute liver failure are adults. In 1992, Ryckman et al., in a general review of the overall experience with pediatric liver transplantation in Cincinnati, mentioned their experience with ten children with acute liver failure. More recently, Dhawan and others from our center presented the results of transplantation for 37 children treated in a ten-year period for acute liver failure (Dhawan et al. 1995). These reports emphasize important differences between adults and children who require liver transplantation for acute liver failure. First, the etiology of liver failure is different in children than in adults. Children have a higher incidence of metabolic diseases as well as infections caused by *Herpes simplex*, *Herpes zoster*, cytomegalovirus, and Epstein–Barr virus. Second, an important subset of children develop aplastic anemia following liver transplantation for what is believed to be acute viral hepatitis (Cattral et al. 1994). In our experience, this has been the major cause of death with four of eight afflicted children dying of sepsis following transplantation.

A third difference is that the progression of coma is likely to be much more rapid in a child than in an adult. In addition, intracranial pressure monitoring is a less reliable prognostic tool in children, particularly in those less than two years of age. Among 12 children under two years of age in our series, six died, three from cerebral death despite low intracranial pressure levels. In these latter children, one possible clue to their deteriorating condition may have been their wide pulse pressure and very low diastolic pressure, yielding a low mean arterial pressure and a relatively low cerebral perfusion pressure despite what were thought to have been satisfactory intracranial pressures.

COMMENTS ON AUXILIARY TRANSPLANTATION

In the absence of aplastic anemia, most of the viral causes of acute liver failure can be expected to resolve following transplantation. This has important implications when considering the use of auxiliary transplantation rather than total hepatectomy. In fact, we believe auxiliary liver transplantation may be the treatment of choice in many patients with acute liver failure who progress to deep coma. In our experience, auxiliary transplantation has resulted in complete recovery of native liver function in six of eight patients treated by this modality. Unfortunately, two of these six patients went on to die of complications related to aplastic anemia associated with non-A non-B non-C hepatitis. All but one of the remaining four have either had their allografts removed or have been withdrawn from immunosuppression.

In all of these cases, a partial hepatectomy of the native liver was performed and either a portion of donor liver or an entire donor liver was placed in an orthotopic position. Our goal for these procedures was to make it possible that, should the native liver not recover, it could be readily removed and the transplant liver left intact in an orthotopic position. This is less likely to be possible when the heterotopic position is used.

The value of histology for predicting recovery remains undocumented. In all of our cases, the native liver was devoid of virtually all viable hepatocytes, yet most of the livers recovered fully. One child had fibrosis on initial biopsy and went on to develop cirrhosis in the native liver. This child also has chronic rejection and fibrosis in the allograft and yet has completely normal liver function studies, no evidence of portal hyertension, and normal growth and development. Nevertheless, we currently view fibrosis as the main histologic contraindication to auxiliary liver transplantation for acute liver failure (see also Chapter 17).

TOTAL HEPATECTOMY: MOSTLY A BAD IDEA

In an effort to address the problem associated with hemodynamic instability and acid–base disturbances associated with acute liver failure, some authors have advocated portocaval shunt with total hepatectomy while awaiting the availability of a donor organ (Ringe et al. 1988; Ringe et al. 1993; Rozga et al. 1993). As criticized by Lee (1994), these experiences are uncontrolled and anecdotal and do not support the routine use of this procedure. In fact, our more recent experience with extracorporeal circulation and with auxiliary transplantation suggests that removing the dying liver is neither necessary nor wise. The patient's metabolic disturbances can be readily corrected with aggressive intensive support and, if it eventually proves effective in more controlled trials, with supplementary support from extracorporeal circulation. Just as importantly, the native liver can recover following auxiliary transplantation, even in the face of massive collapse and necrosis on histologic examination.

EXTRACORPOREAL SUPPORT MEASURES

Extracorporeal support for patients awaiting liver transplantation remains controversial and unproven. Nevertheless, some groups have reported significant extension of survival for those patients whose course appeared to be headed towards certain cerebral death (Rozga et al. 1993; Sussman et al. 1994a; Sussman et al. 1994b). The ready availability of a means of artificial support of patients with liver failure will represent the most significant development in the field of hepatology over the last twenty years and will dramatically change the role of liver transplantation for this disorder. If only short-term support is possible, then at least the time available for obtaining a satisfactory donor organ can be extended, increasing the chances that transplantation can take place at an optimal time. Longer term support may eliminate the need to perform liver transplantation in many of these patients as recovery of the native liver may occur within 1–6 months.

INTO THE HAZE

Here are some predictions about the future treatment of acute liver failure. These are offered at a time when advances in the field are occurring more rapidly than the publication of new book chapters, making such speculation here a dangerous proposition. Nonetheless, sometimes the risk of embarrassment attending crystal ball gazing is outweighed by the relish with which such easy predictions are made.

Over the next several years, increasing experience with auxiliary transplantation will delineate the indications for this procedure, making it the preferred treatment for acute liver failure and obviating the need for lifelong immunosuppression for most of these patients. Before the end of the century, primate xenograft livers will provide the several weeks to months of function needed to allow the native liver to recover.

None of the bioartificial liver support systems (involving the use of semipermeable membrane cartridges) currently undergoing testing will prove to provide life-sustaining liver function to patients with acute liver failure. The membrane pore sizes of all of the current devices are too small, the amount of liver tissue too little and the tremendous metabolic needs of active hepatocytes (particularly their thirst for oxygen) too great to allow the current popular devices to suffice. Nevertheless, before the year 2005, we will have an artificial liver that will support patients with acute and chronic liver failure. It will be based on more sophisticated devices that incorporate immortalized, humanized hepatocytes (and other cells), the delivery of oxygen using hemoglobin or a suitable substitute, and continuous low flow (relative to total cardiac output) perfusion with patient blood (or plasma) separated from the cells by a highly permeable membrane.

Within 15 years, administration of cytoprotectant and hepatotrophic factors (or perhaps hepatocyte preparations) will assume the dominant role in the treatment of acute liver failure, enhancing recovery of the native liver during periods of artificial support and, we hope, reducing the role of transplantation in the treatment of these patients.

The development of artificial liver devices will also see the elucidation of the specific mechanisms by which acute liver failure leads to cerebral edema. This will allow more effective therapy to prevent brain swelling.

SUMMARY

Acute liver failure is a devastating disease, often affecting otherwise young and productive people. When it progresses to the development of stage III–IV hepatic encephalopathy, the chances of spontaneous recovery fall dramatically. Rapidly progressive coma, even in a young patient, is an indication to proceed with rapid transplantation since, in the absence of proven effective artificial support, these patients will have a high risk of succumbing to cerebral edema. The best results of transplantation are achieved when rapid transplantation is available. However, because of the shortage of human donor livers, this is not a practical option for many patients who present with acute liver failure, underscoring the need for alternative means of support. In the next decade, bioartificial devices and xenograft liver tissue will play an increasing role in the treatment of acute liver failure.

REFERENCES

Ascher, N.L., Lake, J.R., Emond, J.C. and Roberts, J.P. 1993. Liver transplantation for fulminant hepatic failure. *Arch Surg* 128: 677–82.

Cattral, M.S., Langnas, A.N., Markin, R.S., Antonson, D.L., Heffron, T.G., Fox, I.J., Sorrell, M.F. and Shaw, B.W. Jr. 1994. Aplastic anemia after liver transplantation for fulminant hepatic failure. *Hepatology* 20: 813–18.

Dhawan, A., Langnas, A.N., Vanderhoof, J.A., Antonson, D.L., Mack, D.R., Kaufman, S.S., Fox, I.J., Heffron, T.G. and Shaw, B.W. Jr. 1995. Outcome of liver transplantation for fulminant liver failure in children: 10 year experience. *Hepatology* 22: 208A.

Ede, R.J. and Williams, R.W. 1986. Hepatic encephalopathy and cerebral edema. *Sem Liver Dis* 6: 107–18.

Friend, P.F., Lim, S., Smith, M., Jamieson, N.V., Rolles, K., O'Grady, J., Williams, R. and Calne, R.Y. 1989. Liver transplantation in the Cambridge/King's College Hospital series – the first 400 patients. *Transpl Proc* 21: 2397–8.

Iwatsuki, S., Esquivel, C.O., Gordon, R.D., Shaw, B.W. Jr., Starzl, T.E., Shade, R.R. and Van Thiel, D.H. 1985. Liver transplantation for fulminant hepatic failure. *Sem Liver Dis* 5: 325–8.

Iwatsuki, S., Stieber, A.C., Marsh, H.W., Tzakis, A.G., Todo, S., Koneru, B., Makowka, L., Gordon, R.D. and Starzl, T.E. 1989. Liver transplantation for fulminant hepatic failure. *Transpl Proc* 21: 2431–4.

Lee, W.M. 1994. Selected summaries: total hepatectomy for acute liver failure: don't take out my liver! *Gastroenterology* 107: 894–7.

Lidofsky, S.D., Bass, N.M., Prager, M.C., Washington, D.E., Read, A.E., Wright, T.L., Ascher, N.L., Roberts, J.P., Scharschmidt, B.F. and Lake, J.R. 1992. Intracranial pressure monitoring and liver transplantation for fulminant hepatic failure. *Hepatology* 16: 1–7.

Potter, D., Peachey, T., Eason, J., Ginsburg, R. and O'Grady, J. 1989. Intracranial pressure monitoring during orthotopic liver transplantation for acute liver failure. *Transpl Proc* 21: 3528.

Ringe, B., Lubbe, N., Kuse, E., Frei, U. and Pichlmayr, R. 1993. Management of emergencies before and after liver transplantation by early total hepatectomy. *Transpl Proc* 25: 1090.

Ringe, B., Pichlmayr, R., Lubbe, N., Bornscheuer, A. and Kuse, E. 1988. Total hepatectomy as temporary approach to acute hepatic or primary graft failure. *Transpl Proc* 20: 552–7.

Rozga, J., Podesta, L., LePage, E., Hoffman, A., Morsiani, E., Sher, L., Woolf, G.M., Makowka, L. and Demetriou, A.A. 1993. Control of cerebral edema by total hepatectomy and extracorporeal liver support in fulminant hepatic failure. *Lancet* 342: 898–9.

Ryckman, F.C., Fisher, R.A., Pedersen, S.H. and Balistreri, W.F. 1992. Liver transplantation in children. *Sem Ped Surg* 1: 162–72.

Schafer, D.F. and Shaw, B.W. Jr. 1989. Fulminant hepatic failure and orthotopic liver transplantation. *Sem Liver Dis* 9: 189–94.

Shaw, B.W. Jr., Wood, R.P., Gordon, R.D., Iwatsuki, S., Gillquist, W.P. and Starzl, T.E. 1985. Influence of selected patient variables and operative blood loss on six-month survival following liver transplantation. *Sem Liver Dis* 5: 385–93.

Sidi, A. and Mahla, M.E. 1995. Noninvasive monitoring of cerebral perfusion by transcranial Doppler during fulminant hepatic failure and liver transplantation. *Anesth Analg* 80: 194–200.

Sussman, N.L., Gislason, G.T. and Kelly, J.H. 1994a. Extracorporeal liver support. Application to fulminant hepatic failure. *J Clin Gastroenterol* 18: 320–4.

Sussman, N.L., Gislason, G.T., Conlin, C.A. and Kelly, J.H. 1994b. The Hepatix extracorporeal liver assist device: initial clinical experience. *Artif Org* 18: 390–6.

Venes, J.L., Shaywitz, B.A. and Spencer, D.D. 1978. Management of severe cerebral edema in the metabolic encephalopathy of Reye–Johnson syndrome. *J Neurosurg* 48: 903–15.

17 Auxiliary liver transplantation

Karim Boudjema, Marie-Pierre Chenard-Neu and Daniel Jaeck

INTRODUCTION

Although conventional orthotopic liver transplantation (OLT), that is, resection of the native entire liver and its replacement by an allograft, is the most effective means of rapidly restoring liver function in patients with acute liver failure (ALF), this procedure still has many drawbacks. In particular, it carries the risks inherent in long-term immunosuppression, such as Ebstein–Barr virus-related lymphoproliferative syndrome and lymphoma, increased incidence and severity of acute infections by common pathogens, and frequent cyclosporin- or FK506-related chronic renal impairment. It also rules out native liver regeneration, yet livers removed from patients with ALF always show clusters of viable hepatocytes that could be the starting point for regeneration. Moreover, because the availability of liver allografts is unpredictable, the fear of losing a patient while waiting for a graft may sometimes lead to unnecessary early transplantation. Finally, in some cases, the severity of neurological status leads to acceptance for transplantation of an ABO-incompatible liver, with an increased risk of mid-term sclerosing cholangitis and subsequent destruction of the graft.

Auxiliary liver transplantation (ALT) has been developed in an attempt to overcome these problems. It consists of implanting an additional liver in the abdominal cavity as a temporary means of restoring liver function. When the native liver has regenerated, then the auxiliary graft can be removed and immunosuppressive therapy stopped.

AUXILIARY LIVER TRANSPLANTATION: NEW INTEREST IN AN OLD CONCEPT

The concept of ALT for acute liver failure is not new. In the 1960s, ALT was attempted in patients with end-stage liver failure (Terpstra, Reuvers and Schalm 1988) and fulminant hepatitis (Marion et al. 1970; Pouyet and Berard 1971; Galmarini et al. 1972; Terpstra et al. 1988). The liver graft (an allograft, or a primate or nonprimate xenograft) was implanted heterotopically, either in the groin on the iliac vessels, or intraperitoneally on the inferior vena cava and aorta. Almost all the patients died, probably because of hyperacute or acute rejection. At all events the auxiliary grafts would not have functioned for long. Later, when immunosuppressive therapy became available and improved long-term allograft tolerance, Starzl and coworkers noticed that, in experimental conditions, systemic venous blood supply to the graft led to its atrophy. Based on the studies of Rous

(Rous and Larimore 1920), they soon established that supplying the graft with portal blood was essential for maintaining its mass and function (Starzl et al. 1975), probably by providing the liver with "hepatotrophic factors" that have still to be clearly identified.

In clinical practice, auxiliary liver transplantations with grafts supplied with splanchnic (portal or splenic) and arterial blood were initially performed on patients with cirrhosis (Starzl 1967; Fortner et al. 1979; Terpstra et al. 1988). The graft (an entire liver) was implanted below the native liver, in the right paravertebral gutter, or in the splenic fossa, while venous drainage was accomplished through a vena cava-to-vena cava anastomosis at the level of the recipient's renal veins. Portal hypertension, present in chronic liver disease, no doubt avoided a 'steal' of portal blood by the native liver and subsequent graft atrophy, a phenomenon which was observed experimentally by Shalm et al. (1956) when the healthy native liver was left in place. The presence of an additional liver in the abdominal cavity was almost always possible, as the abdominal cavity had previously been distended by ascites.

At the start of the cyclosporin era, several patients with acute liver failure underwent heterotopic liver transplantation (Letoublon et al. 1989; Moritz et al. 1990; Metselaar et al. 1990; Stampfl et al. 1990; Moritz et al. 1993; Terpstra 1993) with a graft supplied with portal and arterial blood. In order to avoid competition for portal flow and to perfuse the graft preferentially, the native portal vein was partially or totally occluded (Nagashima et al. 1994). Because of the lack of room for an additional liver, the abdominal cavity was sometimes left open temporarily, or the graft was reduced to its right lobe. Most of these patients died rapidly, while some developed cirrhosis of the native liver, or rapidly underwent conventional orthotopic liver transplantation. Only two patients showed unexpected regeneration of the native liver, allowing immunosuppressive therapy to be withdrawn. The failure of these early clinical attempts, and the simultaneous improvement in conventional orthotopic liver transplantation, led most liver transplant teams to abandon the concept of heterotopic auxiliary liver transplantation.

The first successful ALT performed in an adult with the goal of giving the native liver a chance to regenerate, was performed in 1989 (Gubernatis et al. 1991). A reduced liver graft was implanted not below, but beside a previously reduced native liver, in an orthotopic position. This technique was used to create space in the abdominal cavity and to avoid compression of both the graft and the native liver during closure. It also facilitated venous drainage of the graft by implanting its veins in an anatomical position, and avoided compromising native liver regeneration by partial obstruction of the portal vein. We and others later successfully used this so-called auxiliary partial orthotopic liver transplantation procedure (APOLT) to treat children and adults (Boudjema et al. 1993; Oldhafer et al. 1994).

These anecdotal reports of successful auxiliary liver transplantation have recently revived interest in this approach. Since 1989, at least 36 ALT procedures have been reported in Europe (Auxilary Liver Transplant Registry of the European Auxiliary Liver Transplant Study Group, University Hospital Leiden, The Netherlands), and the list is no doubt far from complete.

TECHNICAL ASPECTS

Auxiliary heterotopic liver transplantation (Figure 17.1)

The procedures we describe here are based on the anatomic classification of Couinaud (Couinaud 1957). This technique is still the preferred method used in Leiden. Because of limited space in the adominal cavity, the auxiliary liver must be small or be reduced to its right lobe. Graft retrieval follows the standard procedure for multiple organ procurement. On the back table

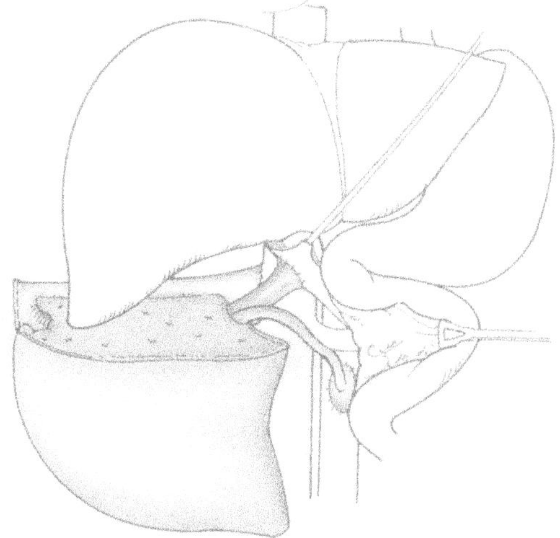

Figure 17.1 Auxiliary partial heterotopic liver transplantation using a right liver graft. Bile is drained through a Roux-en-Y jejunal limb (not shown in the figure).

the graft is reduced by resection of segments 2 and 3. The reduced graft is then implanted below the native diseased liver. In the heterotopic position, pressure in the hepatic veins of the graft is higher than in physiologic conditions and jeopardizes intrahepatic blood flow. For this reason most authors recommend constriction of the native portal vein cephalad to the graft portal vein implantation.

Auxiliary partial orthotopic liver transplantation

The procedures consist of three main steps. First, a right (segments 5 to 8) or a left (segments 1 to 4) hepatectomy of the native liver is performed to prepare a space large enough to accept a right or left liver graft, respectively. During the procedure, total clamping of the portal pedicle should be avoided as it may compromise the viability of remaining hepatocytes and subsequent liver regeneration. Next, the donor liver is reduced to a size compatible with its implantation beside the partially resected native liver. To shorten the cold preservation time of the graft, this step may be undertaken by a second team, while resection of the portion of the native liver is being carried out. The technique of liver reduction (or bipartition) has been extensively described elsewhere (Bismuth and Houssin 1984; Couinaud and Houssin 1991).

Three types of auxiliary liver can be used to perform APOLT: a right liver (segments 5 to 8), a left liver (segments 1 to 4) or a left lobe (segments 2 and 3). The frequent multiplicity of the right hepatic vein, and the need to preserve the median hepatic vein to drain segments 5 and 8, necessitate leaving the retrohepatic segment of the inferior vena cava attached to the right graft. The proximal end of the vena cava is suture-ligated and its distal end is left wide open to be implanted on the recipient inferior vena cava (Figure 17.2). The left liver graft is drained through the median and left hepatic vein, which are harvested with their common stem and a narrow cuff of inferior vena cava. When the graft is a left lobe, the median hepatic vein is ligated distally (Figure 17.3).

Finally, the donor liver segments are implanted orthotopically (Bismuth et al. 1984).

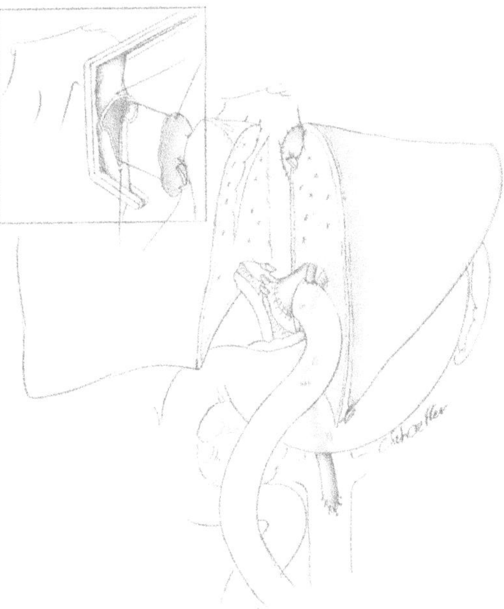

Figure 17.2 Left auxiliary partial orthotopic liver transplantation. The graft has been reduced to segments 2 and 3 (left lobe) of an entire liver.

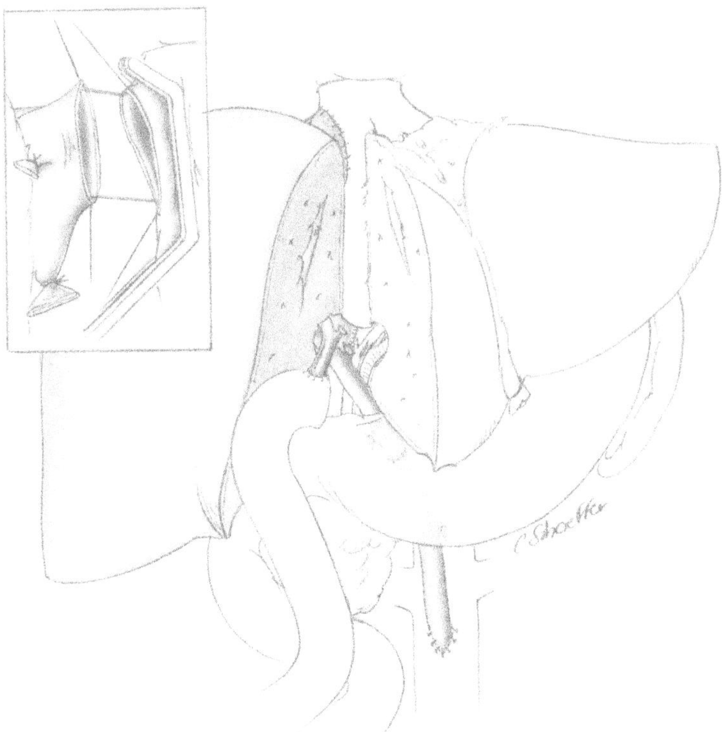

Figure 17.3 Right auxiliary partial orthotopic liver transplantation.

The hepatic veins of a left or right graft are first anastomosed end-to-side to the left and right sides of the native vena cava, respectively, at the origin of the resected hepatic vein. During anastomosis, the graft is flushed with cold (4°C) 5 percent serum albumin. The graft portal vein is then anastomosed end-to-side to the native portal vein. The graft hepatic artery is anastomosed to the native common hepatic artery or extended by means of a segment of donor iliac artery that is anastomosed end-to-side to the infrarenal aorta. A Roux-en-Y choledochojejunostomy is used to reconstruct the biliary tract, and the anastomosis is usually stented with a trancystic drain to collect graft bile production.

APOLT has two theoretical advantages over heterotopic auxiliary liver transplantation. First, the orthotopic position of the graft allows its suprahepatic veins to be implanted on a physiological site, close to the right atrium, which facilitates graft venous outflow. Second, partial resection of both the native liver and the graft reduces the volume of both, sparing intraabdominal space. For this reason, closure of the abdomen does not jeopardize the remaining graft portal flow, which, under these conditions, depends only on parenchymal resistance. This resistance is higher in the necrotic native liver than in the auxiliary graft, at least until the native liver has regained a normal histological structure. Thus, it is not necessary to band the native portal vein distal to the graft portal anastomosis.

There are no firm rules as to which part of the native liver should be resected, or which type of reduced auxiliary graft should replace it. However, in our experience (Boudjema et al. 1995), when the recipient and donor livers are size-matched, a right APOLT should be performed. Indeed, the right lobe represents 60 percent of the parenchyma and thus provides a volume of functional hepatocytes large enough to restore liver function rapidly. Moreover, the segment of native vena cava exposed after the right native liver hepatectomy is large and allows for wide and easy implantation of the graft vena cava. The right graft can lie in the right hypochondrium, thereby avoiding traction on the vascular and biliary anastomosis. When the recipient is a child and the donor an adult (the most frequent situation), we recommend left hepatectomy on the native liver and implantation of the donor left lobe. Such a graft still contains a large volume of hepatocytes (compared to recipient body weight), and it is flat enough to be lodged in the anterior space of the left hypochondrium. In one of our cases, a left lobectomy (segments 2 and 3) was performed on the native liver, and a size-matched left liver (segments 1 to 4) was implanted orthotopically. This resulted in a suprahepatic vein thrombosis of the graft and subsequent graft failure. Persistence of segment 4 on the native liver prevented lateral clamping of the vena cava which is necessary to enlarge the existing orifice of the native left suprahepatic vein.

CLINICAL EXPERIENCE WITH AUXILIARY LIVER TRANSPLANTATION

Between October 1992 and May 1995, nine patients at our unit underwent 10 APOLT procedures for fulminant or subfulminant hepatic failure. One patient was retransplanted again using an auxiliary graft. The patients' characteristics are given in Table 17.1. None of the patients had a past history of liver disease. The decision to transplant was taken when certain well-defined criteria were met. All but one of the patients was comatose and showed clinical or radiological (computed tomography) signs of cerebral edema. Hepatic failure was reflected by a drop in prothrombin time (PT) and (factor V) levels, combined with severe cholestasis. Three patients also had acute renal failure. As soon as transplantation was decided on, the patients were put on the emergency list of the French network for organ procurement and transplantation (*Etablisement Français des Greffes*) with authorization from a national expert. The waiting time for transplantation ranged between 3 and 36 h.

Surgical procedures

All but one of the donors were adults. The livers were retrieved using the standard technique for multiple organ procurement, and flushed and cold stored with UW solution. The donor/recipient blood groups were compatible in seven cases and incompatible (A to O) in two. The decision to perform ALT rather than conventional liver transplantation was taken during the operation, after a frozen-section biopsy had revealed massive hepatocellular necrosis, bloated hepatocytes predominantly in periportal areas above the liver capsule, and the absence of bridging fibrosis. These findings were confirmed later by Trichrome staining of fixed liver tissue. All auxiliary livers were implanted orthotopically. Five patients received a left APOLT, while the remaining four received a right APOLT. The mean graft storage time was 7.8 h and the mean total operating time was 7.5 h. Mean blood loss during the operation was 12 units (1–24 units). Immunosuppression was started perioperatively and included cyclosporin A, azathioprine and methylprednisolone.

Specific follow up

Compared to conventional OLT, ALT necessitates monitoring both the native and the auxiliary liver. Global liver function was evaluated on the basis of neurological status and EEG findings. Laboratory monitoring included daily assays of liver enzymes (AST and ALT), PT, factor V and total bilirubin blood concentrations. During the first postoperative days, these parameters reflected the function of the auxiliary graft. The function of the native and auxiliary livers was also compared. Doppler ultrasound examination was performed every day during the first week to check the patency of the native and graft vessels, and once a week thereafter. Protocol biopsies of both the native liver and graft were

Table 17.1. *Clinical experience with auxiliary liver transplantation. Patient characteristics at time of transplantation*

Transplant no./Patient	1/1	2/2	3/3	4,5/4	6/5	7/6	8/7	9/8	10/9
Age/sex	4/M	12/M	23/F	15/M	65/F	54/F	30/F	35/M	51/M
Cause of hepatic failure	HAV	HAV	NSAI	HAV	HBV	Halot	Imm.	Unkn.	HBV
Jaundice to encephalopathy (days)	45	48	30	50	20	21	14	10	4
Coma (grade)	2	1	3	3	3	–	3	3	3
Prothrombin time (%)	<10	17	10	12	<10	15	<10	<10	18
Factor V (%)	42	24	20	25	20	23	23[a]	23[a]	32[a]
Bilirubin (mmol/l)	650	350	320	430	150	330	320	524	572

[a] Fresh frozen plasma transfusion.
HAV, Hepatitis A virus; NSAI, nonsteroidal anti-inflammatory; HBV, Hepatitis B virus; Halot, Halothane; Imm., Autoimmune; Unkn., Unknown.

performed every week during the first month, then every 3–4 weeks, depending on individual clinical and laboratory findings. Hepatobiliary scintigraphy was performed on day 7, then every 2–4 weeks.

Postoperative course and complications

Seven patients regained normal consciousness and were extubated within 2 weeks of the operation. EEG findings ran parallel to clinical recovery and eventually returned to normal. The patients who had anuria before transplantation began a diuresis within a few hours following graft reperfusion. All the allografts produced bile immediately, and AST and ALT peaked on day one or two, decreased slowly over the first month, then plateaued above normal values for several weeks before returning to normal; PT and factor V reached normal values within 10 days; and total bilirubin concentrations returned to normal within 4 to 6 weeks.

Two patients had persistent encephalopathy. One regained consciousness but showed persistent asterixis. The auxiliary liver produced small amounts of bile. At the end of the first week, while AST and ALT values were decreasing, the PT and factor V levels were still below 50 percent of control values. Doppler ultrasound showed an inversion of graft portal blood flow, and an angiogram confirmed thrombosis of the suprahepatic vein anastomosis. Emergency retransplantation was decided upon on day 10, and was performed on day 13. The graft was removed and auxiliary liver transplantation was again performed with an adult left lobe. The patient regained normal consciousness and was extubated five days after retransplantation. The neurological status of the second patient improved slightly but liver function remained poor. Bile production was absent. Doppler ultrasound did not show vascular thrombosis. The picture was compatible with poor initial graft function. It was then decided to retransplant the patient by conventional complete orthotopic technique. While waiting for a new graft, the native liver was removed. This maneuver did not improve neurological status, which argues against the notion that leaving a necrotic liver in place is deleterious to the graft recipient.

In this series, the auxiliary liver transplantation technique was associated with a high morbidity rate. In addition to graft venous thrombosis or initial dysfunction, four patients had to be re-explored within the first 3 weeks. One patient who received a left lobe graft developed a bile leak from the choledochojejunostomy; this complication was due to devascularization of the left bile duct during the reduction procedure. Another patient was reoperated on on day 10 to correct a small-bowel obstruction due to its intussusception behind the Roux-en-Y jejunal limb. Two other patients developed intraperitoneal bleeding originating from the native liver and graft liver slices, respectively. All these complications could probably have been avoided by using a conventional orthotopic transplantation procedure with an entire liver graft.

Five of the nine patients (55 percent) had at least one acute rejection episode, a rate similar to that of acute rejection after OLT. This argues against the increased risk of rejection that has been shown in experimental conditions, when total removal of the native liver was necessary to induce tolerance of liver grafts (Gugenheim et al. 1981). The diagnosis of acute rejection was readily made on the basis of specific histological features (Snover 1986), combined with abnormal elevations of liver enzyme activities.

Four patients died, three of infectious complications: the patient who was retransplanted by means of ALT developed herpetic bronchiolitis and died 45 days after the first transplantation. A 65-year-old woman with HBV-related fulminant hepatitis developed the Guillain–Barré syndrome necessitating mechanical ventilation. She died of cardiac arrest on day 32. A 51-year-old man whose hepatic failure was also due to HBV died after his native liver had completely regenerated; while immunosuppression was being tapered, a hepatic artery thrombosis of the graft occurred, necessitating removal of the graft. In the third postoperative week, while liver function was normal, he developed a massive pulmonary embolism. The fourth patient died of multiple organ failure after a conventional retransplant for primary nonfunction of the auxiliary graft.

Five out of the nine patients (55 percent) are alive with a follow-up of 12 to 36 months, with normal liver function present in either the auxiliary graft or the regenerated native liver.

Outcome of the native and auxiliary livers

The patients in this group who had HAV-related liver failure and those with drug-induced liver failure showed rapid histological regeneration of their native liver. By the end of the first postoperative month, the parenchyma was almost normal. During the first 2 to 3 weeks, the remaining hepatocytes rapidly grew in number and totally refilled the lobules. At this time, inflammation had disappeared and trabecular arrangement was still absent. The lobular architecture gradually recovered and the morphological pattern became normal by the end of the second postoperative month. The grafted liver was removed in two cases. At the time of surgery, the native and auxiliary liver slices were still separate. However, there were dense adhesions between the graft and surrounding gastrointestinal structures, and its portal pedicle was retracted into the hilum. Retrieval of the graft appeared difficult, with a high risk of bowel perforation and native liver pedicle injury. This led us to leave the auxiliary liver to atrophy in two patients by tapering the immunosuppression over a 6-month period. This was successful in one case but led to hepatic artery thrombosis and intrahepatic abscesses in the second. Three patients have permanently stopped taking immunosuppressive therapy. Histological examination of the excised or atrophied auxiliary graft showed typical signs of chronic rejection. In one patient (HBV-related ALF, 65 years old) the remaining native hepatocytes showed little regenerative activity. Within 3 weeks the collapsed area was replaced by extensive fibrosis, with little inflammation and only nodular foci of hepatocytes. The native liver of a patient with halothane-induced liver failure showed no regenerative activity or fibrotic changes up to the third postoperative month. At that time a new biopsy showed no obvious thickening of the collageneous network of the lobules, which were partly occupied by small cuboid epithelial cells arranged in pseudoglands. Liver function was being performed by the graft under full immunosuppression. Surprisingly, although resistance in the native liver was higher than in the morphologically normal auxiliary liver, an angiogram demonstrated normal arterial and portal flow into the native liver. The native liver of the patient whose hepatic failure was of autoimmune origin is still small one year after transplantation. However, its histological appearance is almost normal, with very few fibrotic zones. Immunosuppression is now being tapered.

REGENERATION OF THE NATIVE LIVER: EUROPEAN EXPERIENCE

All European teams with experience in performing auxiliary liver transplantation were invited to a workshop in Strasbourg in October 1994. The aim was to evaluate the native liver's potential for regeneration and the outcome for patients with acute liver failure (Chenard-Neu et al. 1996). Twelve groups provided data on 30 patients (including the nine patients in our series). The graft was implanted either orthotopically, beside the native liver (n=23) or heterotopically (n=7), below the native liver.

As at October 1994, 19 of the 30 patients (63 percent) were alive after 3–67 months of follow-up. Thirteen of these 19 survivors (68 percent) had recovered normal native liver function and had permanently stopped taking immunosuppressive drugs. The graft had been removed in nine patients and left to atrophy in four with no subsequent deleterious effect on native liver function. Immunosuppression was being tapered in a further three patients, and four patients (21 percent) with normal graft function were still on immunosuppression 5, 6, 9 and 10 months after auxiliary liver transplantation. Eleven patients (37 percent) died due to surgical complications and sepsis (n=9) or because of poor graft function (n=2), leading to retransplantation by conventional or auxiliary approaches in one case each. Biopsy specimens of the native liver were obtained from 22 patients during follow-up (18 survivors and four patients who died more than 1 month after transplantation). Three types of morphological change were seen. Complete regeneration was the most frequent outcome, being observed in 15 patients (15/22, 68 percent). It was more frequent in patients under 40 years old, in those with acute liver failure due to viral hepatitis or acetaminophen overdose, or when ALF was of the hyperacute type (O'Grady et al. 1993). Apparently, regeneration occurred in two phases. First, hepatocytes proliferated and repopulated the lobules, the centrilobular zones being restored last. The trabecular architecture was restored during the second or third month after auxiliary liver transplantation. A few patients showed persistent thin arachnoid, nonbridging, periportal or centrilobular fibrotic scars.

Incomplete regeneration of the native liver with areas of fibrosis occurred in three patients (3/22, 14 percent). In two cases, liver failure was due to 'ecstasy' intoxication and native liver function was not sufficient to allow interruption of immunosuppressive therapy. In the remaining case, the fulminant hepatic failure was of unknown origin. The graft was removed despite significant fibrosis of the native liver, indicating that complete regeneration is not an absolute requirement for withdrawal of the auxiliary graft.

Massive fibrosis occurred in four patients (4/22, 18 percent) in whom normal liver function was provided by the auxiliary liver graft. In two of these cases, the acute liver failure was due to HBV infection. In the two remaining cases the acute liver failure was of autoimmune origin and halothane toxicity, respectively.

CONCLUSIONS

Although ALT appears to be an effective means of reversing life-threatening cerebral edema in patients with acute liver failure, many questions remain to be answered.

The first is the type of auxiliary transplant performed. The heterotopic technique has the major disadvantage of implanting the auxiliary graft in a nonphysiologic position and compromising native liver regeneration by reducing portal flow. This was clearly demonstrated in experimental conditions (Nagashima 1994). However, this technique has the advantage of being simpler to perform, and is theoretically safer than the orthotopic technique. In the European experience reported at the Strasbourg meeting, 57 percent (4 of 7) of the patients who received a heterotopic graft died. Although a small number of patients, this result compares unfavorably with the 30 percent death rate among patients transplanted with an orthotopic auxiliary graft. Since there is still room for improving the surgical technique of APOLT, we believe that this approach is preferable to a heterotopic ALT.

As ALT offers the advantage of being reversible, the question arises as to whether the indications are precisely the same as for conventional OLT, the criteria for which are predictive of death in 90 to 95 percent of nontransplanted patients (Bernuau et al. 1986). However, waiting for these criteria to be fulfilled dangerously reduces the time remaining to find a suitable graft for the patient.

Leaving the host liver in situ may have certain disadvantages compared with conventional OLT. First, when fulminant hepatic failure is due to HBV, the native liver may be more likely to infect the (auxiliary) graft. This risk, however, should be no higher than after conventional OLT for ALF (Samuel et al. 1991), since viral particles are not only located in the necrotic liver but also in other organs and circulating blood cells. There is also the possibility of developing chronic viral hepatitis in the native liver. One of the two patients in our series in whom hepatic failure was due to HBV survived long enough for the serological markers of acute hepatitis B present before transplantation to disappear a few weeks after transplantation. No histological features of acute or chronic infection developed in the regenerated native liver. A similar observation was made by the Leiden group, who performed auxiliary liver transplantation in a patient with fulminant hepatic failure due to HBV despite the fact that the patient did not receive hyperimmune antiHBs globulins (van Hoek et al. 1995). Second, patients with extensive liver necrosis may temporarily improve after removal of their liver, and it has been suggested that, in fulminant hepatic failure, cerebral edema and hemodynamic instability may be worsened by toxic products of the remaining necrotic native liver (Ringe et al. 1993). No such "toxic liver syndrome" could be appreciated during the postoperative course of our patients, which suggests to us that hemodynamic instability and/or cerebral edema may be related to the lack of sufficient viable hepatocytes rather than to the persistence of necrotic liver tissue. Another potential disadvantage is that the native liver may become cirrhotic and negate the long-term benefits of ALT. Permanent immunosuppression may be required to maintain auxiliary graft tolerance and this may introduce the risk of hepatocellular carcinoma in the native cirrhotic liver. This cannot occur in the case of HAV infection, but was observed in four patients in the European experience reported above, with HBV, halothane and ecstasy-related acute liver failure. If these patients survive, it may be optional management to remove the native liver. The possible superiority of ALT over OLT remains dependent on an understanding and interpretation of predictive factors for liver regeneration. Although European experience of ALT is still limited, analysis of the data provided by each center leads us to suspect that patients with acute liver failure whose native liver is likely to sustain complete regeneration are those who are younger than 40 years, and who have viral hepatitis or liver failure due to acetaminophen (paracetamol) overdose as well as those in whom the interval between the onset of jaundice and encephalopathy is shorter than a week. Because ALF is rare, the only way to confirm these assumptions is to perform a multicenter prospective study.

Finally, the value of perioperative histological examination as a predictive factor for hepatocyte regeneration is questionable, since a simple needle biopsy may not be representative of the entire parenchyma; the presence of few viable hepatocytes on biospy may not necessarily reflect the capacity for regeneration. Such biopsies are, however, recom-

recommended, at least to rule out the risk of previous chronic liver disease which would preclude any long-term benefit from ALT.

With the increasing success of conventional OLT for chronic liver failure patients, interest in ALT as a form of temporary liver support has lessened. However, the concept of a "spare wheel" liver remains an attractive procedure for patients with acute liver failure who are often young and previously healthy, and in whom the native liver may well recover completely. Auxiliary partial orthotopic liver transplantation seems to be better than the heterotopic technique for achieving this goal. It is, however, still associated with a high morbidity rate and should thus be considered as an alternative to OLT. Its precise place with respect to OLT and the new bioartificial liver devices remains to be determined.

REFERENCES

Bernuau, J., Goudean, A., Poyhard, T., Dubois, F., Lesage, G., Yvonnet, B., Degott, C., Bezeaud, A., Rueff, B. and Benhamou, J.P. 1986. Multivariate analysis of prognostic factors in fulminant hepatitis B. *Hepatology* 6: 648–51.

Bernuau, J., Samuel, D., Durand, F. et al. 1991. Criteria for emergency liver transplantation in patients with acute viral hepatitis and factor V below 50 percent of normal: a prospective study. *Hepatology* 14: 49A.

Bismuth, H. and Houssin, D. 1984. Reduced-sized orthotopic liver graft in hepatic transplantation in children. *Surgery* 95: 367–70.

Boudjema, K., Cherqui, D., Jaeck, D., Chenard-Neu, M.P., Steib, A., Freis, G., Becmeur, F., Brunot, B., Simeoni, U., Bellocq, J.P. et al. 1995. Auxiliary liver transplantation for fulminant and subfulminant hepatic failure. *Transplantation* 59: 218–23.

Boudjema, K., Jaeck, D., Siméoni, U. et al. 1993. Temporary auxiliary liver transplantation for subacute liver failure in a child. *Lancet* 342: 778–9.

Chenard-Neu, M.P., Boudjema, K., Bernuau, J. et al. 1966. Auxiliary liver transplantation: regeneration of the native liver and outcome in 30 patients with fulminant hepatic failure – a multicenter European study. *Hepatology* 23: 1119–27.

Couinaud, C. 1957. In *Le Foie: Etudes anatomiques et chirurgicales.* Paris: Masson.

Couinaud, C. and Houssin, D. 1991. *Controlled partition of the liver for transplantation: anatomical limitations.* Paris.

Fortner, J.G., Yeh, S.D.J., Kim, D.K. et al. 1979. The case for and technique of liver grafting. *Transpl Proc* 11: 269–72.

Galmarini, D., Riquier, G., Vercesi, G. et al. 1972. Coma hépatique: expérimentation de traitement dans deux cas avec greffe hétérotopique temporaire du foie. *Acta Chir Belg* 71: 145–52.

Gubernatis, G., Pichlmayr, R., Kemnitz, J. et al. 1991. Auxiliary partial orthotopic liver transplantation (APOLT) for fulminant hepatic failure: first successful case report. *World J Surg* 15: 660–6.

Gugenheim, J., Houssin, D., Tamisier, D. et al. 1981. Spontaneous long term survival of liver allografts in inbred rats: influence of the hepatectomy of the recipients own liver. *Transplantation* 32: 445–50.

Letoublon, C., Guignier, M., Barnoud, D. et al. 1989. Transplantation hépatique hétérotopique pour hépatite fulminante. *Chirurgie* 115: 30–5.

Marion, P., Betroye, A., Mikaeloff, P. and Bolot, J.F. 1970. Essai de traitement du coma hépatique par hétérogreffe auxiliaire. *Mem Acad Chir* 96: 152–61.

Metselaar, H.J., Hesselink, E.J., De Rave, S. et al. 1990. Recovery of failing liver after auxiliary heterotopic transplantation. *Lancet* 335: 1156–7.

Moritz, M.J., Jarrell, B.E., Armenti, V. et al. 1990. Heterotopic liver transplantation for fulminant hepatic failure-abridge to recover. *Transplantation* 50: 524–6.

Moritz, M.J., Jarrell, B.E., Muñoz, S.J. and Maddrey, W.C. 1993. Regeneration of the native liver after heterotopic liver transplantation for fulminant hepatic failure. *Transplantation* 55: 952–94.

Nagashima, I., Bergmann, L. and Schweizer, R. 1994. How can we share the portal blood inflow in auxiliary partial heterotopic liver transplantation without portal hypertension? *Surgery* 116: 101–6.

O'Grady, J.G., Schalm, S.W. and Williams, R. 1993. Acute liver failure: redefining the syndromes. *Lancet* 342: 273–5.

Oldhafer, K.J., Gubernatis, G., Schlitt, H.J., Rodeck, B., Böker, K. and Pichlmayr, R. 1994. Auxiliary partial orthotopic liver transplantation for acute liver failure: The Hannover experience. In *Clinical Transplants 1994*, eds. Terasaki and Cecka, 181–7. Los Angeles, California: UCLA Tissue Typing Laboratory.

Pouyet, Y. and Berard, P. 1971. Deux cas de transplantation hétérotopique vraie de foie de babouin au cours d'hépatites aigües malignes. *Lyon Chir* 67: 288–91.

Ringe, B., Lübbe, N., Kuse, E. et al. 1993. Total hepatectomy and liver transplantation as two-stage procedure. *Ann Surg* 218: 3–10.

Rous, P. and Larimore, L.D. 1920. Relation of the portal blood to liver maintenance. A demonstration of liver atrophy conditional on compensation. *J Exp Med* 31: 609–32.

Samuel, D., Bismuth, A., Mathieu, D. et al. 1991. Passive immunoprophylaxis after liver transplantation in HBsAg-positive patients. *Lancet* 337: 813–15.

Shalm, L. Bax, H.R. and Mansens, B.J. 1956. Atrophy of the liver after occlusion of the bile ducts or portal vein and compensatory hypertrophy of the unoccluded portion and its clinical importance. *Gastroenterology* 31: 131–6.

Snover, D.C. 1986. The pathology of acute rejection. *Transpl Proc* 18: 123–7.

Stampfl, D.A., Muñoz, S.J., Moritz, M.J. et al. 1990. Heterotopic liver transplantation for fulminant Wilson's disease. *Gastroenterology* 12: 1834–6.

Starzl, T.E. 1967. Clinical auxiliary transplantation. In *Experience in Liver Transplantation*, ed. T.E. Starzl, 516–27. Philadelphia: W.B. Saunders.

Starzl, T.E., Porter, K.A., Kashigawi, N. and Putnam, C.W. 1975. Portal hepatotrophic factors, diabetes mellitus and acute liver atrophy, hypertrophy and regeneration. *Surg Gynecol Obstet* 141: 843–57.

Terpstra, O.T., 1993. Perspective d'avenir: la

transplantation auxiliaire hétérotopique du foie. In *Insuffisance Hépatique Aiguë Grave et Réanimation*, eds. J.D. Tempé and A. Jaeger, 245–50. Paris: Arnette.

Terpstra, O., Reuvers, C.B. and Schalm, S.W. 1988. Auxiliary heterotopic liver transplantation. *Transplantation* 45: 1003–7.

Terpstra, O.T., Schalm, S.W., Weimar, W. et al. 1988. Auxiliary liver transplantation for end-stage chronic liver disease. *N Engl J Med* 319: 1507–11.

van Hoek, B., Ringers, J., Kroes, A.C., van Krieken, J.H., van Schelven, W.D., Masclee, A.A., van Krikken-Hogenberk, L.G., Haak, H.R., Lamers, C.B. and Terpstra, O.T. 1995. Temporary heterotopic auxiliary liver transplantation for fulminant hepatitis B. *Hepatology* 23: 109–18.

PART FIVE Artificial and Bioartificial Liver Devices

18 Extracorporeal liver support: historical background and critical analysis

Evren O. Atillasoy and Paul D. Berk

INTRODUCTION

Acute liver failure (ALF), the rapid development of severely deranged and relentlessly worsening liver function in the previously healthy individual, progressing to encephalopathy, coma and death, is the most dramatic illness with which the hepatologist is confronted. Historically, the condition seemed uncommon, and most reports in the literature before 1960 described isolated cases or, at most, small series of a few patients (Benhamou et al. 1972). The first systematic effort to accumulate data on a larger experience was the National Fulminant Hepatic Failure Study, stimulated by an apparent ALF epidemic associated with the use of halothane anesthesia, in which investigators assembled data on a large number of cases from multiple institutions (Trey and Davidson 1970). The interest that followed this study, the wave of cases caused by the growing popularity of acetaminophen (paracetamol) overdose as a means of attempting suicide, and the availability of experimental therapeutic technologies led, starting in the 1970s, to the establishment of specialized liver failure units. These units, at first principally in the United Kingdom and in France, developed experience in the care of large numbers of cases. They thus provided the first opportunity to assess new, experimental therapies in significant numbers of patients, and indeed, stimulated the development of successive waves of new therapies. The United States initially lagged in this effort. However, the role of liver transplantation in the treatment of ALF has led increasingly to the referral of such cases to centers which could offer transplantation as a treatment of last resort. Consequently, several centers in the United States now see appreciable numbers of patients, and treat them with increasing expertise. At our own institution, for example, referrals have increased the number of such patients from a historical level of two or three per year to a current experience of three or four per month. This growing experience has been accompanied by improved outcomes, at least for some sub-sets of patients.

The goal of this chapter is to review what has been learned from this larger experience, from efforts to develop hepatic assist devices for the treatment of ALF, and from the clinical use of such devices. To accomplish this goal, we shall review briefly the functions of the normal liver, examine what is known about the pathophysiology of ALF, and examine how various types of hepatic assist devices used historically or currently under development address the critical and life-threatening components of this pathophysiologic state. Since we are not mystery writers, there is no need to save our punch-line for the end. Our view, strengthened by the exercise of preparing this chapter, is that virtually all advances to date in the understanding and treatment of ALF have come from the classical methods of clinical research: meticulous observation of the patient, augmented by the mobilization of the laboratory to enhance and deepen appreciation of what has been observed at the bedside. The research laboratory has for the most part followed rather than guided the clinician. Efforts to apply the methods of bioengineering to the development of liver assist devices have largely failed, principally because they were based on highly simplistic views of the pathophysiologic changes requiring correction. Although current efforts, which incorporate living liver cells into various types of extracorporeal liver assist devices, go appreciably beyond what has been tried in the past, we remain unconvinced that even they address the issues essential to survival in this setting.

FUNCTIONS OF THE LIVER

The liver plays a central role in metabolic homeostasis, and a much less appreciated but no less critical role in host defense mechanisms. The metabolic capabilities of the liver reside mainly in the hepatocyte, aided by the biliary epithelial cell, while host defenses are principally the responsibility of the various nonparenchymal cells. These diverse functions are made possible by numerous specialized features at the level of the whole organ, the hepatocyte, and hepatocytic subcellular organelles (Berk et al. 1995). Examples include the dual vascular supply of the liver; the structural organization of the hepatic acinus, in which one-cell thick plates of hepatocytes and accompanying nonparenchymal cells are bathed on two sides with plasma from the systemic and splanchnic circulations; the unique, fenestrated sinusoidal endothelium; the blood filtration process offered by intrasinusoidal reticuloendothelial phagocytes; the counter-current exchange mechanism provided by the microvasculature surrounding the smallest biliary radicles; and the highly specialized metabolic, transport, and detoxification machinery of the differentiated hepatocyte. All of these features must be preserved if normal "liver function" is to be maintained.

The hepatocyte, which constitutes more than two thirds of the mass of the liver, is the main metabolically functional component of the acinus. It is one of the most complex, metabolically diverse, and highly differentiated cells in the body, having evolved specialized cellular machinery to perform a variety of essential tasks. These include: uptake via specific transport mechanisms of clinically important substances such as bile acids, bilirubin, free fatty acids and other organic anions, amino acids, carbohydrates, lipophilic neutral compounds and amphipathic cations, and sequestration, usually by endocytotic mechanisms, of macromolecules, including plasma proteins; intracellular metabolism and interconversion of carbohydrates, lipids, and amino acids, resulting in de novo synthesis of, for example, glucose, fatty acids, cholesterol, and phospholipids, storage of glycogen and triglycerides in times of excess or release of glucose and fatty acids for peripheral consumption, and generation of ammonia; synthesis of plasma proteins, including albumin, coagulation factors and lipoproteins; biotransformation/detoxification of endo- and xenobiotics; and secretion into sinusoidal blood and bile of essential proteins, enzymes, and cofactors required for normal digestion, bodily function, and waste elimination (Zucker and Gollan 1994). The intensity of each of these activities is regulated to meet physiologic needs, and modified by acute and chronic injury of the liver. The ability of the liver to modify substances progressively as they pass through the sinusoids is made possible by establishment of compartments of functionally different hepatocytes which vary in metabolic activities, gene expression, and replication (Gumucio and Berkowitz 1992). The central control mechanisms responsible for coordination of cellular activity, replication, and organ function are still poorly understood but are thought to involve autocrine, paracrine, and endocrine processes.

In addition to hepatocytes and bile duct cells, nonparenchymal cells such as the Kupffer cell, the sinusoidal endothelial cell, the lipocyte, stellate or Ito cell, and the pit cell make up roughly a third of liver mass and are intimately involved in the normal functioning of the liver (Roll and Friedman 1992). Kupffer cells have important cytokine-mediated regulatory effects on hepatocyte function and are an integral part of the host defense system, being responsible for phagocytosis and clearance of pathogens and other noxious materials, including micro-organisms, endotoxin, immune complexes, tumor cells, lipids, and other particulate matter. They are involved in a complex network of cell–cell interactions that include processing and presentation of antigens to lymphocytes and the release of a host of immunoregulatory compounds. Defects in, or "blockade" of, reticuloendothelial function, or excessive stimulation or activation of Kupffer cells have each been shown to cause hepatocellular injury by several mechanisms, including release of cytokines, proteases, prostaglandins, and toxic oxygen species, and also to have important consequences for susceptibility to infection. Fenestrated sinusoidal endothelial cells have an important filtration role, providing direct access to the hepatocyte surface of various materials as large as lipoprotein molecules for use by hepatocytes, as well as waste products including denatured proteins and connective tissue components for disposition, while excluding particular pathogens. The size of the fenestrae, and hence, access to the surface of the hepatocyte, change both in response to physiologic stimuli and to hepatic injury. Hepatic endothelial cells are capable of modulating various hepatocyte activities, and do this through a variety of mediators, including interleukin-1, interleukin-6, interferons, and nitric oxide. They also have been shown to produce extracellular matrix components and to undergo morphologic and functional changes which encourage both leukocyte adhesion and cytoprotective mechanisms. Stellate cells are increasingly recognized as having a host of cytokine-mediated modulatory functions besides their well recognized participation in the synthesis of extracellular matrix components and in the development of hepatic fibrosis. Apart from cytotoxic activity against virally infected cells and tumor cells, it is not known whether pit cells contribute to liver function.

While the nature of the cellular interactions is poorly understood, these nonparenchymal cells are clearly major regulators of normal hepatocyte function and major mediators of hepatocyte injury in liver disease, including ALF. Indeed, while the loss of hepatocyte function during ALF is undoubtedly very important, many clinical features of ALF appear to reflect more directly a loss of non-parenchymal cell function or disordered cell–cell interaction.

THE SYNDROMES OF ACUTE LIVER FAILURE

Definitions

The terms used to describe the several most common scenarios associated with the rapid development of liver failure have undergone a gradual evolution over the past decade. The definitions which have evolved result from the perception by experienced clinicians that a number of different syndromes, with different clinical features, outcomes, and (perhaps) etiologies, can be dissected out from the now large clinical experience. The classification of these syndromes is dealt with in more detail elsewhere in this book (Chapter 1).

Features of acute liver failure

Patients with typical acute liver failure (ALF) invariably present with a spectrum of biochemical abnormalities, and their clinical consequences, which clearly reflect the loss of well recognized aspects of hepatocellular function. However, the full-blown clinical picture of these syndromes includes a variety of additional features, including the most common causes of death, which cannot so readily be attributed to the loss of particular functions of the hepatocyte.

Derangements of hepatocellular function

A massive loss of hepatocellular function leads to a predictable constellation of metabolic derangements. As examples, defective gluconeogenesis leads to the hypoglycemia which is a common accompaniment of ALF, and defective ureagenesis to a reduced blood urea nitrogen and BUN/creatinine ratio. Impaired protein synthesis leads rapidly to reduced levels of hepatocyte-derived coagulation factors, and to hypoalbuminemia, although the latter may occur only gradually in view of the three week half-life of serum albumin. Impaired hepatocellular uptake, biotransformation, and excretory function contribute to the development of jaundice and to the need to monitor carefully blood levels of therapeutic agents normally detoxified by the liver. The consequences of a sudden and massive loss of hepatocellular function are most clearly seen in anhepatic animal models, in which the liver is removed surgically (Hickman et al. 1992). It is important to note that the clinical picture which develops in these models differs from that in models in which the liver is left in situ after being infarcted by hepatic artery/ portal vein ligation or severely damaged by intoxication with galactosamine or CCl_4 (Potter and Berk 1992). The latter, much more than the former, resembles many aspects of ALF.

Other major features of acute liver failure

The full-blown clinical pictures of these syndromes encompass a constellation of often life-threatening features, including encephalopathy with or without cerebral edema, hemorrhage, electrolyte, and acid–base abnormalities, renal failure, respiratory problems, peripheral vasodilatation, a hyperdynamic circulation, cardiovascular instability, pancreatitis and infection. These features are described in more detail in Part Three. While certain etiologies are especially associated with particular complications (e.g. acetaminophen overdose with renal insufficiency), a high risk for most of these complications characterizes these syndromes in general, and several, if not all, will be found in the majority of cases.

The complications associated with the poorest prognosis continue to be encephalopthy and cerebral edema. The metabolic basis for encephalopathy in ALF is believed to be different from the classical portosystemic encephalopathy of chronic liver disease. Having said that, its precise biochemical/ pathophysiologic basis remains unclear (Blei 1991). Some investigators continue to attribute it to the usual suspects: ammonia, mercaptans, phenols, and short and medium chain fatty acids, acting either alone or in combination. Others have presented intriguing data to implicate stimulation of the GABA-benzodiazepine receptor, possibly by an endogenous benzodiazepine-like agonist, in its pathogenesis. Clearly this crucial issue merits intensive further investigation employing new investigative strategies and methods, as well as an open-minded review of data as they are produced. Encephalopathy may occur without, or at least before, clinically detectable cerebral edema. Nevertheless, data derived from several experimental models suggest that some degree of cerebral edema usually precedes deep coma. Cerebral edema is almost certainly multifactorial in origin. The rapid increase in brain water results from a loss of cell membrane integrity and an alteration in the permeability of the blood brain barrier. As with most complications of acute liver failure, its pathogenesis has been postulated to be the inability of the liver to synthesize or export factor(s) necessary to maintain membrane integrity or blood brain barrier impermeability, or its inability to protect the brain by detoxifying deleterious compounds.

Hemorrhage in ALF is the consequence of a complicated hemostatic defect of which decreased hepatocellular production of clotting factors and of coagulation and fibrinolytic inhibitors is only one aspect. Difficulty in reversing the coagulopathy with clotting factor concentrates suggests that defective factor synthesis may, in fact, be a relatively minor component of the problem. Consumptive phenomena manifested by disseminated intravascular coagulation and hyperfibrinolysis are major contributors to the clinical hemorrhagic manifestations (Preston 1991).

Patients with ALF also have a high incidence of bacterial and fungal infection. These have been attributed to multiple abnormalities which include decreased Kupffer cell phagocytic function, reduced circulating fibronectin, decreased complement levels and activity, faulty polymorphonuclear adherence and locomotion, and altered cell mediated and humoral immunity (Rolando et al. 1993).

Pathophysiology

As indicated above, a contemporary appreciation of the ALF syndromes suggests that they are characterized by a spectrum of complications leading to multiorgan failure. Although a substantial literature and much of the thinking behind current efforts to develop liver support devices ultimately attribute these complications either to a lack of crucial substances normally produced by the hepatocyte or to the accumulation of toxins normally removed by the hepatocyte, in our view, it is difficult to attribute the majority of these severe complications directly to the loss of hepatocellular function. Some aspects, such as the clotting factor deficient aspects of the coagulopathy, clearly result from the loss of the normal synthetic function of the hepatocyte. However, many other features, including cerebral edema, renal insufficiency, ventilatory and acid–base disturbances, disseminated intravascular coagulation and hyperfibrinolysis, and an increased incidence of both bacterial and fungal sepsis, are not as clearly attributed to the loss of normal hepatocellular function. Endotoxemia, reflective of defective Kupffer cell function, and abnormal cytokine cascades (some possibly related to endothelial damage and others to massive cell necrosis) seem likely candidates to explain these aspects of the syndrome. Indeed, evidence in man and animal models of ALF demonstrates that the main cell types within the liver, hepatocytes, endothelial cells, and Kupffer cells, undergo quantitative and qualitative changes in association with ALF. These include alterations in number, morphology, cytosolic, microsomal, and mitochondrial metabolic activity, nuclear activity, and cell to cell interactions, and various measures of functional capability. Nevertheless, over much of the past four decades, investigators have focused on two specific and superficially divergent conceptual constructs which ascribe the syndrome of ALF either to a profound loss of hepatocellular metabolic capacity or to the accumulation of toxins ordinarily detoxified by the healthy liver cell. These two widely discussed theories have been designated the metabolic mass hypothesis and the toxin hypothesis.

The metabolic mass hypothesis

This hypothesis proposes: that a minimum mass of well functioning hepatocytes is required to meet the basic metabolic needs of the body; and that once the functional capacity of the hepatocyte mass falls below this critical threshold, end organ dysfunction and ultimately failure occur due to deficiencies in hepatocellular production of factors required to support peripheral organ function. An implied corollary is the assumption that a hepatocyte which looks healthy on histologic examination functions normally. Early evidence for this concept came from observations that the extent of hepatic tissue injury was inversely related to certain quantifiable measures of hepatocyte activity. For example, patients with massive hepatocyte loss in histopathologic materials had severely diminished levels of hepatocyte-derived coagulation factors (i.e. V, VII) and associated compromise in other hepatocellular functions as measured by clearance studies. Many subsequent attempts to quantify this critical hepatocyte mass yielded somewhat varied results. For example, surgical removal of 80–90 percent of the liver in man leads to an ALF-like syndrome in some, but by no means all, cases (Pack et al. 1962). Liver failure can be induced in some animals following much smaller hepatic resections under specific experimental conditions, but the similarity to the human ALF syndrome is unclear. In human ALF, the hepatocyte volume fraction, that is, the fraction of biopsy specimens comprising of seemingly viable hepatocytes, was found to correlate directly with survival (Donaldson et al. 1993). Likewise, estimation of the functional hepatocyte mass from clearance studies measuring pyrazone and galactose elimination put it at 5–10 percent of normal in nonsurvivors, but at least 15–20 percent in survivors (Ramsoe et al. 1980).

Support for the metabolic mass concept also came from a comparison of enzyme patterns in freshly autopsied liver tissue and sera from patients with ALF with the results in biopsies from nonfatal hepatitis and normal liver. On the whole, enzyme activities were markedly lower in the fatal cases. Analysis of nearly 30 enzyme activities in necropsied ALF liver tissue showed a loss of liver-specific functions in favor of enzyme pathways seen in undifferentiated cells such as fetal or tumor cells. These changes in enzyme systems towards glycolysis, and away from gluconeogenesis (including enzymes linked to amino acid and lipid metabolism) and the hexose monophosphate pathway, a slowing of citric acid cycle and probable impairment of the urea cycle (Taketa et al. 1976; Schmidt and Schmidt 1981) suggest that remaining hepatocytes optimize cell survival strategies to the possible detriment of other cells and organs.

The toxin hypothesis

The rapidity of onset of multiorgan failure and cerebral edema in ALF led other investigators to postulate a toxic phenomenon as central to this syndrome. Starting in the 1960s and 1970s, the finding of elevated levels of ammonia, mercaptans, phenols, and fatty acids in the blood of patients with ALF suggested that portal blood was not being cleared adequately of these gut-derived materials by the liver. Despite conflicting evidence about the separate roles of each of these putative toxins, a considerable body of animal data suggest that these compounds can act synergistically to produce coma (Zieve 1992). Whether this coma bears any relationship to that observed in ALF remains unclear. Thus, cerebral edema occurs essentially only in ALF, and extremely rarely not in comatose patients with chronic liver disease despite similar blood levels of these compounds. Moreover, reduction of these blood levels by administration of nonabsorbable antibiotics improves cerebral function in chronic but not acute encephalopathy. Defenders of the toxin hypothesis attributed these differences to the rapidity of onset of toxemia in ALF, the development of local secondary events in the brain, the deficiency of key liver-derived substrates, and other unspecified factors. Further support for this hypothesis was provided by reported improvements in neurologic status in ALF after detoxification by, for example, extracorporeal sorbent hemoperfusion and polyacrylonitrile hemodialysis and by documentation of deleterious effects of these compounds at the cellular level in the brain and in other organs. However, as discussed later, when the clinical detoxification regimens were subjected to randomized, controlled trials, no benefit was found (O'Grady et al. 1988).

A critique

As we have pointed out, massive hepatic necrosis such as occurs in ALF involves injury to all of the cell types within the liver, as well as disruption of critical anatomic relationships between hepatocytes, bile ductules, reticuloendothelial phagocytes and their blood supply.

The focus of both of the hypotheses just described is entirely on hepatocellular function. Indeed, to the extent that proponents of the toxin hypothesis examined principally the potentially toxic roles of small molecules such as ammonia, mercaptans, phenols or short chain fatty acids metabolized or detoxified by the hepatocyte, the two hypotheses are fundamentally the same. Furthermore, in attributing all of the many features of the ALF syndromes to deficits in either the synthetic or detoxification functions of the hepatocyte, proponents of both of these hypotheses speculated far beyond what could be supported by data.

Although a focus on hepatocellular failure continues to underlie most experimental treatment strategies, by the late 1970s or early 1980s it had become clear that these conceptual constructs did not adequately explain the complexity of the syndrome. Hans Popper observed astutely that the severity and duration of clinical events in ALF were considerably influenced by the cause of the injury and did not correlate neatly with estimates of histopathologic injury (Popper 1976). This has been confirmed by clinical and laboratory studies in which the presence of regenerative foci, elevated mitotic indices, or adequacy of histologically viable hepatocytes (hepatocyte volume fractions ⩾35–40 percent) did not prevent development of end organ complications or prognosticate survival (Gazzard et al. 1975; Tygstrup et al. 1981). Similarly, high hepatocyte growth factor (HGF) levels or efforts to stimulate regeneration of liver mass in small studies using insulin and glucagon have been unsuccessful in enhancing survival (Chapter 10). Increasing skill in the metabolic support of the anhepatic experimental animal has led to a growing recognition of the differences in pathophysiology between these animals and those with massive hepatic necrosis. These observations are supported by the observation that removal of the necrotic liver in ALF actually stabilizes the patient, at least temporarily, while awaiting transplant (Ringe et al. 1988; Olafsson et al. 1995). Finally, careful clinical study of the various complications of ALF has led to increasing focus on the roles of endotoxemia and cytokine cascades, presumably reflecting reticuloendothelial and endothelial cell injury (Izumi et al. 1994; Bhagwandeen 1987). Thus, outcome in ALF is probably tied both to the nature of the underlying injury and to the resulting cascade phenomena. Based on current information, the spectrum of multiorgan failure in ALF can be explained best by a model in which the primary injury results in a chain of events, both in and outside of the liver, which occur and may perpetuate themselves regardless of the state of the liver. Therapeutic strategies in ALF must address a far more complex pathophysiology than can be explained solely by defective hepatocellular function.

An alternative view

To understand more fully the pathobiology of ALF, it is essential, first of all, to examine the role of the hepatocyte in far greater detail. In particular, it is important to scrutinize carefully the implicit assumption that the histologic appearance of viability is equivalent to normal hepatocellular function. Second, the role of injury to nonparenchymal cells requires closer investigation. Finally, the relationship of cellular injury within the liver to a variety of networks and cascades which provide likely explanations for the nonhepatic manifestation of ALF must be integrated into the overall understanding.

Recent technologic advances in molecular and cell biology have yielded considerable new information about cellular dysfunction and injury. It is clear that the progressive evolution of ALF results from complex cellular, biochemical, and molecular events which include not only the failure of metabolic machinery of the cell, but also generation of toxic species, decreased cytoprotective capabilities, and altered cell to cell interaction. As we shall note subsequently, most (but not all) cases of ALF are associated with liver cell necrosis. The mechanisms which lead to liver cell necrosis have recently been reviewed in detail (Rosser and Gores 1995). They include: loss of plasma membrane integrity, including bleb formation and rupture; loss of intracellular ion homeostasis; an imbalance of prooxidant and antioxidant pathways; mitochondrial dysfunction and ATP depletion; and activation of degradative hydrolases. The ability to reverse these processes, once initiated, would represent a major breakthrough in the treatment of ALF. Indeed, preliminary efforts have shown some success both in vitro and in vivo, the most striking examples involving the use of *N*-acetylcysteine. However, the generalized application of this strategy in ALF is still in its infancy.

While it is clear that profound hepatocyte injury leads to metabolic failure including, for example, a failure to clear gut derived toxins, the conventional view of events focuses only on the consequence of a reduction or absence of normal hepatocyte function. The growing recognition that the hepatocyte actively contributes to the syndrome of ALF is a major change in thinking. The "toxemia of liver failure" is proving much more complex than previously conceived. Moreover, there is growing evidence that essential components of this toxemia derive from hepatocytes, including those necrotic, those injured and those still functional, rather than from extrahepatic sources like the gut. Qualitative differences among hepatocytes have been demonstrated by both electron microscopic and biochemical studies which showed morphologic changes in subcellular organelles, including disruption of rough endoplasmic reticulum with loss of attachment and disappearance of ribosomes, and mitochondrial and plasma membrane changes, as well as alterations in phase I and phase II enzymatic processes involved in biotransformation and detoxification (Popper 1976; Holloway 1981). These observations suggest that viable-appearing hepatocytes in a setting of cell injury may exhibit a markedly altered physiology. More recent studies of newly formed cells produced in a toxin-induced regenerative environment suggest that such cells possess fetal phenotypes and do not carry out the differentiated functions of adult hepatocytes (Diehl et al. 1994). Distinguishing the role of actual hepatocellular injury from the effects of viable yet qualitatively altered hepatocytes is not yet possible. However, the occurrence of many features of the ALF syndrome in conditions characterized by microvesicular steatosis emphasizes that aberrant rather than absent cellular metabolic processes may be central to pathogenesis in the absence of necrosis. In the presence of necrosis, however, necrosis itself seems to achieve a pathogenetic role. We have already noted that cerebral edema and (at least initially) hemodynamic compromise are not prominent in anhepatic animal models, in contrast to toxic or ischemic models (Olafsson et al. 1995), and that near terminal patients awaiting liver transplantation often show dramatic improvement in intracranial pressures, hemodynamic and metabolic parameters after hepatectomy (Ringe et al. 1988; Olafsson et al. 1995). How the necrotic liver contributes to cerebral edema and cardiovascular instability is at present entirely speculative.

Apart from the possibly deleterious role of the necrotic or dysfunctional hepatocyte in mediating extrahepatic manifestations of ALF, observations in man and in experimental models of liver failure point to the involvement in pathogenesis of other cell types within and outside of the liver. In the majority of cases of ALF hepatic histopathology reveals the presence of polymorphonuclear cells, T cells, B cells, other mononuclear cells, and activated sinusoidal cells. Molecular biologic advances are illuminating the cellular interactions which are critical in mediating injury, repair, and regeneration. Some of these are discussed in detail in Chapters 7 and 9. The idea that synergistic forces (i.e. endotoxin, cytokines, cells) are critical in the amplification of liver injury characteristic of ALF began to crystallize in the late 1970s as a result of studies of reticuloendothelial function and endotoxemia (Nolan 1981). This work demonstrated that hepatic injury induced by a variety of toxins could be ameliorated by removal of endotoxin by colectomy, antibiotics or genetic manipulation. Investigators speculated that alterations of Kupffer cell function, which had been found to be often decreased in ALF, increased Kupffer cell sensitivity to damage by endotoxin; and that endotoxemia thereby further compromised hepatic detoxification mechanisms, allowing endotoxin to cause direct and indirect, mediator induced damage to hepatocytes, endothelial cells, and extrahepatic sites. Data obtained in several models of acute liver failure (e.g. frog virus 3), forms of acute liver injury such as anoxia/reperfusion, virally mediated diseases, and drug hepatotoxicity also suggest that the Kupffer cell plays a key role in injury and in the recruitment of a host of inflammatory cells (Rosser and Gores 1995). The steps from initial hepatocyte injury to the inflammatory response, and the mechanisms responsible for this synergistic toxicity, are still poorly understood. However, it is clear that both nonparenchymal cells such as sinusoidal endothelial and Ito cells, resident and nonresident macrophages, and migratory inflammatory cells are involved, and that they release toxic oxygen species, proteases, phospholipase A2, mitochondrial radicals, leukotrienes, cytokines including TNF-α, NO, and procoagulants (Spitzer 1994). The actions and functions of these various compounds are likewise incompletely understood, but they are thought collectively to mediate inflammation, B and T cell stimulation, immunosuppression, antiviral and tumor effects, local ischemic injury due to microvascular stasis and thrombosis, and tissue remodeling. Recent studies attempting to clarify these relationships in the galactosamine and CCl_4 models have demonstrated that blockage or depletion of some mediators (e.g. TNF-α, MH-3 prothrombinase musfiblp) or inflammatory cells such as neutrophils and T cells, leads to markedly improved histology and survival compared to control animals (Czaja et al. 1995; Komatsu et al. 1994; Li et al. 1992).

Evidence suggesting modulation of extrahepatic events by these nonparenchymal cells and their mediators has also been accumulating. Similarities between sepsis and ALF, such as the hyperdynamic circulation, abnormalities in tissue oxygen extraction, disseminated intravascular coagulation, and immune coagulation activation, have long raised questions about a similar pathogenesis. Recent evidence of improvement in tissue oxygen extraction, hemodynamic parameters, and cerebral edema after *N*-acetylcysteine administration has highlighted the role of various mediators (Harrison et al. 1996). It has been suggested that the beneficial effects of *N*-acetylcysteine result from inhibition of proinflammatory cytokines, enhanced NO production, and improved microvascular tone. Despite this work, and known disturbances in the levels of cytokines, endotoxin, prostaglandins (e.g. E_1, I_2), and Gc protein in ALF, no single pathogenetic mechanism or mediator thus far explains the various features of the syndrome. Further, the lack of efficacy of various therapies employed in this condition, including steroids, anticoagulants, prostaglandins, and antivirals, emphasizes both the persistent challenge of acute liver failure and the importance of developing relevant animal models.

ANIMAL MODELS

The development of a suitable animal model of ALF which is representative of the human experience has long been recognized as an important goal, since, inter alia, it would provide a system in which to test experimental therapies. The task has been difficult due in part to the diversity of presentations and etiologies in man. Investigators recognized early on that basic requirements for an optimal animal model should include: reversibility of the lesion; reproducibility in the proportion of animals dying and in time of death; death after a coma demonstrably caused by hepatic failure; minimal hazard of causative agent to personnel; and applicability to man, similarity in biocompatibility characteristics as they relate to devices, and ease of serial measurements and treatments (Terblanche et al. 1975).

Several models of hepatic failure and hepatic encephalopathy have been developed, reflecting the diversity of etiologies which culminate in ALF. These include: induction by chemical agents which interfere in part with metabolic pathways in the liver (i.e. galactosamine, thioacetamide, carbon tetrachloride, acetaminophen, anesthetics); surgical models such as the anhepatic state and devascularization procedures (portacaval shunt model with or without modifications including hepatic artery ligation, partial hepatectomy, and/or preoperative dimethylnitrosamine); viral models (adenovirus, HBV, frog virus 3); and immunologic models (e.g. monoclonal antibody directed toward plasma glycoprotein) (Potter and Berk 1992).

To date, no animal model meets all of the desired criteria. Shortcomings include marked variations in mortality not only between species, but even within strains (e.g. galactosamine, portacaval shunt, frog virus 3); lack of uniformity in development of encephalopathy (galactosamine in rats) or in the tempo of its progression; and the recognition of important differences in molecular mechanisms of cell replication and regeneration between partial hepatectomy and cell injury models (see Chapter 9). Most importantly, these animal models do not reproduce the clinical picture of ALF with respect to metabolic and physiologic compromise of the liver or the involvement and failure of other critical organs. Despite their deficiencies, animal models have been helpful to our understanding of pathophysiology and in the development of liver assist technologies.

LIVER ASSIST STRATEGIES AND DEVICES

Against this background, we shall examine both the underlying premises and the experimental and clinical results achieved within various types of extracorporeal liver assist devices and related modalities in the treatment of ALF. In theory, if they were to represent definitive therapy for ALF these strategies had to accomplish four objectives: support of the metabolic function of the hepatocyte; stabilization of other critical organs; prevention or amelioration of extrahepatic complications; and fostering of hepatic regeneration. The last is less important if the device is to be used solely as a short-term bridge to transplantation. The relevant literature is vast, much of it describing techniques that represent only minimal variations on those tried and reported earlier. In view of our Editors' merciful restrictions on the size of the reference list, we cite here only representative examples of the various broad approaches which have been described. It may be of interest to the reader that most of the basic concepts already employed or currently under development had been reported by 1960. The development of various strategies, physicochemical, biological, or hybrid devices which combined physicochemical and biological components, mirrored the theoretical beliefs of their proponents about the underlying abnormalities in ALF which artificial liver support systems would need to address: performance of synthetic and metabolic functions, detoxification, and/or assistance with excretory function. Efforts to develop extracorporeal support systems went on in parallel with other experimental therapeutic approaches including heparinization, cytoprotective therapies, and efforts to stimulate regeneration. It is important to state that, over the past quarter century, the major advances in survival in ALF have come from other quarters: from improvements in the intensive care offered to patients with ALF in specialized centers, and from liver transplantation.

Purely physicochemical extracorporeal liver assist devices

The premise that noxious substances (toxins) are central to the pathophysiology of ALF, as they are in kidney failure and in chronic liver disease, made it plausible to investigate the use in ALF of treatments already being applied in kidney failure (hemodialysis) and drug intoxication (adsorption). Waste products and toxins removed by the kidney are typically small (molecular weight <400 daltons), hydrophilic, water soluble and nonprotein bound, and therefore suitable for ultrafiltration at the glomerulus. Wastes taken up by the liver are more often hydrophobic or amphiphilic, more tightly protein bound, and therefore removed from the circulation by specific plasma membrane transport systems. On theoretical grounds, one would predict that hemodialysis would provide a better analog of glomerular ultrafiltration, and some form of adsorbent system a better model of hepatic uptake. Nevertheless, the observation in the 1950s that hemodialysis could improve encephalopathy in cirrhotics led to attempts in ALF to remove small nitrogenous waste molecules such as ammonia, urea, and other compounds by hemodialysis across standard dialysis membranes (Kiley et al. 1956). After anecdotal successes, lack of improved survival in larger series (Benhamou et al. 1972) led to the conclusion that the toxemia of ALF was not composed simply of soluble low molecular weight compounds, and resulted in the use of modified membranes of greater porosity to allow removal of larger soluble toxins (Opolon et al. 1976a). That toxins could also have differing physicochemical characteristics (hydrophobic rather than hydrophilic), and differing physical states (protein-bound rather than free) was not specifically known but made sense in light of the liver's complex metabolic role. Two markedly differing approaches developed: broad-based detoxification of either water soluble compounds (by dialysis) or both soluble and nonsoluble compounds (by adsorption); and detoxification of specific compounds within a narrower spectrum (e.g. by affinity chromatography, enzyme-carrier systems). It was hoped that any successful treatment would remove unidentified toxins along with successful removal of presumed model compounds. This approach to ALF made the implicit assumption that accumulation of toxins normally removed by the hepatocyte was at the root of the ALF syndrome.

Middle molecules

The middle molecule (MM) hypothesis became a major focus of investigation in ALF as a result of evidence that removal of soluble but otherwise uncharacterized compounds in the molecular weight range of 400 to 1500 daltons (so-called middle molecules) resulted in an improvement in encephalopathy in patients with both kidney failure and chronic liver disease (Oules et al. 1978). Several groups subsequently identified unique or greatly augmented chromatographic peaks within the middle-molecule size range in the plasma of patients with acute and chronic liver disease, using gel filtration, as seen in Figure 18.1 (Leber et al. 1981). Similar peaks were observed in animal models such as the galactosamine intoxicated rat. Isolation of several individual peaks and further analysis by thin layer chromatography, as seen in Figure 18.2, identified a number of particular peptides among the components of these peaks (Leber et al. 1981). Despite finding that there were major increases in specific fractions in liver failure which differed from the fractions that were increased in uremia, and that some of these liver failure related fractions and their peptide components could be corrected either by dialysis using a special large pore polyacrylonitrile (PAN) membrane or by sorbent hemoperfusion (Leber et al. 1981; Nikolaev et al. 1992), few further attempts were made to determine the makeup of these peaks, or the nature of protein bound macromolecules also found to be increased. The failure to characterize the makeup of the toxemia in acute liver failure was in contrast to the extensive efforts made to characterize the biochemical composition of uremic plasma. Moreover, several investigators had established that specific test molecules could be removed from plasma with very high efficiency either by affinity chromatography over specifically designed gel

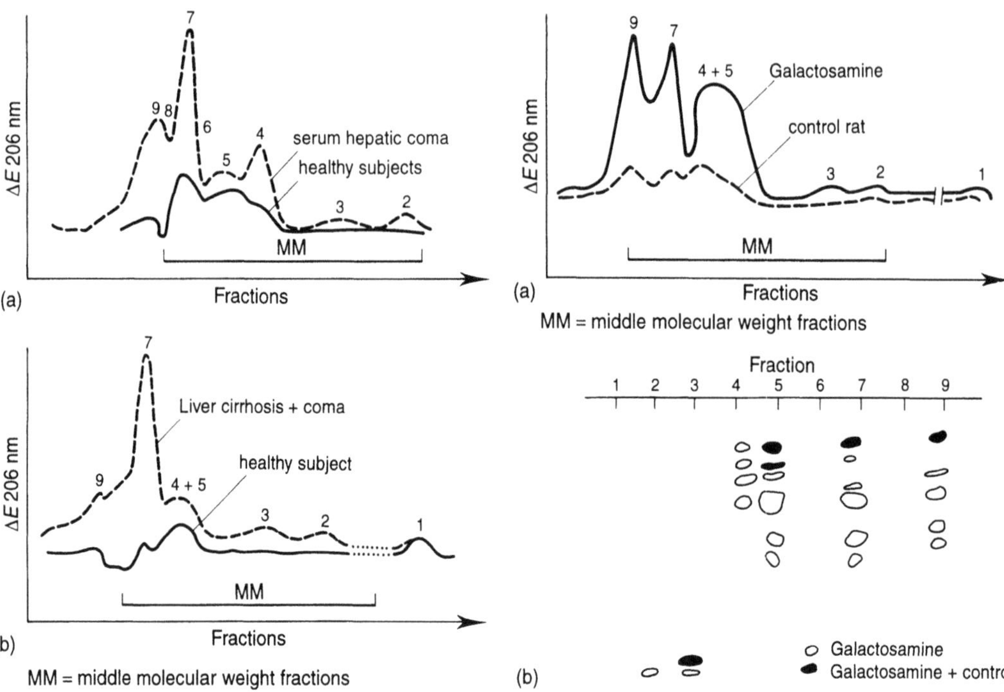

Figure 18.1 Sephadex GS gel filtration studies of plasma obtained from a patient with hepatic coma associated with (a) fulminant viral hepatitis and (b) cirrhosis. Peaks seen in the absorbance measurements suggest increased quantities of discrete compounds in patient plasma compared to healthy controls. In larger numbers of patients the pattern of abnormal peaks in ALF differed in some respects from that in chronic portosystemic encephalopathy. Modified from Leber et al. 1981 with permission.

Figure 18.2 (a) Sephadex gel filtration pattern of plasma from a rat with galactosamine-induced acute liver failure and a normal control animal. (b) Thin layer chromatographic analysis of peptides in the fractions identified in (a). Peptides were identified by ninhydrin staining. Those indicated in black were present in samples from both normal and galactosamine treated animals; those shown in outline were found only in the plasma of galactosamine treated animals. Modified from Leber et al. 1981 with permission.

matrices (Plotz et al. 1974), or with the use of artificial carrier or gel entrapped immobilized enzyme(s) (Grunwald and Chang 1979). In the absence of data about the particular toxins which need removal in ALF, the strategy of specific detoxification largely fell by the wayside. Instead, investigators generated a large body of literature on the ability of various relatively nonspecific sorbents or different hemodialysis membranes to remove a variety of model compounds. Compounds of interest included a variety of water soluble middle and low molecular weight molecules (e.g. ammonia, various amino acids, including phenylalanine, tyrosine, and tryptophan, which are the precursors of both true neurotransmitters and false neurotransmitter compounds such as octopamine) as well as more lipophilic, protein bound compounds (e.g. certain mercaptans, phenols, and fatty acids).

Sorbent hemoperfusion

The prototypical sorbent is charcoal. Because of its enormous surface area, a consequence of its porosity, it has an enormous if quite nonspecific adsorptive capacity. Several studies compared the adsorptive properties of charcoals from different sources. Although coconut charcoal came to be relatively favored, little firm data suggested that it had any significant clinical advantages. Possibly because of its surface area, or its many jagged edges, untreated charcoal particles proved not to be biocompatible; that is, when perfused with blood they caused a significant loss of formed elements, particularly platelets and neutrophils, initiated complement activation, and precipitated a number of other problems which limited their clinical applicability. To improve biocompatibility, activated charcoal granules coated with albumin (ACAC) or encapsulated in cellulose nitrate or a variety of hydrophilic gels were investigated. To some extent, the nature of the coating modified the spectrum of molecules adsorbed, leading to a further expansion of this literature. So great was the optimism about the potential effectiveness and biocompatibility of coated charcoal that it was discussed in the literature as the basis for "artificial cells," and as a component of a future "artificial liver device" for use in ALF. In contrast to charcoal, neutral synthetic resins were expected to have fewer problems with biocompatibility and to be more effective in removing lipophilic compounds. Positively charged (anion exchange) resins were of interest because of the hope that they would have an advantage in the selective removal of negatively charged species.

Ultimately, three major classes of sorbents were employed in laboratory and/or clinical hemoperfusion studies: various forms of charcoal, with a variety of coatings; synthetic resins, including both neutral resins such as XAD-2, XAD-4, XAD-7 and anion exchange resins, for example, dowex-1; and agarose gels to which compounds with specific binding affinities had been coupled (e.g. albumin: agarose affinity chromatography). Many of these sorbents were tested in hemoperfusion experiments in various animal models, almost in the hope that comparison of sorbents with somewhat differing specificity might identify, or rather stumble on, the right spectrum of model compounds to have a clinical impact. Biocompatibility was repeatedly compared, although it was clearly established that choice of species and experimental conditions could markedly modify the results of biocompatibility studies (Berk et al. 1982).

Comparisons of these sorbents did reveal some broad differences in the spectrum of materials adsorbed. ACAC had a high capacity for removal of a wide range of materials, with relatively little specificity. Thus, it fairly efficiently removed various middle molecules in the 1000–1500 daltons molecular weight range, polypeptides, mercaptans, GABA, other neurotransmitter metabolites, phenols, aromatic amino acids, endotoxin, and inhibitors of hepatic regeneration and cerebral Na-K ATPase (Losgen et al. 1992), but removed ammonia poorly and did not remove protein-bound molecules at all. As predicted, resins had a superior ability to remove lipid soluble organic molecules (uncharged resins) or various high molecular weight materials including cytokines and complex side chain anions, which are normally bound to proteins (anion exchange resins).

Hemodialysis

Development of modified hemodialysis membranes increased their permeability to permit efficient passage of molecules with molecular weights of up to 15,000 daltons. Unlike sorbents, use of these membranes was not associated with major biocompatibility issues or the generation of particulate matter and hence was assumed to be safer. As with various hemoperfusion systems, dialysis studies with the polyacrylonitrile (PAN) membrane in irreversible animal models reported that it could prolong survival, improve neurologic function as judged clinically and by electroencephalogram, and also improve measurements of plasma and brain amino acids and neurotransmitters (Opolon et al. 1976b).

Clinical efficacy

The development of liver failure centers in the 1970s in the UK and France allowed for the first time testing of PAN hemodialysis and sorbent hemoperfusion in appreciable numbers of patients. Typical of this period, widespread enthusiasm for these purely physicochemical devices was based on temporary improvements in levels of putative toxins and depth of coma discussed in reports of isolated cases, small series, and uncontrolled trials in patients, as well as improvements in survival reported both in patients and in animal models (Tabata and Chang 1980). Thus, a relatively extensive series of patients treated at King's College Hospital, London, with coated charcoal hemoperfusion showed appreciably better outcomes than did historical controls (Gazzard et al. 1974). This enthusiasm failed to take into account the major improvements in survival achieved by simultaneous advances in liver failure intensive care, most of which also emanated from this same unit at King's. When the charcoal hemoperfusion regimen was eventually subjected to a randomized, controlled comparison with contemporaneous controls, no beneficial effect on survival was observed (O'Grady et al. 1988). Similarly, a study of PAN hemodialysis in 24 patients showed a statistically significant improvement in neurologic status compared to historical controls but no improvement in survival. Lengthening duration of PAN hemodialysis or combining PAN hemodialysis with correction of abnormal amino acid profiles by various methods was not associated with improved outcome (Losgen et al. 1981).

A post mortem

These failures to show a survival benefit of either charcoal hemoperfusion or PAN hemodialysis represented a major setback to proponents of a purely physicochemical approach to artificial liver support systems. They suggested that, while the nonspecific removal of a variety of substances might improve metabolic encephalopathy, it did not alter survival.

Failure of these detoxification approaches had in fact been predicted (Berk and Goldberg 1988). It was suggested that crucial gaps in knowledge made these approaches a shot in the dark, which were unlikely to succeed without a firmer scientific basis. The specific concerns raised included: the biochemical nature of the toxemia of ALF had been characterized only superficially; causal relationships between particular, known biochemical abnormalities and acute hepatic encephalopathy were entirely speculative; the pathogenesis of the various extrahepatic manifestations of ALF, which as noted earlier are the principal causes of death, were largely unknown; and the possible negative impact of removal of unrecognized stimulatory factors, hormones, and other beneficial compounds had not been considered adequately. Moreover, even if correction of toxemia was a theoretically valid strategy, the absence of critical information about the internal distribution and kinetics of relevant toxins compromised the development of logical treatment protocols (Berk et al. 1980). Despite these concerns, which remain equally valid today, efforts using modified broad spectrum detoxification devices based on sorbents and newly designed membranes are ongoing (Chapter 22).

Biological support

Failure of mechanical devices to improve survival reinforced the concept that replacement of deficient substrates and/or lost hepatic synthetic and metabolic capabilities might be critical to any treatment strategy. In its earliest forms, this approach simply involved exchange transfusion or plasma exchange. More advanced forms of biologic support involve providing the patient with the support of an extracorporeal, functioning liver, or a means of perfusing the patient's blood or plasma through a system incorporating viable, functioning hepatocytes. Irrespective of the pathogenesis of the extrahepatic manifestation of ALF, an optimized biologic support device should be able to provide an interim replacement for many aspects of hepatocyte function.

Exchange blood transfusion/plasma exchange

This form of therapy dates back to the 1950s,

with a brief renewal of interest a decade later, when continuous flow centrifuges greatly increased the efficiency of the procedure. Removal of large volumes of the patient's plasma theoretically accomplished the removal of middle molecules and protein bound toxins. Exchange with fresh blood or plasma combined this effect with the provision of essential circulating substances, including clotting factors and other, unidentified hepatocyte products. Unfortunately these forms of treatment are not risk free. They also have not been shown to alter survival (Chapter 21).

Biological extracorporeal liver assist devices

Extracorporeal whole organ perfusion

In parallel with physicochemical detoxification efforts, other investigators studied the effectiveness of extracorporeal liver tissue in liver failure. In 1957, cross-hemodialysis between man and dog, in which a semipermeable cellophane membrane separated two blood filled circuits, led to rapid recovery from coma accompanied by ammonia clearance (Hori 1982). Subsequent experimental studies of the extracorporeal perfusion of pig livers with human blood demonstrated bile flow, galactose elimination, clearance of ammonia, bilirubin and BSP, but no significant improvement in survival (Eiseman et al. 1965). Many reports, from the 1960s to the 1990s, virtually all uncontrolled, described extracorporeal perfusion of blood from patients with ALF or with chronic liver disease through either cadaveric or live organs from baboons, pigs, and calves. While evidence of effective function, as measured by clearance techniques, has commonly been reported, these studies have not convincingly demonstrated a survival benefit, except possibly as a bridge to transplantation (Chari et al. 1994). Issues of rapid organ availability, safety, simplicity, hyperacute rejection in nonprimates and other aspects of immunologic incompatibility, as well as recent issues of animal welfare, have hindered the further development of this approach.

Liver assist devices containing liver elements or isolated liver cells

In vitro experiments as long as 40 years ago with devices containing canine and porcine derived fresh liver homogenate, slices, and freeze-dried "granules" showed beneficial effects on glucose levels, hyperammonemia, and lactic acidemia (Nose et al. 1963). The first clinical studies of this approach, in 1959, used freeze-dried liver granules and slices in a small number of patients (Mikami et al. 1959). Subsequent extracorporeal perfusion studies using liver slices in anhepatic pigs (Soyer et a. 1973), while not improving survival, did demonstrate improvement in EEG tracings, bilirubin conjugation, and ureagenesis. The failure of these early efforts to exploit liver cells/tissue for extracorporeal support has been attributed to the limited durability of the liver components and to the use of relatively impermeable dialysis membranes separating these components from the patient's circulation. During the next two decades, the ability to isolate, preserve, and maintain the functional integrity of hepatocytes or liver-derived cell lines, including their long term storage in cartridges for extracorporeal perfusion, has been instrumental in development of biologically based liver assist devices (LADs). Prototypes consisting of such biological components alone, or as hybrid devices which also incorporate nonbiological methods of detoxification, are described in detail elsewhere (Chapters 19, 20, and Rozga et al. 1994). The devices with which the largest recent clinical experience has been gained incorporate either primary pig hepatocytes or a transformed human hepatoblastoma cell line (C3A), respectively.

The results of historical in vitro experimental studies with prototype "bioreactor" systems demonstrated protein synthesis, gluconeogenesis, ureagenesis, and phase I and phase II biotransformation activities

(Table 18.1). The comparable in vivo experience in toxic, devascularized, and anhepatic animal models of ALF (Table 18.2), using isolated hepatocytes in a variety of "bioreactors," also demonstrated variable degrees of metabolic function, including gluconeogenesis, albumin production, ureagenesis, and ornithine production from arginine; p450 function (production of MEGX from lidocaine) and other biotransformation activities; and detoxification (ammonia clearance) (Rozga et al. 1994). Variable improvements in survival and neurologic function have been seen. The anhepatic model, while unassociated with the necrotic phenomena seen in most cases of human ALF, has been useful in determining the appropriate number of hepatocytes required in different experimental LADs to sustain useful metabolic function. Direct comparison of the efficacy of these two systems has been difficult because of, inter alia, differences in the design and bioengineering of the units themselves, differences in the procedures which have been used to assess their respective functional activities, differences in the clinical spectrum of liver failure associated with the different animal models tested, the relatively small number of animals used per group in each experiment, as well as the variation in outcome among control animals.

Role of LAD in the 1990s

Apart from a controlled clinical study from Latvia, which did not substantiate function of a small suspension of porcine hepatocytes in a charcoal column (Margulis et al. 1989), there

Table 18.1. *Historical results with bioartificial livers in vitro. Modified from Rozga et al. 1994 with permission*

Author	Hepatocytes	Bioreactor	Effect
Wolf and Munkelt (1975)	Reuber hepatoma	Hollow-fiber	Bilirubin uptake and conjugation
Hager et al. (1978)	Mouse	Hollow-fiber	Ureagenesis, protein synthesis, diazepam metabolism, cytidine deamination
Kasai et al. (1980)	Dog	Hollow-fiber	Cytotoxicity of post-perfusion pig serum to dog hepatocytes, maintenance of ATP
Demetriou et al. (1986)	Rat, microcarrier-attached	Chromatography column	Bilirubin synthesis and conjugation, protein synthesis
Yanagi et al. (1989)	Rat and rabbit, gel-entrapped	Rotating discs	Ammonium removal, urea synthesis
Moscioni et al. (1990)	Human, micro-carrier-attached	Hollow-fiber metabolism	Cyclosporin
Shatford et al. (1992)	Rat	Hollow-fiber	Albumin synthesis, amino acid and lidocaine clearance, oxygen consumption
Sussman et al. (1992)	C3A (hepatoma-derived) cells	Hollow-fiber	Glucose utilization, albumin synthesis
Nyberg et al. (1993b)	Rat	Hollow-fiber	Synthesis of albumin urea and ornithine, O_2 uptake, lidocaine metabolism, arginine clearance
Li et al. (1993)	Rat	Pyrex glass beads in a glass vessel	Urea and albumin synthesis
Rozga et al. (1993b)	Rat	Hollow-fiber	Cyclosporin and 19-*Nor*-testosterone metabolism

Table 18.2. *Historical results with bioartificial livers in vivo. Modified from Rozga et al. 1994 with permission*

Author	Hepatocytes	Bioreactor	Animal model	Effect
Matsumura (1973)	Rat	Hemodialyzer	CCl_4-induced liver failure in rats	Clearance of BSP, bilirubin, NH_3, albumin synth.
Olumide et al. (1977)	Pig	Parallel plate membranes	Anhepatic pig	Neurologic improvement
Kasai et al. (1984)	Dog	Hollow-fiber	Gal-induced liver failure in dogs	Improved survival time
Uchino et al. (1988)	Pig	Glass plates	Anhepatic pig	Improved survival time
Yanagi et al. (1989)	Rabbit (gel-entrapped)	Rotating discs	Ischemic liver failure in cats	Ammonium clearance
Arnaout et al. (1990)	Rat	Hollow-fiber	Hyperbilirubinemic (Gunn) rat	Bilirubin conjugation
Shnyra et al. (1991)	Rat (microcarrier-attached)	Unspecified column	CCl_4 and D-Gal-induced liver failure in rats	Improved survival
Nyberg et al. (1992 and 1993a)	Rat	Hollow-fiber rabbit	Anhepatic rabbit	Albumin synthesis, clearance of amino acids, NH_3 and lactate
Sussman et al. (1992)	C3A (hepatoma-derived) cells	Hollow-fiber	Acetaminophen-induced liver failure in dogs	Two of three dogs survived
Takahashi et al. (1992)	Porcine	50 glass plates	Anhepatic rabbit	Improved survival time?
Fremond et al. (1993)	Rat	Hollow-fiber	Gunn rat	Conjugation of bilirubin
Rozga et al. (1993a)	Dog, porcine, cryopreserved and fresh, microcarrier-attached	Hollow-fiber	Ischemic liver failure in dogs	Normoglycemia, clearance of NH_3 lactate, normal PT, hemodynamic stability

have been no large clinical trials of LADs. The devices receiving the most attention have been the pig hepatocyte-based bioartificial liver (BAL) device developed by Demetriou's group (Rozga et al. 1994) and the extracorporeal liver assist device (ELAD) described by Sussman et al. (Sussman et al. 1994). The major differences between these devices include: the nature of the cells employed to provide hepatocellular function; the nature of the perfusate (plasma in the BAL, blood in the ELAD); inclusion of a nonbiologic charcoal column in the system (only with BAL); and length and pattern of treatment (continuous or repeated pulse). These differences, and the most up to date review of the in vivo experience in animals and man, are discussed elsewhere (Chapter 20; Rozga, Podesta et al. 1994).

Preliminary testing of both the BAL and ELAD in humans is still very limited, but suggests overall safety and, possibly, some efficacy. Specifically, in a noncontrolled series of seven patients, treatment with the BAL was accompanied by a significant reduction of intracranial pressure (ICP), increase in cerebral perfusion pressure, improvement in the ratio of branched chain to aromatic amino acids in plasma and reduced circulating ammonia. These changes were accompanied by an improvement in neurologic status. All of these patients underwent orthotopic liver transplantation as donor organs became available, and the effect of BAL on outcome, except possibly as a bridge to transplantation, cannot be assessed. What role, if any, the entire BAL or the hepatocytes it contains played in the reductions in ICP cannot be determined from the available data in this small experience. The ELAD has recently been tested in a small controlled pilot study at the King's. While showing evidence of metabolic function, it did not significantly influence survival, either with or without transplantation.

TREATMENT OF ACUTE LIVER FAILURE

Contemporary management

The history of therapies for acute liver failure is one of repeated cycles of great enthusiasm based on a limited, uncontrolled but always positive published experience. It was this history which led to the apt advice of Benhamou and colleagues (1972) to sufferers of ALF: "Be published or perish." However, such enthusiasm has, until now, inevitably been followed by disillusionment as more rigorous data are produced. Thus, more meticulous evaluations of the efficacy of many previously accepted therapies, such as steroids, heparin, prostaglandins, exchange transfusion, and charcoal hemoperfusion, have led to their abandonment. During this same period, as the pathophysiology of ALF and its complications have become better understood, significantly better survival has been achieved with meticulous improvements in standard liver failure intensive care. This improved care has increased mean survival in ALF from 15 percent to 50 percent in certain patient groups by providing metabolic support and prevention or treatment of numerous associated and predictable complications (Atillasoy and Berk 1995).

The basis for a rational approach to treatment was provided by Tygstrup (Tygstrup et al. 1975). According to his model (Figure 18.3), ALF patients with stage III–IV encephalopathy can be divided into three groups. Group I comprises patients whose residual liver function, although reduced to a degree that results in neurological dysfunction, does not fall below a hypothetical survival limit. For those patients, conventional intensive care to prevent or manage life threatening complications should assure survival. In Group II are those patients whose residual function becomes inadequate to sustain life but whose livers nevertheless have the potential to regenerate if they can be kept alive long enough. Temporary liver support systems, future cytoprotective therapies, and growth factors to stimulate regeneration would all be of potential benefit in this population. Group III comprises patients with liver damage sufficient to preclude effective regeneration and whose only hope for survival is transplantation.

If it were possible to accurately classify patients into Groups I, II, or III, a menu of general medical, liver-specific and surgical options could be called upon to customize the approach to the individual patient. Accurate

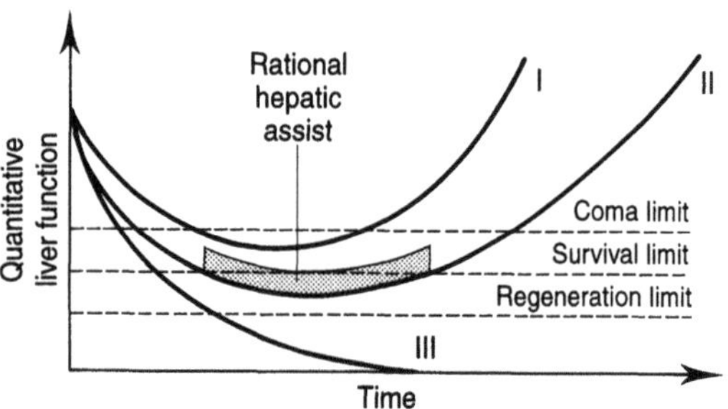

Figure 18.3 Hypothetical courses of patients with fulminant hepatic failure, classified according to residual hepatic function. The extent of residual function, if it could be clinically determined with sufficient precision, would define the therapeutic approach in each case. Patients in group I would be candidates for intensive medical therapy in a specialized liver failure unit, while those in group III should be referred for early liver transplantation. Group II patients represent candidates for artificial liver support. Reproduced from Tygstrup et al. 1975 with permission.

classification would not only be therapeutically valuable, but would also dramatically improve the ability to assess the value of new treatments. Unfortunately, the lack of biochemical, clinical, or pathologic variables which are consistently predictive of outcome for an individual patient early in the course of ALF has made application of Tygstrup's conceptual basis for treatment strategies difficult to implement.

Proven available therapies are, therefore, meticulous liver failure intensive care (described in Chapter 10) and liver transplantation. Calls for a multicenter trial comparing medical therapy and transplantation, including cases with intermediate levels of illness, are not merely premature, but probably misguided. In appropriately categorized and prognosticated patient populations, the two should be mutually exclusive.

What about LADs? As stated above, we see them ultimately as one aspect of a bridge to transplantation. Before they can achieve even this limited role, numerous technical and bioengineering issues must be solved, not the least of which is the fundamental question of how large a cell mass is required to provide meaningful metabolic support in humans? Once this and other issues have been solved in the context of a much improved understanding of the biology of the normal liver and of ALF, large randomized controlled trials will still be necessary to determine their efficacy. Unless such trials can be conducted in appropriately selected populations as described by Tygstrup, their interpretation will remain fraught with uncertainty.

Future strategies

Fundamental questions about the pathophysiology of ALF, posed previously (Berk and Goldberg 1988; Berk 1978), remain largely unanswered. Provision of an adequate metabolic mass which can produce necessary substrates and possibly detoxify a still undefined spectrum of toxins remains, so to speak, a stab in the dark. This quasi-strategy does not address the complexity of parenchymal and nonparenchymal hepatic and extrahepatic events. Areas requiring considerable further attention include cellular and immunologic mechanisms of injury, full characterization of the nature and consequences of hepatic toxemia, the pathogenesis of the extrahepatic manifestations of ALF, the potential of cytoprotective strategies, and regulation of hepatocellular repair and regeneration. Further work on prognostic indicators and relevant animal models would in our view also pay large dividends. We would argue that without therapies having the potential of ending primary injury, stimulating cellular cytoprotective defenses, repairing early and reversible subcellular damage, and stimulating regeneration, the role of present day LADs will be limited, at best, to short term pretransplant support.

CONCLUSIONS

As we have indicated above, it is our view that each of the major cell populations within the liver makes a crucial contribution to normal homeostasis, and that ALF reflects the loss of the contribution of at least the endothelial and Kupffer cell populations as well as the hepatocyte. Indeed, many of the clinical features which dominate the syndrome of ALF and frequently lead to death, including cerebral edema, renal failure, infection and coagulopathy, probably reflect nonparenchymal cell dysfunction, endotoxemia, and cytokine cascades resulting from massive tissue necrosis to a far greater extent than they reflect the loss of hepatocellular function. The corollary to this view is that strategies for liver assist devices that focus solely on restoring hepatocellular function are likely to fail.

Survival in ALF of certain etiologies has increased substantially over the past two decades, as careful bed-side observation and good clinical science have led to management strategies which stave off, or at least delay, potentially fatal complications. The etiologies which have benefited presumably are those in which affected livers have the greatest potential for early regeneration. For those without this potential, survival in the absence of transplantation has changed relatively little. We have argued for some time that more science, both basic and clinical, and improved understanding of fundamentals such as regeneration, rather than the application of increasingly complex devices bioengineered on the basis of an inadequate knowledge base, are the strategies most likely to optimize outcomes in this dramatic and frightening illness.

REFERENCES

Arnaout, W.S., Moscioni, A.D., Barbour, R.L., et al. 1990. Development of bioartificial liver: bilirubin conjugation in Gunn rats. *J Surg Res* 48: 379–82.

Atillasoy, E. and Berk, P.D. 1995. Fulminant hepatic failure: pathophysiology, treatment, and survival. *Ann Rev Med* 46: 181–91.

Benhamou, J.P., Rueff, B. and Sico, C. 1972. Severe hepatic failure: a critical study of current therapy. In: *Liver and Drugs*, eds. F. Orlandi and A.M. Jezequel, 213–28. New York: Academic Press.

Berk, P.D. 1978. Artificial liver: a baby delivered prematurely. *Gastroenterology* 74: 789–90.

Berk, P.D. and Goldberg, J.D. 1988. Charcoal hemoperfusion: plus ça change, plus c'est la même chose. *Gastroenterology* 94: 1228–30.

Berk, P.D., Schafer, D.F., Blitzer, B.L. and Jones, E.A. 1980. Computer models and animal models: A rational stepwise approach to the development of artificial hepatic support systems for the treatment of fulminant hepatic failure. In: *Hemoperfusion: Kidney and Liver Support and Detoxification*, eds. S. Sideman and T.M.S. Chang. Hemisphere Publishing Corp., Washington, 151–74.

Berk, P.D., Schafter, D., Baruch, J., Kulshretha, V.K. and Jones, E.A. 1982. Sorbent biocompatibility is a function of species and parameter studied, and choice of anticoagulant. *Artifical Organs: Proceedings of the III Meeting of the International Society for Artificial Organs*, Vol. 5 (Supplement). pp. 542–46.

Berk, P.D., Sorrentino, D. and Van Ness, K. 1995. Whole organ, hepatocellular and subcellular specialization of the liver with respect to its role in bile secretion and the transport of small molecules: An overview. In: *Methods in Biliary Research*, ed. M. Muraca, 1–19. Boca Raton: CRC Press.

Bhagwandeen, S.B., Apte, M., Manwarring, L. and Dickeson, J. 1987. Endotoxin induced hepatic necrosis in rats on an alcohol diet. *J Pathol* 152: 47–53.

Blei, A. 1991. Cerebral edema and intracranial hypertension in acute liver failure: distinct aspects of the same problem. *Hepatology* 13: 376–9.

Chari, R.S., Collings, B.H., Magee, J.C., DiMaio, J.M., Kirk, A.D., Harland, R.C., McCann, R.S., et al. 1994. Brief report: treatment of hepatic failure with ex-vivo pig liver perfusion followed by liver transplantation. *N Engl J Med* 331: 234–7.

Czaja, M.J., Xu, J. and Alt, E. 1995. Prevention of carbon tetrachloride-induced rat liver injury by soluble tumor necrosis factor receptor. *Gastroenterology* 108: 1849–54.

Demetriou, A.A., Whiting, J., Levenson, A.M., et al. 1986. New method of hepatocyte transplantation and extracorporeal liver support. *Ann Surg* 204: 259–71.

Diehl, A., Yin, M., Fleckenstein, J., Yang, S., Lin, H., Brenner, D., Westwick, J., Bagby, G. and Nelson, S. 1994. Tumor necrosis factor – alpha induces c-jun during the regenerative response to liver injury. *Am J Physiol* 267: G552–61.

Donaldson, B.W., Gopinath, R., Wanless, I.R., Phillips, M.J., Cameron, R., Roberts, E.A., Greig, P.D., Levy, G. and Blendis, L.M. 1993. The role of transjugular liver biopsy in fulminant liver failure: relation to other prognostic indicators. *Hepatology* 18: 1370–4.

Eiseman, B., Liem, D.S. and Raffucci, F. 1965. Heterologous liver perfusion in treatment of hepatic failure. *Ann Surg* 162: 329–45.

Fremond, B., Malandain, C., Guyomard, C., et al. 1993. Correction of bilirubin conjugation in the Gunn rat using hepatocytes immobilized in alginate gel beads as an extracorporeal bioartificial liver. *Cell Transpl* 2: 453–60.

Gazzard, B.G., Portmann, B., Murray-Lyon, I.M. and Williams, R. 1975. Causes of death in fulminant hepatic failure and relationship to quantitative histologic assessment of parenchymal damage. *Q J Med.* 175: 615–26.

Grunwald, J. and Chang, T.M.S. 1979. Microencapsulated multienzyme system and the recycling of NAD^+ bound to soluble dextran. In: *Hemoperfusion: Kidney and Liver Support and Detoxification*, eds. S. Sideman and T.M.S. Chang. Hemisphere Publishing Corp., New York, 389–98.

Gumucio, J.J. and Berkowitz, C.M. 1992. Structural organization of the liver and function of the hepatic acinus. In: *Liver and Biliary Diseases*, ed. N. Kaplowitz, 2–17. Baltimore: Williams & Wilkins.

Hager, J.C., Carman, R., Stroller, R., et al. 1978. A prototype for a hybrid artificial liver. *ASAIO J* 24: 250–3.

Harrison, P., Wendon, J. and Williams, R. 1996. Evidence of increased guanylate cyclase activation by acetylcysteine in fulminant hepatic failure. *Hepatology* 23: 1067–72.

Hickman, R., Bracher, M., Tyler, M., Lotz, Z. and Fourie, J. 1992. Effect of total hepatectomy on coagulation and glucose homeostasis in the pig. *Dig Dis Sci* 37: 328–34.

Holloway, C.J. 1981. The biochemistry of hepatic detoxification. In: *Artificial Liver Support*, eds. G. Brunner and F.W. Schmidt. Springer-Verlag, New York, 32–38.

Hori, M. 1982. Artifical liver: the concept and working hypothesis of hybrid organs from a 25-year-old anecdote to the 21st century model. *ASAIO J* 28: 639–41.

Izumi, S., Hughes, R.D., Langley, P.G., Pernambuco, J.R.B. and Williams, R. 1994. Extent of the acute phase response in fulminant hepatic failure. *Gut* 35: 982–6.

Kasai, S., Ohno, M., Asakawa, M., et al. 1980. Studies on hybrid artifical liver metabolic activity of isolated hepatocytes after cryopreservation. *Jpn J Artif Organs* 9: 390–3.

Kasai, S., Oikawa, I., Asakawa, H., Yamamoto, T., Sawa, M., Sakata, H., et al. 1984. Evaluation of an artificial liver support device using isolated hepatocytes. In:

Progress in Artificial Organs – 1983, eds. K. Atsumi, M. Maekawa, K. Ota. ISAO Press, Cleveland, 732–8.

Kiley, J.E., Welch, H.F., Pender, J.C. and Welch, C.S. 1956. Removal of blood ammonia by hemodialysis. *Proc Soc Exp Biol Med* 91: 489–90.

Komatsu, Y., Shiratori, Y., Kawase, T., Hashimoto, N., Han, K., Shiina, S., Matsumura, M., Niwa, Y., Kato, N., Tada, M., Ikeda, Y., Tanaka, M. and Omata, M. 1994. Role of polymorphonuclear leukocytes in galactosamine hepatitis: mechanism of adherence to hepatic endothelial cells. *Hepatology* 20: 1548–56.

Leber, H.W., Klausmann, J., Goubeaud, G. and Shutterle, G. 1981. Middle molecules in the serum of patients and rats with liver failure: influence of sorbent-hemoperfusion. In: *Artifical Liver Support*, eds. G. Brunner and F.W. Schmidt. Springer-Verlag, New York, 96–102.

Li, A.P., Barker, G., Beck, D., et al. 1993. Culturing of primary hepatocytes as entrapped aggregates in a packed bed bioreactor; a potential bioartificial liver. *In Vitro Cell Dev Biol* 29A: 249–54.

Li, C., Fung., L.S., Crow, A., et al. 1992. Monoclonal anti-prothrombinase (3D4.3) prevents mortality from murine hepatitis virus infection (MHV-3). *J Exp Med* 1763: 689–97.

Losgen, H. 1992. Absorption therapy in acute liver failure: a critical resume. In: *Artificial Liver Support – Concepts, Methods, Results*, eds. G. Brunner and M. Mito. Springer-Verlag, New York, 175–80.

Losgen, H., Neumann, E., Eisenbach, G., Schmidt, F.W. and Brunner, G. 1981. Correction of increased plasma amino acid levels by dialysis with amino-acid-electrolyte-glucose solutions. In: *Artificial Liver Support*, eds. G. Brunner and F.W. Schmidt. Springer-Verlag, New York, 153–58.

Margulis, M.S., Erukhimov, E.A., Andreiman, L.A. and Viksna, L.M. 1989. Temporary organ substitution by hemoperfusion through suspension of active donor hepatocytes in a total complex of intensive therapy in patients with acute hepatic insufficiency. *Resuscitation* 18: 85–94.

Matsumura, K.N. 1973. Method and device for purifying blood. US Patent No. 3734851. US Patent Office, Washington, DC.

Matsumura, K.N., Guevara, G.R., Huston, H., Hamilton, W.L., Rikamuru, M., Yamasaki, G. and Matsumara, M.S. 1987. Hybrid bioartificial liver in hepatic failure: Preliminary clinical report. *Surgery* 101: 151–7.

Mikami, J., Moto, M., Nishimuro, A., et al. 1959. Surgical treatment of acute liver failure II: an experimental study of extracorporeal metabolism in the artificial liver using slices of canine liver. *Jpn J Gastroenterol* 56: 1022.

Moscioni, A.D., Backisch, G., Black, D. and Demetriou, A.A. 1990. Long term cryopreserved human hepatocytes maintain drug metabolizing activity. *Surg Forum* 41: 3–4.

Nikolaev, V.G., Sarnatskaya, V.V., Ivanyuk, A.A. and Yushko, L.A. 1992. Thermodynamic criteria for the removal of certain hepatic insufficiency markers from protein containing solutions. In: *Artificial Liver Support: Concepts, Methods, Results*, eds. G. Brunner and M. Mito. Springer-Verlag, New York, 197–210.

Nolan, J.P. 1981. Endotoxin, reticuloendothelial function, and liver injury. *Hepatology* 1: 458–65.

Nose, Y., Mikami, J., Kasai, Y., et al. 1963. An experimental artificial liver utilizing extracorporeal metabolism with sliced and granulated canine liver. *ASAIO J* 358–62.

Nyberg, S.L., Payne, W.D., Amiot, B., Shirabe, K., Remmel, R.P., Hu, W.S. and Cerra, F.B. 1993. Demonstration of biochemical function by extracorporeal xeno-hepatocytes in an anhepatic model. *Transl Proc* 25: 1944–5.

Nyberg, S.L., Platt, J.L., Shirabe, K., Payne, W.D., Hu, W.S. and Cerra, F.B. 1992. Immunoprotection of xenocytes in a hollow fiber bioartificial liver. *ASAIO J* 38: M463–7.

Nyberg, S.L., Shatford, R.A., Peshwa, M.V., et al. 1993a. Evaluation of a hepatocyte entrapment hollow fiber bioreactor: a potential artificial liver. *Biotechnol Bioeng* 41: 194–203.

Nyberg, S.L., Mann, H.J., Remmel R.P., et al. 1993b. Pharmacokinetic analysis verifies P450 function during in vitro and in vivo application of a bioartificial liver. *ASAIO J* 39: M252–6.

Nyberg, S.L., Shirabe, K., Peshwa, M.V., et al. 1993. Extracorporeal application of gel-entrapped bioartificial liver: demonstration of drug metabolism and other biochemical functions. *Cell Transpl* 2: 441–52.

O'Grady, J.G., Gimson, A.E.S., O'Brien, C.J., Pucknell, A., Hughes, R.D. and Williams, R. 1988. Controlled trials of charcoal hemoperfusion and prognostic factors in fulminant hepatic failure. *Gastroenterology* 94: 1186–92.

Olaffson, S., Gottstein, J. and Blei, A.T. 1995. Brain edema and intracranial hypertension in rats after total hepatectomy. *Gastroenterology*. 108: 1097–103.

Olumide, F., Eliashiv, A., Kralios, N., Norton, L. and Eiseman, B. 1977. Hepatic support with hepatocyte suspensions in a permeable membrane dialyzer. *Surgery* 82: 599–606.

Opolon, P., Lavallard, M.C., Huguet, C., Bidallier, M., Granger, A., Gallot, D. and Bloch, P. 1976a. Hemodialysis versus cross hemodialysis in experimental liver coma. *Surg Gynecol Obstet* 142: 845–54.

Opolon, P., Rabin, J.R., Huquet, C., Granger, A., Delorme, J.L., Boschat, M. and Sausse, A. 1976b. Hepatic failure coma treated by polyacrylonitrile membrane hemodialysis. *ASAIO J* 22: 701–10.

Oules, R., Asaba, H., Meuhausser, M., Yahiel, V., Baehrendtz, S., Gunnarsson, B., Bergstrom, J. and Furst, P. 1978. Hemoperfusion and removal of endogenous uremic middle molecules. In: *Artificial Kidney, Artifical Liver, and Artificial Cells*, ed. T.M.S. Chang. Plenum Press, New York, 153–64.

Pack, G.T., Islami, A.H., Hubbard, J.C. and Brasfield, R.D. 1962. Regeneration of human liver after hepatectomy. *Surgery* 52: 617–22.

Plotz, P.H., Berk, P.D., Scharchmidt, B.F., Gordon, J.K. and Vergalla, J. 1974. Removing substances from blood by affinity chromatography. 1. Removing bilirubin and other albumin bound substances from plasma and blood with albumin-conjugated agarose beads. *J Clin Invest* 53: 778–85.

Popper, H. 1976. Pathogenesis of hepatic failure. *Kidney Int* 10: S225–8.

Potter, B.J. and Berk, P.D. 1992. Animal models of hepatic failure and encephalopathy. In: *Artificial Liver Support*, eds. G. Brunner and M. Mito, 94–120. New York: Springer-Verlag.

Preston, F.E. 1991. Haemorrhagic diathesis and control. In: *Acute Liver Failure; Improved Understanding and Better Therapy*, eds. R. Williams and R.D. Hughes, 36–9. London: Miter Press.

Ramsoe, K., Andreasen, P.B. and Ranek, L. 1980. Functioning liver mass in uncomplicated and fulminant acute hepatitis. *Scan J Gastroenterol*. 15: 65–72.

Ringe, B., Pichlmayr, R., Lubbe, N., Bornscheuer, A. and Kuse, E. 1988. Total hepatectomy as temporary approach to acute hepatic or primary graft failure. *Transpl Proc* 20 (Suppl. 1): 552–7.

Rolando, N., Gimson, A., Wade, J., Philpott-Howard, J., Casewell, M. and Williams, R. 1993. Prospective controlled trial of selective parenteral and enteral antimicrobial regimen in fulminant liver failure. *Hepatology* 17: 196–201.

Roll, F.J. and Friedman, S.L. 1992. Role of sinusoidal endothelial cells, lipocytes, Kupffer cells, and pit cells in the liver. In: *Liver and Biliary Diseases*. ed. N. Kaplowitz, 2–17. Baltimore: Williams & Wilkins.

Rosser, B.G. and Gores, G.J. 1995. Liver cell necrosis: cellular mechanisms and clinical implications. *Gastroenterology* 108: 252–75.

Rozga, J., Holzman, M.D., Ro, M.S., et al. 1993a. Hybrid artificial liver support – treatment of animals with severe ischemic liver failure. *Ann Surg* 217: 502–11.

Rozga, J., LePage, E., Morsiani, E. and Demetriou, A.A. 1994. Liver support system development. In: *Support of the Acutely Failing Liver*, ed. A.A. Demetriou. R.G. Landes Co., Austin, 60–81.

Rozga, J., Podesta, L., LePage, E., Morsiani, E., Moscioni, A.D., Hoffman, A., Sher, L., Villami, F., Woolf, G., McGrath, M., Kong, L., Rosen, H., Lanman T., Vierling, J., Makowka, L. and Demetriou, A.A. 1994. A bioartificial liver to treat severe acute liver. *Ann Surg* 219: 538–46.

Rozga, J., Williams, F., Ro, M.S., et al. 1993b. Development of a bioartificial liver: properties and function of a hollow fiber module inoculated with liver cells. *Hepatology* 17: 258–65.

Schmidt, E. and Schmidt, F.W. 1981. Enzyme patterns in liver failure. In: *Artificial Liver Support*, eds. G. Brunner and F.W. Schmidt. Springer-Verlag, New York, 8–17.

Shatford, R.A., Nyberg, S.L., Meier, S.J., White, J.G., Payne, W.D., Hu, W.S. and Cerra, F.B. 1992. Hepatocyte function in a hollow fiber bioreactor; a potential artificial liver. *J Surg Res* 53 (6): 549–57.

Shnyra, A., Bocharov, A., Bochkova, N., et al. 1991. Bioartificial liver using hepatocytes on Biosilon microcarriers: treatment of chemically induced acute hepatic failure in rats. *Artif Org* 15: 189–97.

Soyer, T., Lempinen, M., Walker, J., et al. 1973. Extracorporeal assist of anhepatic animals using liver slice perfusion. *Am J Surg* 126: 20–4.

Spitzer, J. 1994. Cytokine stimulation of nitric oxide formation and differential regulation in hepatocytes and nonparenchymal cells of endotoxemic rats. *Hepatology* 19: 217–28.

Sussman, N.L., Chong, M.G., Koussayir, T., He, D.E., Shong, T.A., Whisennand, H.H. and Kelly, J.H. 1992. Reversal of fulminant hepatic failure using an extracorporeal liver assist device. *Hepatology* 16: 60–5.

Sussman, N.L., Gislason, G.T., Conlin, C.A. and Kelly, J.H. 1994. The *Hepatix* extracorporeal liver assist device: initial clinical experience. *Artif Org* 18: 390–6.

Tabata, Y. and Chang, T.M.S. 1980. Comparison of six artificial liver support regimes in fulminant hepatic coma rat. *ASAIO J* 26: 394–99.

Takahashi, M., Matsue, H., Matsushita, M., et al. 1992. Does a porcine hepatocyte hybrid artificial liver prolong the survival time of anhepatic rabbits? *ASAIO J* 38: M468–72.

Taketa, K., Shimamura, J., Taesue, A., Tanaka, A. and Konsake, K. 1976. Undifferentiated patterns of key carbohydrate-metabolizing enzymes in injured livers. *Enzyme* 21: 200–10.

Terblanche, J., Hickman, R., Miller, D.J. and Saunders, S.J. 1975. Animal experience with support systems: are there appropriate animal models of fulminant hepatic necrosis? In: *Artificial Liver Support*, eds. R. Williams and I.M. Murray-Lyon. Pitman Publishing Corp., New York, 163–72.

Trey, C. and Davidson, C. 1970. The management of fulminant hepatic failure. *Pro Liver Dis* 3: 282–90.

Tygstrup, N., Andreasen, P.B. and Ranek, L. 1975. Liver failure and quantitative liver function. In: *Artificial Liver Support*, eds. R. Williams and I.M. Murray-Lyon. Pitman Medial, Tunbridge Wells, UK, 286–90.

Tygstrup, N., Gaub, J. and Ranek, L. 1981. Determination of liver function and liver regeneration in fulminant hepatic failure. In: *Artificial Liver Support*, eds. G. Brunner and F.W. Schmidt. Springer-Verlag, New York, 39–45.

Uchino, J., Tsuburaya, T., Kumagai, F., et al. 1988. A hybrid bioartificial liver composed of multiplated hepatocyte monolayers. *ASAIO J* 34: 972–7.

Wolf, C.F.W. and Munkelt, B.F. 1975. Bilirubin conjugation by an artificial liver composed of cultured cells and synthetic capillaries. *Trans ASAIO J* 21: 16–27.

Yanagi, K., Ookawa, K., Mizuno, S. et al. 1989. Performance of a new hybrid artificial liver support system using hepatocytes entrapped within a hydrogel. *Trans ASAIO J* 35: 570–2.

Zieve, L. 1992. Biochemistry of liver failure. In: *Artificial Liver Support – Concepts, Methods, Results*. Brunner G., Mito M., eds. Springer-Verlag, New York, 21–31.

Zucker, S.D. and Gollan, J.L. 1994. Physiology of the liver. In: *Bockus Gastroenterology. Fifth edition, Vol. 3 (Liver)*, eds. W.S. Haubrich, F. Schaffner and J.E. Berk, 1858–1905. Philadelphia: Saunders.

19 Hepatocyte culture and bioreactor design for liver support systems

Jörg C. Gerlach

INTRODUCTION

Massive necrosis of hepatocytes in acute liver failure destroys synthesis, metabolism, and elimination pathways of the liver. For the past 20 years, artificial liver systems have been under development with the aim of providing temporary extracorporeal liver support (Wolf and Munkelt 1975). Most recently, development of "bioartificial" liver support systems has utilized liver cells cultivated in bioreactors to provide the biological activity of liver cells in extracorporeal systems (Pappas 1988). In this review, liver cell culture systems, bioreactor design and construction, animal experiments with hybrid liver support systems, and initial clinical applications are described.

In vitro studies have demonstrated the long-term external metabolic function of primary isolated hepatocytes within bioreactors. These cell systems are capable of supporting essential liver functions. Animal experiments have verified the possibility of scaling-up the bioreactors for use in man. However, since there is no reliable animal model in which the treatment of acute liver failure can be properly assessed, results obtained from experimental studies to date, however promising, have limited relevance. The small number of clinical studies performed so far is not sufficient to allow conclusions to be drawn on improvements in the therapy of acute liver failure. Although important progress has been made in the development of these systems, the multiple different hepatocyte culture models and bioreactor constructions which are being described in the literature are an indication of the competition (and perhaps the limited successes) in this field of medical research.

The bioreactor construction designed by the author incorporates utilization of both hepatocytes and sinusoidal endothelial cells. The reactor is based on capillaries for hepatocyte aggregate immobilization, coated with biomatrix. Four separate capillary membrane systems, each permitting a different function, are woven in order to create a three-dimensional network. Cells are perfused via independent capillary membrane compartments. Decentralized oxygen supply and carbon dioxide removal with low gradients is possible. There is a decentralized co-culture compartment for nonparenchymal liver cells. The use of identical parallel units to supply smaller numbers of hepatocytes facilitates the scale-up to clinical use.

HEPATOCYTE CULTURE MODELS

Based upon advances in cell biology, several different culture models for maintenance of hepatocytes in vitro have been developed. These developments used basic cell culture methods in the construction of bioreactors for large-scale investigations in extracorporeal liver support (Figures 19.1–4). At least four types of cell culture designs or methods have been used. The differences relate variously to two important features, mainly the method of cell adhesion to the bioreactor, and the relation of cells to each other. Cells floating suspended in medium do not function effectively (Clayton et al. 1985). However, cells may be immobilized upon artificial membranes or capillaries (Figure 19.1). Earlier studies utilized immobilized cells on synthetic polymer capillaries (Wolf and Munkelt 1975), or polystyrene Amicon XM-50 capillaries (Amicon, Beverly, MA) (Jauregui et al. 1983). This usually implies a single cell sheet, and the cell-to-cell communication may be of value as well as providing close proximity of each cell to the membrane surface for interchange within plasma.

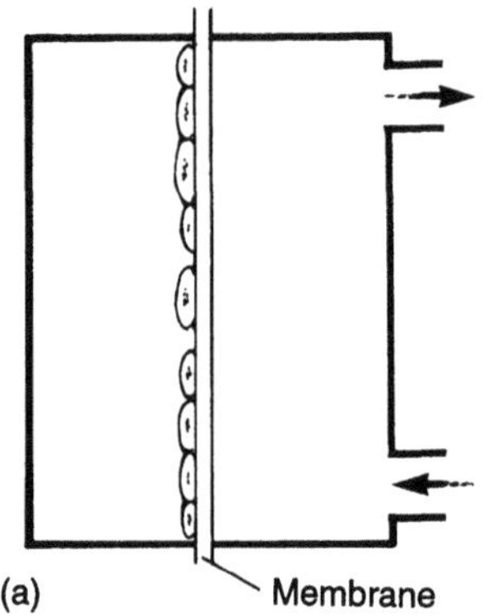

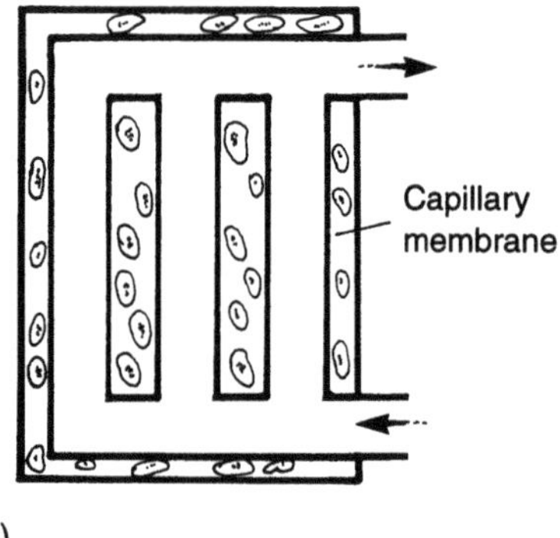

Figure 19.1 A bioreactor can be regarded as a chamber in which cells are maintained in order to support their survival, or in order to use their functions. The simplest way to do this is with the use of a suspension reactor in which the cells move freely in the culture medium. A more sophisticated construction which prevents loss of cells across the outlets is the use of a flat sheet (a) or capillary membranes (b). These membranes may be used in addition to enhance mass exchange to and from the cells.

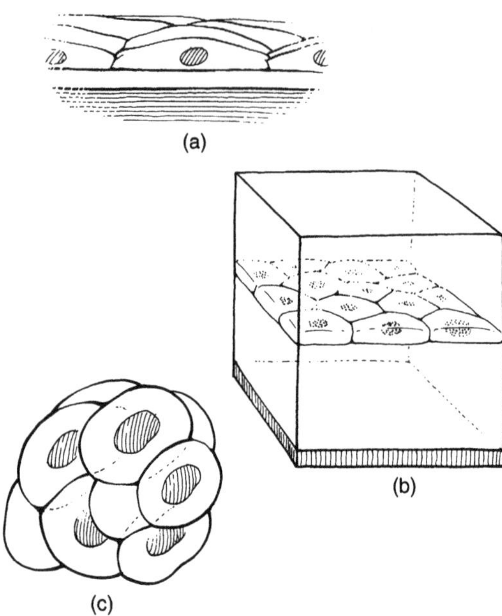

Figure 19.2 It is difficult to maintain hepatocytes in suspension, since they grow better on a substrate matrix. Immobilization may be accomplished by adhesion of cells to the surface of an artificial substrate (a), within a biological matrix (b) or by self-aggregation of hepatocytes (c).

A second approach employs microcarriers, artificial spherical bodies made from different materials including dextran, polystyrene and glass (Cunningham and Hodgson 1992), to which cells can adhere (Figure 19.2a). The carriers themselves can be cultured in suspension. The advantage of this technique (Kasai et al. 1992; Shynra et al. 1990), when compared with the standard monolayer culture in plastic flasks, is a larger surface for cell adhesion. Co-culturing of microcarriers with different cell types has also been investigated (Voss and Seibert 1991).

A third method of hepatocyte immobilization is the encapsulation of cells within

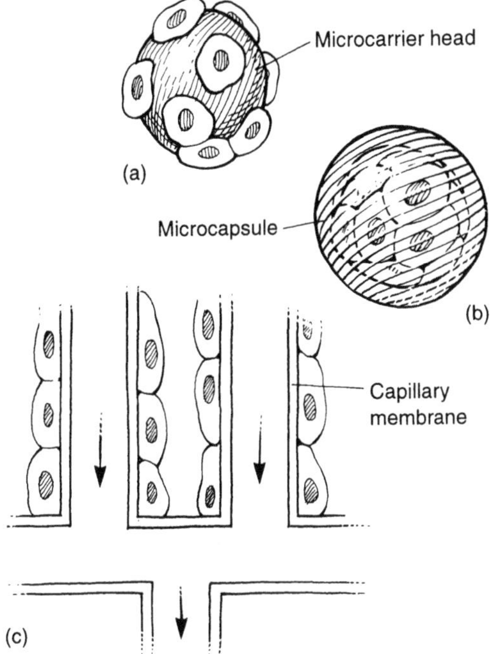

Figure 19.3 Microcarrier beads (a) represent a common method for immobilization to artificial substrates. Another possibility is the use of specially-developed microcapsules to encapsulate the cells prior to loading them into the reactor (b). The most common way is the use of the capillary membrane itself for hepatocyte immobilization (c).

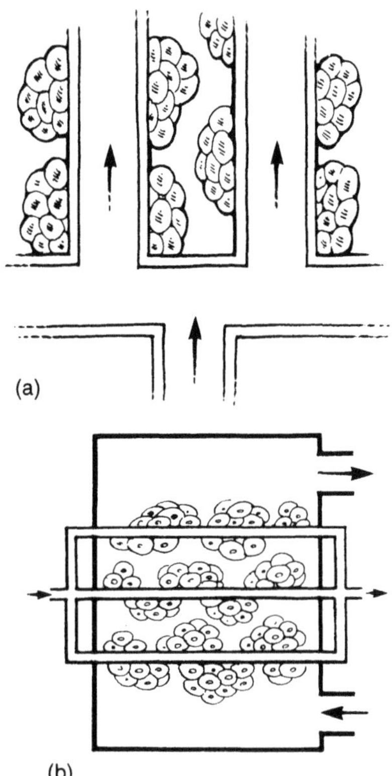

Figure 19.4 Hepatocytes can immobilize themselves under defined conditions by binding to each other and forming aggregates. One advantage of the capillary membrane technique is that it is possible to bind cell self-aggregates to capillaries. This diminishes the amount of artificial surface necessary for cell immobilization (a). Capillaries in reactors can also be used to enhance other technical functions like cell oxygenation (b). An even more promising bioreactor construction would be the use of several capillary systems for cell immobilization and additionally for nutrient exchange. Two capillary systems are show here – three independent systems are also feasible.

semipermeable membranes (Figure 19.2b). With this technique, cells are protected from mechanical damage. Additionally, the encapsulation provides immunoisolation from xenogeneic cells (Chang 1992; Sugamori et al. 1986). Some groups use alginate–polylysine as a capsule material (Sun et al. 1986; Sun et al. 1987). Results have also been reported with Matrigel® as an additional adhesion substrate (Dixit et al. 1992). Other groups have used polyacrylate (Sugamori et al. 1986) or sodium cellulose acetate and polymethylammonium-chloride (Stange et al. 1993).

A fourth method utilizes a culture model which is described as a "collagen sandwich culture" (Dunn et al. 1989). Cells are spread on a monolayer and then covered with another collagen layer. The long-term maintenance of function (Dunn et al. 1992) and integrity of the cytoskeleton (Ezzel et al. 1993) found by these workers have been attributed to the more physiological cell-to-cell interactions which take place in this model. The metabolizing capacity of liver-specific drugs in this type of cell culture can be measured (Bader et al. 1994). Koebe et al. have made the sandwich culture easier to handle with their "immobilization gel" technique showing comparable results (Koebe et al. 1994a) while at the same time offering greater stability of the cell culture in perfused systems with flow-induced shear stresses (Koebe et al. 1994b).

The aggregate culture technique involves

the immobilization of cells without the use of artificial matrix materials (Gerlach et al. 1995). Active self-aggregation of hepatocytes has been used (Landry et al. 1985) with neonatal hepatocytes, and with adult hepatocytes, respectively (Tong et al. 1990). A further refinement of the aggregate system uses a culture technique in which supplementary proteoglycans from reticular fibers of the rat liver are used (Shinji et al. 1988). In this system, cells are maintained in spherical aggregates with a diameter of approximately 120 μm. This culture model has the advantage that a suspension of cells as free aggregates in the medium is possible, avoiding further artificial adhesion materials (Koide et al. 1990). A number of factors influence cell growth and development in these systems. Glycosaminoglycans (Spray et al. 1987) in combination with insulin, epidermal growth factor (Kawaguchi et al. 1992) and other uncharacterized factors secreted by cells (Sakaguchi et al. 1991) were reported to influence cell morphology in these aggregates. Electron-microscopy of these multicellular spheroids reveals a well-differentiated cytoplasmic architecture and multiple bile canaliculi-like structures. In addition, nonparenchymal cells and a newly synthesized extracellular matrix could be observed (Asano et al. 1989).

Aggregate methods appear to have several advantages. While albumin production decreases in normal monolayer culture after four days, this cell culture method maintains a steady albumin synthesis for 14 days (Koide et al. 1989). Others have measured a reduced DNA-synthesis expression rate by increased synthesis of albumin in spheroid culture when compared to the monolayer techniques (Yuasa et al. 1993). Spherical aggregates can be encapsulated or used in a bioreactor over several weeks (Takabatake et al. 1991).

Other culture models have been developed. For example, calcium alginate has been used for immobilization (Miura et al. 1986), and protein synthesis has been demonstrated with this system. Detoxification (Miura et al. 1990; Tompkins and Carter 1988) has also been demonstrated in an alginate matrix system. A further refinement is the use of retained hepatocytes in reticular sponge structures (Yanagi et al. 1989).

Implantable systems utilizing microcarriers, microcapsules or aggregates have also been the subject of considerable work (see Chapter 23). Transplantation into the peritoneum or the spleen has been performed. However, a number of technical problems to transplantation of cells occur (Henne-Bruns et al. 1991). If a sufficient cell mass is to be provided, space for the transplanted cells is needed and the location as well as viability of transplanted cells becomes a problem (Henne-Bruns 1993). Additionally, peritonitis and subsequent intra-abdominal adhesions may develop with the accompanying threat of mechanical ileus. The present chapter, therefore, is limited to devices which can be used as extracorporeal systems.

BIOREACTOR CONSTRUCTION

Bioreactors enable the culture models described above to be used on a large scale (Vanholder and Ringoir 1991a; 1991b). They permit the potential of hybrid-type extracorporeal liver support systems to be developed.

The first capillary membrane liver cell bioreactor was constructed in 1972 by Knazek et al. (Knazek et al. 1972; 1974) with some semipermeable capillary membranes for cell adhesion and metabolite exchange. Since then, three general categories of hepatocyte bioreactors have emerged: bioreactors for suspension culture without cell immobilization; bioreactors based on cell immobilization; and bioreactors with membranes which provide both mass transfer and cell immobilization functions.

Most early bioreactors incorporated a concept of cells being nonanchorage dependent, although they were intended for anchorage-dependent liver cells. Olumide et al. developed a two-chamber system which was divided by flat sheet cuprophane membranes (Olumide et al. 1977) (Figure 19.1a). An early clinical trial (Matsumura et al. 1987) was based upon a similar construction. One side of the reactor contained rabbit hepatocytes, and on the other, patient blood was circulated. A large clinical study was performed (Margulis et al. 1989; 1990) in which 20 ml capsules filled with pig hepatocytes in suspension were used.

The advantage of hepatocyte suspension bioreactors is their ability to incorporate a large number of cells in constructions which are simple to build and operate. However, since hepatocytes are anchorage-dependent cells, their viability and function is limited to a few hours after isolation from the donor-organ (Gerlach, Klöppel et al. 1989). This means that such systems are not very practical for clinical treatment, since the cells would have to be exchanged for new ones several times each day.

To address this problem, some bioreactor constructions integrate certain materials for cell attachment (Figure 19.2a). Biosolon® microcarriers may be used to immobilize hepatocytes inside a blood perfused column (Shynra et al. 1991). A similar approach aimed at producing a high adhesion surface area was taken by Uchino (Tuburaya et al. 1989). In a reactor, glass plates with a diameter of 20 × 10 cm were used to culture cells (Uchino et al. 1988; 1991). Others have used a flat sheet model with 40 rotating discs, where hepatocytes were immobilized in calcium alginate hydrogel (Yanagi et al. 1989; Yanagi 1990). The aggregate culture model produces self-immobilized cells. Takabatake et al. used this in an extracorporeal perfusion system (Takabatake et al. 1991) in which some 200 aggregates were perfused and oxygenated in a glass cylinder.

Capillary membrane devices are commonly used in other fields of medicine, e.g. in hemodialysis. Since hepatocytes can be immobilized upon membranes, such reactors offer a large hepatocyte attachment surface (Figure 19.2c). Membranes with different chemical and physical properties have been used (Jauregui et al. 1983; Demetriou et al. 1993). The capillaries of these membranes each generate an intra- and extraluminal compartment with connection of the two compartments by pores of defined size. Hepatocytes are normally attached to the outer capillary wall (Wolf and Munkelt 1975) or in combination with microcarriers (Arnaout et al. 1990; Rozga, Holzmann et al. 1993). Cells may also be attached to coated polysulfone capillaries which are used for cell nutrition and are located adjacent to neighboring cellulose acetate capillaries for blood circulation (Dixit 1994). Intraluminal hepatocyte seeding is also possible (Hu et al. 1991; Nyberg et al. 1993; Shatford et al. 1992; Scholz and Hu 1991).

Most of the more complex culture models described above can be reproduced within hollow fiber bioreactors. Some techniques, such as microencapsulation (Matthew et al. 1991) (Figure 19.2b) or the incorporation of special biological matrix layers (Akaike et al. 1993) may be applicable to use in membrane bioreactors. It remains to be seen whether it is essential for reactors to have an artificial surface for the immobilization of all inoculated hepatocytes. The aforementioned aggregate technique might possibly negate this requirement (Figure 19.3a). In addition to cell immobilization, selective exchange of solutes between two compartments is possible with artificial membranes, so further technical functions can be provided inside a membrane reactor (Figure 19.3b and Figure 19.3c). Our own construction utilizes capillary membrane technology for immobilization of cells which subsequently reorganize to aggregates. These designs also incorporate different types of membrane to effect different functions.

DEVELOPMENT OF BIOREACTOR SYSTEM

Available culture models still produce a remarkable change in the local conditions of cells in comparison to their in vivo situation. It seems important that a culture model ensure high cell densities (Clayton et al. 1985) as well as providing a free three-dimensional cell rearrangement of the microenvironment of hepatocytes. At that point, hepatocyte self-aggregation, the reconstruction of junctional complexes, and the organization of cells into three-dimensional structures should facilitate the cooperative function of cells to maximize their effectiveness.

Most culture models rely on diffusion for substrate exchange, while hepatocytes in vivo operate under perfusion conditions. The in vivo gradients of oxygen, carbon dioxide and metabolites are not usually given sufficient consideration. As a result, the metabolite transfer vectors in such models are often greatly distorted when compared to the in vivo situation. A culture technique which allows the cells to operate under more physiologic conditions, for example flow conditions with low metabolite gradients, may result in a cell macroenvironment more closely related to the physiologic situation.

A culture model has been developed which addresses these requirements. Additional benefits such as high culture densities (Gerlach, Smith et al. 1994), decentralized metabolite exchange and direct membrane contact oxygenation (Gerlach, Klöppel et al 1990) are also incorporated. In this novel bioreactor construction, hepatocyte immobilization is achieved via cell attachment to supporting capillaries (Gerlach et al. 1990; Gerlach, Stoll et al. 1990), use of a biomatrix and a cell compatible capillary potting material (Gerlach, Schauwecker et al. 1989). One specific feature of the model is that the woven capillaries enter and leave the reactor in sorted, discrete bundles so that they can serve different functions. Independent plasma inflow, plasma outflow and oxygen supply as well as carbon dioxide removal are therefore possible. Each of many identical, parallel capillary units supplies only a few hepatocytes, resulting in perfusion with low gradients. Inclusion of a further capillary system allows intraluminal co-culture with sinusoidal endothelial cells to prevent the negative side effects of the hepatocytes over-growing in the intercapillary compartment.

Results of in vitro investigations (Gerlach and Neuhaus 1994; Gerlach, Encke et al. 1994; Gerlach, Encke, Hole, Müller, Courtney et al. 1994; Fuchs et al. 1994) demonstrate that primary hepatocyte cultures can be maintained over a period of several weeks in vitro and that they reorganize themselves to give tissue-like structures within the artificial system. The cells spontaneously form aggregates on and between the capillaries, and reorganize into a three-dimensional array. Rebuilt cell junctions and the reconstitution of bile canaliculi-like structures were demonstrated in all reactors under investigation. Even after seven weeks of perfusion, the cells display a relatively intact ultra-structure (Gerlach, Schnoy et al. 1995).

SIDE EFFECTS OF THERAPY WITH LIVER SUPPORT SYSTEMS

If blood or plasma is perfused through one compartment of a membrane reactor, this membrane can serve as an immunological barrier between the cells cultured on one side, and the patient on the other (Sullivan et al. 1991). In such an application, immunosuppression during and after a treatment with heterologous cells may be less important (Nyberg et al. 1992). Incorporation of a plasmapheresis system in the extracorporeal circuit and the consequent perfusion of reactors with plasma only, avoids direct contact between the patient's immunologically competent blood cells and the bioreactors. This may further prevent activation of the patient's white blood cells. However, movement of cytokines or other plasma factors across membranes may still invoke an inflammatory response.

During one set of experimental applications of hybrid liver support in pigs, evidence of such side effects were not observed. In this study, TNF-α liberation, as one marker of the activation of the cytokine system, was comparable with values obtained from therapy with other extracorporeal systems such as hemodialysis (Gerlach, Jörres, et al. 1993). Other studies may be necessary to further assess the role of activation of inflammatory mediators by bioreactor systems.

CLINICAL TRIALS

The first clinical trial of an artificial liver support system was reported in 1987 by Matsumura et al. (Matsumura et al. 1987). In one patient, metabolic encephalopathy was treated temporarily with rabbit hepatocytes. In two controlled studies, Margulis et al. (Margulis et al. 1989; 1990) utilized a hybrid artificial liver support system based on porcine hepatocytes. More recently, two American groups have reported their results (Sussman et al. 1992; Rozga, Holzman et al. 1993; Neuzil et al. 1993; Rozga, Podesta et al. 1993; Sussman and Kelly, 1993; Wood et al. 1993). Applications differed in terms of the other modes of additional treatment (e.g. charcoal perfusion, or hypothermia) as well as in the overall duration and the mode (i.e. frequency of application) of the treatment. Recent studies by both groups have reported successful application of their systems in larger numbers of patients (see Chapters 20 and 21). The type of cells used may be very important. Sussman et al. used tumor-derived C3A-hepatoma cells (Gislason et al. 1994; Kelly and Sussman 1994), whereas Demetriou et al. (Rozga et al. 1994) used primary cultures of pig hepatocytes. In the clinical applications reported so far, signs of acute immunological reactions were not observed. In particular, there were no hypersensitivity reactions even after repeated therapy sessions in the same patient.

The effect of human plasma exposure on the bioreactor hepatocytes has not been thoroughly studied. Experiments with pig hepatocytes and human serum demonstrated that some human sera contain pre-formed anti-pig antibodies (Takahashi et al. 1993) which, if they prove to be cytotoxic to pig hepatocytes (Haas et al. 1981; Gove et al. 1982), might result in bioreactor failure.

FUTURE PROSPECTS

In conclusion, issues such as the ideal bioreactor configuration, mode of use and the cell source are still being debated. In addition to further development of hybrid liver support devices, workers should also focus on the question of which cell types are of value and whether nonautologous cells in bioreactors cause side effects during clinical use.

In order to obtain sufficient "net" biological activity in bioreactors, rigorous analysis of the culture models is necessary. This is a prerequisite for the construction of scaled-up systems (Langer and Vacanti 1993). Investigations of cell-perfusate mass transfer performance by diffusion and/or convective flow, the cell mass to reactor volume ratio, the distribution of medium and gas and their respective gradients, and the availability of oxygen for the cells are all important parameters (McLimans et al. 1968; Gerlach et al. 1990). Hollow fiber reactors should provide a good ratio of perfusate flow (Wolf and Lauffer 1986), adhesion surface/substrate exchange surface (Davis and Watson 1985; Schonberg and Belfort 1987), oxygen supply (Giorgio et al. 1993), and bioreactor volume. Finally, standardization of techniques and methods in evaluating quantitative bioreactor systems (Hughes and Williams 1994) before and during clinical use will be a very important part of future work.

REFERENCES

Akaike, T., Tobe, S., Kobayashi, A., Goto, M. and Kobayashi, K. 1993. Design of hepatocyte-specific extracellular matrices for hybrid artificial liver. *Gastroenterol Jpn* 28 (Suppl 4): 45–56.

Arnaout, W.S., Moscioni, A.D., Barbour, R.L. and Demetriou, A.A. 1990. Development of bioartificial liver: bilirubin conjugation in Gunn-rats. *J Surg Res* 48: 379–82.

Asano, K., Koide, N. and Tsuji, T. 1989. Ultrastructure of multicellular spheroids formed in the primary culture of adult rat hepatocytes. *J Clin Electr Microsc* 22: 243–52.

Bader, A., Zech, K., Crome, O., Christians, U., Pichlmayr, R. and Sewing, K.F. 1994. Use of organotypical cultures of primary hepatocytes to analyze drug biotransformation in man and animals. *Xenobiotica* 24: 623–33.

Chang, T.M. 1992. Hybrid artificial cells: microencapsulation of living cells. *ASAIO J* 38: 128–30.

Clayton, D.F., Harrelson, A.L. and Darnell, J.E. 1985. Dependence of liver-specific transcription on tissue organization. *Mol Cell Biol* 5: 2623–32.

Cunningham, J.M. and Hodgson, H.J. 1992. Microcarrier culture of hepatocytes in whole plasma for use in liver support bioreactors. *Int J Artif Org* 15: 162–7.
Davis, M.E. and Watson, L.T. 1985. Analysis of a diffusion-limited hollow fiber reactor for the measurement of effective substrate diffusivities. *Biotechnol Bioeng* 27: 182–6.
Demetriou, A.A., Arnaout, W.S., Backfisch, G. and Moscioni, A.D. 1993. Immobilized isolated liver cells on a biomatrix. In: *Artificial Liver Support*, eds. G. Brunner and M. Mito, 283–95. Berlin: Springer.
Dixit, V. 1994. Development of a bioartificial liver using isolated hepatocytes. *Artif Org* 18: 371–84.
Dixit, V., Arthur, M., Reinhardt, R. and Gitnick, G. 1992. Improved function of microencapsulated hepatocytes in a bioartificial liver support system. *Artif Org* 16: 336–41.
Dunn, J.C., Tompkins, R.G. and Yarmush, M.L. 1992. Hepatocytes in collagen sandwich: evidence for transcriptional and translational regulation. *J Cell Biol* 116: 1043–53.
Dunn, J.C.Y., Yarmush, M.L., Koebe, H.G. and Tompkins, R.G. 1989. Hepatocyte function and extracellular matrix geometry: long-term culture in a sandwich configuration. *FASEB J* 3: 174–7.
Ezzel, R.M., Toner, M., Hendricks, K., Dunn, J.C., Tompkins, R.G. and Yarmush, M.L. 1993. Effect of collagen gel configuration on the cytoskeleton in cultured rat hepatocytes. *Exp Cell Res* 208: 442–52.
Fuchs, M., Gerlach, J., Unger, J., Encke, J., Smith, M., Neuhaus, P. and Riedel, E. 1994. Amino acid metabolism by hepatocytes in a hybrid liver support bioreactor. *Int J Artif Org* 17: 663–70.
Gerlach, J., Encke, J., Hole, O., Müller, C., Courtney, J. and Neuhaus, P. 1994. Hepatocyte culture between three dimensional arranged biomatrix-coated independent artificial capillary systems and sinusoidal endothelial cell co-culture compartments. *Int J Artif Org* 17: 301–6.
Gerlach, J., Encke, J., Hole, O., Müller, C., Ryan, C.J. and Neuhaus, P. 1994. Bioreactor for large scale hepatocyte in vitro perfusion. *Transplantation* 58: 984–8.
Gerlach, J., Jörres, A., Vienken, J., Gahl, G.M. and Neuhaus, P. 1993. Side effects of hybrid liver support therapy: TNF liberation in pigs, connected with extracorporeal bioreactors. *Int J Artif Org* 16: 604–8.
Gerlach, J., Klöppel, K., Müller, C., Schnoy, N., Smith, M.D. and Neuhaus, P. 1993. Hepatocyte aggregate culture technique in liver support systems. *Int J Artif Org* 16: 785–8.
Gerlach, J., Klöppel, K. and Schauwecker, H.H. 1989. Use of hepatocytes in adhesion and suspension cultures for liver support bioreactors. *Int J Artif Org* 12: 788–92.
Gerlach, J., Klöppel, K., Stoll, P., Vienken, J., Müller, C. and Schauwecker, H.H. 1990. Gas supply across membranes in liver support bioreactors. *Artif Org* 14: 328–33.
Gerlach, J. and Neuhaus, P. 1994. Culture model for primary hepatocytes. *In Vitro Cell Dev Biol* 30A: 640–2.
Gerlach, J., Schauwecker, H.H., Hennig, E. and Bücherl, E.S. 1989. Endothelial cell seeding on different polyurethanes. *Artif Org* 13: 144–7.
Gerlach, J., Schnoy, N., Encke, J., Müller, C., Smith, M. and Neuhaus, P. 1995. Improved hepatocyte in vitro maintenance in a culture model with woven multicompartment capillary systems: Electron microscopic studies. *Hepatology* 22: 546–52.
Gerlach, J., Smith, M. and Neuhaus, P. 1994. Hepatocyte culture between woven capillary systems – a microscopy study. *Artif Org* 18: 226–30.
Gerlach, J., Stoll, P., Schnoy, N. and Bücherl, E.S.B. 1990. Membranes as substrate for hepatocyte adhesion in liver support bioreactors. *Int J Artif Org* 13: 436–41.
Giorgio, T.D., Moscioni, A.D., Rozga, J. and Demetriou, A.A. 1993. Mass transfer in a hollow fiber device used as a bioartificial liver. *ASAIO J* 39: 886–92.
Gislason, G.T., Lobdell, D.D., Kelly, H.J. and Sussman, N.L. 1994. A treatment system for implementing an extracorporeal liver assist device. *Artif Org* 18: 385–9.
Gove, C.D., Hughes, R.D. and Williams, R. 1982. Rapid inhibition of DNA synthesis in hepatocytes from regenerating rat livers by serum from patients with fulminant hepatic failure. *Br J Exp Pathol* 63: 547–61.
Haas, T.H., Holloway, C.J., Osterhuss, V. and Trautschold, I. 1981. Hepatotoxic effects of sera from patients with fulminant hepatitis B on isolated rat hepatocytes in culture. *J Clin Chem Clin Biochem* 19: 283–90.
Hughes, R. and Williams, R. 1994. Assessment of bioartificial liver support in acute liver failure. *Int J Artif Org*: in press.
Henne-Bruns, D. 1993. Problems and controversies with transplantation of isolated hepatocytes for artificial liver support. In: *Artificial Liver Support*, eds. G. Brunner and M. Mito, 2nd edn., 313–23. Berlin: Springer.
Henne-Bruns, D., Kruger, U., Sumpelmann, D., Lierse, W. and Kremer, B. 1991. Intraperitoneal hepatocyte transplantation: morphological results. *Virchows Arch A Pathol Anat Histopathol* 419: 45–50.
Hu, W.S., Nyberg, S.L. and Shatford, R.A. 1991. Cultivation of hepatocytes in a new entrapment reactor: a potential bioartificial liver. In: *Animal Cell Culture and Production of Biologicals*, eds. R. Sasaki and K. Ikura, 75–80. Dordrecht, The Netherlands: Kluwer.
Jauregui, H.O., Naik, S., Driscoll, J.L., Soloman, B.A. and Galletti, P.M. 1983. Adult rat hepatocyte cultures as the cellular component of an artificial hybrid liver. In *Biomaterials in Artificial Organs*. Proceedings of a seminar on biomaterials held at the University of Strathclyde, Glasgow, eds. J.P. Paul, J.D.S. Gaylor, J.M. Courtney and T. Gilchrist. 130–40.
Jauregui, H.O., Naik, S., Solomon, B.A., Duffy, R.L., Lipsky, M. and Galetti, P.M. 1983. Attachment of adult rat hepatocytes to modified Amicron XM-50 membranes. *ASAIO J* 19: 698–702.
Kasai, S., Sawa, M., Nishida, Y., Onodera, K., Hirai, S., Yamamoto, T. and Mito, M. 1992. Cellulose microcarrier for high density-culture of hepatocytes. *Transpl Proc* 24: 2933–4.
Kawaguchi, M., Koide, N., Sagaguchi, K., Shinji, T. and Tsuji, T. 1992. Combination of epidermal growth factor and insulin is required for multicellular spheroid formation of rat hepatocytes in primary culture. *Acta Med Okayama* 46: 195–201.
Kelly, J.H. and Sussman, H.L. 1994. The hepatic extracorporeal liver assist device in the treatment of fulminant hepatic failure. *ASAIO J* 1: 83–5.
Knazek, R.A., Gullino, P.M., Kohler, P.O. and Dedrick, R.L. 1972. Cell culture on artificial capillaries: an approach to tissue growth in vitro. *Science* 178: 65–7.
Knazek, R.A., Kohler, P.O. and Gullino, P.M. 1974. Hormone production by cells grown in vitro on artificial capillaries. *Exp Cell Res* 84: 251–4.
Koebe, H.G., Pahernik, S., Eyer, P. and Schilberg, F.W. 1994a. Collagen gel immobilization: a useful cell culture technique for long-term metabolic studies on human hepatocytes. *Xenobiotica* 24: 95–107.

Koebe, H.G., Wick, M., Cramer, U., Lange, V. and Schildberg, F.W. 1994b. Collagen gel immobilization provides a suitable cell matrix for long term human hepatocyte cultures in hybrid reactors. *Int J Artif Org* 17(2): 95–106.

Koide, N., Sakagucci, K. and Koide, Y. 1990. Formation of multicellular spheroids composed of adult rat hepatocytes in dishes with positive charged surfaces and under other nonadherent environments. *Exp Cell Res* 186(2): 227–35.

Koide, N., Shinji, T., Tanabe, T., Asano, K., Kawaguchi, M., Sakaguchi, K., Koide, Y., Mori, M. and Tsuji, T. 1989. Continued high albumin production by multicellular spheroids of adult rat hepatocytes in the presence of liver derived proteoglycans. *Biochem Biophys Res Comm* 161: 385–91.

Langer, R. and Vacanti, J.P. 1993. Tissue engineering. *Science* 260: 920–5.

Landry, J., Bernier, D. and Ouellet, C. 1985. Spheroidal aggregate culture of rat liver cells: Histiotypic reorganization, biomatrix deposition, and maintenance of functional activities. *J Cell Biol* 101: 914–23.

Margulis, M.S., Erukhimov, E.A. and Andreiman, L.A. 1989. Temporary organ substitution by hemoperfusion through suspension of active donor hepatocytes in a total complex of intensive therapy in patients with acute hepatic insufficiency. *Resuscitation.* 18: 85–94.

Margulis, M.S., Erukhimov, E.A., Andreiman, L.A., Kuznetsov, K.A., Viksna, L.M., Kuznetsov, A.I. and Devyatov, V.V. 1990. Hemoperfusion through suspension of cryopreserved hepatocytes in a treatment of patients with acute liver failure. *Res Surg* 2: 99–102.

Matsumura, K.N., Guevara, F.R., Huston, H., Hamilton, W.L., Rikimaru, M., Yamasaki, G. and Matsumura, M.S. 1987. Hybrid bioartificial liver in hepatic failure: Preliminary clinical report. *Surgery* 101: 99–103.

Matthew, H.W., Salley, S.O., Peterson, W.D., Deshmukh, D.R., Mukhopadhyay, A. and Klein, M.D. 1991. Microencapsulated hepatocytes. Prospects for extracorporeal liver support. *ASAIO Trans* 37(3): 328–30.

McLimans, W.F., Blumenson, L.E. and Tunnah, K.V. 1968. Kinetics of gas diffusion in mammalian cell culture systems. *Biotechnol Bioeng* 10: 741–63.

Miura, Y., Akimoto, T., Kanazawa, H. and Yagi, K. 1986. Synthesis and secretion of protein by hepatocytes entrapped within calcium alginate. *Artif Org* 10: 460–5.

Miura, Y., Akimoto, T., Yoshikawa, N. and Yagi, K. 1990. Characterization of immobilized hepatocytes as liver support. *Biomater Artif Cells Artif Org* 18: 549–54.

Neuzil, D., Rozga, J., Moscioni, A.D., Ro, M.S., Hakim, R., Arnaout, W.S. and Demetriou, A.A. 1993. Use of a novel bioartificial liver in a patient with acute liver insufficiency. *Surgery* 113: 340–3.

Nyberg, S.L., Platt, J.L., Shirabe, K., Payne, W.D., Hu, W.S. and Cerra, F.B. 1992. Immunoprotection of xenocytes in a hollow fiber bioartificial liver. *ASAIO J* 38: M463–67.

Nyberg, S.L., Russel, A., Shatford, R.A., Madhusudan, V., Peshwa, M.V., White, J.G., Cerra, F.B. and Hu, W.S. 1993. Evaluation of a hepatocyte-entrapment hollow fiber bioreactor: a potential bioartificial liver. *Biotechnol Bioeng* 41: 194–203.

Olumide, F., Eliashiv, A., Kralios, N., Norton, L. and Eisenman, B. 1977. Hepatic support with hepatocyte suspension in a permeable membrane dialyzer. *Surgery* 82: 599–606.

Pappas, S.C. 1988. Fulminant hepatic failure and the need for artificial liver support. *Mayo Clin Proc* 63: 198–200.

Piret, T.D., Moscioni, A.D., Rozga, J. and Demetriou, A.A. 1993. Mass transfer in a hollow fiber device used as a bioartificial liver. *ASAIO J* 39: 886–92.

Rozga, J., Holzmann, M.D., Ro, M.S., Griffin, D.W., Neuzil, D.F., Giorgio, T., Moscioni, A. and Demetriou, A.A. 1993. Development of a hybrid bioartificial liver. *Ann Surg* 217: 502–11.

Rozga, J., Podesta, L., LePage, E., Hoffman, A., Morsiani, E., Sher, L., Woolf, G.M., Makowka, L. and Demetriou, A.A. 1993. Control of cerebral edema by total hepatectomy and extracorporeal liver support in fulminant hepatic failure. *Lancet* 342: 898–99.

Rozga, J., Podesta, L., LePage, E., Morsiani, E., Moscioni, A.D., Hoffman, A., Sher, L., Villamil, F., Woof, G., McGrath, M., Kong, L., Rosen, H., Lanman, T., Vierling, J., Makowka, L. and Demetriou, A.A. 1994. A bioartificial liver to treat severe acute liver failure. *Ann Surg* 219: 538–46.

Sakaguchi, K., Koide, N., Asano, K., Takabatake, H., Matsushima, H., Takenami, T., Ono, R., Sasaki, S., Mori, M. and Koide, Y. 1991. Promotion of spheroid assembly of adult rat hepatocytes by some factors present in the initial 6-hour conditioned medium of the primary culture. *Pathobiology* 59: 351–6.

Scholtz, M. and Hu, W.S. 1991. A two compartment cell entrapment bioreactor with three different holding times for cells, high and low molecular weight compounds. *Cytotechnology* 4: 127–37.

Schonberg, J.A. and Belfort, G. 1987. Enhancement nutrient transport in hollow fiber perfusion bioreactors: a theoretical analysis. *Biotechnol Prog* 3: 80–9.

Shatford, R.A., Nyberg, S.L., Meier, S.J., White, J.G., Payne, W.D., Hu, W.S. and Cerra, F.B. 1992. Hepatocyte function in a hollow fiber bioreactor: a potential bioartificial liver. *J Surg Res* 53: 649–57.

Shinji, T., Koide, N. and Tsuji, T. 1988. Glycosaminoglycans partially substitute for proteoglycans in spheroid formation of adult rat hepatocytes in primary culture. *Cell Struct Funct* 13: 179–88.

Shynra, A., Bocharov, A., Bochkova, N. and Spirov, V. 1990. Large-scale production and cultivation of hepatocytes on Biosolon microcarriers. *Artif Org* 14: 421–8.

Shynra, A., Bocharov, A., Bochkova, N. and Spirov, V. 1991. Bioartificial liver using hepatocytes on biosolon microcarriers: treatment of chemically induced acute hepatic failure in rats. *Artif Org* 15: 189–97.

Spray, D.C., Fujita, M., Saez, J.C., Choi, H., Watanabe, T., Hertzberg, E., Rosenberg, L.C. and Reid, L.M. 1987. Proteoglycans and glycosaminoglycans induce gap junction synthesis and function in primary liver culture. *J Cell Biol* 105: 541–51.

Stange, J., Mitzner, S., Dautzenberg, H., Ramlow, W., Knippel, M., Steiner, M., Ernst, B., Schmidt, R. and Klinkman, H. 1993. Prolonged biochemical and morphological stability of encapsulated liver cells – a new method. *Biomater Artif Cells Immobil Biotechnol* 21: 343–52.

Sugamori, M., Boag, A.H., Broughton, R.L. and Sefton, M.V. 1986. Microencapsulation of mammalian cells in polyacrylate membranes for metabolic prostheses. In

Progress in Artificial Organs, eds. Y. Nose, C. Kjellstrand and P. Ivanovich, 630–4. ISAO Press.

Sullivan, S.J., Maki, T. and Borland, K.M. 1991. Biohybrid artificial pancreas: long-term implementation studies in diabetic, pancreatectomized dogs. *Science* 252: 718–21.

Sun, A.M., Cai, Z., Shi, Z., Ma, F. and O'Shea, G.M. 1987. Microencapsulated hepatocytes: An in vitro and in vivo study. *Biomat Art Cells Art Org* 15: 483–96.

Sun, A.M., Cai, Z., Shi, Z., Ma, F., O'Shea, G.M., and Gharapetian, H. 1986. Microencapsulated hepatocytes as a bioartificial liver. *ASAIO J* 32: 39–41.

Sussman, N.L., Finegold, M.J. and Kelly, J.H. 1992. Recovery from syncytial giant-cell hepatitis (SCGH) following treatment with an extracorporeal liver assist device (ELAD). *Hepatology* 16: 51A.

Sussman, N.L. and Kelly, J.H. 1993. Improved liver function following treatment with an extracorporeal liver assist device. *Artif Org* 17: 27–30.

Takabatake, H., Koide, N. and Tsuji, T. 1991. Encapsulated multicellular spheroids of rat hepatocytes produce albumin and urea in a spouted bed circulating culture system. *Artif Org* 15(6): 474–80.

Takahashi, M., Ishikura, H., Takahashi, C., Nakajiama, Y., Matsushita, H., Matsue, H., Sato, K., Noto, H., Taguchi, K., Koike, M., Nishikawa, M., Kamachi, H., Kon, H., Uchino, J. and Yoshiki, T. 1993. Immunologic considerations in the use of cultured porcine hepatocytes as a hybrid artificial liver. Anti-porcine hepatocyte human serum. *ASAIO J* 39: M242–6.

Tompkins, R.G. and Carter, E.A. 1988. Enzymatic function of alginate immobilized rat hepatocytes. *Biotechnol Bioeng* 31: 11–18.

Tong, J.Z., Bernard, O. and Alvarez, F. 1990. Long term culture of rat liver cell spheroids in hormonally defined media. *Exp Cell Res* 189: 87–92.

Tuburaya, T., Uchino, J. and Komai, T. 1989. Can hepatocytes contribute to an advance of artificial liver? *Artif Org* 13: 381.

Uchino, J., Matsue, H., Takahashi, M., Kahajima, Y., Matsushita, M., Hamada, T. and Hashimura, E. 1991. A hybrid artificial liver. Function of cultured monolayer pig hepatocytes in plasma from hepatic failure patients. *ASAIO J* 37: 337–8.

Uchino, J., Tsuburaya, T., Kumagai, F., Hase, T., Hamada, T., Komai, T., Funatsu, A., Hashimura, E., Makamura, K. and Kon, T. 1988. A hybrid bioartificial liver composed of multiplated hepatocyte monolayers. *ASAIO J* 34: 972–7.

Vanholder, R. and Ringoir, S. 1991. Bioartificial pancreas and liver: a review. *Artif Org* 14: 398–402.

Vanholder, R. and Ringoir, S. 1991. Artificial organs: an overview. *Artif Org* 14: 613–18.

Voss, J.U. and Siebert, H. 1991. Microcarrier-attached rat hepatocytes as a xenobiotic-metabolizing system in cocultures. *Cell Biol Toxicol* 7: 387–99.

Wolf, C.F. and Lauffer, L.L. 1986. Design and fabrication of a capillary cell culture chambers for study of convective flow. *Int J Artif Org* 9: 25–32.

Wolf, C.F.W. and Munkelt, B.E. 1975. Bilirubin conjugation by an artificial liver composed of cultured cells and synthetic capillaries. *ASAIO J* 21: 16–27.

Wood, R.P., Katz, S.M., Ozaki, C.F., Monsour, H.P., Gislason, G.T., Kelly, J.H. and Sussman, N.L. 1993. Extracorporeal liver assist device (ELAD): a preliminary report. *Transpl Proc* 25: 53–4.

Yanagi, K., Mizuno, S. and Ohshima, N. 1990. A high density culture of hepatocytes using a reticulated polyvinyl formol resin. *ASAIO J* 36: M727–9.

Yanagi, K., Ookawa, K., Mizuno, S. and Oshima, N. 1989. Performance of a new hybrid artificial liver support system using hepatocytes entrapped within a hydrogel. *ASAIO J* 35: 570–2.

Yuasa, C., Tomita, Y., Shono, M., Ishimura, K. and Ichihara, A. 1993. Importance of cell aggregation for expression of liver functions and regeneration demonstrated with primary cultured hepatocytes. *J Cell Physiol* 156: 522–30.

20 Clinical experience with an extracorporeal liver assist device

Antony J. Ellis, Norman L. Sussman, James H. Kelly and Roger Williams

INTRODUCTION

Acute liver failure (ALF) results in failure of the body to sustain vital metabolic functions such as energy production, protein synthesis, and detoxification–excretion of metabolic by-products. In addition, experimental evidence suggests that plasma from patients with ALF is cytotoxic (Seda et al. 1984a), possibly as the result of cytokine and free radical release from the necrotic liver (Nagaki et al. 1991). This combination of decreased metabolic reserve and increased levels of cytotoxic compounds determines the severity of the clinical syndrome which follows.

Development of liver support has been ongoing for at least 30 years, and has included techniques such as hemodialysis, blood and plasma exchange, xenogeneic and allogeneic liver perfusion, and blood "purification" with charcoal and ion exchange resins (Sussman and Kelly, 1995a and Chapters 18 to 21). Despite a number of promising preliminary reports with various techniques, the results of clinical studies in man have been disappointing, that is, no mode of treatment appears to improve survival after ALF. Although non-biological systems such as charcoal hemoperfusion are capable of reducing levels of ammonia (Schechter et al. 1984), "middle molecules" (Opolon 1979) and other putative deleterious compounds (Seda 1984b; Nagaki et al. 1991), these systems do not provide the requisite metabolic support to sustain a patient with ALF until regeneration of the native liver can occur.

Extracorporeal perfusion of a whole liver theoretically provides a complete form of organ replacement. The unavailability of compatible organs as well as inconvenience, inconsistent function, and the risk of infections all limit the use of this mode of therapy. For example, human organs appear to function well ex vivo (Fox et al. 1993), but are generally not available because they are needed for transplantation. On the other hand, animal livers, especially those of non-primate origin, are subject to hyperacute rejection, and have a useful functional life of several hours at most (Chari et al. 1994; Sussman and Kelly 1995b). Primate livers appear to function for somewhat longer periods, but the lack of availability as well as the risk of introducing new pathogens into human hosts are severe limitations.

Biological liver support devices attempt to provide liver support without the difficulties observed with whole liver perfusion. Liver cells grown or suspended in a synthetic housing can be perfused with either blood or plasma, and provide the metabolic functions essential for survival. Furthermore, the synthetic membrane which separates the patient's bodily fluids from the cells protects them from immune attack. Such devices have the potential to maintain metabolic function in patients with ALF until the native liver regenerates or until a liver transplant can be performed. The patient is likely to benefit in either case; a stable preoperative course improves the outcome of liver transplantation (Ascher et al. 1993), and recovery of the native liver as a result of liver regeneration represents a complete healing process with a normal life expectancy (Karvountzis et al. 1974).

THE CONCEPTUAL BASIS OF LIVER ASSIST

A variety of approaches to biological liver assistance have been suggested, with major variations in the source of the liver cells, the geometry of the support matrix, and the nature of the perfusate (blood or plasma). However, before discussing specific devices it is worth considering the basic principles of organ assist and the necessary properties of the ideal liver assist device. Table 20.1 summarizes these features.

EXTRACORPOREAL LIVER ASSIST DEVICES: CURRENT STATUS

The extent to which extracorporeal liver assist devices (ELADs) fulfil the requirements outlined in Table 20.1 are discussed briefly below. A point-by-point discussion has recently been published (Sussman and Kelly 1995b).

The C3A cell line

To be effective, cell-based therapy must provide sufficient liver function to meet the metabolic needs of the patient. The liver weighs approximately 1,500 g of which 1,200 g is hepatocyte mass. If encephalopathy occurs when hepatocyte function falls below 15–30 percent, then an ELAD must be capable of providing the functional equivalent of at least several hundred grams of liver. This is an important concept, and it adds a second tier to our thinking about the nature of the metabolic requirements. The cells which are used to populate an ELAD must be comparable to normal hepatocytes, and they must be available in sufficient quantities to support the patient with near-total liver necrosis or absent liver function. When taken in the context of the world-wide population of patients with ALF, thousands of kilograms of liver cells would be required annually to make ELADs.

Primary hepatocytes (cells isolated from fresh liver) have been shown to function well in vitro, and they provide measurable benefits in animal studies (see below). The problem lies in the "scale-up." The harvesting procedure is complex, costly, and labor-intensive, and it is not suited to bulk manufacturing. For example, one group has used $1–6 \times 10^9$ cells (an estimated 1–12 g) to treat patients (Rozga et al. 1994; Demetriou et al. 1995), and other research groups have described the use of 5×10^7 to 5.6×10^8 cells (Wolf and Munkelt 1975; Shatford et al. 1992; Li et al. 1993; Jauregui et al. 1995). When added to the problems of lot-to-lot inconsistency and sterility issues, primary hepatocyte cultures appear inadequate if ELADs are to become widely available.

A logical alternative in liver assist devices to the use of primary hepatocytes is the use of immortalized cell lines (Wolf and Munkelt 1975; Melkonian et al. 1994). Cell lines offer a number of advantages including the ability to create a highly characterized master cell bank, the ease of maintenance, and the possibility of indefinite clonal expansion. The main problem encountered previously has been one of verifying cellular differentiation; established cell lines have not performed at the level of normal hepatocytes (Nyberg et al. 1994). With this in mind, a highly differentiated clonal population was isolated from the human hepatoblastoma cell line, HepG2. The new cell line, C3A, performs normal liver-specific metabolic functions including ureagenesis, gluconeogenesis, and inducible P-450 activity (J.H.K. unpublished observations). In

Table 20.1. *Basic elements of the ideal liver assist device*

Feature	Rationale
Minimally invasive	Acute liver failure is reversible and the patients are unstable; trauma should be minimized. Extracorporeal treatment is preferred.
Sufficient metabolic capacity	Liver support requires about 30% of liver function, i.e. 300–400 g of hepatocytes.
Continuous treatment	Liver support must be provided around-the-clock for several days to maximize chance of regeneration.
Available on short notice	Patients are often very unstable; irreversible deterioration may result if treatment is delayed.
Easy to operate	Should be managed by ICU nurses or technicians, i.e. comparable in complexity to hemodialysis.
Safe	Neither the patient nor the device should suffer during treatment.
Cost-effective	Increasing world attention on health care costs.

addition, this cell line secretes liver-specific proteins and clotting factors, and its growth is strongly contact-regulated. Finally, extensive testing has failed to reveal any infectious agents to be present. These in vitro indicators of cell function were subsequently confirmed in animal studies which are described later in this chapter.

The support matrix

The structure which supports the growth of the cells and provides the interface between the cells and the patient's blood/plasma is critical to the function of an ELAD. The matrix must support an adequate cell mass and must provide an adequate cell/fluid interface. Important characteristics of the interface include permeability to important molecules, optimal surface area, and the exclusion of immunoregulatory agents which might damage the cells. In practical terms, the exclusion of white cells is sufficient to prevent immune-mediated damage to cultured cells of all types.

Most of the ELADs currently in development utilize some variant of a hollow fiber dialysis cartridge (Kelly et al. 1992; Sussman et al. 1992; Nyberg et al. 1993; Rozga et al. 1993; Gerlach et al. 1995; Jauregui et al. 1995). For example, our device is a hemodialysis cartridge which contains approximately 10,000 hollow fibres with a surface area of 2 m^2. Cells are grown in the extracapillary space, and culture media (during growth) or blood (during treatment) flow through the interior of the fibers (Figure 20.1). The individual fibers are generally less than four cells apart so that most cells receive adequate oxygenation during blood perfusion (Figure 20.2). The membranes have a molecular weight cutoff of 70,000 so that leukocytes and immunoglobulins do not come into contact with the cells. At the same time, middle molecules and ammonia can move freely across the membrane.

Perfusion of the ELAD with blood

We (Sussman et al. 1992; Sussman et al. 1994) and others (Nyberg et al. 1992; 1993) have elected to perfuse the ELAD with whole blood (as opposed to plasma) during treatment for several reasons. First, the oxygen requirements of the cells are met more easily with blood; plasma perfusion would require in-line oxygenation and a very high flow rate. Second, plasma separation cannot be done for more than a few hours at a time, and therefore limits the length of treatment. Third, continuous plasma separation makes the procedure considerably more complicated. A comparison between a blood perfusion circuit and a plasma perfusion circuit is shown in Figure 20.3.

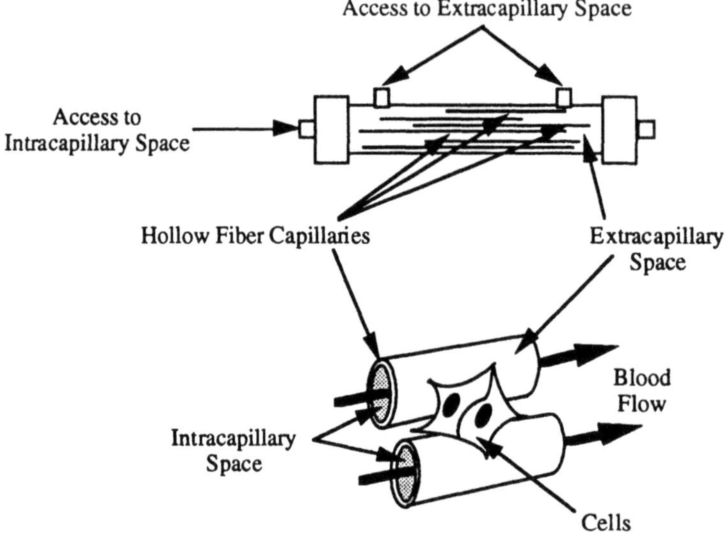

Figure 20.1 Diagram of a hollow fiber cartridge. Access to the intracapillary space is via the end ports, and the extracapillary space is accessed via the side ports. The close-up view shows cells attached to the external surface of the fibers.

MANUFACTURE OF THE ELAD

In order to make an ELAD, we inoculate 2 g of C3A cells into the extracapillary space of a hollow fiber dialyzer and incubate the cells within the cartridge under appropriate conditions for 3–4 weeks. During the growth phase, fresh culture medium is supplied continuously and glucose, pH, and Po_2 are controlled. Maturity of each device is determined by albumin synthesis and glucose consumption. At maturity, each device synthesizes 4–5 g of albumin and utilizes 8 g of glucose daily and has the metabolic capacity of 200 g of normal liver. Once mature, the cartridges have a practically unlimited life-span as long as culture conditions are maintained; cartridges have been held in culture for up to 8 months without a decline in biochemical activity. In fact, it is not cost-effective to keep cartridges in culture for prolonged periods of time, and the devices which are used to treat patients are always 4–8 weeks old.

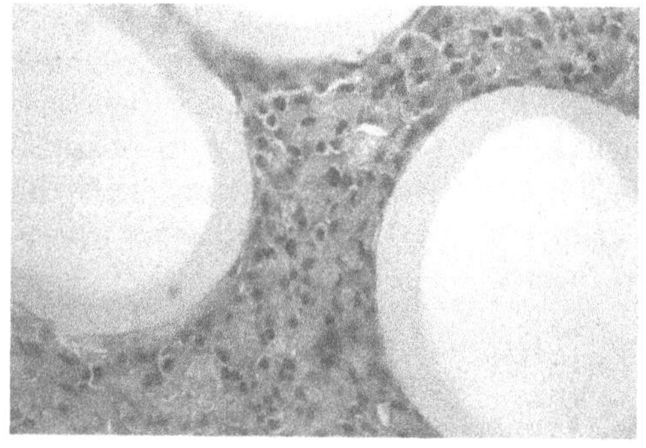

Figure 20.2 Micrograph showing C3A cells attached to the outside surface of hollow fibers.

ANIMAL STUDIES

Initial studies of the Hepatix ELAD were performed in anhepatic animals (Kelly et al. 1992). Six male beagles underwent a portacaval shunt and total hepatectomy. Vascular access for perfusion of the ELAD was gained via the carotid artery and external jugular vein. Bolus doses of thiamylal sodium were given in the postoperative period to maintain sedation. $NaHCO_3$ in increments of 10 mEq every 30 min was given to keep the blood bicarbonate above 12 mEq/l, and 5 percent dextrose was infused at 30 ml/h to maintain euglycemia. Blood flow through the ELAD was estimated at 80–100 ml/min, and was

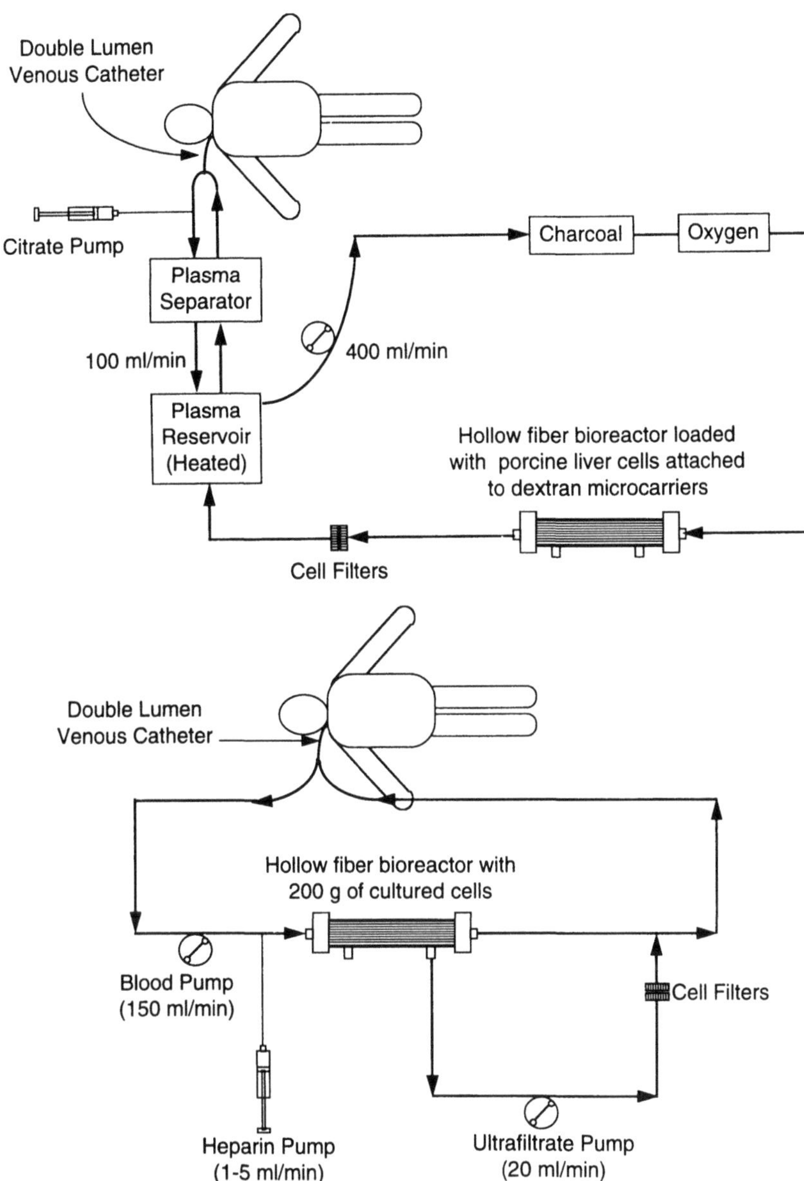

Figure 20.3 ELAD perfusion; plasma versus blood. Perfusion with plasma is more complicated than with blood because it requires on-line plasma separation, a heated reservoir, oxygenator, and, in this case, a charcoal column. The top figure is modified from Rozga et al. 1994. The bottom figure is from Gislason et al. 1994.

driven solely by arterial pressure. Heparin was infused into the proximal side of the device to keep the whole blood clotting time above 18 min, and control dogs received 1000 unit boluses to maintain a similar clotting time.

The three control animals and two of the three ELAD-treated animals lived for 3–5 h after surgery. The third treated dog lived for 125 h, more than twice the survival time seen in our controls and in a series of similarly treated animals previously reported (Daloze et al. 1990). None of the control dogs awoke from anesthesia, but two of the three ELAD dogs required further sedation, the longest survivor requiring four extra doses of thiamylal sodium. In addition, this particular dog required additional heparin to keep the whole blood clotting time above 18 min. Following surgery, the plasma ammonia stabilized for a short period and then rose in the control dogs in the preterminal period. This secondary rise was not seen in the treated group. Human albumin was detectable in the bloodstream of the treated dogs.

In order to test the ELAD in a setting which more closely resembled human ALF, an animal model of acute liver failure based on acetaminophen and buthionine sulfoximine was developed (Kelly et al. 1992). Control animals developed ALF with hypoglycemia, encephalopathy, prolonged prothrombin time, elevated alanine amino transferase (ALT), and decreased serum albumin. Death was universal, and occurred 15–30 h after the ALT began to rise. ELAD therapy was started in the treatment group when the ALT reached 7,000 units/l, a level which signified lethal liver damage in control animals. Two of an initial three dogs survived despite the presence of a severe coagulopathy and peak ALT levels of 9,000 and 31,000 units/l respectively (Sussman et al. 1992). With the addition of two more treated dogs, overall survival was 80 percent, and ELAD therapy was discontinued after 42–48 h (Sussman and Kelly 1993). The dogs remained fully conscious during treatment, and ELAD therapy appeared to reduce the extent of liver necrosis. Human proteins (albumin, α-fetoprotein, and transferrin) were detected in dog serum, confirming the ongoing function of the ELAD.

CLINICAL TRIALS IN MAN

For use in humans, the treatment format was modified in several ways. Blood access was gained via the femoral artery and vein in the first patient, and by venovenous access in the remaining patients. The switch to venovenous perfusion necessitated an active pumping system which was developed for this purpose (Gislason et al. 1994; see Figure 3, bottom figure). In addition to blood perfusion at 125–200 ml/min, the system generates a negative pressure in the extracapillary space. This results in the continuous formation of an ultrafiltrate which passes over the cells and through a set of filters prior to its return to the patient's blood stream. The filters prevent detached C3A cells from escaping downstream, and the transfiber pressure gradient assures that retrograde flow of cells will not occur in the event of a ruptured fiber. The ultrafiltrate has two additional functions; it delivers high molecular weight proteins which are unable to pass through the wall of the hollow fibers (cutoff 70,000), and it prevents the accumulation of toxic levels of bile acids in the extracapillary space. Anticoagulation of the system is achieved by the infusion of heparin into the afferent limb of the circuit.

Initially, ten patients with ALF and one who had undergone a total hepatectomy following primary graft failure were treated for a total of 579 h using 36 cartridges (Sussman et al. 1994) (for details of patients see Table 20.2). The patients were treated at four centers over a period of two years with the aim of assessing biocompatibility and safety. All patients were in Grade III or IV encephalopathy and nine required mechanical ventilation at the commencement of therapy.

Only one adverse event, transient hypotension, was attributed to ELAD therapy. Other instances of hypotension, acidosis, thrombocytopenia, and worsening of central nervous system function were thought to represent disease progression (Sussman et al. 1994). The mental status improved in eight of the eleven patients; one improved within an hour of starting ELAD treatment (Sussman et al. 1992) and in one improvement was delayed for three days (Sussman et al. 1994). Most patients remained hemodynamically stable throughout the study, and renal function was preserved in those patients who were not anuric at the commencement of treatment. In several cases the clinical effect of the ELAD was seen only in retrospect when perfusion was discontinued prematurely.

Table 20.2. *Summary of eleven patients treated with the Hepatix^{TM} ELAD*

Pt No.	Date	Location	Age (years)	Sex	Etiology	Rx (h)	Carts	Outcome
1	Jun '91	Houston	67	F	Idiopathic	144	8	Died post-Rx
2	Apr '92	Houston	12	F	SGCH	58	1	Alive
3	Oct '92	Houston	9	M	NANB	28	3	Died – CE
4	Oct '92	Houston	33	F	ACAP/EtOH	90	5	Died – CE
5	Dec '92	Houston	27	F	ACAP/EtOH	36	2	Died – CE
6	Jan '93	Houston	43	F	INH	24	3	Died – CE
7	Jun '93	Pittsburgh	46	M	NANB	35	5	Died – CE
8	Jul '93	Pittsburgh	44	M	FIAU	75	3	OLT
9	Jul '93	Charlottesville	42	M	FIAU	21	2	OLT
10	Jul '93	Charlottesville	37	F	FIAU	58	2	OLT
11	Aug '93	San Francisco	63	M	Anhepatic	9	2	OLT

The first patient recovered from liver failure, but died of sepsis several days after weaning from the ELAD. The second patient is alive and healthy more than 2 years after treatment. Patients 3–7 died of cerebral edema, usually after an unforeseen event which interrupted ELAD therapy. The last four patients were successfully bridged to orthotopic liver transplantation. Patient 11 was treated with two cartridges in series. Carts = number of cartridges used, SGCH = syncytial giant cell hepatitis, NANB = non-A non-B hepatitis, CE = cerebral edema, ACAP = acetaminophen (paracetamol), EtOH = alcohol, INH = isoniazid, FIAU = fialuridine, OLT = orthotopic liver transplantation.
From Sussman, Gislason, Conlin and Kelly, 1994.

Several tests of liver function including factor V and VII activity, whole blood ammonia levels, galactose elimination capacity (GEC), lidocaine metabolism, and caffeine clearance were performed. Measurement of clotting factors was not a useful assay because of the intermittent infusion of fresh frozen plasma. Caffeine clearance was negligible in all patients, and lidocaine metabolism proved to be poorly reproducible. The only test which proved reliable and correlated well with clinical status was the galactose elimination capacity (GEC).

GEC values below 10 μmol/min/kg represent nonlinear (i.e. nonhepatic clearance of galactose, and values below 12.8 μmol/min/kg are thought to be incompatible with recovery (Ranek et al. 1976). In this study a GEC above 18 (8 μmol/min/kg hepatic clearance) correlated with clinical neurological improvement. Hepatic GEC is shown in Figure 20.4. Several observations can be made concerning this finding. First, the initial GEC was generally below the survival threshold in all patients. Second, the patients with the higher GECs were those with fialuridine (FIAU) toxicity (see below). Third, the patient in whom the GEC did not change was later found to have very low levels of inorganic phosphate. It is likely that she was unable to form high energy phosphate bonds because of lack of substrate.

The cause of ALF in three of the patients was fialuridine (FIAU), an experimental nucleoside analogue which was undergoing testing as an anti-viral agent (McKenzie et al. 1995). The drug caused a diffuse mitochondrial toxicity, and the patients initially were observed to have severe lactic acidosis. ELAD therapy was instituted with the assumption that mitochondrial recovery would take place, and to provide a rationale for liver transplantation if the toxicity did not remit. Although the lactic acidosis improved dramatically in two of the three patients, the devices eventually lost effect. Despite the fact that all three patients were able to be supported until transplantation could be accomplished, all died later of various complications unrelated to ELAD treatment (Sussman et al. 1994).

CONTROLLED PILOT STUDY

With the evidence of clinical efficacy described above, a controlled pilot study was undertaken. The aim was to further establish the safety and biocompatibility of the device and

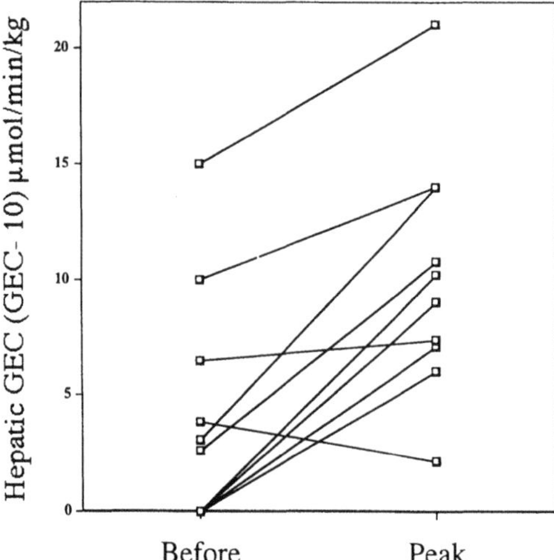

Figure 20.4 Pretreatment and peak hepatic GEC values in ten patients. Galactose (500 mg/kg) was injected over 3–5 min, and blood samples were taken at 20, 30, 40, 50, and 60 min. Serum galactose was plotted, and the elimination capacity was extrapolated from the linear portion of the curve. GEC values below 10 µmol/min/kg are nonlinear, and therefore represent nonhepatic clearance. Hepatic GEC (GEC-10) is shown in order to display only hepatic clearance. From Sussman et al. (1994).

to develop a protocol suitable for use in a multicenter study. Because of the inevitable heterogeneity of the study population with respect to etiology and severity, stratification into two groups was performed. Group I consisted of patients thought to have a 50 percent chance of recovery, and Group II were those who fulfilled transplant criteria (O'Grady et al. 1989) at the time of enrolment. The need for such stratification is essential if future studies are to determine: whether extracorporeal liver support can be used to prolong the interval during which the patient is stable enough for spontaneous recovery to occur; and whether liver support improves outcome in those patients who progress to liver transplantation.

Initial data from this pilot study has been reported in abstract form (Ellis et al. 1994). Of 14 patients enrolled in Group I, nine received ELAD therapy and five were entered as controls. Three ELAD patients (33 percent) progressed to fulfil transplant criteria, two were subsequently transplanted, and the overall survival for Group I was 8/9 (89 percent). Of the five controls, one deteriorated and was transplanted, but died, giving an overall survival of 4/5 (80 percent). Of the six patients in Group II, three received ELAD therapy, and three were treated as controls. One patient in each limb of the study proceeded to transplantation and both survived (Figure 20.5). A further case who fulfilled transplant criteria but for whom surgery was contraindicated for psychiatric reasons, was maintained on ELAD therapy continuously for 168 h, a time period unique in the field of liver support. In this case, the INR which had been greater than 15 for 48 h fell to 4.8 after 96 h of treatment.

Function of the device was assessed by a combination of clinical parameters which were measured hourly, and biochemical assays which were performed before the start of ELAD therapy, six h and 24 h after institution of therapy, and daily thereafter until the end of therapy. A final assay was also performed six h after the end of treatment. Measurement of intracranial pressure was undertaken in one ELAD patient, a 21-year-old with acetaminophen overdose who demonstrated signs of raised intracranial pressure prior to the start of ELAD therapy. She subsequently died before a donor organ became available, but her ICP fell from a mean value of 30 mmHg to 4 mmHg after 20 h of treatment with maintenance of her cerebral perfusion pressure.

Galactose elimination capacity (GEC) rose after six h of ELAD treatment, and was significantly higher than in control patients. After this point there was no difference in GEC (Figure 20.6). Factor V levels rose during the treatment period from a mean of 15 percent to 37 percent. This was not significantly different from control patients in whom levels rose from 9 percent to 41 percent. Initial whole blood ammonia was raised in both patient groups, and declined in the treated group (106–100 µmol/l) while rising in the control group (107–110 µmol/l). This difference failed to achieve statistical significance because of the

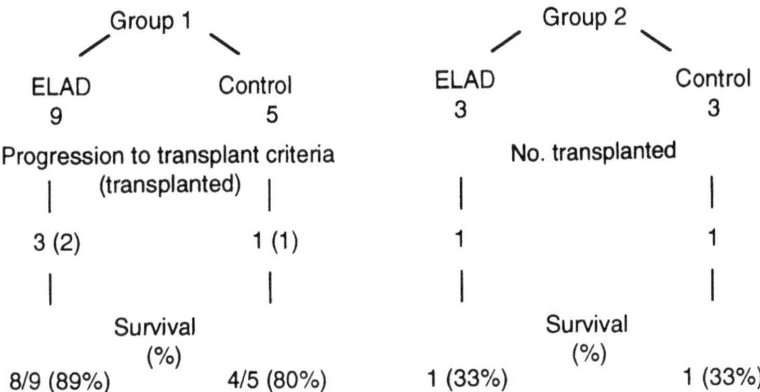

Figure 20.5 Survival data from controlled pilot study, separated by likelihood of recovery. Group I represented those patients thought on admission to have a 50 percent chance of recovery; Group II represented those patients who met criteria for transplantation on admission.

small number of patients treated. The arterial ketone body ratio, a measure of the hepatic redox potential, was no different in the two groups at any point of the study. Serum bilirubin fell in some patients, but median values were not affected.

With respect to biocompatibility, platelet counts fell in both groups. Although two patients in the ELAD group experienced significant declines, mean values were not significantly different compared to controls. There was a significant fall in fibrinogen in the ELAD group after six hours, but this was not sustained and probably represented bonding to the plastic tubing of the ELAD circuit. There was no hypotension associated with the commencement of treatment, but two patients were withdrawn from the study; one following worsening of pre-existing disseminated intravascular coagulation with hematemesis and bleeding from line sites, and a second who developed wheezing and tachycardia, apparently an allergic reaction to a component of the device.

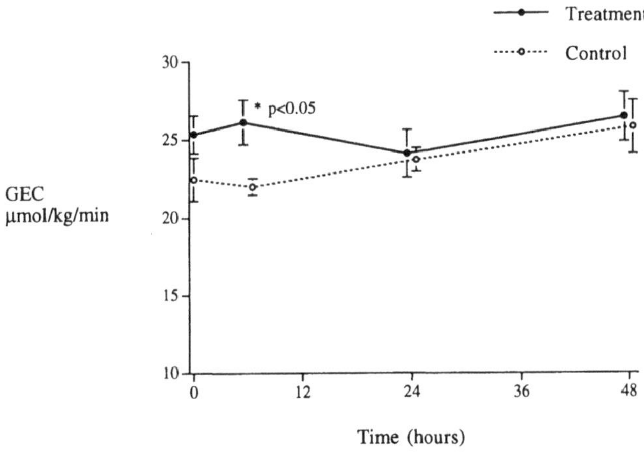

Figure 20.6 Serial estimates of galactose elimination capacity (GEC) in patients enrolled in the pilot study.

THE FUTURE

Metabolically active liver assist devices are now a feasible method of providing temporary liver support in acute liver failure. Those devices which utilize a dialysis cartridge as a support matrix represent the configuration most likely to achieve successful clinical use. Depending on the nature of the device, clinical trials of approximately 200 patients will have to be performed before formal conclusions about efficacy can be drawn. A multicenter trial, despite the inherent inconsistencies in patient selection and treatment, is the only feasible method of enrolling such a large cohort within a reasonable time frame.

If an improvement in survival can be demonstrated in ALF, it may be possible to broaden the use of liver support to include patients with initial poor function of a liver graft, patients who have undergone hepatic resection, those with temporary decompensation of chronic liver disease, and possibly even the routine treatment of decompensated cirrhotic patients. More work is required to establish whether ELAD treatment has a role in the enhanced liver recovery seen in animal experiments. Possible mechanisms such as the production of growth factors and the removal of inhibitory substances will be worth exploring if this proves to be the case.

REFERENCES

Ascher, N.L., Lake, J.R., Emond, J.C. and Roberts, J.P. 1993. Liver transplantation for fulminant hepatic failure. *Arch Surg* 128: 677–82.

Chari, R.S., Collins, B.H., Magee, J.C., DiMaio, J.M., Kirk, A.D., Harland, R.C., McCann, R.L., Platt, J.L. and Meyers, W.C. 1994. Brief report: treatment of hepatic failure with ex vivo pig–liver perfusion followed by liver transplantation. *N Engl J Med* 331: 234–7.

Daloze, P., Des Rosiers, C., Arnoux, R., Daloze, T., Smeesters, C. and Brunengraber, H. 1990. One-stage hepatectomy in the dog. *J Surg Res* 48: 33–7.

Demetriou, A.A., Rozga, J., Podesta, L., LePage, E., Morsiani, E., Moscioni, A.D., Hoffman, A., McGrath, M., Kong, L., Rosen, H., Villamil, F., Woolf, G., Vierling, J. and Makowka, L. 1995. Early clinical experience with a hybrid bioartificial liver. *Scand J Gastroenterol* 30 (Supp. 208): 111–17.

Ellis, A.J., Wendon, J., Hughes, R., Langley, P., Sussman, N.L., Kelly, J.H., Gislason, G.T. and Williams, R. 1994. A controlled trial of the Hepatix extracorporeal liver assist device (ELAD) in acute liver failure [Abstract]. *Hepatology* 20: 140A.

Fox, I.J, Langnas, A.N., Fristoe, L.W., Shaefer, M.S., Vogel, J.E., Antonson, D.L., Donovan, J.P., Heffron, T.G., Markin, R.S., Sorrell, M.F. and Shaw, B.W. 1993. Successful application of extracorporeal liver perfusion: a technology whose time has come. *Am J Gastroenterol* 88: 1876–81.

Gerlach, J.C., Schnoy, N., Encke, J., Smith, M.D., Muller, C. and Neuhaus, P. 1995. Improved hepatocyte in vitro maintenance in a culture model with woven multicompartment capillary systems: electron microscope studies. *Hepatology* 22: 546–52.

Gislason, G.T., Lobdell, D.D., Kelly, J.H. and Sussman, N.L. 1994. A treatment system for implementing an extracorporeal liver assist device. *Artif Org* 18: 385–9.

Jauregui, H.O., Mullon, C.J.-P., Trenkler, D., Naik, S., Santangini, H., Press, P., Muller, T.E. and Solomon, B.A. 1995. In vivo evaluation of a hollow fiber liver assist device. *Hepatology* 21: 460–9.

Karvountzis, G.G., Redeker, A.G. and Peters, R.L. 1974. Long term follow up studies of patients surviving fulminant viral hepatitis. *Gastroenterology* 67: 870–7.

Kelly, J.H., Koussayer, T., He, D., Chong, M.G., Shang, T.A., Whisennand, H.H. and Sussman, N.L. 1992a. Assessment of an extracorporeal liver assist device in anhepatic dogs. *Artif Org* 16: 418–22.

Kelly, J.H., Koussayer, T., He, D.E., Chong, M.G., Shang, T.A., Whisennand, H.H. and Sussman, N.L. 1992b. An improved model of acetaminophen-induced fulminant hepatic failure in dogs. *Hepatology* 15: 329–35.

Li, A.P., Barker, G., Beck, D., Colburn, S., Monsell, R. and Pellegrin, C. 1993. Culturing of primary hepatocytes as entrapped aggregates in a packed bed bioreactor: a potential bioartificial liver. *In Vitro Cell Dev Biol* 29A: 249–54.

McKenzie, R., Fried, M.W., Sallie, R., Conjeevaram, H., Di Bisceglie, A.M., Park, Y., Savarese, B., Kleiner, D., Tsokos, M., Luciano, C., Pruett, T., Stotka, J.L., Straus, S.E. and Hoofnagle, J.H. 1995. Hepatic failure and lactic acidosis due to fialuridine (FIAU), an investigational nucleoside analogue for chronic hepatitis B. *N Engl J Med* 333: 1099–105.

Melkonian, A.D., Gaylor, J.D., Cousins, R.B. and Grant, M.H. 1994. Culture of a differentiated liver cell line, Hep G2, in serum with application to a bioartificial liver: effect of supplementation of serum with amino acids. *Artif Org* 18: 611–17.

Nagaki, M., Hughes, R.D., Lau, J.Y. and Williams, R. 1991. Removal of endotoxin and cytokines by adsorbents and the effect of plasma protein binding. *Int J Artif Org* 14: 43–50.

Nyberg, S.L., Platt, J.L., Shirabe, K., Payne, W.D., Hu, W.S. and Cerra, F.B. 1992. Immunoprotection of xenocytes in a hollow fiber bioartificial liver. *ASAIO J* 38: M463–7.

Nyberg, S.L., Remmel, R.P., Mann, H.J., Peshwa, M.V., Hu, W.S. and Cerra, F.B. 1994. Primary hepatocytes outperform Hep G2 cells as the source of biotransformation functions in a bioartificial liver. *Ann Surg* 220: 59–67.

Nyberg, S.L., Shirabe, K., Peshwa, M.V., Sielaff, T.D., Crotty, P.L., Mann, H.J., Remmel, R.P., Payne, W.D., Hu, W.S. and Cerra, F.B. 1993. Extracorporeal application of a gel-entrapment, bioartificial liver: demonstration of drug metabolism and other biochemical functions. *Cell Transpl* 2: 441–52.

O'Grady, J.G., Alexander, G.J., Hayllar, K.M. and Williams, R. 1989. Early indicators of prognosis in fulminant hepatic failure. *Gastroenterology* 97: 439–45.

Opolon, P. 1979. High-permeability membrane hemodialysis and hemofiltration in acute hepatic coma: experimental and clinical results. *Artif Org* 3: 354–60.

Ranek, L., Andreasen, P.B. and Tygstrup, N. 1976. Galactose elimination capacity as a prognostic index in patients with fulminant liver failure. *Gut* 17: 959–64.

Rozga, J., Holzman, M.D., Ro, M.S., Griffin, D.W., Neuzil, D.F., Giorgio, T., Moscioni, A.D. and Demetriou, A.A. 1993. Development of a hybrid bioartificial liver. *Ann Surg* 217: 502–11.

Rozga, J., Podesta, L., LePage, E., Morsiani, E., Moscioni, A.D., Hoffman, A., Sher, L., Villamil, F., Woolf, G., McGrath, M., Kong, L., Rosen, H., Lanman, T., Vierling, J., Makowka, L. and Demetriou, A.A. 1994. A bioartificial liver to treat severe acute liver failure. *Ann Surg* 218: 538–6.

Schecter, D.C., Nealon, T.F. and Gibbon, J.H. 1985. A simple extracorporeal device for reducing elevated blood ammonia levels. *Surgery* 44: 892–7.

Seda, H.W., Hughes, R.D., Gove, C.D. and Williams, R. 1984a. Inhibition of rat brain Na^+,K^+-ATPase activity by serum from patients with fulminant hepatic failure. *Hepatology* 4: 74–9.

Seda, H.W., Hughes, R.D., Gove, C.D. and Williams, R. 1984b. Removal of inhibitors of brain Na^+,K^+-ATPase by hemoperfusion in fulminant hepatic failure. *Artif Org* 8: 174–8.

Shatford, R.A., Nyberg, S.L., Meier, S.J., White, J.G., Payne, W.D., Hu, W.S. and Cerra, F.B. 1992. Hepatocyte function in a hollow fiber bioreactor: a potential bioartificial liver. *J Surg Res* 53: 549–57.

Sussman, N.L. and Kelly, J.H. 1993. Extracorporeal liver assist in the treatment of fulminant hepatic failure. [Review]. *Blood Purif* 11: 170–4.

Sussman, N.L. and Kelly, J.H. 1995a. Temporary liver support: theory, practice, predictions. *Xenobiotica* 3: 63–7.

Sussman, N.L. and Kelly, J.H. 1995b. Temporary hepatic support systems. In *Transplantation of the Liver*, eds. W.C. Maddrey and M.F. Sorrell, 357–69. Appleton & Lange: New York.

Sussman, N.L., Chong, M.G., Koussayer, T., He, D.E., Shang, T.A., Whisennand, H.H. and Kelly, J.H. 1992. Reversal of fulminant hepatic failure using an extracorporeal liver assist device. *Hepatology* 16: 60–5.

Sussman, N.L., Finegold, M.J., Barish, J.P. and Kelly, J.H. 1994. A case of syncytial giant-cell hepatitis treated with an extracorporeal liver assist device. *Am J Gastroenterol* 89: 1077–82.

Sussman, N.L., Gislason, G.T., Conlin, C.A. and Kelly, J.H. 1994. The Hepatix extracorporeal liver assist device: initial clinical experience. *Artif Org* 18: 390–6.

Sussman, N.L., Gislason, G.T. and Kelly, J.H. 1994. Extracorporeal liver support. Application to fulminant hepatic failure. [Review]. *J Clin Gastroenterol* 18: 320–4.

Wolf, C.F.W. and Munkelt, B.E. 1975. Bilirubin conjugation by an artificial liver composed of cultured cells and synthetic capillaries. *Trans ASAIO* 21: 16–26.

PART SIX Other Applications

21 Treatment of acute liver failure by high volume plasmapheresis

Niels Tygstrup, Fin Stolze Larsen and Bent Adel Hansen

INTRODUCTION

When ammonia intoxication was believed to be the dominant cause of hepatic encephalopathy, and hemodialysis was introduced for treatment of renal failure, the idea of dialyzing patients with hepatic failure seemed obvious (Kiley et al. 1956). When hemodialysis proved to have little or no effect on hepatic encephalopathy, it became apparent that encephalopathy is not caused by high blood concentrations of dialyzable substances.

Other possible causal mechanisms would include an accumulation of harmful non-dialyzable substances (the intoxication concept) or a lack of production of compounds essential for cerebral metabolism (the fallout concept). The intoxication concept remains the more popular one, probably because of the analogy to renal failure.

Discrimination between these possibilities has not been possible so far. Instead, attempts have been made to develop support systems combining both concepts. Several systems have been tried including exchange blood transfusion, plasmapheresis, and the most complete system, perfusion of the patient's blood through an extracorporeal liver. No liver support system to date (except orthotopic liver transplantation) has demonstrated convincing and reproducible beneficial effects. Possible explanations for the limited success with support systems include that the procedures mainly have been used in cases with irreversible brain damage, or that they have been quantitatively insufficient. In the latter case the solution might be to increase the capacity of the system being used.

PLASMAPHERESIS

Plasmapheresis satisfies the condition of both removing potentially toxic compounds from the blood, independent of molecular weight (unless they are bound to blood cells), and of providing required compounds from healthy subjects (unless they are short-lived). Plasmapheresis for hepatic coma was first suggested by Lepore and Martel in 1967, and this group has published results in a series of nine patients treated for one to 12 days with exchange of 10–83 l of plasma (Lepore and Martel 1967; Lepore et al. 1972). In two patients the degree of coma was reduced, but neither survived. Haapanen and Tiula in 1972 proposed exchange with human albumin, and in 1973 Buckner et al. treated four patients, exchanging ten liters per day for three to 36 days, with three patients surviving.

The introduction of membrane cell separators simplified the procedure and expanded the use of plasmapheresis. Inoue et al. (1981)

reported three survivors of seven patients with fulminant hepatic failure exchanging five liters, one to sixteen times. Freeman et al. (1986), by repeated (mean 4.5) exchange of three liters, obtained an improvement in seven, and survival in five of nine patients (Splendiani et al. 1990). These authors exchanged 50–60 percent of the plasma volume one to five times in eight patients of whom three recovered. Brunner et al. (1992) performed 61 exchanges in ten patients with survival in seven.

At about the same time, liver transplantation became the treatment of choice for acute liver failure (ALF), and plasmapheresis was then studied by Winikoff as a "bridge" to liver transplantation (Winikoff et al. 1985). Muñoz et al. (1989) performed 33 exchanges in 19 patients of whom five survived without, and seven with, liver transplantation. Treatment did not influence blood requirements during surgery, but facilitated preoperative preparation by correction of the coagulopathy.

HIGH VOLUME PLASMAPHERESIS

In spite of the greater biochemical facility provided by the membrane cell separator, most studies performed to date have been based on the conventional exchange of a volume corresponding to the plasma volume. However, the effect of increasing the volume of exchange had not been considered. Since the capacity actually needed to compensate for failing liver function is unknown, estimates have been made on the basis of the "intoxication concept", that is, the amount of exchange needed to clear a protein-bound compound from the circulation. By computer simulation, assuming that a toxic substance represented by unconjugated bilirubin is distributed in a volume corresponding to the extracellular space, Berk (1977) demonstrated the theoretical benefit to be obtained by prolonging and/or repeating the periods of hemoperfusion.

Applying a similar concept to plasmapheresis (Kondrup et al. 1992) with an exchange rate of 1 l/h, and ignoring the transfer rate from extra- to intravascular beds (Keller et al. 1984), we planned a study in which we would use this treatment on three consecutive days when necessary (if the patient did not recover) and if possible (if the patient did not die or receive a transplant).

THE COPENHAGEN STUDY

Patients

From January 1987 to December 1994, 52 of 111 patients admitted with acute liver failure were treated with high volume plasmapheresis (HVP). In Table 21.1, the 52 patients are grouped according to etiologic factors: Group A, acetaminophen ingestion (16 patients); Group B, hepatitis (18 patients including two with HAV, three with HBV, two autoimmune and 11 non-ABCDE); and Group C (miscellaneous, including eight drug-induced [six disulfiram, two halothane], one primary graft dysfunction, one hypoxic injury, one *Amanita* intoxication).

Patients with acetaminophen intoxication were treated with *N*-acetylcysteine (NAC) and standard supportive treatment in the liver intensive care unit. Volume-controlled mechanical ventilation, without muscle relaxation, was instituted simultaneously with recording of arterial and central venous pressures. None or minimal positive end expiratory pressure (PEEP) was used with peak inspiratory pressure less than 40 mmHg and $Paco_2$ was initially maintained above 4.5 kPa. Subdural intracranial pressure (Camino Lab., California) with a 20° head/neck elevation was recorded after development of coma grade IV. If intracranial pressure increased to >25 mmHg, mannitol, thiopental, and mild hyperventilation were gradually initiated in stepwise fashion, according to the response.

Bilirubin, hemoglobin, platelets, white blood cell count, and electrolytes in blood and urine were determined by standard methods, prothrombin index by SPA reagents (Diagnostica Stago, Ashieres-sur-Seine, France);

Table 21.1. *Group A – acetaminophen intoxicated patients; Group B – patients with viral hepatitis; Group C – miscellaneous (for details of B and C see text)*

Group	Male/ Female	Age (range)	Days of symptoms before admission	Coma grade on admission	Number of deaths	Number of OLT	Deaths after OLT
A	5/16	34.8 (17–49)	2.7 (0–5)	2.1 (0–4)	9	4	1
B	8/10	36.2 (1–60)	38.3 (4–175)	1.4 (0–4)	10	9	2
C	9/4	38.5 (12–67)	16.0 (3–75)	2.2 (0–4)	5	8	1

galactose elimination capacity (Tygstrup 1966) and Glasgow coma score (in nonsedated patients) were measured before and after each plasmapheresis.

As changes in cerebral perfusion may provide more accurate prognostic information than intracranial pressure with regard to development of brain death (Aggarwal et al. 1994), cerebral perfusion was monitored by internal jugular vein saturation ($Svjo_2$) in 19 patients, transcranial Doppler mean flow velocity in the middle cerebral artery (V_{mean}) in 32 patients, and in six patients also by the ^{133}Xenon injection technique for cerebral blood flow (CBF). In order to maintain cerebral perfusion within physiologic values, i.e. $Svjo_2$ 55–75 percent, $V_{mean} < 100$ cm s^{-1}, CBF <60 ml 100 g^{-1} min^{-1}, $Paco_2$ was adjusted prior to start of high volume plasmapheresis via the respiratory and/or arterial pressure by volume regulation and vasopressor agents. Plasmapheresis was started when the patients were in coma grade III to IV.

Methods

An Excorim (Gambro, Copenhagen, DK) plasmapheresis apparatus and disposable plasma separators with a pore size of 0.65 μm were used. Exchange was performed through a double lumen catheter (Vascath, Gambro Co., Sweden) inserted either via a subclavian or femoral vein. Heparin was used during the start of the program, but avoided later. The apparatus pumps the blood of the patient through the separator, removing about 60 percent of the plasma which is quantitatively replaced by preheated fresh, frozen plasma which is returned to the patient. Alkalosis produced by citrated plasma was prevented by infusion of isotonic hydrochloric acid, usually about 200 mg per hour to maintain standard base excess below 6 mmol/l. Reduction of the blood level of ionized calcium was prevented by infusion of calcium leavulate, usually 5 mmoles for each liter of plasma exchanged, guided by hourly determinations.

Intracranial pressure was monitored by a subdural transducer inserted through a parietal burr hole (Camino, Camino Laboratories, San Diego, CA). Catheters were also inserted into a radial artery for blood sampling and mean arterial pressure measurement, and in the right internal jugular vein, with the position in the superior jugular bulb assured by radiographic examination (Wendon et al. 1994).

The CBF was measured by intravenous injection of 15–25 mCi ^{133}Xenon followed by external detection of cerebral uptake and washout by a ten stationary detector system (Cerebrograph 10A, Simonsen Medical, Hadsund, DK). Since hematocrit influences the partition coefficient (lambda) for ^{133}Xenon, CBF was corrected.

Transcranial Doppler sonography (Multi Dop X, DWL, Ulden, Germany), assessed flow (V_{mean}) in the middle cerebral artery and cerebral arteriojugular venous oxygen content differences ($AVDo_2$) were recorded by insonation of the middle cerebral artery with a 2 MHz pulsed Doppler probe fixated in the left temporal "window" by a headband (Larsen, Olsen, Hansen, Paulson and Knudsen 1994). Cerebral oxygen consumption ($CMRo_2$) was calculated as $AVDo_2$ times CBF, and the oxygen extraction fraction as the ratio between $AVDo_2$ and the arterial oxygen content (Wendon et al. 1994). Systemic hemodynamic variables were determined by a Swan–Ganz catheter.

Results

Figure 21.1 shows data on plasmapheresis, and outcome (transplantation and death) in all 52 patients in consecutive order in relation to admission. Case No. 16 was the first to have a transplant (in 1990). Twenty-eight patients survived (54 percent), 17 after liver transplantation. Four patients died in spite of liver transplantation, one each in groups A and C, two in group B (Table 21.1). The mortality was not significantly different in the three etiologic groups, but significantly fewer in group A received a transplant (20 percent versus 50 percent and 62 percent). Three patients >60 years old and one <10 years of age all died; otherwise no relation between age and mortality was evident. No patient with a galactose elimination capacity below 10 mmol/kg on admission survived (Figure 21.2).

The effect of high volume plasmapheresis on the Glasgow coma score (in nonsedated patients), prothrombin and bilirubin concentration is shown in Figure 21.3. The mean effect on coma score was greater in surviving than in nonsurviving patients but, in both instances, cases with no effect or a marked effect were found. The effect on prothrombin concentration was highly consistent, nonsurvivors differing from survivors by a greater fall from the end of one to the start of the next treatment. Bilirubin was higher in nonsurvivors than in survivors prior to high volume plasmapheresis and showed a similar or greater fall during treatment.

High volume plasmapheresis appears to increase V_{mean}, CBF and $CMRo_2$ in patients with acute liver failure (unpublished data; Figure 21.4). Furthermore, mean arterial pressure (MAP) and cerebral perfusion pressure (CPP) appear to increase during plasmapheresis while intracranial pressure remains unchanged. Systemic vascular resistance (SVR) increases in parallel with MAP and CPP while cardiac output decreases (Larsen, Hansen, Ejlersen, Mogensen et al. 1995b).

Discussion

When compared with other "liver assist" procedures, the effect of high volume plasmapheresis in acute liver failure remains uncertain and will remain so until randomized clinical trials can give a certain answer. However, adequate controlled clinical trials are impossible in most centers because too few patients can be accrued, and most of the procedures proposed are too complex to ensure uniform protocols for multicenter trials. Historical controls are of limited value because of several small, but probably significant, developments in intensive care, and changes in the pattern of diseases and referral. Two-thirds of the patients in the present study were referred during the last half of the period of inclusion, i.e. after liver transplantation became available, which may explain the shorter time course in that period (Figure 21.1).

The introduction of liver transplantation represents a further methodological complication due to the unpredictable availability of donor livers. Among the surviving patients in the present patient group, all of whom had been placed on the waiting list for a transplant and were treated with high volume plasmapheresis, 11 of 31 (35 percent) have survived without a transplant being performed, compared with 17 of 21 (81 percent) who did get transplanted. This does not prove the absolute

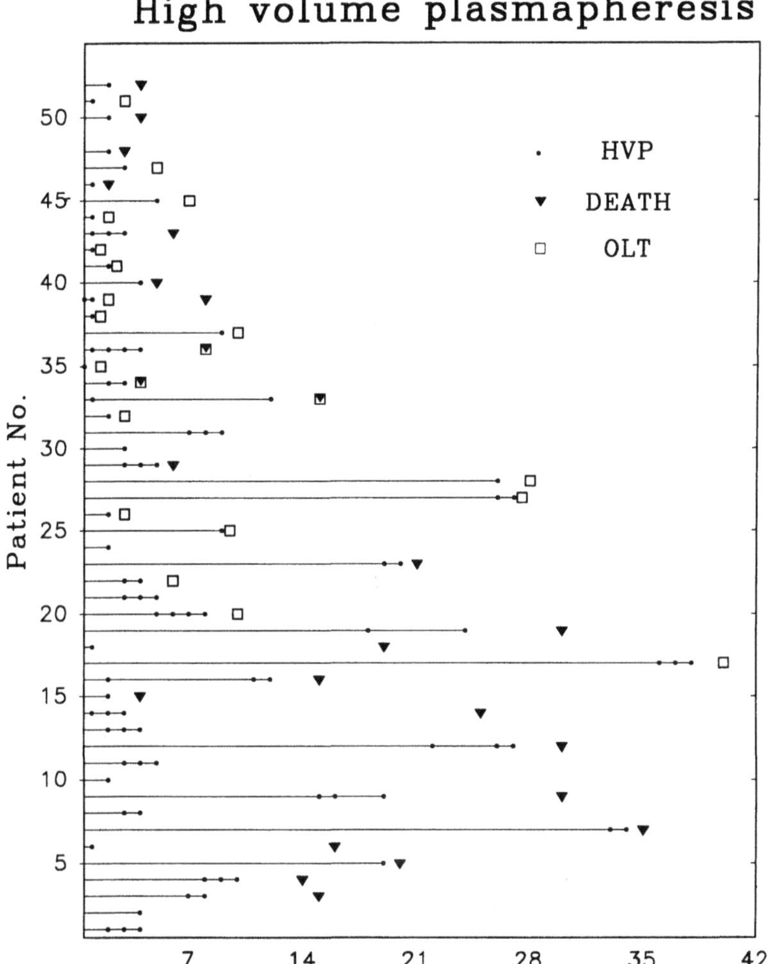

Figure 21.1 High volume plasmapheresis (HPV), death, and liver transplantation (OLT) in relation to days after admission in 52 consecutive patients.

value of high volume plasmapheresis but is reassuring enough in our view to retain it as a "bridge" to transplantation, and as alternative treatment in the absence of a donor liver.

An increased survival of treated patients not expected to survive according to low galactose elimination capacity (Tygstrup and Ranek 1986) with high volume plasmapheresis was not demonstrable (Figure 21.2). Even if the effect of such plasmapheresis on survival from acute liver failure may be limited, other effects may not be negligible. The transient recovery of consciousness in some patients during the procedure may be a clue to the pathogenesis of hepatic encephalopathy, and the lesser effect in its nonsurviving group may be an indication of irreversible brain damage. Furthermore, the elimination of coagulopathy may prevent hemorrhagic complications, especially during transplantation, even if a significant effect of (low volume) plasmapheresis on the need for blood transfusions was not demonstrable (Muñoz et al. 1989).

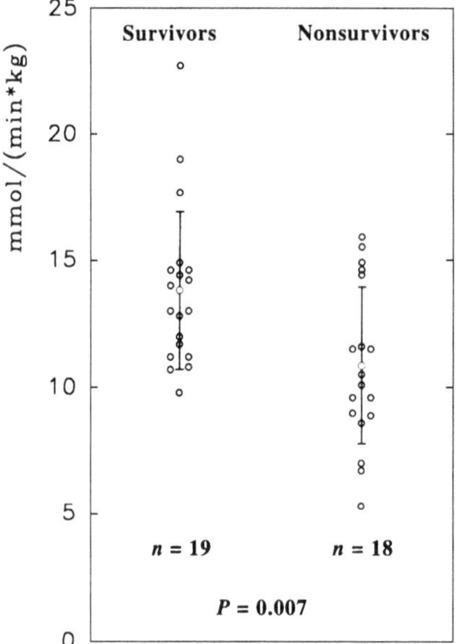

Figure 21.2 Galactose elimination capacity in patients with acute liver failure before high volume plasmapheresis, with mean and standard deviation for surviving and nonsurviving patients.

EFFECT ON HEMODYNAMICS

Central volume depletion may lead to arterial hypotension and decreased preload. Insufficient perfusion of vital organs not improved by intervention with inotropic agents may contribute to a poor prognosis. When organ perfusion decreases, the ability to increase oxygen extraction is impaired, and oxygen consumption then depends directly on oxygen delivery, that is on cardiac output.

In most of the patients, the mean arterial pressure was low prior to, and increased during plasmapheresis, whereas cardiac output decreased (Figure 21.4). Thus, systemic vascular resistance increased, and total oxygen delivery decreased. Nevertheless, oxygen consumption remained constant, indicating improved oxygen extraction by the organs (Larsen et al. 1995b). The effect on systemic vascular resistance lasted for about 12 h, suggesting that arterial hypotension in acute liver failure is caused by one or more vasodilator substances with a rapid turnover. This suggests that high volume plasmapheresis can improve microcirculatory function in patients with ALF.

High volume plasmapheresis increased cerebral blood flow (CBF), V_{mean} and cerebral oxygen metabolism ($CMRo_2$). The increase in CBF probably reflects preservation of the coupling between CBF and brain metabolism, as seen in the normal brain and supported by previous observations in acute liver failure (Larsen, Olsen et al. 1994; Larsen, Knudsen et al. 1994). According to the toxin concept, we assume that high volume plasmapheresis increases $CMRo_2$ by removal of toxic plasma substances responsible for deranged neuronal metabolism resulting in a subsequent increase in CBF.

Intracranial hypertension and sepsis are among the most important factors determining the outcome of acute liver failure (Larsen, Hansen et al. 1994). Although cerebral perfusion pressure increases, manifest intracranial hypertension cannot be reversed by high volume plasmapheresis. Of 40 patients with intracranial hypertension due to acute liver failure evaluated during the period 1991 to 1995, 25 were treated with high volume plasmapheresis, and 12 (48 percent) survived (8 after liver transplantation), while 13 died. Of the remaining 15 patients not treated by high volume plasmapheresis, three survived (20 percent) and 12 died.

It has been suggested that cerebral swelling is particularly prominent in patients with a high CBF (Larsen, Knudsen et al. 1994). In seven patients with intracranial hypertension, CBF was found to be severely elevated before high volume plasmapheresis and associated with jugular oxygen saturation values above 75 percent, that is "luxury-perfusion" syndrome (Lassen 1966). The syndrome is associated with a very poor prognosis, with cerebral perfusion reaching a peak approximately 10 h before development of brain death (Larsen, Pott et al. 1995). A state of dissociated vasoparalysis, for example,

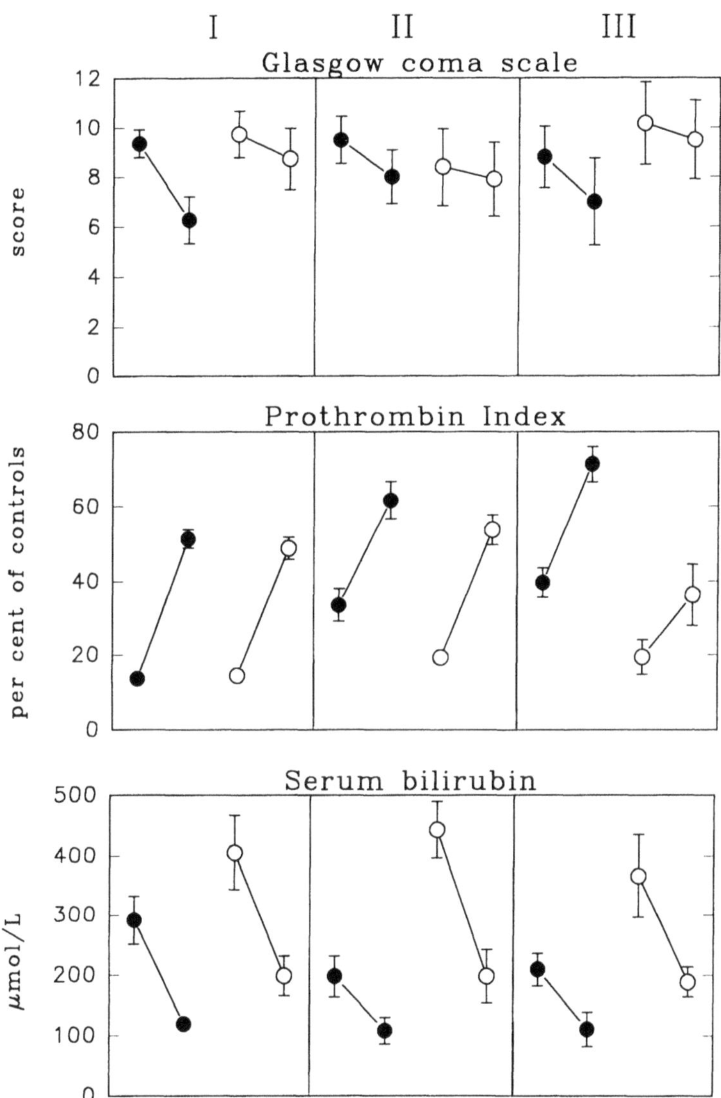

Figure 21.3 Effect of first, second, and third high volume plasmapheresis on consciousness (in non-sedated patients) as estimated by the Glasgow Coma Scale (upper panel), prothrombin concentration (middle panel), and serum bilirubin (lower panel) in surviving and nonsurviving patients, as mean and standard error of the mean.

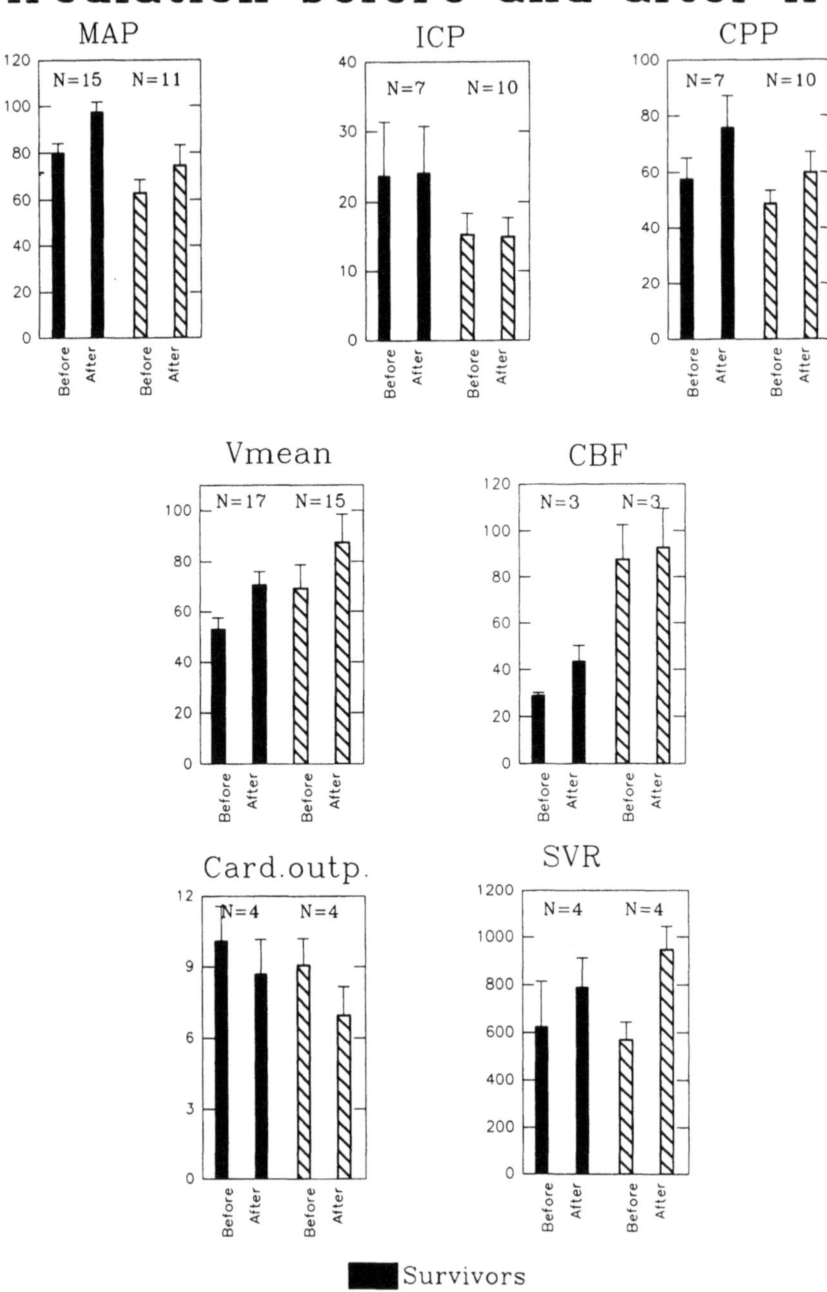

Figure 21.4 The effect of high volume plasmapheresis on circulation variables before and after high volume plasmapheresis in surviving and nonsurviving patients, as mean and standard error of the mean: MAP = mean arterial pressure (mmHg), ICP = intracranial pressure (mmHg), CCP = cerebral perfusion pressure (mmHg), V_{mean} = mean flow velocity in middle cerebral artery (cm sec^{-1}), CBF = cerebral blood flow (ml 100 g^{-1}), Card.outp. = cardiac output (1 min^{-1}), SVR = systemic vascular resistance (mmHg (1 $min^{-1})^{-1}$).

impaired autoregulation with preserved CO_2 reactivity in acute liver failure patients has been suggested and may be assumed to precede the luxury-perfusion syndrome (Larsen, Hansen et al. 1995).

Our data do not elucidate the mechanism by which the procedure may compensate for failing liver function, that is, whether it eliminates toxins or adds compounds in demand. On the former assumption, using bilirubin as a marker of a toxic substance, our data have been compared with a model describing the clearance of a compound from the extracellular volume by high volume plasmapheresis as aimed at in the present study, that is, exchange of 1 l per hour for eight hours on three consecutive days (Figure 21.5). The outcome depends on the rate with

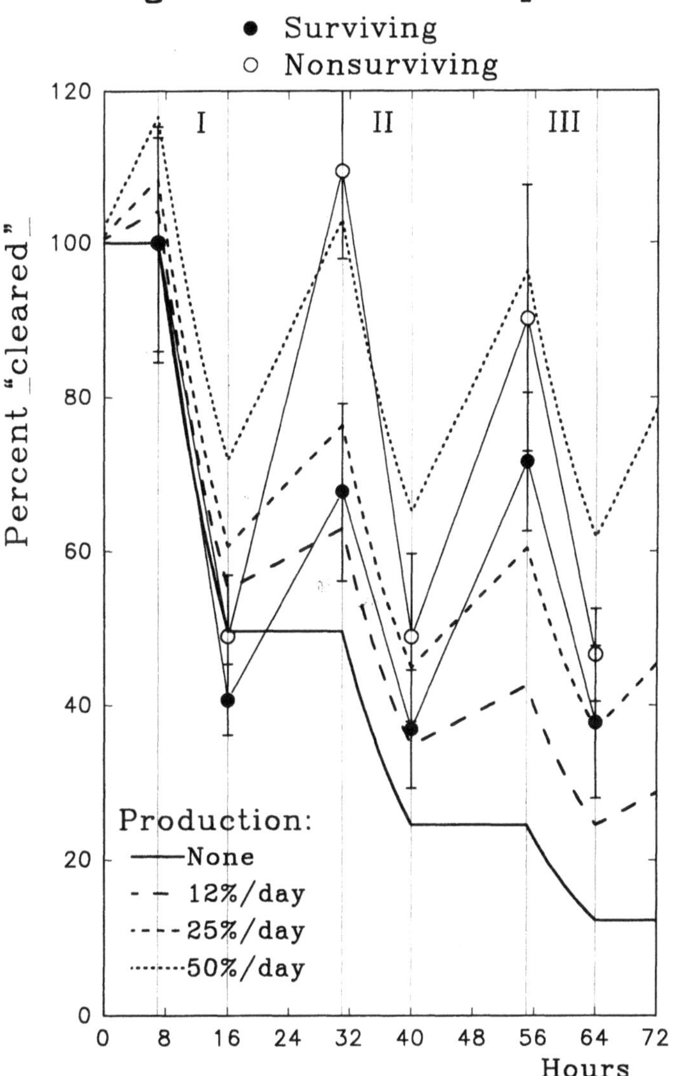

Figure 21.5 Simulated effect of high volume plasmapheresis (1 liter per hour for 8 hours) on three consecutive days, assuming clearance from the extracellular volume. Normalized data for bilirubin (lower panel in Figure 21.3) are plotted. See text for comments.

which the compound is produced. The bilirubin data do not fit the simulated curves precisely. Both the fall in bilirubin levels during treatment and the increase observed between treatments is steeper, indicating elimination from a smaller volume and rapid redistribution from extracellular to vascular volume during the intervals. It seems, however, that the bilirubin production rate in nonsurvivors is about twice as high as in survivors.

COMPLICATIONS OF HIGH VOLUME PLASMAPHERESIS

Some real and possible disadvantages of high volume plasmapheresis cannot be ignored. Although the cost of the equipment is moderate in relation to other medical appliances, the expense of the large amount of plasma required and the need for personnel for surveillance may be a problem in some units.

Microemboli in the pulmonary circulation have previously been described as a complication of plasmapheresis in patients with acute liver failure (Akamatsu and Ohta 1992), and a venous arterial circulation has been recommended to avoid this. In our cases, clinical signs of pulmonary microemboli have not been observed, and the pulmonary vascular resistance remained unchanged during high volume plasmapheresis even when the systemic vascular resistance increased.

The invasive procedures together with heparinization present a risk of hemorrhage. We have reduced heparin treatment to 0–2000 units for a 10 l plasmapheresis which is sufficient if the procedure is performed by experienced personnel and with few interruptions of the extracorporeal circulation.

Saibara et al. (1994) have suggested that plasmapheresis causes citrate intoxication and suppression of hepatocyte regeneration. However, the complete recovery observed in several patients with severe acute liver failure treated with high volume plasmapheresis who did not receive a liver transplant argues against such a toxic effect on the liver.

The possibility of an increased risk of infection (sepsis) after high volume plasmapheresis is also present. However, a recent retrospective analysis has shown that only about 5 percent of the patients with acute liver failure treated by plasmapheresis later developed sepsis (Clemmesen et al. 1995). No direct relationship with the procedure was found, but a prospective study is needed to evaluate the risk.

The likelihood that the plasma exchange removes useful compounds such as hormones, cytokines, growth factors or other compensatory substances from the circulation must be kept in mind and further investigated.

CONCLUSION

Published studies and the results presented from the Copenhagen experience fail to show a marked beneficial effect of plasmapheresis on survival from acute liver failure. The effects of high volume plasmapheresis on several variables indicate, however, that it may be a useful part of conservative case management. Furthermore, it may help in the evaluation and understanding of several important components of the liver failure syndrome, in particular the role of cerebral hemodynamics and metabolism. The procedure is relatively simple to standardize and perform, and is thus a promising candidate for a multicenter trial.

REFERENCES

Aggarwal, S., Kramer, D., Yonas, H. et al. 1994. Cerebral hemodynamic and metabolic changes in fulminant hepatic failure: A retrospective study. *Hepatology* 19: 80–7.

Akamatsu, K. and Ohta, Y. 1992. Pulmonary microembolism due to plasma exchange replaced by fresh frozen plasma. In *Artificial Liver Support*, eds. G. Brunner and M. Mito, 235–47. New York: Springer Verlag.

Berk, P.D. 1977. A computer simulation study to the treatment of fulminant hepatic failure by hemoperfusion. *Proc Soc Exp Biol Med* 155: 535–9.

Brunner, G., Bahlmann, J. and Eisenbach, G.-M. 1992. Improved plasma exchange for the treatment of fulminant hepatic failure by plasma replacement into the femoral artery. In *Artificial Liver Support*, eds. G. Brunner and M. Mito, 244–8. New York: Springer Verlag.

Buckner, C.D., Clift, R.A., Volwiler, W. et al. 1973. Plasma exchange in patients with fulminant hepatic failure. *Arch Intern Med* 132: 487–92.

Clemmesen, J.O., Larsen, F.S., Rasmussen, A. and Hansen, B.A. 1995. Antimicrobial therapy in patients with fulminant hepatic failure prior to liver transplantation. *Transpl Proc.*

Freeman, J.G., Matthewson, K. and Record, C.O. 1986. Plasmapheresis in acute liver failure. *Int J Artif Org* 9: 433–8.

Haapanen, E. and Tiula, E. 1972. Plasmapheresis with albumin as main substitute in acute hepatic coma. *Scand J Gastroenterol* 7: 75–83.

Inoue, N., Yoshiba, M., Yamazaki, Z. et al. 1981. Continuous flow membrane plasmapheresis utilizing cellulose acetate hollow fiber in hepatic failure. In *Artificial Liver Support*, eds. G. Brunner and F.W. Schmidt, 175–80. Berlin: Springer Verlag.

Keller, F., Offermann, G. and Scholle, J. 1984. Kinetics of the redistribution phenomenon after extracorporeal elimination. *Int J Artif Org* 7: 181–8.

Kiley, J.E., Welch, H.F., Pender, J.C. and Welch, C.S. 1956. Removal of blood ammonia by hemodialysis. *Proc Soc Exp Biol Med* 91: 489–90.

Kondrup, J., Almdal, T., Vilstrup, H. and Tygstrup, N. 1992. High volume plasma exchange in fulminant hepatic failure. *Int J Artif Org* 15: 669–76.

Larsen, F.S., Hansen, B.A., Jorgensen, L.G., et al. 1994. Cerebral blood flow velocity during high volume plasmapheresis in fulminant hepatic failure. *Int J Artif Org* 17: 353–61.

Larsen, F.S., Hansen, B.A., Ejlersen, E., Secher, N.H., Tygstrup, N. and Knudsen, G.M. 1995a. Functional loss of cerebral blood flow autoregulation in patients with fulminant hepatic failure. *J Hepatol* 23: 212–17.

Larsen, F.S., Hansen, B.A., Ejlersen, E., Mogensen, T., Tygstrup, N. and Secher, N.H. 1995b. The effect of high volume plasmapheresis on systemic haemodynamics in patients with fulminant hepatic failure. *Eur J Gastoenterol Hepatol* 7: 887–92.

Larsen, F.S., Knudsen, G.M., Paulson, O.B. and Vilstrup, H. 1994. Cerebral blood flow autoregulation is absent in rats with thioacetamide-induced hepatic failure. *J Hepatol* 21: 491–5.

Larsen, F.S., Olsen, K.S., Hansen, B.A., Paulson, O.B. and Knudsen, G.M. 1994. Transcranial Doppler is valid for determination of the lower limit of cerebral blood flow autoregulation. *Stroke* 25: 1985–8.

Larsen, F.S., Pott, F., Hansen, B.A., et al. 1995. The value of transcranial Doppler mean flow velocity and intracranial pressure to predict brain death in patients with fulminant hepatic failure. *Transpl Proc* 27: 3519–20.

Lassen, N.A. 1966. The luxury-perfusion syndrome and its possible relation to acute metabolic acidosis localized within the brain. *Lancet* 2: 1113–15.

Lepore, M.J. and Martel, A.J. 1967. Plasmapheresis in hepatic coma. *Lancet* ii: 771–2.

Lepore, M.J., Stutman, L.J., Bonanno, C.A., Conklin, E.F., Robilotti, J.G. and McKenna, P.J. 1972. Plasmapheresis with plasma exchange in hepatic coma. II. Fulminant viral hepatitis as a systemic disease. *Arch Intern Med* 129: 900–7.

Muñoz, S.J., Ballas, S.K., Moritz, M.J. et al. 1989. Perioperative management of fulminant and subfulminant hepatic failure with therapeutic plasmapheresis. *Transpl Proc* 21: 3535–6.

Saibara, T., Maeda, T., Onishi, S. and Yamamoto, Y. 1994. Plasma exchange and the arterial blood ketone body ratio in patients with acute hepatic failure. *J Hepatol* 20: 617–22.

Splendiani, G., Tancredi, M., Daniele, M. and Giammaria, U. 1990. Treatment of acute liver failure with hemodetoxification techniques. *Int J Artif Org* 13: 370–4.

Tygstrup, N. 1966. Determination of the hepatic elimination capacity (Lm) of galactose by single injection. *Scand J Clin Lab Invest* 18 (Suppl. 92): 118–25.

Tygstrup, N. and Ranek, L. 1986. Assessment of prognosis in fulminant hepatic failure. *Sem Liver Dis* 6: 129–37.

Wendon, J.A., Harrison, P.M., Keays, R. and Williams, R. 1994. Cerebral blood flow and metabolism in fulminant liver failure. *Hepatology* 19: 1407–13.

Winikoff, S., Glassman, M.S. and Spivak, W. 1985. Plasmapheresis in a patient with hepatic failure awaiting liver transplantation. *J Pediatr* 107: 547–9.

22 Dialysis/adsorption techniques for acute liver failure

Robin D. Hughes and James M. Courtney

INTRODUCTION

The basis for the application of membranes or adsorbents in the treatment of acute liver failure is that benefit can be derived from the removal of circulating toxic substances, which have accumulated as a result of the loss of liver function, by extracorporeal blood purification procedures. This approach to detoxification, sometimes termed artificial or nonbiological liver support (Malchesky 1994) is dependent for success on the nature of the substances to be removed, the properties of membranes or adsorbents, and the utilization of membranes or adsorbents in an appropriate extracorporeal circuit (Giordano 1980; Konstantin et al. 1992; Hughes and Williams 1993; Uchino and Matsushita 1994).

Consideration of potential toxins has led to the implication of ammonia, amino acids, fatty acids, mercaptans, bilirubin, bile acids, phenols, middle molecules and endotoxin as being involved with the possibility of synergistic effects. This wide range of substances requires the use of nonspecific adsorbents rather than detoxification systems with a high specificity; the application of membranes or adsorbents must also take into account protein-bound and lipophilic toxins.

The options for the application of membranes or adsorbents (Table 22.1) have been examined in terms of hemodialysis-related procedures, membrane plasmapheresis, adsorbent treatment of blood or plasma and biocompatibility aspects, with the emphasis on the current situation.

Table 22.1. *Options for toxin removal by membranes or adsorbents*

Procedure	Variations
Hemodialysis	High permeability membranes, sorbent suspension dialysate
Hemofiltration	Continuous use, postdilutional filtration
Hemoperfusion	Selective adsorbents
Membrane plasmapheresis/plasma exchange	Large volume
Membrane plasmapheresis/plasma perfusion	Uncoated multisorbents, small particle size adsorbents
Centrifugal plasmapheresis	(as membrane)

HEMODIALYSIS-RELATED PROCEDURES

The clinical success of hemodialysis in the treatment of chronic renal failure encouraged interest in its relevance for the treatment of acute liver failure. However, hemodialysis is suitable only for the removal of low molecular weight solutes by a diffusive process. Improved solute removal can be achieved from the replacement of the generally used regenerated cellulose membranes by more permeable synthetic polymer membranes, eg. polyacrylonitrile, polysulfone, or from the replacement of hemodialysis by the convective process of solute removal in hemofiltration. This improved solute removal is insufficient to deal with protein-bound and lipophilic substances. Therefore, the application of hemodialysis in the treatment of acute liver failure (other than for the management of the associated renal failure) requires modifications to the standard procedure. Proposed modifications are the use of liquid membranes and dialysate suspensions.

Liquid membranes

A liver support system utilizing a liquid membrane (Konstantin et al. 1992) has focused on the removal of lipophilic toxins while preventing the elimination of physiological substances, such as hormones, which could have detrimental effects. The system contains a selective lipophilic liquid membrane filter and a hydrophilic membrane. Both types of membrane are in hollow fiber form. The liquid membrane filter consists of a hydrophobic polysulfone membrane with large voids that contain a paraffin oil. Blood is passed through the liquid membrane filter with a sodium hydroxide acceptor solution on the other side. Protein-bound toxins contacting the membrane are released into the oily layer, diffuse through the membrane and become water-soluble through reaction with the acceptor solution. The hydrophilic membrane module is a polysulfone dialysis membrane and the water-soluble solutes are eliminated by dialysis. This liquid membrane system has been assessed in vitro and with pigs and in initial clinical use: the system was reported to improve the coma state of a patient with liver failure.

Dialysate suspensions

The addition of adsorbents to the dialysate is not new (Giordano 1980). However, the original applications were directed towards dialysate regeneration and the development of portable and wearable artificial kidneys. With respect to liver support, the introduction of adsorbents into the dialysate is intended to enhance toxin removal, while avoiding the biocompatibility problems caused by direct blood-adsorbent contact in hemoperfusion. Another advantage over hemoperfusion is that the rate of solute removal can be increased by the use of small particle adsorbents.

In artificial liver support, the use of adsorbent suspensions in the dialysate is the basis of the BioLogic-DT system (HemoCleanse Inc. West Lafayette, IN) (Ash et al. 1992; 1993). The BioLogic-DT device contains a flat bed or parallel plate dialyser with cellulose membranes. A sorbent suspension is passed from a bag through the dialyser and back to the bag by positive and negative pressure applied to an accumulator near the top of the dialyser. Expansion and compression of the membranes forces blood through the dialyser and mixes the sorbent suspension at the membrane surface.

The sorbent suspension of the BioLogic-DT device comprises a powdered charcoal and a sodium-loaded cation exchange resin. The charcoal can also be preloaded with substances which are transferred to the patient during treatment. Examples of such substances are glucose and branched-chain amino acids. The cation exchange resin has functional binding for ammonium which is important in the context of liver failure. The detoxification procedure is described as hemodiabsorption (Ash 1994) on the basis that it is a combination of hemodialysis and absorption, although it is really only adsorption which is taking place.

The BioLogic-DT device can only remove solutes which are permeable through the cellulose membranes. Therefore, it cannot eliminate endotoxin or protein-bound solutes such as unconjugated bilirubin. It was reported (Ash et al. 1992) that the BioLogic-DT device can be used clinically in the absence of an anticoagulant and produced a neurological improvement in patients with liver failure, though mainly these were patients with chronic liver disease. However, these potential advantages were less clear-cut in patients with acute liver failure (Hughes et al. 1994). The BioLogic-DT system is under evaluation at different centers.

It is obvious that the purification procedure used in the BioLogic-DT system could be modified by the selection of different sorbent suspensions. However, this would not address the problem of removing protein-bound solutes, though plans have been made for enhancing the effectiveness of the procedure by the inclusion of a plasmapheresis membrane in the circuit. Consideration of the removal of protein-bound solutes which are generally considered to be important in liver failure and, in particular, the role of albumin has led to the concept of dialysis against a recycled albumin solution and the development of the Molecular Absorbents Recirculating System (MARS) system (Stange, Mitzner et al. 1993; Stange, Ramlow et al. 1993; Stange & Mitzner 1995). In this approach, an asymmetric polysulfone membrane is impregnated on both sides with albumin, and dialysis takes place against a closed loop dialysate containing albumin. The presence of albumin in the dialysate enhances the removal of albumin-bound toxins. To reduce the cost of this procedure, albumin can be regenerated from dialysate containing albumin-bound toxins by passage over charcoal and anion exchange resin. It is reported that use of the MARS-system leads to a clinical improvement in liver patients and that this is evidence of a key role in liver failure for albumin-bound toxins. This system needs to be evaluated in a controlled clinical trial.

MEMBRANE PLASMAPHERESIS

Improvements in membrane technology have promoted the clinical utilization of membrane plasmapheresis (Kambic and Nose 1993) and interest in membrane plasmapheresis followed by plasma exchange as a liver failure treatment. A summary of the Japanese experience (Matsubara 1994) suggests that plasma exchange can be beneficial for the removal of bilirubin, bile acids and endotoxin, improves the coagulation profile and contributes to the recovery of the lowered host defense mechanism. These advantages are reported to be offset by an ineffective clearance of low molecular weight solutes.

With respect to the status of membrane plasmapheresis followed by plasma exchange, it has been proposed as an acceptable bridge to liver transplantation (Agishi et al. 1994). There is interest in high volume plasma exchange (Kondrup et al. 1992; Larsen et al. 1994 and Chapter 21) and possibilities exist for improving the effectiveness of the procedure by reducing hemolysis (Philp et al. 1993). Improving toxin removal by combining plasma exchange with hemofiltration using high performance membranes has been reported to maintain patients for long periods of time (Yoshiba et al. 1993). An additional option for improved toxin removal remains membrane plasmapheresis followed by on-line adsorbent treatment of plasma.

ADSORBENT TREATMENT OF BLOOD OR PLASMA

With the exception of plasma exchange, nonbiological liver support systems generally utilize adsorbents. These adsorbents can be considered in terms of selection, development, utilization, and evaluation.

Adsorbent selection

Adsorbents for blood or plasma contact in artificial liver support fall into two broad categories. These are nonspecific or broad-based adsorbents, such as charcoal, and adsorbents directed towards the removal of particular substances such as bilirubin or endotoxin.

Activated charcoal or carbon is a highly porous material prepared by carbonization and activation of a source material, with variations in the source material and activation process offering scope for varying the properties of the finished product. With respect to adsorption from a liquid phase, based on the general rule of mutual affinity of substances with similar polarity, charcoal (a nonpolar adsorbent) will preferentially adsorb nonpolar solutes from a polar solvent. In the treatment of acute liver failure, a system based on charcoal adsorption alone is not considered to be sufficient, which is supported from results of clinical trials (O'Grady et al. 1988), although charcoal is likely to form a component of a liver support system.

Nonionic macroreticular resins are porous materials with a polymeric structure often based on polystyrene. The adsorptive properties are derived from the porosity, surface area, and the selection of a comonomer for styrene. Macroreticular resins offer the possibility of removing lipid-soluble and protein-bound substances. An example of a nonionic macroreticular resin is Amberlite XAD-7 (Rohm & Hass Ltd., Croydon, Surrey, UK) which was shown to remove protein-bound substances from patients with liver failure (Bihari et al. 1983). An ion exchange resin can be regarded as a matrix containing diffusible ions capable of exchange. The properties of the ion exchange resin are influenced by the nature of the matrix and the nature of the exchangeable ions. Ion exchange resins may have an organic or inorganic matrix and, depending on the nature of the functional groups, are termed strong, intermediate, or weak exchangers. Both cation and anion exchange resins have been utilized in artificial liver support, however, considerable care is required to prevent deleterious effects on blood electrolytes. As previously considered, a cation exchange resin can be used in a sorbent suspension dialysate (Ash et al. 1992). Anion exchange resins, in uncoated form, are generally applied in plasma purification (Malchesky 1994). Charcoal and resins represent the starting point in designing a sorbent-based artificial liver support system. Additional options come from the preparation of sorbents with a more specific action.

Adsorbent development

As stated, charcoal is a common component of nonbiological liver support systems. In principle, improved charcoal sorbents could result from chemical modification of the charcoal surface or improvements in sorbent pretreatment. This development could be directed towards enhanced biocompatibility or toxin removal.

An important objective for adsorbent development has been bilirubin removal and this is exemplified by a nonionic macroporous resin (Chen and Yu 1991) and an anion exchange resin (Usami et al. 1995). Another approach utilized the ability of the basic polypeptide polylysine to bind bilirubin (Zhu et al. 1990) in the preparation of a bilirubin adsorbent based on polylysine-immobilized chitosan beads (Chandy and Sharma 1992).

Another more recent objective in artificial liver support has been the development of an adsorbent for endotoxin removal. Successful removal has been reported for the antibiotic polymyxin B immobilized on polystyrene fibers (Hanasawa et al. 1989). However, the nephrotoxicity and neurotoxicity of polymyxin B make immobilization critical and the influence on blood makes the selection of a suitable antithrombotic agent difficult. An alternative to polymyxin B is the utilization of a cationic polymer and success has been reported for polyethyleneimine immobilized on cellulose spheres (Mitzner et al. 1993; Weber et al. 1994; Weber et al. 1995). This combination of polyethyleneimine and cellulose leads to materials with promising blood compatibility and there is evidence that the combination is important for endotoxin removal (Falkenhagen et al. 1993). In addition removal of cytokines, e.g. interleukins and interferons released in response to endotoxin or other inflammatory stimuli, may also be worthwhile. Existing adsorbents can remove cytokines (Nagaki et al. 1992), but more specific materials could be developed.

Adsorbent utilization

The utilization of adsorbents in artificial liver support must take into account biocompatibility and effectiveness. The direct purification of blood by hemoperfusion offers the advantage of simplicity but this is offset by the adverse alteration to blood components and the need to consider multisorbent systems. While an improved blood response can be achieved by coating an adsorbent with polymer, this reduces the rate of removal and where there is more than one adsorbent, purification of plasma is the preferred option.

Plasma purification by adsorbents not only reduces blood compatibility problems, but it also enhances the effectiveness of toxin removal by enabling the use of multiple sorbents, which extend the rate of removal, and the use of small particle sorbents, which increase the rate of removal. An example of adsorbent utilization with a potential benefit in artificial liver support is the recirculation of small particle sorbents in the extracapillary compartment of a membrane plasma separator with a centrifugal pump (Weber et al. 1994).

Adsorbent evaluation

The preclinical evaluation of adsorbents can be either simple in the case of in vitro single solute removal, or complex in the case of animal studies involving models of liver failure. Because of the complexity of toxins involved, an animal model offers advantages. In this respect, rats have been used as a convenient model to investigate the role of multisorbents and the influence of sorbents on liver regeneration (Ryan et al. 1991) and could be relevant for evaluating the influence of sorbents on the progression of hepatic coma (Ryan et al. 1990).

BIOCOMPATIBILITY

Blood component alterations

In contact with the artificial surfaces of membranes and adsorbents, alteration to blood components is inevitable (Forbes and Courtney 1994). Blood–material contact can induce protein adsorption, platelet reactions, activation of the intrinsic coagulation, fibrinolytic activity, complement activation, and alterations to erythrocytes and leukocytes. Despite the stated advantages of plasma perfusion, a number of these effects can still occur on interaction of plasma proteins with an adsorbent material. In extracorporeal procedures (Courtney et al. 1993), the blood response can be considered as coming under the influence of the materials involved, the nature of the application, the disease state of the blood and the influence of antithrombotic agents.

Material–antithrombotic agent relationship

For biomaterials generally, there is an overall relationship between the blood, the biomaterial, and the antithrombotic agent (Courtney et al. 1993), with an altered blood response coming from alteration to the biomaterial, the antithrombotic agent or both. Consideration has been given to the replacement of the anticoagulant heparin by low molecular weight heparin or by the protease inhibitor nafamostat mesilate (Abe et al. 1992) and the addition of prostacyclin as a platelet inhibitor. However, the ability of membranes to adsorb anticoagulants (Vienken and Bowry 1993; Inazaki et al. 1992), with a consequent influence on pharmacologic activity, makes the adsorbent–antithrombotic agent relationship a relevant topic in the development of nonbiological artificial liver support systems. However, as most biological systems also involve the use of membranes to separate liver cells from direct contact with blood, the same concerns arise about blood compatibility with the additional possibility of release of synthesized procoagulant proteins at membrane surfaces and of anticoagulants being metabolized by the liver cells.

FUTURE ASPECTS

Although there has been a recent tendency to "write off" systems of liver support for liver failure using adsorbents or dialysis in favor of bioartificial systems, there have been few proper clinical trials and, though not reviewed here, there is a reasonable amount of supportive data from animal experiments. Artificial systems are still being developed, particularly to utilize the powerful effects of adsorbents with a small particle size. Bioartificial systems do have the potential advantage of metabolic and synthetic function, but may lack the important excretory function which can readily be supplied by adsorbents or high performance hemodialysis. In fact one group has already incorporated a charcoal column into the perfusion circuit to reduce the load of toxic metabolites on the hepatocytes in the device (Rozga et al. 1993) and this may have accounted for some of the positive effects observed on cerebral function. It is highly likely that a successful liver support system will be a multicomponent system.

With greater knowledge of the metabolic abnormalities of liver failure, the key toxic substances can be better identified, and adsorbents could then be designed to specifically remove these substances and therefore play an important role. In relationship to this, one area where this could soon be possible is the development of materials for the removal of substances inhibitory to liver regeneration.

REFERENCES

Abe, H., Tani, T., Numa, K., Endo, Y., Yoshioka, T. and Kodama, M. 1992. Efficacy of nafomostat mesilate as a regional anticoagulant in experimental direct hemoperfusion and plasma exchange in humans. *Artif Org* 16: 206–12.

Agishi, T., Nakagawa, Y., Teraoka, S., Kubo, K., Nakazato, S. and Ota, K. 1994. Plasma exchange as a rescue strategy for hepatic failure. *ASAIO J* 40: 77–9.

Ash, S.R. 1994. Hemodiabsorption in the treatment of acute hepatic failure and chronic cirrhosis with ascites. *Artif Org* 18: 355–62.

Ash, S.R., Blake, D.E., Carr, D.J., Carter, C., Howard, T. and Makowka, L. 1992. Clinical effects of a sorbent suspension dialysis system in treatment of hepatic coma (the BioLogic-DT). *Int J Artif Org* 15: 151–61.

Ash, S.R., Carr, D.J., Blake, D.E., Rainier, J.B., Demetriou, A.A. and Rozga, J. 1993. Effect of sorbent-based dialytic therapy with the BioLogic-DT on an experimental model of hepatic failure. *ASAIO J* 39: M675–80.

Bihari, D., Hughes, R.D., Gimson, A.E.S., Langley, P.G., Ede, R.J., Eder, G. and Williams, R. 1983. Effects of resin haemoperfusion in fulminant hepatic failure. *Int J Artif Org* 6: 299–302.

Chen, C-Z. and Yu, Y-T. 1991. Clinical trials for removal of bilirubin by high capacity adsorbent in hemoperfusion. *Artif Org* 15: 295.

Chandy, T. and Sharma, C.P. 1992. Polylysine-immobilized chitosan beads as adsorbent for bilirubin. *Artif Org* 16: 568–76.

Courtney, J.M., Irvine, L., Jones, C., Mosa, S.M., Robertson, L.M. and Srivastava, S. 1993. Biomaterials in medicine – a bioengineering perspective. *Int J Artif Org* 16: 165–71.

Courtney, J.M., Sundaram, S. and Forbes, C.D. 1993. Extracorporeal situations: biocompatibility of biomaterials. In *Management of Bleeding Disorders in Surgical Practice*, eds. C.D. Forbes, A. Cushieri, 236–76. Oxford: Blackwell Scientific.

Falkenhagen, D., Mitzner, S., Loth, F., Courtney, J.M. and Klinkmann, H. 1993. Endotoxin removal by polymeric adsorbents-potential application in medicine. In *Polymers in Medicine and Surgery*. eds. R.L. Kronenthal, Z. Oser, E. Martin, 165–71. London: Plenum Press.

Forbes, C.D. and Courtney, J.M. 1994. Thrombosis and artificial surfaces. In *Haemostasis and Thrombosis*, 3rd Edn, eds. A.L. Bloom, C.D. Forbes, D.P. Thomas, E.G.D. Tuddenham, 1301–24. Edinburgh: Churchill Livingstone.

Giordano, C. ed. 1980. *Sorbents and Their Clinical Applications*. New York: Academic Press.

Hanasawa, K., Tani, T. and Kodama, M. 1989. New approach to endotoxic and septic shock by means of polymyxin B immobilized fiber. *Surg Gynecol Obstet* 168: 323–31.

Hughes, R.D., Pucknell, A., Routley, D., Langley, P.G., Wendon, J.A. and Williams, R. 1994. Evaluation of the BioLogic-DT sorbent-suspension dialyser in patients with fulminant hepatic failure. *Int J Artif Org* 17: 657–62.

Hughes, R.D. and Williams, R. 1993. Use of sorbent columns and haemofiltration in fulminant hepatic failure. *Blood Purif* 11: 163–9.

Inazaki, O., Nishian, Y., Iwaki, R., Nakagawa, K., Takamitsu, Y. and Fujita, Y. 1992. Adsorption of nafomostat mesilate by hemodialysis membranes. *Artif Org* 16: 553–8.

Kambic, H.E. and Nose, Y. 1993. Plasmapheresis: historical perspective, therapeutic applications, and new frontiers. *Artif Org* 17: 850–81.

Kondrup, J., Almdal, T., Vilstrup, H. and Tygstrup, N. 1992. High volume plasma exchange in fulminant hepatic failure. *Int J Artif Org* 15: 669–76.

Konstantin, P., Chang, J., Otto, V. and Brunner, G. 1992. Artificial liver. *Artif Org* 16: 235–42.

Larsen, F.S., Hansen, B.A., Jørgensen, L.G., Secher, N.H., Bondesen, S., Linkis, P., Hjortrup, A., Kirkegaard, P., Agerlin, N., Kondrup, J. and Tygstrup, N. 1994. Cerebral blood flow velocity during high volume plasmapheresis in fulminant hepatic failure. *Int J Artif Org* 17: 353–61.

Malchesky, P.S. 1994. Nonbiological liver support: historical overview. *Artif Org* 18: 342–7.

Matsubara, S. 1994. Combination of plasma exchange and

continuous hemofiltration as temporary metabolic support for patients with acute liver failure. *Artif Org* 18: 363–6.

Mitzner, S., Schneidewind, J., Falkenhagen, D., Loth, F. and Klinkmann, H. 1993. Extracorporeal endotoxin removal by immobilized polyethyleneimine. *Artif Org* 17: 775–81.

Nagaki, M., Hughes, R.D., Keane, H.M., Lau, J.Y.N. and Williams, R. 1992. In vitro plasma perfusion through adsorbents and plasma ultrafiltration to remove of endotoxin and cytokines. *Circ Shock* 38: 182–8.

O'Grady, J.G., Gimson, A.E.S., O'Brien, C.J., Pucknell, A., Hughes, R.D. and Williams, R. 1988. Controlled trials of charcoal hemoperfusion and prognostic factors in fulminant hepatic failure. *Gastroenterology* 94: 1186–92.

Philp, J., Jaffrin, M.Y. and Ding, L.H. 1993. Hemolysis reduction in plasmapheresis by module design: operating with pulsed flow filtration enhancement. *Int J Artif Org* 16: 100–7.

Rozga, J., Holzman, M.D., Ro, M-S., Griffin, D.W., Neuzil, D.F., Giorgio, T., Moscioni, A.D. and Demetriou, A.A. 1993. Development of a hybrid bioartificial liver. *Ann Surg* 217: 502–11.

Ryan, C.J., Aslam, M. and Courtney, J.M. 1990. Transference of hepatic coma to normal rats from galactosamine treated donors by reverse plasma exchange. *Biomater Artif Cells Artif Org* 18: 477–82.

Ryan, C.J., Aslam, M. and Courtney, J.M. 1991. Experimental procedures for the assessment of artificial liver support. In *Acute Liver Failure. Improved Understanding and Better Therapy*, eds. R. Williams, R.D. Hughes, 60–6. London: British Society of Gastroenterology.

Stange, J. and Mitzner, S. 1995. Mass transfer of albumin bound toxins through membranes – comparison between hemofiltration and the MARS-system. *ASAIO J* 41: 11.

Stange, J., Mitzner, S., Ramlow, W., Gliesche, T., Hickstein, H. and Schmidt, R. 1993. A new procedure for the removal of protein bound drugs and toxins. *ASAIO J* 39: M621–5.

Stange, J., Ramlow, W., Mitzner, S., Schmidt, R. and Klinkmann, H. 1993. Dialysis against a recycled albumin solution enables the removal of albumin-bound toxins. *Artif Org* 17: 809–13.

Uchino, J. and Matsushita, M. 1994. Strategies for the rescue of patients with liver failure. *ASAIO J* 40: 74–7.

Usami, M., Nomura, H., Nishimatsu, S., Shiroiwa, H., Kasahara, H., Takeyama, Y. and Saitoh, Y. 1995. In vivo and in vitro evaluation of bilirubin removal in postoperative hyperbilirubinemia patients. *Artif Org* 19: 102–5.

Vienken, J. and Bowry, S. 1993. Optimisation in anticoagulation. *European Dialysis Transplantation Nurses Association European Renal Care Association Journal* 19: 12–17.

Weber, C., Rajnoch, C., Loth, T. and Falkenhagen, D. 1995. Development of cationically modified cellulose adsorbents for the removal of endotoxins. *ASAIO J* 41: 87.

Weber, C., Rajnoch, C., Loth, F., Schima, H. and Falkenhagen, D. 1994. The microspheres based detoxification system (MDS). A new extracorporeal blood purification procedure based on recirculated microspherical adsorbent particles. *Int J Artif Org* 17: 595–602.

Yoshiba, M., Sekiyama, K., Iwamura, Y. and Sugata, F. 1993. Development of reliable artificial liver support (ALS) - plasma exchange in combination with hemodiafiltration using high-performance membranes. *Dig Dis Sci* 38: 469–76.

Zhu, X.X., Brown, G.R. and St-Pierre, L.E. 1990. Adsorption of bilirubin with polypeptide-coated resins. *Biomater Artif Cells Artif Org* 18: 75–93.

23 Hepatocyte transplantation in liver failure and inherited metabolic disorders

Ira J. Fox, Namita Roy Chowdhury and Jayanta Roy Chowdhury

INTRODUCTION

Although orthotopic liver transplantation has markedly improved the prognosis for patients with acute and chronic liver failure or inherited metabolic disorders of the liver, a world-wide shortage of donor organs significantly limits the universal use of this procedure. The whole liver can be stored for only 24–48 h, necessitating rapid transport of the organ. The technical and financial resources required for orthotopic liver transplantation will keep routine use of this procedure impractical in many parts of the world for a long time. Transplantation of isolated liver cells could address many of these problems. In many conditions, transplantation of a fraction of hepatocytes derived from a single liver would be sufficient, permitting the use of a single donor organ in the treatment of several patients. Cryopreservation of hepatocytes can make the cells readily available, averting the problem of organ transport. Isolated liver cells have been used also as vehicles for liver-directed ex vivo gene therapy for metabolic liver diseases. Recently, techniques of conditional immortalization of hepatocytes have opened another potential avenue to grow hepatocytes in culture, thereby increasing the availability of the cells for therapeutic use. However, as in whole organ transplantation, immune rejection limits the survival of transplanted hepatocytes, requiring prolonged immunosuppression. Active research is going on in several laboratories for abrogating allograft rejection. Here, we wish to present a brief discussion of critical aspects of hepatocyte transplantation and the work currently in progress.

DEVELOPMENT OF HEPATOCYTE TRANSPLANTATION SYSTEMS

Effective methods for obtaining viable isolated hepatocytes by collagenase perfusion of the liver were developed three decades ago (Berry and Friend 1969; Seglen 1976). Studies of hepatocyte transplantation began in the 1970s (Rugstad et al. 1970). Infusion of hepatocytes into the portal vein in Gunn rats (that have unconjugated hyperbilirubinemia due to the lack of hepatic bilirubin glucuronidation) resulted in the amelioration of jaundice for several weeks (Rugstad et al. 1970; Matas et al. 1976; Groth et al. 1977). However, inability to distinguish the host liver parenchymal cells from the engrafted cells made it difficult to prove engraftment of the transplanted cells. Therefore, several investigators examined the fate of hepatocytes transplanted at extrahepatic sites. Injection into muscles or subcutaneous tissue did not result in significant survival of hepatocytes (Rugstad et al. 1970; Groth et al. 1977). Initial studies also suggested that hepatocytes injected alone into the intraperitoneal cavity did not survive. However, when hepatocytes were anchored to microcarriers or synthetic fibers, or encapsulated in biocompatible materials (Demetriou, Levenson, et al. 1986; Bosman et al. 1989; Thompson et al. 1989; Cai et al. 1989; Dixit et al. 1990) before transplantation, prolonged survival and function were demonstrated after injection into the peritoneal cavity. Limited survival of hepatocytes was also reported after injection into interscapular fat pads (Jirtle et al. 1980; Gebhardt et al. 1989), beneath the renal capsule (Ricordi et al. 1989), in pancreas (Jaffe et al. 1988; Vroemen et al. 1988) in the pulmonary vascular bed (Selden et al. 1984) or in the lung parenchyma (Then et al. 1991). Hepatocytes do not survive after intra-arterial infusion into splanchnic or renal vascular beds (Mito et al. 1978).

In contrast to other extrahepatic sites, excellent hepatocyte survival and function was noted when the cells were injected into the splenic pulp (Kusano and Mito 1982; Woods et al. 1982; Lee et al. 1983; Nordlinger et al. 1985; Darby et al. 1986). Later investigations using genetically marked hepatocytes demonstrated that following intrasplenic injection, hepatocytes migrate to the liver, where they survive and function throughout the life of recipient rodents.

SITES OF HEPATOCYTE TRANSPLANTATION

Hepatocyte transplantation into the peritoneal cavity

Because of its accessibility and large capacity, the peritoneal cavity has been explored as a site of liver cell transplantation. Initial studies suggested that intraperitoneal transplantation of isolated hepatocytes failed to produce engraftment. However, when rat hepatocytes were attached to collagen-coated microcarriers prior to intraperitoneal injection, a vascularized conglomerate formed within a few days (Demetriou, Levenson, et al. 1986; Bosman et al. 1989; Demetriou, Whiting, et al. 1986). Similarly, hepatocytes encapsulated in alginate–polylysine capsules are also rapidly organized (Dixit et al. 1990). The microcarrier-attached hepatocytes contained large peroxisomes characteristic of hepatocytes and formed bile canaliculi (Demetriou, Levenson, et al 1986). After transplantation of congeneic normal hepatocytes into Gunn rats in this manner, serum bilirubin levels were reduced and bilirubin glucuronides were excreted in bile (Rugstad et al. 1970; Matas et al. 1976; Groth et al. 1977). Similarly, albumin appeared in the serum of Nagase analbuminemic rats (NAR) (Demetriou, Levenson, et al. 1986; Demetriou, Whiting, et al. 1986) and serum low-density lipoprotein levels were decreased in Watanabe heritable hyperlipidemic (WHHL) rabbits that lack the LDL receptor (Wilson et al. 1991) after transplantation of normal liver cells. However, although the peritoneal cavity is a potentially useful site for hepatocyte engraftment, survival of the transplanted cells was limited to several months.

In more recent studies, large numbers of hepatocytes were transplanted into the peritoneal cavity of mice along with a mixture of nonparenchymal cells (Selden et al. 1995). This procedure also resulted in the formation of conglomerates and excellent metabolic function of the transplanted cells. These studies were confirmed in transplantation experiments in Gunn rats (Kim et al. 1995). Transplanted normal hepatocytes were found to start functioning within hours and to continue functioning for two to three months, as demonstrated by the excretion of bilirubin glucuronides in bile (Kim et al. 1995).

Other ectopic sites

Liver cells injected into the dorsal fat pads of rats display features of differentiated hepatocytes for a limited time (Jirtle et al. 1980; Gebhardt et al. 1989). Although liver cells transplanted beneath the renal capsule survive only for a few days, survival improves if hepatocytes are cotransplanted with pancreatic islets (Ricordi et al. 1989). Hepatocytes also survive after injection into the pancreas although this route has not been studied thoroughly (Jaffe et al. 1988; Vroemen et al. 1988; Motokina and Kanematsu 1992). Hepatocytes lodged in the pulmonary vascular bed following intravenous injection die shortly after the injection (Selden et al. 1984). However, limited survival has been reported after direct injection into the lung parenchyma (Sandbichler et al. 1992).

Hepatocyte transplantation by intrasplenic injection

It has been known for a long time that injection of hepatocytes into the splenic pulp leads to superior hepatocyte survival (Kusano and Mito 1982; Woods et al. 1982; Lee et al. 1983; Nordlinger et al. 1985; Darby et al. 1986; Saito et al. 1992). The reason for this became clear from studies using genetically marked hepatocytes which showed that a large fraction of the hepatocytes transplanted into the spleen migrates to the liver (discussed in the next paragraph). However, the small number of hepatocytes that remain in the spleen proliferate eventually replacing up to 40 percent of the spleen in several months (Kusano and Mito 1982). The transplanted cells or their progeny survive in the spleen throughout the life-span of small animals. These cells contain glycogen, albumin, glucose-6-phosphatase, and urea cycle enzymes (Kusano and Mito 1982; Darby, Gupta, et al. 1986; Maganto et al. 1990; Lamers et al. 1990) and clear organic anions, such as ^{99m}Tc-HIDA (Vroemen et al. 1987).

Engraftment within the liver

The liver parenchyma provides an optimal environment for survival of the transplanted hepatocytes because of the interaction with nonparenchymal liver cells and hepatic extracellular matrix, and availability of paracrine growth factors. Infusion of hepatocytes into the portal vein has been shown to ameliorate inherited metabolic disorders of the liver in mutant animals and to dramatically improve survival in experimentally induced acute hepatic failure (Rugstad et al. 1970; Matas et al. 1976; Groth et al. 1977; Sutherland et al. 1977; Sommer et al. 1979). This transplantation method has been used also as a vehicle for liver-directed ex vivo gene therapy. Transplantation of radiolabeled or fluorescently labeled hepatocytes has demonstrated excellent engraftment of the transplanted cells within the liver parenchyma (Gupta et al. 1994; Soriano et al. 1992). Biodistribution of transplanted hepatocytes injected into the splenic pulp by whole body gamma scanning using ^{111}Indium-labeled cells showed that approximately 50 percent of the hepatocytes injected into the spleen migrate immediately into the liver, about 10 percent remain in the spleen, and approximately 3 percent each migrate into the lungs or the pancreas (Gupta et al. 1994). Similarly, transplantation of hepatocytes derived from transgenic mice secreting hepatitis B virus surface antigen (HBsAg) (Gupta et al. 1990), or human α-1 antitrypsin (hAAT) or expressing *E. coli* β-galactosidase (Ponder et al. 1991) into congeneic recipients has shown life-long survival of the transplanted cells in the liver. Such massive migration of intrasplenically injected hepatocytes to the liver explains the superiority of the splenic pulp as a site for ectopic hepatocyte transplantation. Transplantation of normal rat hepatocytes into the liver of dipeptidylpeptidase IV-deficient rats has shown that the transplanted cells become integrated with the liver cords of the recipient within 72 h (Gupta et al. 1991). These cells are morphologically identical to the host liver cells, but can be identified by histochemical staining for dipeptidylpeptidase.

TOLERANCE TO FOREIGN ANTIGENS SECRETED BY HEPATOCYTES TRANSPLANTED INTO THE LIVER PARENCHYMA

After intrasplenic injection of hepatocytes from hepatitis B transgenic mice into congeneic normal mice, the transplanted cells persist within the liver parenchyma throughout the life of the recipient. However, despite the continuous secretion of HBsAg by these cells, no antibody response occurred despite rechallenge with HBsAg in an immunizing regimen (Vemuru et al. 1992). In contrast, when the hepatocytes were transplanted into the peritoneal cavity, there was an anti-HBs response with further increase in titers after rechallenge. Thus, intrahepatic transplantation may be an advantage for hepatic gene therapy in subjects that lack a protein and could conceivably mount an immune response to the transgene. The tolerance is specific for defined heterologous antigens and the host immune response to other antigens remains normal.

HEPATOCYTE TRANSPLANTATION FOR ACUTE LIVER FAILURE

Acute liver failure is associated with extremely high mortality, orthotopic liver transplantation (OLT) being the only treatment that significantly improves survival. Further improvement in results is encumbered by difficulties in early identification of suitable recipients and timely procurement of donor livers. Because in acute liver failure the major problem is the loss of hepatocytes, rather than a deficiency of proliferation of the surviving liver cells (Wolf and Michalopoulos 1992), liver repopulation is a rational approach to salvaging damaged liver. As hepatocytes can be cryopreserved, the cells should be available for transplantation at short notice. Transplantation of cells from a single donor into several recipients could alleviate organ shortage for OLT (Rijntes et al. 1986; Loretz et al. 1989; Lawrence and Benford 1991). Hepatocyte transplantation is also attractive because it does not require removal of the host liver. In communities where routine use of OLT is not available because of limited resources or for social reasons, hepatocyte transplantation may be a more pragmatic approach.

The repopulating potential of transplanted hepatocytes has been elegantly illustrated in albumin–urokinase (ALB-uPA) transgenic mice. These mice express an hepatotoxic transgene which creates defective hepatocytes. In young mice, in a small number of hepatocytes the transgene is deleted; these cells selectively expanded during regeneration. When hepatocytes from congeneic normal adult mice were transplanted into the liver of ALB-uPA transgenic mice, 80 percent of the native liver cells were replaced with donor hepatocytes (Rhim et al. 1994). Similarly, when immunodeficient ALB-uPA/nude mouse hybrids were transplanted with rat hepatocytes, the liver parenchyma of the recipient mice was replaced almost entirely with xenogeneic hepatocytes (Rhim et al. 1995).

The efficacy of hepatocyte transplantation in altering the mortality associated with acute liver failure has been investigated in laboratory animals for more than two decades. In early studies, dimethylnitrosamine (DMNA), was used as a selective hepatotoxin. When 1.5–2.0 g of hepatocytes were transplanted by intraportal or intraperitoneal injection 24 h after administration of 20 mg/kg of the toxin, 60–70 percent of rats survived three weeks, whereas only 6 percent and 17 percent of untreated rats and saline injected controls, respectively, survived (Sutherland 1977). In later studies, intrasplenic injection of as few as 6×10^6 syngeneic or allogeneic hepatocytes was shown to improve survival in rats administered 30 mg/kg DMNA. However, transplantation of xenogeneic hepatocytes did not improve survival (Contini et al. 1983).

The most common hepatotoxin used to induce acute liver failure has been D-galactosamine (D-gal). As in studies using DMNA, trans plantation with 30×10^6 hepatocytes into the peritoneal cavity, the portal vein or the spleen resulted in 63, 83 or 80 percent survival, respectively, which was significantly better than the 10 percent survival in saline treated control rats (Sommer et al. 1979). Intraperitoneal transplantation of 40 million syngeneic or allogeneic rat hepatocytes, or xenogeneic hepatocytes from rabbit or pig given up to 60 h after D-gal administration, increased survival of recipient rats to 60–70 percent compared to zero in untransplanted controls (Makowka et al. 1980; Makowka et al. 1981). Transplantation of syngeneic and xenogeneic fetal liver fragments into the omentum has also been shown to improve survival following D-gal induced acute hepatic failure (Makowka et al. 1980). Kawai et al. (1987) used a slightly different dose of D-gal to produce a subacute form of liver failure. When as few as 5 × 10^6 hepatocytes were transplanted into the spleen 48 h after D-gal administration, these investigators demonstrated that 50–60 percent of animals survived two weeks after the induction of liver failure compared to a survival of less than 10 percent in control rats. In this system, allogeneic hepatocyte transplantation produced no significant prolongation in survival unless the hepatocytes were modified with UV-B irradiation. Transplantation with UV-B irradiated allogeneic hepatocytes increased survival to 27–66 percent (Kawai et al. 1987).

Thus, if hepatotoxins are used to create liver insufficiency, transplantation has consistently improved survival when performed after the induction of acute liver failure. However, the great variability in the doses of DMNA and D-gal (0.75 to 2.6 g/kg) used by various investigators to induce hepatic failure raise questions regarding reproducibility of these methods. In addition, some of the benefits of hepatocyte transplantation could be obtained also by the injection of irradiated hepatocytes, bone marrow cells, hepatocyte supernatants and homogenates. Therefore, it is not clear whether the beneficial effects observed in the toxin-induced liver failure experiments resulted from engraftment of viable cells or from substances contained within them (Makowka et al. 1981; Baumgartner et al. 1983; Makowka, Falk, et al. 1980). These questions prompted investigators to use more reproducible surgical techniques for the evaluation of hepatocyte transplantation in acute liver failure.

For many investigators, near total or 90 percent hepatectomy has provided a reliable model for the study of hepatocyte transplantation. Following hepatectomy, animals became acutely hypoglycemic and uniformly died within 48 h when allowed only 5 percent dextrose orally ad lib following resection. Forty percent of rats undergoing 90 percent hepatic resection survived when 10 × 10^6 microcarrier-attached hepatocytes were transplanted three days before surgical resection. When liver cells alone or attached to microcarriers were injected intraperitoneally immediately after 90 percent partial hepatectomy, all rats became hypoglycemic and died within 48 h, suggesting that vascularization of the transplant was required for function of the transplanted hepatocytes. Because the onset of acute liver failure cannot be predicted in a clinical setting, therapeutic application of this method is apparently limited. However, other investigators have demonstrated that this limitation can be overcome. Cotransplantation of 10 × 10^6 hepatocytes with 400 pancreatic islet cells into the spleen at the time of 90 percent hepatectomy has proven to be effective in reducing mortality from acute liver failure (Xiangdong et al. 1991). The cooperative effect of the cotransplanted pancreatic islets is supported by data indicating that pancreatic islets improve the viability of hepatocytes when transplanted together (Ricordi et al. 1989).

Because of the ready accessibility of the pulmonary vascular bed and its high oxygen tension, the lung has been investigated as a site for hepatocyte transplantation. Hepatocyte transplantation into the lung parenchyma was found to be effective when acute liver failure is induced by 75–80 percent hepatectomy and portacaval shunt in rats. Without treatment, this form of liver failure is associated with a mortality of greater than 90 percent. Following transplantation, the mortality was reduced to less than 10 percent. However, 50 percent of animals injected with hepatocyte supernatant also survived in this study, raising questions about whether the results can be interpreted as evidence for successful engraftment of the cells. Histologic examination of lung tissue from surviving animals revealed apparently well preserved hepatocytes within the alveolar spaces three days after transcutaneous injection, but six months later only a scar could be found at the injection site (Sandbichler et al. 1992; 1994).

Hepatocyte transplantation was also shown to be of benefit in experimental acute ischemic liver failure. In this model, acute liver failure is produced by occlusion of the portal vein and hepatic artery immediately following a portafemoral venous bypass. Injection of hepatocytes into the spleen 48 h before the procedure significantly lowered serum ammonia concentrations and supported blood glucose levels in animals that received hepatocyte transplantation, compared to those that did not (Takeshita et al. 1993). Thus, with the exception of experiments using cotransplantation of pancreatic islets, hepatocyte transplantation has improved survival in surgically induced acute liver failure only when the cells are transplanted before the induction of liver failure.

HEPATOCYTE TRANSPLANTATION FOR CHRONIC LIVER INSUFFICIENCY

Hepatocyte transplantation has been used to improve liver function and ameliorate symptoms of experimentally induced chronic liver failure. In rats treated chronically with carbon tetrachloride, transplantation of syngeneic fetal liver fragments into the omentum reduced serum AST and ALT levels compared with controls (Hagihara et al. 1994). Hepatocellular transplantation also improved symptoms of hepatic encephalopathy when chronic liver insufficiency was induced in rats by end-to-side portacaval shunt. Following portacaval shunt, rats have a reduction in spontaneous activity and nose poke exploration when assessed by a behavior score. Intrasplenic transplantation with 10×10^6 million hepatocytes significantly increased their spontaneous activity after two months and their level of nose poke exploration after three weeks (Ricordi et al. 1989). Increases in plasma ammonia levels after portacaval shunt were not reversed by hepatocyte transplantation, but amino acid imbalances and bile acid concentrations were partially corrected. Additional studies have confirmed the functional capacity of transplanted hepatocytes by demonstrating inducible cytochrome P-450 gene expression six to ten weeks after fetal liver cell transplantation in the spleen (Kato et al. 1995). It should be noted that in the presence of cirrhosis of the liver, the liver is not a suitable site for hepatocyte transplantation. Hepatocytes may obstruct branches of the portal vein acutely and permanently increase portal pressure (Gupta, Yerneni, et al. 1993). Moreover, cells translocating to the pulmonary vascular bed via systemic collaterals may result in pulmonary hypertension (Gupta, Yerneni, et al. 1993). Therefore, in these cases transplantation at ectopic sites appears to be the only practical way of increasing the functional liver mass.

TRANSPLANTATION OF CONDITIONALLY-IMMORTALIZED HEPATOCYTES

Because of the limited availability of human livers for either whole organ or hepatocyte transplantation, investigators have conditionally immortalized hepatocytes by transferring the gene for a thermolabile SV40 T antigen (Fox et al. 1995). These cells proliferate in culture at permissive temperatures (33°C). But at 37–39°C, these cells stop growing and exhibit characteristics of differentiated hepatocytes. To assess their potential for developing into tumors, these cells were transplanted into syngeneic rats and SCID mice and did not produce tumors up to one year following transplantation. When transplanted into the spleens of 90 percent hepatectomized rats, survival improved to 50 percent, which was equivalent to that observed with primary hepatocytes. Again, the improved survival occurred only when the immortalized cells were transplanted prior to hepatectomy (Okamoto et al. 1995). However, when 200×10^6 primary or conditionally immortalized hepatocytes were transplanted into the peritoneal cavity at the time of 90 percent hepatectomy, survival was increased to greater than 50 percent (I.J. Fox and J. Roy Chowdhury, unpublished observations).

Intrasplenic transplantation of conditionally-immortalized hepatocytes was also evaluated in chronic hepatic insufficiency models produced by total portacaval shunting in rats. These rats develop high serum ammonia levels and exhibit signs of hepatic encephalopathy after ammonium acetate administration. Following intrasplenic transplantation of the conditionally immortalized hepatocytes, in the portacaval shunted (PCS) rats, the increase of serum ammonia level was abated and the recipients were protected from ammonium acetate-induced encephalopathy. As the portal flow is diverted from the liver in this model, intrasplenically injected cells cannot migrate to the liver. The transplanted hepatocytes could be identified morphologically in the spleen, and were shown to produce albumin mRNA and bile. Upon removal of the spleen, which contained the resident liver cells, PCS rats were no longer protected from ammonium acetate-induced hepatic encephalopathy (Schumacher et al. 1994).

HEPATOCYTE TRANSPLANTATION IN CLINICAL SETTINGS

Based on these laboratory studies, two institutions have used hepatocyte transplantation clinically to treat patients with liver failure. Ten patients in Japan had either chronic hepatitis or cirrhosis and received hepatocytes recovered from the left lateral segment of their own livers (Mito and Kusano 1993). Four patients underwent hepatic artery ligation, in addition to hepatocyte transplantation, to control ascites. Patients were injected with $0.15–6 \times 10^8$ hepatocytes into their spleens, either by direct splenic puncture or via the splenic artery or the portal vein. Graft survival was assessed by ^{99}Tc-PMT radioisotope uptake by intrasplenic hepatocytes and was detected up to eleven months after transplantation in one patient. In this patient, the ascites and encephalopathy eventually resolved, but the improvement was not felt to be a consequence of hepatocyte transplantation. The second study was reported from India where seven patients with acute liver failure were transplanted with human fetal hepatocytes pooled from blood group-matched, 26–34 week gestational age fetuses. The hepatocyte suspension was administered into the peritoneum through a peritoneal dialysis catheter in a single dose of 60×10^6 cells/kg body weight. The overall survival of patients receiving hepatocyte transplantation was 43 percent compared with 33 percent in matched controls. In this report, fetal hepatocyte transplantation had its most dramatic effect in patients with grade III and grade IV-A hepatic encephalopathy. No improvement in survival was found in patients admitted with grade IV-B hepatic encephalopathy (Habibullah et al. 1994). For patients admitted in grade III hepatic encephalopathy, 100 percent of patients in the transplantation group survived compared with 50 percent survival in matched controls. Clinical recovery from encephalopathy following hepatocyte transplantation was observed within 48 h.

HEPATOCYTE-DIRECTED EX VIVO GENE THERAPY

Exciting recent advances in the techniques of gene introduction into mammalian cells has made it practical to attempt precise reconstitution of genetic defects. Liver-directed gene therapy received a major impetus from the advances in liver cell transplantation. Viral vectors have been used with variable degrees of efficiency for transducing a large proportion of target cell populations with a therapeutic gene (Wilson et al. 1988). Recombinant murine, avian and primate retroviruses, as well as DNA viruses, such as adenoviruses or adenoassociated parvoviruses have been used successfully in gene transfer. For expression, recombinant retroviruses require integration into the host genome, which in turn needs cell division. Because of its integrating property, cell transduction via retroviral agents is permanent and persists in the progeny of the transduced cell. In contrast, recombinant adenoviruses express from episomal sites and do not require cell division. However, integration is rare with adenoviral agents, and although the transduction efficiency is extremely high, the duration of transgene expression is limited. Adeno-associated parvoviruses integrate at several specific sites in the host genome, and therefore, the expression is expected to be long-term. These agents are being vigorously explored as vehicles for gene therapy.

One approach to liver-directed gene therapy consists of harvesting hepatocytes from the mutant, establishing the primary hepatocytes in culture, transducing them with a therapeutic gene and transplanting the genetically modified cells into a mutant recipient. This method, termed ex vivo gene therapy, has been applied to the experimental treatment of genetic metabolic diseases (Hatzoglou et al. 1990; Armentano et al. 1990). The first inherited metabolic disorder treated by this method was inherited LDL receptor (LDLR) deficiency. This genetic disorder results in familial hypercholesterolemia (FH) in human subjects (Brown and Goldstein 1986) and an identical metabolic disorder in mutant Watanabe heritable hyperlipidemic (WHHL) rabbits (Yamamoto et al. 1986). Subjects homozygous for FH have extremely high plasma LDL cholesterol levels and develop premature atherosclerosis with a high incidence of serious cardiovascular complications, such as ischemic heart disease, congestive heart failure and cerebrovascular accidents early in life. Liver transplantation has been used successfully in ameliorating hypercholesterolemia in this disorder (Bilheimer et al. 1984; Hoeg et al. 1989). LDL cholesterol levels were also reduced by transplantation of normal rabbit hepatocytes into WHHL rabbits (Wilson et al. 1990; Wilson et al. 1991). However, the duration of effect was limited by allograft rejection.

Studies mentioned above provided the impetus to develop a method for gene therapy of this disorder. To circumvent the problem of allograft rejection, hepatocytes harvested from a surgically removed liver segment from a WHHL rabbit were cultured and transduced with recombinant retroviruses expressing a normal LDL receptor gene (Roy Chowdhury et al. 1991). The genetically modified WHHL hepatocytes were then transplanted into the rabbit from which the cells were harvested (Grossman et al. 1994). Expression of the transgene was demonstrated in the livers of WHHL recipients by in situ hybridization. This procedure resulted in 25–30 percent reduction in serum LDL cholesterol levels, which persisted throughout the duration of the study (24 weeks). In contrast, serum cholesterol levels in control WHHL rabbits, which received autologous hepatocytes, retrovirally transduced with an *E. coli* β-galactosidase gene, remained unaltered. The strategy described above is being evaluated in a clinical trial. A 29-year-old woman with familial hypercholesterolemia underwent hepatocyte-directed ex vivo gene therapy in June 1992 (Versland et al. 1992). Approximately 10 percent of the liver was removed to isolate hepatocytes, which were genetically reconstituted in vitro and then transplanted into the liver. This first human trial of liver-directed gene therapy resulted in modest reduction of hypercholesterolemia (20 percent to 40 percent of the preoperative values) without the assistance of cholesterol-lowering drugs. A subsequent liver biopsy demonstrated that the introduced LDLR gene was being expressed in the liver.

Other strategies for gene delivery to the liver utilize in vitro transduction using recombinant viruses or introduction of therapeutic genes specifically into hepatocytes using endocytosis mediated by liver-specific receptors (Wilson et al. 1988) or via recombinant viruses (Grossman et al. 1994; Versland et al. 1992). Receptor-directed in vivo gene therapy has the potential advantage of being noninvasive. However, presently the method results in only short duration and low level of transgene expression, and more research is needed before determining its place in practical gene therapy.

THE PROBLEM OF ALLOGRAFT REJECTION AND POTENTIAL APPROACHES TO ITS SOLUTION

A major problem in organ transplantation in humans is immune rejection of allografts. Studies in rats, mice and rabbits comparing the effects of liver cell transplantation using congeneic versus allogeneic donors have shown that allograft rejection is also a major issue in liver cell transplantation. Preventing rejection of allogeneic hepatocytes by drugs such as cyclosporin, has shown only limited success (Makowka et al. 1986; Darby, Selden and Hodgson 1986; Maganto et al. 1988). One approach to avoid this problem in hepatocyte-directed gene therapy is to obtain liver cells from a mutant for transduction with a therapeutic gene before transplantation back into the donor (see above). However, this autografting procedure requires a potentially hazardous partial liver resection. Therefore, development of methods for abrogation of allograft rejection would be a major progress in liver cell transplantation and ex vivo gene therapy. Several lines of strategies for circumventing allograft rejection are being developed by various laboratories. Some of these are discussed briefly below.

Shielding the transplanted cells from the host immunological system

Encapsulation of hepatocytes in selectively permeable synthetic membranes has allowed the survival of hepatocytes in culture and in vivo. When alginate–polylysine encapsulated hepatocytes were implanted into the peritoneal cavity of Gunn rats, function of the hepatocytes was demonstrated by a decline of serum bilirubin levels (Dixit et al. 1990). However, the synthetic membrane provokes an intense fibrotic reaction around the capsules, thereby limiting duration of survival and function of the transplanted cells. Other encapsulation systems have utilized chitosan (unbranched chains of $\beta(1\rightarrow4)$ 2-amino-2-deoxy-D-glucan obtained by deacetylation of chitin) (Gupta, Kim, et al. 1993). Chitosan, electrostatically bound to anionic sodium alginate creates an outer biopolymer membrane around the capsule. In culture, the encapsulated hepatocytes derived from HBsAg transgenic mice remained viable and secreted HBsAg into the medium. After intraperitoneal transplantation of encapsulated hepatocytes in congeneic recipients, peak serum HBsAg level occurred two weeks after transplantation. Hepatocytes recovered from chitosan capsules contained HBsAg mRNA. However, the chitosan membranes failed to prevent the rejection of the hepatocytes transplanted into allogeneic recipients, as shown by disappearance of serum HBsAg in one week and absence of hepatocytes in recovered capsules.

Depletion of antigen presenting cells

Hepatocytes express MHC class I, which is a very weak stimulant of the host immune reaction. However, most cell preparations contain contaminating "passenger" leukocytes, which by virtue of their MHC class II expression, serve as antigen-presenting cells. When pancreatic islet cell preparations were subjected to ultraviolet irradiation followed by culturing at high oxygen tension before transplantation into allogeneic recipient rodents, the cells were not rejected (Lau et al. 1984), presumably due to the depletion of MHC class II-containing dendritic cells. Based on this observation, hepatocytes isolated from normal rats were attached to collagen-coated microcarriers, irradiated with long-wave length ultraviolet light, cultured for 24 h and then transplanted into allogeneic genetically analbuminemic rats by intraperitoneal injection. This resulted in appearance and persistence of albumin in the serum of the recipients for several months (Patel et al. 1989). Although the presumed reason of tolerance of the transplanted liver cells is depletion of putative antigen presenting cells (dendritic cell equivalents) in the hepatocyte preparation, such cells have not been identified and characterized. Therefore, the precise mechanism of allograft tolerance in this model is not understood. Whether this strategy will be useful in other species remains to be verified.

Induction of alloantigen-specific tolerance in the host

Development of methods to abrogate allograft rejection, without the need for chronic immunosuppression would be of major importance in transplantation biology. An intriguing recent approach to abrogation of allograft rejection utilizes prior injection of donor cells into the thymus of the recipient. Considering the strategies used to tolerize the host to donor cells, it is necessary to have a basic understanding of the mechanism by which the body recognizes "self" from "foreign" antigens.

The thymus is the site at which such recognition occurs. Immature progenitor T lymphocytes originating in the bone marrow "home" to the thymus, where they mature into phenotypes expressing either $CD4^+$ or $CD8^+$ (Schwartz 1989). T cells that recognize "self" antigens that are already present in the thymus, are clonally deleted or anergized. Only a small fraction of the progenitor cells entering the thymus are released as mature T cells. Alternatively, negative regulatory cells produced in the thymus may induce unresponsiveness to antigens recognized as "self" (Gassel et al. 1987). Once the T cells leave the thymus, they rarely return to it. Waksman and colleagues developed a concept that this physiologic phenomenon might be mimicked by a direct injection of antigens into the thymus, thereby inducing an immune unresponsiveness to the injected antigen (Staples et al. 1966). In these studies, peripheral lymphocytes were depleted by irradiation, shielding the spleen or the thymus. Specific antigens were then injected into the spleen or thymus. Subsequent injections of the antigen in foot pads did not produce an immune response only when the antigen was first injected into the thymus. These results indicate that intrathymic inoculation of soluble antigens can result in antigen-specific immune tolerance. Extending these concepts, Naji and associates injected allogeneic pancreatic islet cells into the thymus and used an antilymphocyte serum to deplete peripheral lymphocytes (Posselt et al. 1990) Subsequently, transplantation of pancreatic islets was accepted. Recently, unresponsiveness to heart or liver allografts has been reported following intrathymic inoculation of bone marrow cells (Kamada 1985; Kamada et al. 1988). It is hypothesized that following the depletion of peripheral lymphocytes, the newly formed progenitor cells from the bone marrow "home" to the thymus to mature into functional T cells, identifying the inoculated histocompatibility antigens as "self". When an allograft expressing the same histocompatibility antigens is transplanted at an extrathymic site, the new T cells do not respond to the alloantigen.

Abrogation of hepatocyte allograft rejection by thymic re-education

Experiments have been performed to test the hypothesis that intrathymic injection of splenocytes in peripheral lymphocyte-depleted adult rats should result in the abrogation of rejection of allografted hepatocytes

(Fabrega et al. 1995). Nagase analbuminemic rats (NAR) (200 g) were used as hepatocyte transplant recipients and allogeneic normal Brown Norway (BN) served as donors. All recipients were injected with one ml of antirat lymphocyte serum (Sigma, St. Louis, MO) intraperitoneally, 14 days and seven days before hepatocyte transplantation. The rats in the experimental group received an intrathymic inoculation of donor splenocytes (5×10^7). Two weeks later, hepatocytes (10^7) were transplanted by intrasplenic injection. In NAR rats that were inoculated intrathymically with BN rat splenocytes, hepatocytes isolated from BN rats survived and functioned in the spleen and the liver of the recipients on a long-term basis. DNA polymerase chain reaction studies (PCR) using primer pairs which recognize the wildtype albumin gene were used to demonstrate the persistence of the transplanted hepatocytes in the liver, spleen and pancreas. Expression of albumin mRNA by the transplanted cells was shown by in situ hybridization for the duration of the experiment (154 days). The transplanted hepatocytes were integrated into the liver cords and were histologically indistinguishable from the host liver cells. Serum albumin levels increased by 0.5 to 1.2 mg/ml in 5 to 14 days after HC transplantation and remained unattenuated throughout the study.

To evaluate whether induction of tolerance requires intrathymic inoculation of splenocytes from the same strain as that of the hepatocyte donors, another group received splenocytes from Wistar rats and hepatocytes from BN rats. In this group, serum albumin levels peaked at 0.1 to 0.2 mg/ml on day 5, but returned to baseline in 14 days, indicating that donor-specific splenocytes are required for immune abrogation.

To determine whether intrathymic inoculation has an advantage over intravenous infusion of splenocytes, another group received an intravenous infusion of isolated splenocytes from BN rats, followed by hepatocytes also from BN rats. In this group also, serum albumin levels peaked at 0.2 mg/ml on day 5, but returned to baseline in 14 days, indicating that intrathymic injection is more effective than the intravenous route.

A possible role of a liver allograft in maintaining tolerance

In some strain combinations, but not others, rat liver allografts exhibit spontaneous immune unresponsiveness. In these situations, following an initial phase of acute cell-mediated rejection, the allograft is accepted (Kamada 1985). Although it is not clear whether such spontaneous unresponsiveness occurs by mechanisms similar to those involved in the induction of tolerance by intrathymic inoculation of antigens, these observations raise the possibility that the liver allograft may secrete soluble factors that have a role in the maintenance of immune tolerance (Kamada et al. 1988). Alternatively, some cells present in the liver allograft may enter the circulation, migrate to the thymus (Michie et al. 1988), thereby maintaining tolerance. Starzl and colleagues have demonstrated the persistence of donor strain lymphocytes in recipients who have developed delayed tolerance to liver allografts (Starzl et al. 1993). In these patients, it was possible to discontinue immune suppression several years after transplantation of livers from allogeneic donors, without immune rejection. The coexistence of two different tissue types of lymphocytes, termed chimerism, has been observed in various organs, including the thymus. Whether such chimerism is necessary or sufficient for induction of tolerance is not known. Following injection of allogeneic splenocytes into rodent thymus, microchimerism has been observed for two to three weeks only (Odorico et al. 1992). However, failure to find microchimerism at subsequent time points could be related to insensitivity of the fluorescence activated cell sorting (FACS) method used in these studies. Recently, using a highly sensitive PCR-based detection method, persistence of microchimerism following intrathymic injection of splenocytes has been demonstrated (J. Roy Chowdhury and A. Davidson, unpublished observation).

Adoptive transfer of allograft tolerance

To evaluate whether allograft tolerance is mediated by circulating cells or soluble factors, several investigators have performed adoptive transfer studies. Adoptive transfer of lymphocytes into sublethally irradiated naive recipients have yielded conflicting evidence regarding putative suppressor cells that maintain a tolerant state. The failure to induce tolerance by injection into only one lobe of the thymus argues against suppressor cell induction as a mechanism of allograft tolerance (Odorico, Barker, et al. 1993). Some investigators have found no evidence for suppression using T cell mixing experiments (Shimonkevitz and Bevan 1988). In contrast, other investigators have been able to induce tolerance with peripheral blood cells or splenocytes from tolerized allografted animals, but not from nongrafted animals (Odorico, Posselt, et al. 1993), suggesting that a continuing source of donor antigen is required to maintain tolerance, and that some type of regulatory cells are induced in the tolerized grafted animals. The reasons for such conflicting data may be related to the temporal relationship of grafting to the adoptive transfer experiments, as these cells appear not to develop until at least two weeks after grafting. Thus, the development of the negative regulatory cells may be a late mechanism for maintaining tolerance.

A summary of possible mechanisms of induction/maintenance of tolerance

Evidence has been presented for transplantation across MHC class 1, MHC class II or mixed lymphocyte system barriers that supports induction either of clonal deletion or clonal anergy of alloreactive T cells. There is conflicting data as to whether a state of microchimerism of donor cells in the thymus or the periphery is involved in the maintenance of tolerance, or whether secretion of soluble factors or recirculating cells from the allograft are sufficient. Intensive investigation is under way at various laboratories to determine the mechanism of induction of specific allograft tolerance. These studies are beginning to provide answers that may pave the path for future application of recent exciting findings in the transplantation of human organs or cells.

SUMMARY

Hepatocyte transplantation has a great, albeit unrealized, therapeutic potential. Gaps in our knowledge regarding the assimilation, fate and proliferative potential of transplanted hepatocytes remain. One to five percent of the host hepatic mass has been reconstituted by transplanted hepatocytes in rodents and additional strategies are being developed for even more massive reconstitution of the host liver. It may be possible to achieve more efficient repopulation of the liver using liver cell progenitors or conditionally immortalized hepatocytes. Finally, the ability to induce host tolerance to specific alloantigens should provide a major boost to the application of liver cell transplantation in the treatment of liver failure and inherited metabolic liver diseases, as well as hepatocyte-directed ex vivo gene therapy.

Acknowledgments

This work was partly supported by the following NIH grants: RO1-DK 46057 (to J.R.C.); RO1-DK 39137 (to N.R.C.), and the Liver Research Core Center (P30-DK 41296) of Albert Einstein College of Medicine.

REFERENCES

Armentano, D., Thompson, A.R., Darlington, G. and Woo, S.L. 1990. Expression of human factor IX in rabbit hepatocytes by retrovirus-mediated gene transfer: potential for gene therapy of human hemophilia B. *Proc Natl Acad Sci USA* 87: 6141–5.

Baumgartner, D., LaPlante-O'Neill, P.M., Sutherland, D.E.R. and Najarian, J.S. 1983. Effects of intrasplenic injection of hepatocytes, hepatocyte fragments, and hepatocyte culture supernatants on D-galactosamine-induced liver failure in rats. *Eur Surg Res* 15: 129–35.

Berry, M.N. and Friend, D.S. 1969. High yield preparation of isolated rat liver parenchymal cells. A biochemical and fine structural study. *J Cell Biol* 43: 506–20.

Bilheimer, D.W., Goldstein, J.L., Grundy, S.M., Starzl, T.E. and Brown, M.S. 1984. Liver transplantation to provide low-density lipoprotein receptors and lower plasma cholesterol in a child with homozygous familial hypercholesterolemia. *N Engl J Med* 311: 1658–64.

Bosman, D.K., de Haan, J.G., Smit, J., Jorning, G.G.A., Maas, M.A.W. and Chamuleau, A.F.M. 1989. Metabolic activity of microcarrier attached liver cells after intraperitoneal transplantation during severe liver insufficiency in the rat. *J Hepatol* 9: 49–58.

Brown, M.S. and Goldstein, J.L. 1986. A receptor-mediated pathway for cholesterol homeostasis. *Science* 232: 34–47.

Cai, Z., Shi, Z., Sherman, M. and Sun, A.M. 1989. Development and evaluation of a system of microencapsulation of primary rat hepatocytes. *Hepatology* 10: 855–60.

Contini, S., Pezzarossa, A., Sansoni, P., Mazzoni, M.P. and Botta, G.C. 1983. Hepatocellular transplantation in rats with toxic induced liver failure: results of iso-, allo- and xenografts. *Ital J Surg Sci* 13: 25–30.

Darby, H., Gupta, S., Johnstone, R., Selden, A.C. and Hodgson, H.J.F. 1986. Observations on rat spleen reticulum during the development of syngeneic hepatocellular implants. *Br J Exp Pathol* 67: 329–39.

Darby, H., Selden, C. and Hodgson, H.J. 1986. Prolonged survival of cyclosporine-treated allogeneic hepatocellular implants. *Transplantation* 42: 325–6.

Demetriou, A.A., Levenson, S.M., Novikoff, P.M., Novikoff, A.B., Roy Chowdhury, N.R., Whiting, J., Reisner, A. and Roy Chowdhury, J. 1986. Survival, organization and function of microcarrier-attached hepatocytes transplanted in rats. *Proc Natl Acad Sci USA* 83: 7475–9.

Demetriou, A.A., Whiting, J., Levenson, S.M., Roy Chowdhury, N., Schechner, R., Michalski, S., Feldman, D. and Roy Chowdhury, J. 1986. New method of hepatocyte transplantation and extracorporeal liver support. *Ann Surg* 204: 259–71.

Demetriou, A.A., Whiting, J.F., Feldman, D., Levenson, S.M., Roy Chowdhury, N., Moscioni, A.D., Kram, M. and Roy Chowdhury, J. 1986. Replacement of liver function in rat by transplantation of microcarrier-attached hepatocytes. *Science* 233: 1190–2.

Dixit, V., Darvasi, R., Arthur, M., Brezina, M., Lewin, K. and Gitnick, G. 1990. Restoration of liver function in Gunn rats without immunosuppression using transplanted microencapsulated hepatocytes. *Hepatology* 12: 1342–9.

Fabrega, A.J., Bommineni, V.R., Blanchard, J., Tetali, S., Rivas, P.A., Pollak, R., Sengupta, K., Roy Chowdhury, N. and Roy Chowdhury, J. 1995. Amelioration of analbuminemia by transplantation of allogeneic hepatocytes in tolerized rats. *Transplantation* 59: 1362–4.

Fox, I.J., Roy Chowdhury, N., Gupta, S., Kondapalli, R., Schilsky, M., Stockert, R.J. and Roy Chowdhury, J. 1995. Conditional immortalization of Gunn rat hepatocytes: An ex vivo model for phenotypic correction of bilirubin-UDP-glucuronosyltransferase deficiency by gene transfer. *Hepatology* 21: 837–46.

Gassel, H.J., Hutchinson, I.V., Engmann, R. and Morris, P.J. 1987. Demonstration of donor-specific T suppressor lymphocytes in rats accepting orthotopic liver allograft. *Transpl Proc* XIX: 4207–8.

Gebhardt, R., Jirtle, R., Moorman, A.F., Lamers, W.H. and Michalopoulos, G. 1989. Induction of glutamine synthetase and transient co-expression with carbamoylphosphate synthetase in hepatocytes transplanted into fat pads of syngeneic hosts. *Histochemistry* 92: 337–42.

Grossman, M., Raper, S.E., Kozarsky, K., Stein, E.A., Englehardt, J.F., Muller, D., Lupien, P.J. and Wilson, J.M. 1994. Successful ex vivo gene therapy directed to liver in a patient with familial hypercholesterolemia. *Nat Genet* 6: 335–41.

Groth, C.G., Arborgh, B., Bjorken, C., Sundberg, B. and Lundgren, G. 1977. Correction of hyperbilirubinemia in the glucuronyltransferase-deficient rats by intraportal hepatocyte transplantation. *Transpl Proc* 9: 313–16.

Gupta, S., Lee, C-D., Vemuru, R.P. and Bhargava, K.K. 1994. ^{111}Indium-labeling of hepatocytes for analyzing biodistribution of transplanted cells. *Hepatology* 19: 750–7.

Gupta, S., Roy Chowdhury, R., Jagtiani, R., Gustin, K., Shafritz, D.A., Roy Chowdhury, J. and Burk, R.D. 1990. A novel system for transplantation of isolated hepatocytes utilizing HBsAg producing transgenic donor cells. *Transplantation* 50: 472–5.

Gupta, S., Aragona, E., Vemuru, R.P., Bhargava, K., Burk, R.D. and Roy Chowdhury, J. 1991. Permanent engraftment and function of hepatocytes delivered to the liver: implications for gene therapy and liver repopulation. *Hepatology* 14: 144–9.

Gupta, S., Kim, S., Vemuru, R.P., Aragona, E., Yerneni, P., Burk, R.D. and Rha, C.K. 1993. Hepatocyte transplantation: An alternative system for evaluating cell survival and immunoisolation. *Int J Artif Org* 16: 71–9.

Gupta, S., Yerneni, P., Vemuru, R.P., Lee, C.D., Yellin, E.L. and Bhargava, K.K. 1993. Studies on the safety of intrasplenic hepatocyte transplantation: relevance to ex vivo gene therapy and liver repopulation in acute hepatic failure. *Hum Gene Ther* 4: 249–57.

Habibullah, C.M., Syed, I.H., Qamar, A. and Taher-Uz, Z. 1994. Human fetal hepatocyte transplantation in patients with fulminant hepatic failure. *Transplantation* 58: 951–2.

Hagihara, M., Shimura, T., Takebe, K., Munkhbat, B. and Tsuji, K. 1994. Effects of iso- and xeno-fetal liver fragments transplantation on acute and chronic liver failure in rats. *Cell Transpl* 3: 283–90.

Hatzoglou, M., Lamers, W., Bosch, F., Wynshaw-Boris, A., Wade Clapp, D. and Hanson, R.W. 1990. Hepatic gene transfer in animals using retroviruses containing the promoter from the gene for phosphoenolpyruvate carboxykinase. *J Biol Chem* 265: 17285–93.

Hoeg, J.M., Starzl, T.E. and Brewer, H.B. Jr. 1989. Liver transplantation for treatment of cardiovascular disease: Comparison with medication and plasma exchange in homozygous familial hypercholesterolemia. *Arteriosclerosis* (Suppl 1) I-33–8.

Jaffe, V., Darby, H., Selden, S. and Hodgson, H.J.F. 1988. The growth of transplanted liver cells within the pancreas. *Transplantation* 45: 497–8.

Jirtle, R.L., Biles, C. and Michalopoulos, G. 1980. Morphologic and histochemical analysis of hepatocytes transplanted into syngeneic hosts. *Am J Pathol* 101: 115–26.

Kamada, N. 1985. The immunology of experimental liver transplantation in the rat. *Immunology* 55: 369–85.
Kamada, N., Brons, G. and Davies, H.F.F.S. 1988. Fully allogeneic liver allografting in rats induces a state of systemic nonreactivity to donor transplantation antigens. *Transplantation* 29: 429–34.
Kato, K., Hodgson, W., Abraham, N., Kasai, S., Onodera, K., Matsuda, M. and Mito, M. 1995. Long-term developmental expression and inductivity of cytochrome P450s within intrasplenically transplanted fetal hepatocytes from spontaneously hypertensive rats. *Cell Transpl* 4: S33–6.
Kawai, Y., Price, J.B. and Hardy, M.A. 1987. Reversal of liver failure in rats by ultraviolet-irradiated hepatocyte transplantation. *Transpl Proc* 19: 989–91.
Kim, B.H., Roy Chowdhury, J. and Roy Chowdhury, N. 1995. Primary hepatocytes transplanted intraperitoneally in Gunn rats start functioning immediately. *Hepatology* 22: A419.
Kusano, M. and Mito, M. 1982. Observations on the fine structure of long survived isolated hepatocytes inoculated into rat spleen. *Gastroenterology* 82: 616–28.
Lamers, W.H., Been, W., Charles, R. and Moorman, A.F.M. 1990. Hepatocytes explanted in the spleen preferentially express carbamoylphosphate synthetase rather than glutamine synthetase. *Hepatology* 12: 701–9.
Lau, H., Reemtsma, K. and Hardy, M.A. 1984. Prolongation of rat islet allograft survival by direct ultraviolet irradiation of the graft. *Science* 223: 607–9.
Lawrence, J.N. and Benford, D.J. 1991. Development of an optimal method for the cryopreservation of hepatocytes and their subsequent monolayer culture. *Toxicol In Vitro* 5: 39–51.
Lee, G., Medline, A., Finkelstein, S., Tatematsu, M., Makowka, L. and Farber, E. 1983. Transplantation of hepatocytes from normal and preneoplastic livers into spleens of syngeneic host rats. *Transplantation* 36: 218–21.
Loretz, L.J., Li, A.P., Flye, M.W. and Wilson, A.G.E. 1989. Optimization of cryopreservation procedures for rat and human hepatocytes. *Xenobiotica* 19: 489–98.
Maganto, P., Cienfuegos, J.A., Santamaria, L., Codesal, J., Tendillo, F. and Castillo-Olivares, J.L. 1988. Effect of cyclosporin on allogeneic hepatocyte transplantation: a morphological study. *Eur Surg Res* 20: 248–53.
Maganto, P., Traber, P.G., Rusnell, C., Dobbins III, W.O., Keren, D. and Gumucio, J.J. 1990. Long-term maintenance of the adult pattern of liver-specific expression for P-450b, P-450e, albumin and α-fetoprotein genes in intrasplenically transplanted hepatocytes. *Hepatology* 11: 585–92.
Makowka, L., Lee, G., Cobourn, C.S., Farber, E., Falk, J.A. and Falk, R.E. 1986. Allogeneic hepatocyte transplantation in the rat spleen under cyclosporine immunosuppression. *Transplantation* 42: 537–41.
Makowka, L., Rotstein, L., Falk, R., Falk, J., Langer, B., Nossal, N., Blendis, L. and Phillips, M. 1980. Reversal of toxic and anoxic induced hepatic failure by syngeneic, allogeneic and xenogeneic hepatocyte transplantation. *Surgery* 88: 244–53.
Makowka, L., Rotstein, L., Falk, R., Falk, J., Zuk, R., Langer, B., Blendis, L. and Phillips, M. 1981. Studies into the mechanism of reversal of experimental acute hepatic failure by hepatocyte transplantation. *Can J Surg* 24: 39–44.
Makowka, L., Falk, R.E., Rotstein, L.E., Falk, J.A., Nossal, N., Langer, B., Blendis, L.M. and Phillips, M.J. 1980. Cellular transplantation in the treatment of experimental hepatic failure. *Science* 210: 901–3.
Matas, A.J., Sutherland, D.E.R., Steffes, M.W., Mauer, S.M., Lowe, A., Simmons, R.L. and Najarian, J.S. 1976. Hepatocellular transplantation for metabolic deficiencies: Decrease of plasma bilirubin in Gunn rats. *Science* 192: 892–4.
Michie, S.A., Kirkpatrick, E.A., Rouse, R.V. et al. 1988. Rare peripheral T-cells migrate to and persist in normal mouse thymus. *J Exp Med* 168: 1929–35.
Mito, M., Kusano, M., Onishi, T., Saito, T. and Ebata, H. 1978. Hepatocellular transplantation. *Gastroenterol Jpn* 13: 480–90.
Mito, M. and Kusano, M. 1993. Hepatocyte transplantation in man. *Cell Transpl* 2: 65–74.
Motokina, K. and Kanematsu, T. 1992. Bile secretion and histology of liver autotransplanted into the pancreatic parenchyma. *Transplantation* 54: 784–9.
Nordlinger, B., Bouma, M.E., Wang, S.R. et al. 1985. High-yield preparation of porcine hepatocytes for long survival after transplantation in the spleen. *Eur Surg Res* 17: 377–82.
Odorico, J.S., Barker, C.F., Markmann, J.F., Posselt, A.M. and Naji, A.M. 1993. Prolonged survival of rat cardiac allograft after intrathymic inoculation of donor thymocytes. *Transpl Proc* XXV: 295–6.
Odorico, J.S., Barker, C.F., Posselt, A.M. et al. 1992. Induction of donor-specific tolerance to rat cardiac allografts by intrathymic inoculation of bone marrow. *Surgery* 112: 370–7.
Odorico, J.S., Posselt, A.M., Naji, A. et al. 1993. Promotion of rat cardiac allograft survival by intrathymic inoculation of donor splenocytes. *Transplantation* 55: 1104–15.
Okamoto, T., Schumacher, I.K., Roy Chowdhury, N., Roy Chowdhury, J. and Fox, I.J. 1995. Treatment of acute liver failure induced in rats with 90% hepatectomy by transplantation of conditonally-immortalized hepatocytes. *J Invest Med* 43: 400A.
Patel, A., Hardy, M., Roy Chowdhury, N., Wajsman, R., Sandoval, M., Wilson, J.M. and Roy Chowdhury, J. 1989. Long-term correction of genetic defect of liver function in rat by transplantation of liver cells after ultraviolet irradiation. *Mol Biol Med* 6: 187–96.
Ponder, K.P., Gupta, S., Leland, F., Darlington, G., Finegold, M., DeMayo, J., Ledley, F.D., Roy Chowdhury, J. and Woo, S.L.C. 1991. Mouse hepatocytes migrate to liver parenchyma and function indefinitely after intrasplenic transplantation. *Proc Natl Acad Sci USA* 88: 1217–21.
Posselt, A.M., Barker, C.F., Tomaszewski, J.E. et al. 1990. Induction of donor-specific unresponsiveness by intrathymic islet transplantation. *Science* 249: 1293–300.
Rhim, J.A., Sandgren, E.P., Degen, J.L., Palmiter, R.D. and Brinster, R.L. 1994. Replacement of diseased mouse liver by hepatic cell transplantation. *Science* 263: 1149–53.
Rhim, J.A., Sandgren, E.P., Palmiter, R.D. and Brinster, R.L. 1995. Complete reconstitution of mouse liver with xenogeneic hepatocytes. *Proc Natl Acad Sci USA* 92: 4942–6.
Ricordi, C., Lacey, P.E., Callery, M.P., Park, P.W. and Flye, M.W. 1989. Trophic factors from pancreatic islets in combined hepatocyte-islet allografts enhance hepatocellular survival. *Surgery* 105: 218–23.
Rijntes, P.J.M., Moshage, H.J., Van Gemert, P.J.L., De Waal, R. and Yap, S.H. 1986. Cryopreservation of adult

human hepatocytes. The influence of deep freezing storage on the viability, cell seeding, survival, fine structure and albumin synthesis in primary cultures. *J Hepatol* 3: 7–18.

Roy Chowdhury, J., Grossman, M., Gupta, S., Roy Chowdhury, N., Baker, J.R. and Wilson, J.M. 1991. Long-term improvement of hypercholesterolemia after ex vivo gene therapy in LDL receptor deficient rabbits. *Science* 254: 1802–5.

Rugstad, H.E., Robinson, S.H., Yamoni, C. et al. 1970. Transfer of bilirubin uridine-5-diphosphate-glucuronyltransferase to enzyme deficient rats. *Science* 170: 553–5.

Saito, S., Sakagami, K., Matsuno, T., Tanakaya, K., Takaishi, Y. and Orita, K. 1992. Long-term survival and proliferation of spheroidal aggregate cultured hepatocytes transplanted into the rat spleen. *Transpl Proc* 24: 1520–1.

Sandbichler, P., Erhart, R., Herbst, P., Vogel, W., Herold, M., Dietze, O., Schmid, T.H., Klima, G. and Margreiter, R. 1994. Hepatocellular transplantation into the lung in chronic liver failure following bile duct obstruction in the rat. *Cell Transpl* 3: 409–12.

Sandbichler, P., Then, P., Vogel, W., Erhart, R., Dietze, O., Philadelphy, H., Fridrich, L., Klima, G. and Margreiter, R. 1992. Hepatocellular transplantation into the lung for temporary support of acute liver failure in the rat. *Gastroenterology* 102: 605–9.

Schumacher, I.K., Okamoto, T., Chowdhury, N.R., Chowdhury, J.R. and Fox, I.J. 1994. Transplantation of SV40 conditionally immortalized hepatocytes to treat hepatic encephalopathy. *Hepatology* 20: 139A.

Schwartz, R.H. 1989. Acquisition of immunologic self-tolerance. *Cell* 57: 1073–7.

Seglen, P.O. 1976. Preparation of isolated rat liver cells. *Meth Cell Biol* 13: 29–83.

Selden, C., Colman, D., Morgan, N., Wilcox, H., Carr, E. and Hodgson, H.J.F. 1995. Histidinemia in mice: a metabolic defect treated using a novel approach to hepatocellular transplantation. *Hepatology* 21: 1405–12.

Selden, A.C., Gupta, S., Johnstone, R. and Hodgson, H.F. 1984. The pulmonary vascular bed as a site for implantation of isolated liver cells in inbred rats. *Transplantation* 38: 81–3.

Shimonkevitz, R.P. and Bevan, M.J. 1988. Split tolerance induced by the intrathymic adoptive transfer of thymocyte stem cells. *J Exp Med* 168: 143–56.

Sommer, B.G., Sutherland, D.E., Matas, D.J., Simmons, R.L. and Najarian, J.S. 1979. Hepatocellular transplantation for treatment of D-galactosamine induced acute liver failure in rats. *Transpl Proc* 11: 578–84.

Soriano, H.E., Lewis, D., Legner, M., Brandt, M., Baley, P., Darlington, G., Finegold, M. and Ledley, F.D. 1992. Use of DiI marked hepatocytes to demonstrate orthotopic, intrahepatic engraftment following hepatocellular transplantation. *Transplantation* 54: 717–23.

Staples, P.J., Gery, I., Waksman, B.H. et al. 1966. Role of the thymus in tolerance III. Tolerance to bovine gammaglobulin after direct injection of antigen into the shielded thymus of irradiated rats. *J Exp Med* 124: 127–32.

Starzl, T.E., Demetris, A.J., Trucco, M. et al. 1993. Chimerism after liver transplantation for type IV glycogen storage disease and type I Gaucher's disease. *N Engl J Med* 328: 745–55.

Sutherland, D.E.R., Numate, M., Matas, A.J., Simmons, R.L. and Najaran, J.S. 1977. Hepatocellular transplantation in acute liver failure. *Surgery* 82: 124–32.

Takeshita, K., Ishibashi, H., Suzuki, M. and Kodama, M. 1993. Hepatocellular transplantation for metabolic support in experimental acute ischemic liver failure in rats. *Cell Transpl* 2: 319–24.

Then, P., Sandbichler, P., Erhart, R., Dietze, O., Klima, G., Vogel, W. and Margreiter, R. 1991. Hepatocyte transplantation into the lung for treatment of acute hepatic failure in the rat. *Transpl Proc* 23: 892–3.

Thompson, J.A., Handenschild, C.C., Anderson, K.D., DiPietro, J.M., Anderson, W.F. and Maciag, T. 1989. Heparin-binding growth factor 1 induces the formation of organoid neovascular structures in vivo. *Proc Natl Acad Sci USA* 86: 7928–32.

Vemuru, R.P., Davidson, A., Aragona, E., Burk, R.D., Roy Chowdhury, J. and Gupta, S. 1992. Immune tolerance to a defined heterologous antigen following intrasplenic hepatocyte transplantation: Implications for human gene therapy. *FASEB J* 6: 2836–82.

Versland, M.R., Wu, C.H. and Wu., G.Y. 1992. Strategies for gene therapy in the liver. *Sem Liver Dis* 12: 332–9.

Vroemen, J.P., Buurman, W.A., van der Linden, C.J., Visser, R., Heirwegh, K.P. and Koostra, G. 1988. Transplantation of isolated hepatocytes into the pancreas. *Eur Surg Res* 20: 1–11.

Vroemen, J., van der Linden, C., Buurman, W., Coenegracht, J., Heirwegh, K. and Koostra, G. 1987. In vivo dynamic 99M Tc-HIDA scintigraphy after hepatocyte transplantation: a new method for monitoring graft function. *Eur Surg Res* 19: 140–50.

Wilson, J.M., Jefferson, D.M., Roy Chowdhury, J., Novikoff, P.M., Johnstone, D.M. and Mulligan, R.C. 1988. Retrovirus mediated transduction of adult hepatocytes. *Proc Natl Acad Sci USA* 85: 3014–18.

Wilson, J.M., Roy Chowdhury, N., Grossman, M., Gupta, S., Jeffers, J., Huang, T-J. and Roy Chowdhury, J. 1991. Transplantation of allogeneic hepatocytes into LDL receptor deficient rabbits leads to transient improvement in hypercholesterolemia. *Clin Biotechnol* 3: 21–6.

Wilson, J.M., Roy Chowdhury, N., Grossman, M., Wajsman, R., Epstein, A., Mulligan, R.C. and Roy Chowdhury, J. 1990. Temporary amelioration of hyperlipidemia in low density lipoprotein receptor-deficient rabbits transplanted with genetically modified hepatocytes. *Proc Natl Acad Sci USA* 87: 8437–41.

Wolf, H.K. and Michalopoulos, G.K. 1992. Hepatocyte regeneration in acute fulminant and subfulminant hepatitis: a study of proliferating cell nuclear antigen expression. *Hepatology* 15: 707–13.

Woods, R.J., Fuller, B.J., Attenburro, V.D., Nutt, L.H. and Hobbs, K.E.F. 1982. Functional assessment of hepatocytes after transplantation into rat spleen. *Transplantation* 33: 123–6.

Xiangdong, W., Ar'Rajab, A., Ahren, B., Andersson, R. and Bengmark, S. 1991. Improvement of the effects of intrasplenic transplantation of hepatocytes after 90% hepatectomy in the rat by cotransplantation with pancreatic islets. *Transplantation* 52: 462–6.

Yamamoto, T., Bishop, R.W., Brown, M.S., Goldstein, G.L. and Russell, D.W. 1986. Deletion in cysteine-rich region of LDL receptor impedes transport to cell surface in WHHL rabbit. *Science* 232: 1230–7.

Index

For EU product safety concerns, contact us at Calle de José Abascal, 56–1°, 28003 Madrid, Spain or eugpsr@cambridge.org.

www.ingramcontent.com/pod-product-compliance
Ingram Content Group UK Ltd.
Pitfield, Milton Keynes, MK11 3LW, UK
UKHW050730090726
473066UK00013B/1095
* 9 7 8 0 5 2 1 1 8 8 9 4 4 *